PHYSICAL THERAPY CASE FILES® Sports

Jason Brumitt, PT, PhD, ATC, CSCS
Assistant Professor
George Fox University
Newberg, Oregon

Series Editor: Erin E. Jobst, PT, PhD
Associate Professor
School of Physical Therapy
College of Health Professions
Pacific University
Hillsboro, Oregon

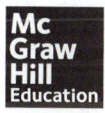

New York Chicago San Francisco Athens London Madrid Mexico City
Milan New Delhi Singapore Sydney Toronto

Physical Therapy Case Files®: Sports

Copyright © 2016 by McGraw-Hill Education. All rights reserved. Printed in the United States of America. Except as permitted under the United States Copyright Act of 1976, no part of this publication may be reproduced or distributed in any form or by any means, or stored in a data base or retrieval system, without the prior written permission of the publisher.

Case Files® is a registered trademark of McGraw-Hill Education. All rights reserved.

1 2 3 4 5 6 7 8 9 0   DOC/DOC   19 18 17 16 15

ISBN 978-0-07-182153-7
MHID 0-07-182153-8

> **Notice**
>
> Medicine is an ever-changing science. As new research and clinical experience broaden our knowledge, changes in treatment and drug therapy are required. The authors and the publisher of this work have checked with sources believed to be reliable in their efforts to provide information that is complete and generally in accord with the standard accepted at the time of publication. However, in view of the possibility of human error or changes in medical sciences, neither the editors nor the publisher nor any other party who has been involved in the preparation or publication of this work warrants that the information contained herein is in every respect accurate or complete, and they disclaim all responsibility for any errors or omissions or for the results obtained from use of the information contained in this work. Readers are encouraged to confirm the information contained herein with other sources. For example and in particular, readers are advised to check the product information sheet included in the package of each drug they plan to administer to be certain that the information contained in this work is accurate and that changes have not been made in the recommended dose or in the contraindications for administration. This recommendation is of particular importance in connection with new or infrequently used drugs.

This book was set in Adobe Jenson Pro by Cenveo® Publisher Services.
The editors were Catherine A. Johnson and Christina M. Thomas.
The production supervisor was Catherine H. Saggese.
Project management was provided by Anupriya Tyagi, Cenveo Publisher Services.
RR Donnelley was the printer and binder.

Library of Congress Cataloging-in-Publication Data

Physical therapy case files. Sports / [edited by] Jason Brumitt.
    p. ; cm.
  Sports
  Includes bibliographical references and index.
  ISBN 978-0-07-182153-7 (pbk.)—ISBN 0-07-182153-8
  I. Brumitt, Jason. editor. II. Title: Sports.
  [DNLM: 1. Athletic Injuries—therapy—Case Reports. 2. Physical Therapy Modalities—Case Reports. 3. Needs Assessment—Case Reports. WB 460]
  RD97
  617.1'027—dc23

2015020335

McGraw-Hill Education books are available at special quantity discounts to use as premiums and sales promotions, or for use in corporate training programs. To contact a representative please visit the Contact Us pages at www.mhprofessional.com.

CONTENTS

Contributors / v
Acknowledgments / xi
Introduction to Series / xiii

Section I
Introduction 1

Section II
Listing of Cases 3
Listing by Case Number... 5
Listing by Health Condition (Alphabetical)... 6

Section III
Twenty-Six Case Scenarios... 7

Index / 461

CONTRIBUTORS

Jaynie Bjornaraa, PhD, MPH, PT, SCS, ATC, CSCS
Associate Professor
Doctor of Physical Therapy Program
St. Catherine University
Minneapolis, Minnesota

Jason Brumitt, PT, PhD, ATC, CSCS
Assistant Professor
George Fox University
Newberg, Oregon
Adjunct Faculty
Rocky Mountain University
Provo, Utah
Adjunct Online Faculty
University of Medical Sciences Arizona
Avondale, Arizona

Kari Brown Budde, PT, DPT, SCS
Owner, Endurance Athletes Physical Therapy
and Sport Performance, LLC
Faculty, Ohio State University
Sports Physical Therapy Residency Program
Lecturer, Ohio State University Doctor of Physical Therapy Program
Columbus, Ohio

Kaan Celebi, PT, DPT, OCS, SCS, CSCS
Lead Therapist
St. Charles Sports Medicine
Port Jefferson, New York

Daniel Cooper, PT, DPT
Progressive Rehabilitation Associates
Portland, Oregon

Todd E. Davenport, PT, DPT, OCS
Associate Professor
Thomas J. Long School of Pharmacy & Health Sciences
University of the Pacific
Stockton, California

Contributors

Todd S. Ellenbecker, DPT, MS, SCS, OCS, CSCS
Clinic Director, Physiotherapy Associates Scottsdale Sports Clinic
National Director of Clinical Research, Physiotherapy Associates
Senior Director Medical Services, ATP World Tour
Scottsdale, Arizona

Jonathan Eng, PT, DPT, CSCS
PACE Therapeutic Associates
Portland, Oregon

Mathew Failla, PT, MSPT, SCS
Biomechanics and Movement Science
University of Delaware
Newark, Delaware

Kevin R. Ford, PhD, FACSM
Associate Professor
Department of Physical Therapy
School of Health Sciences
High Point University
High Point, North Carolina

Amanda Gallow, PT, DPT
Physical Therapist, Sports Rehabilitation
University of Wisconsin Health Sports Medicine
Madison, Wisconsin

Craig Garrison, PhD, PT, SCS, ATC
Texas Health Ben Hogan Sports Medicine
Fort Worth, Texas

Judy Gelber, PT, DPT, OCS, CSCS
Assistant Professor
Physical Therapy and Neurology
Washington University Program in Physical Therapy
St Louis, Missouri

Joseph Hannon, PT, DPT, CSCS
Texas Health Ben Hogan Sports Medicine
Fort Worth, Texas

Bryan Heiderscheit, PT, PhD
Professor, Departments of Orthopedics and Rehabilitation
and Biomedical Engineering
Director, University of Wisconsin Health Runners' Clinic
Director, Badger Athletic Performance Research
University of Wisconsin-Madison
Madison, Wisconsin

CONTRIBUTORS

Airelle O. Hunter-Giordano, PT, DPT, OCS, SCS
Associate Director of Clinical Services,
University of Delaware Physical Therapy
Director of Sports and Orthopedic Physical Therapy Residencies
Assistant Professor
Newark, Delaware

Christopher J. Ivey, PT, MPT, OCS, SCS, ATC, MS
Assistant Professor
University of St. Augustine for Health Sciences
San Marcos, California

Jason James, PT DPT
Northwest Rehabilitation Associates
Salem, Oregon

Larry Lauer, PhD, CC-AASP
Mental Skills Specialist
USTA Player Development Incorporated
Boca Raton, Florida

B.J. Lehecka, DPT
Assistant Professor
Wichita State University
Department of Physical Therapy
Orthopedic and Sports Physical Therapist
Via Christi Health
Wichita, Kansas

David Logerstedt, PT, PhD, MPT, SCS
Assistant Professor
Department of Physical Therapy
Samson College of Health Sciences
University of the Sciences in Philadelphia
Philadelphia, Pennsylvania

Robert C. Manske, DPT, SCS, MEd, ATC, CSCS
Professor
Department of Physical Therapy
Wichita State University
Via Christi Orthopedic and Sports Physical Therapy
Wichita, Kansas

Timothy Mansour, PT, DPT
Active Life Physical Therapy
Port Ludlow, Washington

Emily Ohlin, PT, SCS
Kinetic Integration
Portland, Oregon

Christine Panagos, PT, SCS, CSCS
Black Diamond Physical Therapy
Portland, Oregon

Phil Plisky, PT, DSc, OCS, ATC, CSCS
Assistant Professor of Physical Therapy
Sports Residency Program Director
University of Evansville & ProRehab-PC
Evansville, Indiana

Daniel Quillin, DPT, ATC
Via Christi Orthopedic and Sports Physical Therapy
Wichita, Kansas

William I. Rubine, MS, PT
Lead Physical Therapist
Comprehensive Pain Center
Oregon Health & Science University
Portland, Oregon

Anthony G. Schneiders, PT, PhD, MSc, PGDipManipTh, PGCertTerTch, DipPhty
Professor and Discipline Lead-Physiotherapy
Central Queensland University
Bundaberg, Australia

Christopher Seagrave, PT, SCS, ATC, CSCS
Emergency Responders Health Center
Boise, Idaho

Marc Sherry, PT, DPT, LAT, CSCS, PES
Physical Therapist, Sports Rehabilitation
University of Wisconsin Health Sports Medicine
Madison, Wisconsin

Angela H. Smith, PT, DPT, OCS, SCS, ATC
Physical Therapist and Assistant Professor
University of Delaware
Newark, Delaware

Jeffrey B. Taylor, PT, DPT, OCS, SCS, CSCS
Assistant Professor
Director of Clinical Education
Department of Physical Therapy
School of Health Sciences
High Point University
High Point, North Carolina

Jill Thein-Nissenbaum, PT, DSc, SCS, ATC
Associate Professor
Doctor of Physical Therapy Program
University of Wisconsin-Madison
Madison, Wisconsin

Jonathan Warren, MHSc, PGD Sports Med, Dip MT, MNZCP
Assistant Professor
University of St. Augustine for Health Sciences
San Marcos, California

ACKNOWLEDGMENTS

I would like to thank each of the authors who contributed cases for this book. Your participation in this project has helped me to create what I believe will be an invaluable book for entry-level students, residents and fellows, and seasoned clinicians. I know that much of my work has been inspired and influenced by your research and clinical practice. We (Erin and I) are fortunate to have your participation.

Next, it can't be said enough, but "we" (the contributors and myself) are fortunate to have Erin Jobst, PT, PhD as our Series Editor. Her tireless efforts have helped us all in the development and editorial process of our cases.

Finally, I would like to thank my family for their support. To my parents—thank you for instilling in me the value of education and life-long learning. I am also forever grateful to my wife Renee and our children Rex, Halsey, and Stone for your patience, love, and support.

Jason Brumitt, PT, PhD, ATC, CSCS

INTRODUCTION TO SERIES

As the physical therapy profession continues to evolve and advance as a doctoring profession, so does the rigor of the entry-level physical therapist education. Students must master fundamental foundation courses while integrating an understanding of new research in all areas of physical therapy. Evidence-based practice is the use of current best evidence in conjunction with the expertise of the clinician and the specific values and circumstances of the patient in making decisions regarding assessment and treatment. Evidence-based practice is a major emphasis in both physical therapy education and practice. However, the most challenging task for students is making the transition from didactic classroom-based knowledge to its application in developing a physical therapy diagnosis and implementing appropriate evidence-based interventions. Ideally, instructors who are experienced and knowledgeable in every diagnosis and treatment approach could guide students at the "bedside," and students would supplement this training by self-directed independent reading. While there is certainly no substitute for clinical education, it is rare for clinical rotations to cover the scope of each physical therapy setting. In addition, it is not always possible for clinical instructors to be able to take the time necessary to guide students through the application of evidence-based tests and measures and interventions. Perhaps an effective alternative approach is teaching by using clinical case studies designed with a structured clinical approach to diagnosis and treatment. At the time of writing the *Physical Therapy Case Files* series, there were no physical therapy textbooks that contain case studies that utilize and reference current literature to support an illustrated examination or treatment. In my own teaching, I have designed case scenarios based on personal patient care experiences, those experiences shared with me by my colleagues, and searches through dozens of textbooks and websites to find a case study illustrating a particular concept. There are two problems with this approach. First, neither my own nor my colleagues' experiences cover the vast diversity of patient diagnoses, examinations, and interventions. Second, designing a case scenario that is not based on personal patient care experience or expertise takes an overwhelming amount of time. In my experience, detailed case studies that incorporate application of the best evidence are difficult to design "on the fly" in the classroom. The two-fold goal of the *Physical Therapy Case Files* series is to provide resources that contain multiple real-life case studies within an individual physical therapy practice area that will minimize the need for physical therapy educators to create their own scenarios and maximize the students' ability to implement evidence into the care of individual patients.

The cases within each book in the *Physical Therapy Case Files* series are organized for the reader either to read the book from "front to back" or to randomly select scenarios based on current interest. A list of cases by case number and by alphabetical listing by health condition is included in Section II to enable the reader to review his or her knowledge in a specific area. Sometimes a case scenario may include a more abbreviated explanation of a specific health condition or clinical test than was provided in another case. In this situation, the reader will be referred to the case with the more thorough explanation.

Every case follows an organized and well-thought-out format using familiar language from both the World Health Organization's International Classification of Functioning, Disability, and Health (ICF) framework[1] and the American Physical Therapy Association's *Guide to Physical Therapist Practice*.[2] To limit redundancy and length of each case, we intentionally did not present the ICF framework or the *Guide's* Preferred Practice Patterns within each case. However, the section titles and the language used throughout each case were chosen to guide the reader through the evaluation, goal-setting, and intervention process and how clinical reasoning can be used to enhance an individual's activities and participation.

The front page of each case begins with a patient encounter followed by a series of open-ended questions. The discussion following the case is organized into seven sections:

1. **Key Definitions** provide terminology pertinent to the reader's understanding of the case; **Objectives** list the instructional and/or terminal behavioral objectives that summarize the knowledge, skills, or attitudes the reader should be able to demonstrate after reading the case; **PT Considerations** provides a summary of the physical therapy plan of care, goals, interventions, precautions, and potential complications for the physical therapy management of the individual presented in the case.
2. **Understanding the Health Condition** presents an abbreviated explanation of the medical diagnosis. The intent of this section is *not* to be comprehensive. The etiology, pathogenesis, risk factors, epidemiology, and medical management of the condition are presented in enough detail to provide background and context for the reader.
3. **Physical Therapy Patient/Client Management** provides a summary of the role of the physical therapist in the patient's care. This section may elaborate on how the physical therapist's role augments and/or overlaps with those of other healthcare practitioners involved in the patient's care, as well as any referrals to additional healthcare practitioners that the physical therapist should provide.
4. **Examination, Evaluation, and Diagnosis** guides the reader how to organize and interpret information gathered from the chart review (in inpatient cases), appreciate adverse drug reactions that may affect patient presentation, and structure the subjective evaluation and physical examination. Not every assessment tool and special test that could possibly be done with the patient is included. For each outcome measure or special test presented, the reliability, validity, sensitivity, and specificity are discussed. When available, a minimal clinically important difference (MCID) for an outcome measure is presented because it helps the clinician to determine the "the minimal level of change required in response to an intervention before the outcome would be considered worthwhile in terms of a patient/client's function or quality of life."[3]
5. **Plan of Care and Interventions** elaborates on a few physical therapy interventions for the patient's condition. The advantage of this section and the previous section is that each case does *not* exhaustively present every outcome measure,

special test, or therapeutic intervention that *could be* performed. Rather, only selected outcome measures or examination techniques and interventions are chosen. This is done to simulate a real-life patient interaction in which the physical therapist uses his or her clinical reasoning to determine the *most appropriate* tests and interventions to utilize with that patient during that episode of care. For each intervention that is chosen, the evidence to support its use with individuals with the same diagnosis (or similar diagnosis, if no evidence exists to support its use in that particular patient population) is presented. To reduce redundancy, standard guidelines for aerobic and resistance exercise have not been included. Instead, the reader is referred to guidelines published by the American College of Sports Medicine,[4] Goodman and Fuller,[5] and Paz and West.[6] For particular case scenarios in which standard guidelines are deviated from, specific guidelines are included.

6. **Evidence-Based Clinical Recommendations** includes a minimum of three clinical recommendations for diagnostic tools and/or treatment interventions for the patient's condition. To improve the quality of each recommendation beyond the personal clinical experience of the contributing author, each recommendation is graded using the Strength of Recommendation Taxonomy (SORT).[7] There are more than 100 evidence-grading systems used to rate the quality of individual studies and the strength of recommendations based on a body of evidence.[8] The SORT system has been used by several medical journals including *American Family Physician, Journal of the American Board of Family Practice, Journal of Family Practice,* and *Sports Health*. We have also chosen to use the SORT system for 2 reasons: it is simple, and its rankings are based on patient-oriented outcomes. The SORT system has only three levels of evidence: A, B, and C. Grade A recommendations are based on consistent, good-quality patient-oriented evidence (*e.g.,* systematic reviews, meta-analysis of high-quality studies, high-quality randomized controlled trials, high-quality diagnostic cohort studies). Grade B recommendations are based on inconsistent or limited-quality patient-oriented evidence (*e.g.,* systematic review or meta-analysis of lower-quality studies or studies with inconsistent findings). Grade C recommendations are based on consensus, disease-oriented evidence, usual practice, expert opinion, or case series (*e.g.,* consensus guidelines, disease-oriented evidence using only intermediate or physiologic outcomes). The contributing author of each case provided a grade based on the SORT guidelines for each recommendation or conclusion. The grade for each statement was reviewed and sometimes altered by the editors. Key phrases from each clinical recommendation are bolded within the case to enable the reader to easily locate where the cited evidence was presented.

7. **Comprehension Questions and Answers** include two to four multiple-choice questions that reinforce the content or elaborate and introduce new, but related concepts to the patient's case. When appropriate, detailed explanations about why alternative choices would not be the best choice are also provided.

My hope is that these real-life case studies will be a new resource to facilitate the incorporation of evidence into everyday physical therapy practice in various settings and patient populations. With the persistent push for evidence-based healthcare to promote quality and effectiveness[9] and the advent of evidence-based reimbursement guidelines, case scenarios with evidence-based recommendations will be an added benefit because physical therapists continually face the threat of decreased reimbursement rates for their services and will need to demonstrate evidence supporting their services. We hope physical therapy educators, entry-level physical therapy students, practicing physical therapists, and professionals preparing for Board Certification in clinical specialty areas will find these books helpful to translate classroom-based knowledge to evidence-based assessments and interventions.

Erin E. Jobst, PT, PhD

1. World Health Organization. International classification of functioning, disability and health (ICF). http://www.who.int/classifications/icf/en/. Accessed August 7, 2012.
2. American Physical Therapy Association. *Guide to Physical Therapist Practice*. Alexandria, VA: APTA; 1999.
3. Jewell DV. Guide to Evidence-based physical therapy practice. Sudbury, MA: Jones and Barlett; 2008.
4. American College of Sports Medicine. *ACSM's Guidelines for Exercise Testing and Prescription*. 8th ed. Philadelphia, PA: Wolters Kluwer/Lippincott Williams & Wilkins; 2010.
5. Goodman CC, Fuller KS. *Pathology: Implications for the Physical Therapist*. 3rd ed. Philadelphia, PA: W.B. Saunders Company; 2009.
6. Paz JC, West MP. *Acute Care Handbook for Physical Therapists*. 3rd ed. St. Louis, MO: Saunders Elsevier; 2009.
7. Ebell MH, Siwek J, Weiss BD, et al. Strength of recommendation taxonomy (SORT): a patient-centered approach to grading evidence in the medical literature. *Am Fam Physician*. 2004;69: 548-556.
8. Systems to rate the strength of scientific evidence. Summary, evidence report/technology assessment: number 47. AHRQ publication no. 02-E015. March 2002. http://www.ahrq.gov/clinic/epcsums/strengthsum.htm. Accessed August 7, 2012.
9. Agency for Healthcare Research and Quality. www.ahrq.gov/clinic/epc/. Accessed August 7, 2012.

SECTION I

Introduction

Physical therapists have numerous active and passive treatment options available to administer or prescribe to a patient with a sport-related musculoskeletal injury. In the age of evidence-based practice, physical therapists must be able to justify the use of an examination technique or intervention based on the best available research evidence, their clinical experience (based on sound clinical reasoning), and the individual patient's values. The purpose of this text is to illustrate how evidence-based practice principles can guide the examination, evaluation, and treatment of the patient with a sport-related musculoskeletal injury. This text contains 26 sports medicine cases from a selection of leaders in physical therapy research, education, and clinical practice. Cases include a spectrum of diagnoses including spine and extremity injuries, postoperative cases, and non-musculoskeletal conditions. Each case presents the best practice patterns supported by the strongest available research for the examination and management of their diagnoses. We hope that the cases presented here help improve the ability of students, new therapists, and experienced clinicians to examine, evaluate, and treat patients. Our hope is that these cases inspire reflections on clinical practice, incite new questions to be asked, and push physical therapists to continually pursue new knowledge.

SECTION II

Listing of Cases

Listing by Case Number

Listing by Health Condition (Alphabetical)

SECTION II: LISTING OF CASES

Listing by Case Number

CASE NO.	HEALTH CONDITION	CASE PAGE
1	Overuse Shoulder Injury in Elite Junior Tennis Player	9
2	Acute Anterior First-Time Shoulder Dislocation	41
3	Glenohumeral Joint Dislocation: Postsurgical Management	59
4	Rehabilitation and Return to Sport After a SLAP Repair in a College Baseball Player	75
5	Ulnar Collateral Ligament Reconstruction	91
6	Spondylolysis in a Gymnast	107
7	Acute Low Back Pain: Spinal Manipulation and Manual Therapy Intervention	121
8	Athletic Pubalgia	139
9	Quadriceps Contusion	153
10	Acute Hamstring Strain	163
11	Hamstring Tendinopathy: Postoperative Management	187
12	Patellofemoral Pain in a Cross-Country Runner	203
13	Patellofemoral Pain in the Cyclist	215
14	Patellar Tendinosis in Volleyball Player With Female Athlete Triad	239
15	Knee Anterior Cruciate Ligament: Injury Prevention	261
16	Knee Anterior Cruciate Ligament: Reconstruction	277
17	Functional Testing to Return Athlete Back to Sport After ACL Reconstruction	297
18	Return to Rugby Following Posterior Cruciate Ligament Reconstruction	309
19	Postsurgical Rehabilitation After Knee Articular Cartilage Repair	325
20	Early (Stages I and II) Posterior Tibial Tendon Dysfunction	337
21	Stress Fracture in Middle-Aged Runner	349
22	Lateral Ankle Sprain	365
23	Preseason Testing to Assess Athletic Readiness and Risk of Injury in a Soccer Player	385
24	Concussion	401
25	Peripheral Neuropathic Pain	415
26	Iron Deficiency in an Endurance Athlete	449

Listing by Health Condition (Alphabetical)

CASE NO.	HEALTH CONDITION	CASE PAGE
2	Acute Anterior First-Time Shoulder Dislocation	41
10	Acute Hamstring Strain	163
7	Acute Low Back Pain: Spinal Manipulation and Manual Therapy Intervention	121
8	Athletic Pubalgia	139
24	Concussion	401
20	Early (Stages I and II) Posterior Tibial Tendon Dysfunction	337
17	Functional Testing to Return Athlete Back to Sport After ACL Reconstruction	297
3	Glenohumeral Joint Dislocation: Postsurgical Management	59
11	Hamstring Tendinopathy: Postoperative Management	187
26	Iron Deficiency in an Endurance Athlete	449
15	Knee Anterior Cruciate Ligament: Injury Prevention	261
16	Knee Anterior Cruciate Ligament: Reconstruction	277
22	Lateral Ankle Sprain	365
1	Overuse Shoulder Injury in Elite Junior Tennis Player	9
14	Patellar Tendinosis in Volleyball Player With Female Athlete Triad	239
12	Patellofemoral Pain in a Cross-Country Runner	203
13	Patellofemoral Pain in the Cyclist	215
25	Peripheral Neuropathic Pain	415
19	Postsurgical Rehabilitation After Knee Articular Cartilage Repair	325
23	Preseason Testing to Assess Athletic Readiness and Risk of Injury in a Soccer Player	385
9	Quadriceps Contusion	153
4	Rehabilitation and Return to Sport After a SLAP Repair in a College Baseball Player	75
18	Return to Rugby Following Posterior Cruciate Ligament Reconstruction	309
6	Spondylolysis in a Gymnast	107
21	Stress Fracture in Middle-Aged Runner	349
5	Ulnar Collateral Ligament Reconstruction	91

SECTION III

Twenty-Six Case Scenarios

Overuse Shoulder Injury in Elite Junior Tennis Player

Todd S. Ellenbecker
Larry Lauer

CASE 1

A 14-year-old elite junior tennis player presented to the physical therapy clinic with a 2-week history of right posterior shoulder pain. The patient has been playing tennis since the age of 8 and has no previous history of shoulder pain. The patient plays tennis daily with an occasional day off from training (1-2 days per month). Her pain occurs primarily during serving in the contact and early follow-through phases, as well as during high forehands. She uses a semi-western grip on her forehand (*i.e.*, modern grip in which the hand is rotated slightly behind the racquet handle compared to the more traditional eastern grip). She denies any recent changes in technique or training volume. She is preparing for a series of high-level tournaments that begin in one month. She reports no neurologic symptoms in her distal right upper extremity, and she has no pertinent medical history or complications. She rates her pain as consistently 8/10 (on 0-10 numerical pain rating scale) during forehands and serves and 0/10 at rest. She reports that her shoulder feels very weak and tired during serves and overhead activities. At the gym, she has started traditional weightlifting including bench press, lateral raises, bicep curls, and push-ups. The patient was referred to physical therapy by her pediatric orthopaedist after standard radiographs were performed. The x-rays were unremarkable with normal growth plate orientation based on the patient's developmental age.

▶ What examination signs may be associated with the suspected diagnosis?
▶ What are the examination priorities?
▶ What are the most appropriate physical therapy interventions?
▶ What is her rehabilitation prognosis?
▶ How would this individual's contextual factors influence or change your patient/client management?

KEY DEFINITIONS

BEIGHTON'S HYPERMOBILITY INDEX: Screen proposed by Beighton and Horan[1] to determine an individual's underlying mobility status; the 5 measurements include hyperextension beyond neutral of the fifth metacarpophalangeal joints, hyperextension of elbows beyond neutral, hyperextension of knees beyond neutral, ability to passively move thumbs to flexor surface of forearms, and ability to touch the floor with both hands flat whilst keeping the knees in full extension. In general, individuals with hypermobility in 3 of the 5 areas are considered to have underlying hypermobility.

FLIP SIGN: Presence of scapular winging or dissociation of the scapula away from the thorax during a manual muscle test (MMT) of glenohumeral external rotation (ER) at the side; observation of the medial border of the scapula during the MMT indicates poor scapular stabilization.

GIRD: Acronym for glenohumeral joint internal rotation deficit; describes a loss of shoulder internal rotation (IR) range of motion

TROM: Acronym for total rotation range of motion; obtained by measuring shoulder IR and ER and adding these 2 values together

Objectives

1. List the phases of the tennis serve that cause the largest activation of the rotator cuff muscles.
2. Describe the most appropriate examination tests and musculoskeletal findings associated with an individual with a tennis-related overuse shoulder injury.
3. Describe evidence-based rehabilitation exercises that are specific for the tennis player.
4. Describe key progressions of therapeutic exercise and range of motion (ROM) for shoulder rehabilitation.
5. Outline a return-to-sport program (*i.e.*, interval tennis program).
6. Understand some of the psychological ramifications of injury in an elite junior tennis player.

Physical Therapy Considerations

PT considerations during management of the young tennis player with posterior shoulder pain:

- **General physical therapy plan of care/goals:** Decrease pain; increase shoulder joint active and passive ROM; increase rotator cuff and scapular strength
- **Physical therapy interventions:** Patient education regarding functional anatomy and injury pathomechanics; modalities and manual therapy to decrease pain;

mobilization and passive stretching to improve joint mobility; resistance exercises to increase muscular strength and endurance of the rotator cuff and scapular stabilizers (lower trapezius, serratus anterior, and rhomboids); home instruction consisting of an exercise program and stretching

▶ **Precautions during physical therapy:** Monitor vital signs; address precautions or contraindications for exercise based on patient's pre-existing condition(s)

▶ **Complications interfering with physical therapy:** Noncompliance with home exercise program; inability to discontinue tennis for a period of time to allow sufficient healing

Understanding the Health Condition

As is commonly observed with overuse shoulder injuries in elite junior tennis players, this player's primary offending activity is the overhead serving motion. Analysis of the tennis serve[2,3] shows high levels of rotator cuff activity during arm cocking and follow-through phases. Given that more than 75% of the typical shots hit in the modern game of tennis are forehands and serves,[4] this player should limit participation in competition at this time because competing without serving is not possible. Once the condition improves, it is imperative that the patient follow an interval return-to-tennis program that limits the initial number of serves to minimize the risk of re-injury.[5]

Physical Therapy Patient/Client Management

The priorities of the physical therapy examination for the overhead athlete with overuse shoulder pain include identification of scapular dysfunction, presence of underlying glenohumeral (GH) joint instability, muscular imbalance, and IR ROM deficiency often referred to as GIRD.[6,7] A common overuse injury in elite junior tennis players is rotator cuff tendonitis.[8] The repetitive loading of the rotator cuff, particularly the supraspinatus and infraspinatus, leads to overuse injury due to the repetitive eccentric muscular activation.[3,8] A recent study by the United States Tennis Association[9] reported overuse injuries occurring in 41% of players in the year studied. This survey of 861 junior players found shoulder injuries to be the second most common injury location in elite players. To perform at the highest level, competitive tennis players have year-round schedules that require ongoing training and competition schedules.[10] One of the biggest challenges to providing physical therapy for this type of athlete is the lack of available time in the patient's schedule to accommodate a period of rest and recovery and *limited* tennis play. In some cases, the patient may need to cease competitive play to allow adequate time for healing and implementation of a therapeutic exercise program to increase strength and endurance of the rotator cuff and scapular muscles. Some of the physical limitations that can remain after rehabilitation can be summarized by the term "the unfinished shoulder." By this, we mean that incomplete restoration of GH joint ROM (*i.e.*, alleviation of GIRD), inadequate scapular stabilization, and incomplete restoration of strength balance often lead to re-injury. This would appropriately be deemed an unsuccessful rehabilitation of this injury. Therefore, the therapist needs to plan and modify the player's rehabilitation program to allow for tendon healing and structural improvements in muscle function and stabilization before the player returns to full tennis activity.

Examination, Evaluation, and Diagnosis

Outcomes that can be used to identify key limitations at the shoulder include measurements of scapular dysfunction, shoulder ROM, and muscular strength. Visual observation of scapular motion with small external loads can accurately identify scapular dysfunction via bilateral comparison of upper extremity movement in the scapular, sagittal, and coronal planes.[11-13] From the posterior view, the physical therapist observed that the patient had a lower dominant right shoulder, prominent inferior angle of the right scapula, and mild atrophy in the infraspinous fossa. These characteristics are associated with what has been described by Kibler et al.[14] as inferior scapular dysfunction. This occurs when there is inadequate muscular stabilization of the scapula and increased anterior tilting, making the inferior angle of the scapula very prominent.[14-16] Placement of the shoulders in the hands-on-hips position exaggerated the prominence of the scapula and highlighted the mild atrophy in the infraspinous fossa (Fig. 1-1). When the patient was asked to raise both arms in forward flexion and scapular plane elevation holding a 1-kg weight, she demonstrated a loss of eccentric control of the right (injured side) scapula

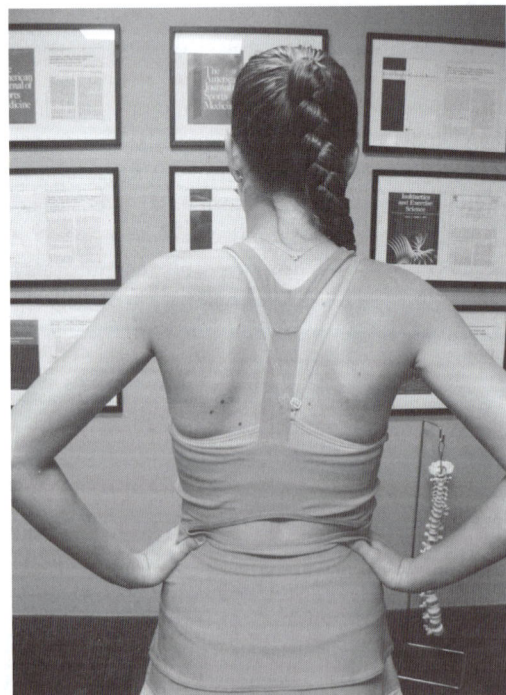

Figure 1-1. Posterior view of elite junior tennis player in hands-on-hips position showing lower right dominant shoulder with mild infraspinatus atrophy and inferior angle prominence.

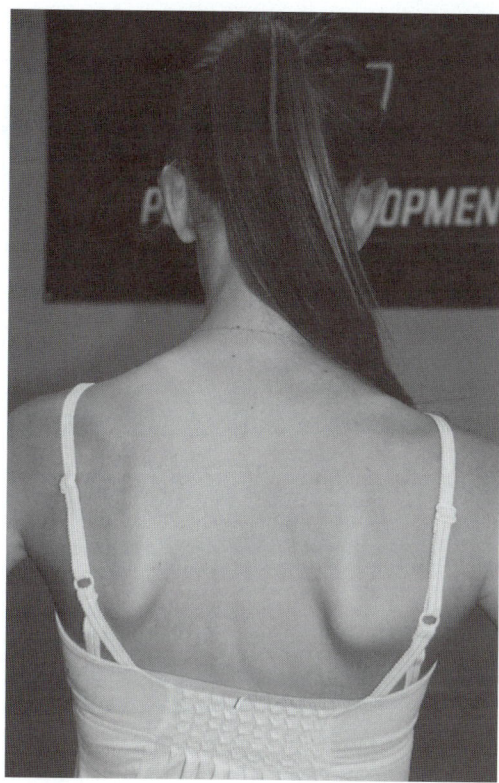

Figure 1-2. Type I Kibler scapular dyskinesis pattern demonstrated by loss of eccentric control upon return from overhead elevation of the right scapula.

when lowering her arm. This increased anterior tilting of the scapula, noted by the prominence of the inferior angle of the scapula, is known as a type I pattern[14] (Fig. 1-2). To determine the effect that scapular stabilization would have, the therapist decided to perform the scapular assistance test (SAT; Fig. 1-3). For this test, the therapist places one hand on the inferior medial aspect of the patient's scapula and the second hand on the superior aspect of the scapula. Next, the clinician provides an upward rotation assistance motion while the patient actively elevates the arm in either the scapular or sagittal plane. A positive SAT occurs when greater arm elevation or decreased pain occurs during the examiner's assistance of the scapula. Kibler et al.[17] have shown that during application of the clinician's stabilization of the scapula, the posterior tilt increases by an average of 7° and this movement was associated with a mean decrease in pain ratings of 56%. This study demonstrated that favorable changes in scapular kinematics could decrease pain in patients with shoulder pain. Rabin et al.[18] tested the inter-rater reliability of the SAT and found coefficient of agreements ranging between 77% and 91% (kappa range 0.53-0.62) for flexion and scapular plane movements. They concluded that the SAT is an acceptable clinical test with moderate test-retest reliability.

Typical of many young overhead athletes, the current patient had negative results (*i.e.*, no reproduction of symptoms) on traditional impingement tests including Neer, Hawkins-Kennedy, coracoid, cross-arm, and Yocum's.[19] Several

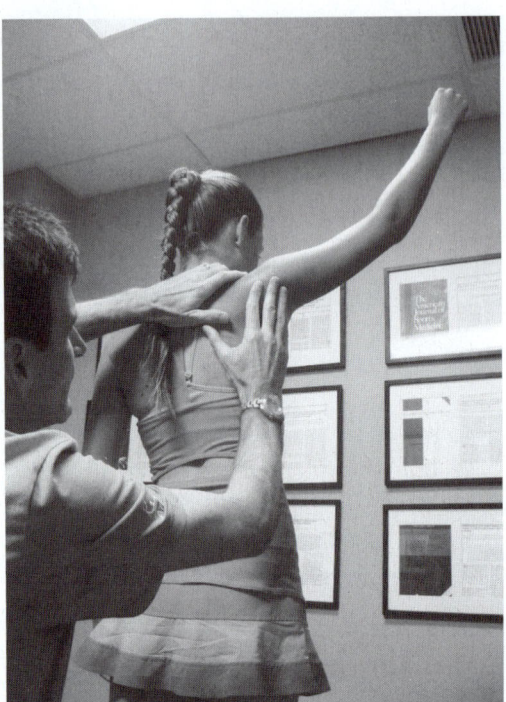

Figure 1-3. Scapular assistance test. Therapist uses his hands to assist the scapula into upward rotation while the patient actively raises her arm.

tests were used to assess the patient's shoulder and general tissue mobility. Based on Beighton's hypermobility index, the patient had all the characteristic signs of hypermobility in her hands, fingers, elbows, and knees.[1] A positive multidirectional instability (MDI) sulcus sign was noted on the right shoulder (see Fig. 2-1), indicating mild instability. The patient had negative O'Brien's and Speeds tests, decreasing the likelihood of superior labral and biceps pathology.[5,19,20] In supine, humeral head translation tests (in 90° abduction in the scapular plane) showed 2^+ anterior translation and 1^+ posterior translation bilaterally. However, no gross apprehension was noted during testing. On the right, the Jobe subluxation/relocation test (Fig. 1-4)[21,22] was positive for reproduction of posterior shoulder pain, highlighting the presence of mild anterior instability.

Gross MMT revealed 5/5 strength bilaterally with no pain reproduction during flexion, abduction, and IR. On the right shoulder, MMT for ER was $4^-/5$ in adduction and at 90° of abduction with immediate pain reproduction. Similar testing of the left shoulder was 5/5 and unremarkable. During MMT of the right shoulder muscles, a positive scapular flip sign was noted. The scapular flip sign is marked by the entire medial border of the scapula protruding away from the thoracic wall, demonstrating a loss of scapular muscle control and stabilization.[23] Strength assessment of the rotator cuff can also be performed using dynamometry. Instrumented[24,25] or isokinetic[25] dynamometry measures both static and dynamic muscle function with the highest level of accuracy. This type of testing can be used for bilateral strength comparisons, unilateral strength ratios (ER/IR), and comparison to normative data.[25]

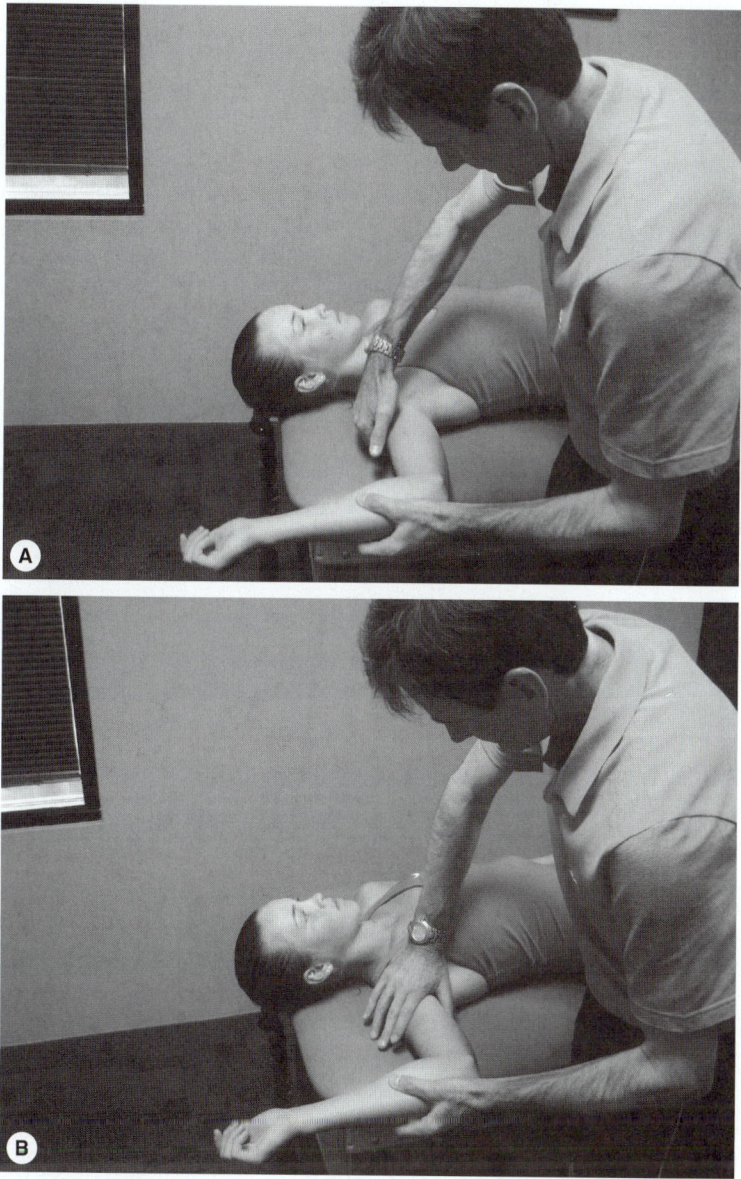

Figure 1-4. Jobe subluxation/relocation test. **A.** Subluxation **B.** Relocation performed in end range external rotation at 90° glenohumeral joint abduction.

Goniometric assessment of shoulder rotation ROM with scapular stabilization provides objective and valid representation of GH joint motion.[26-28] Wilk et al.[26] have demonstrated the importance of using a "C"-shaped scapular stabilization method (Fig. 1-5) to optimize reliability and limit the scapular contribution to GH rotational movement during measurement of rotation ROM. To do so, the therapist places his thumb on the coracoid and his fingers on the scapular spine, thus

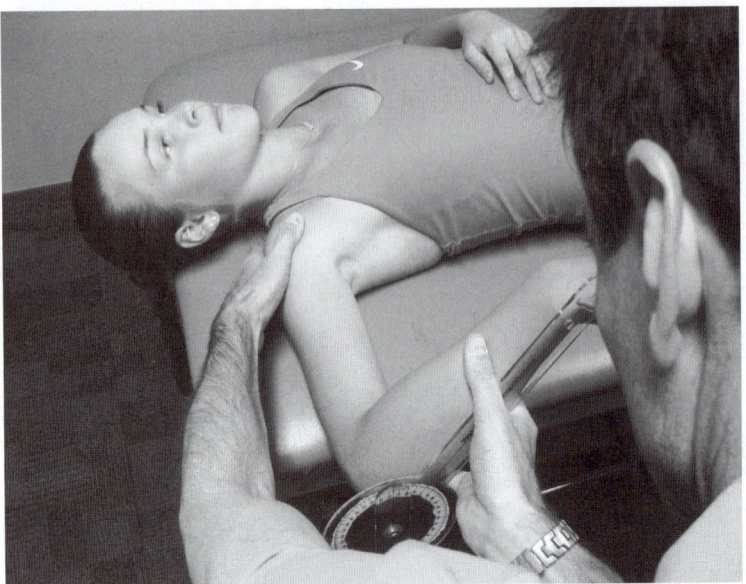

Figure 1-5. "C"-shaped scapular stabilization method to measure glenohumeral joint internal rotation ROM at 90° abduction.

forming a "C" shape to help stabilize the scapula. Research in overhead athletes has highlighted the importance of not only examining IR and ER, but also *total* rotation.[28-30] Total rotation is simply the addition of the IR and ER measurements to form a composite "total rotational profile." Research in overhead athletes has consistently identified the presence of significantly greater ER and less IR on the dominant arm.[28-30] Profiles in elite junior tennis players are slightly different, in that no increase in dominant arm ER has been found. However, in healthy uninjured players, descriptive studies still show decreases of 5° to 10° in total rotation in the dominant arm.[30-32] The player in this case had a 25° loss of IR on the right and a concomitant loss of 20° of total rotation. To assess cross-arm adduction in the supine position with scapular stabilization according to the procedure outlined by Laudner et al.,[33] use of a digital inclinometer is recommended (Fig. 1-6). Recent research has shown 5° to 8° mean decreases in dominant arm cross-arm adduction in healthy uninjured elite junior tennis players.[34] This player had a limitation of 18° on her dominant injured shoulder. Table 1-1 summarizes the passive ROM for the current patient (without overpressure) in the supine position with scapular stabilization.

Thus far in the clinical examination, the therapist identified several critical impairments that have enormous ramifications regarding the development of the plan of care for an elite junior tennis player with an overuse shoulder injury. This patient presents with underlying GH joint instability, loss of shoulder IR (GIRD), scapular pathology, and focal posterior rotator cuff weakness. Each of these factors has been identified as a contributing factor for rotator cuff injury in repetitive overhead athletes.[7] Thus, each contributing factor must form the basis for targeted physical therapy interventions that will address these deficiencies in an attempt to

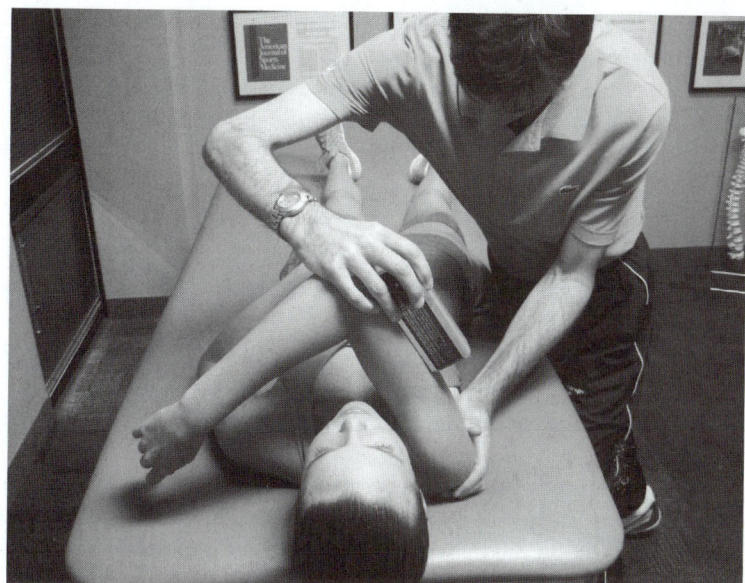

Figure 1-6. Cross-arm adduction measured with a digital inclinometer.

return the patient to full function and sport. The identification of scapular dysfunction indicates the need for early scapular stabilization exercises using specific movement patterns that have been shown to activate scapular muscles.[35-37] Recent studies have reported activation of scapular stabilizers and improved strength following training periods using resistive exercise targeting these muscles.[38,39] The identification of decreased IR and total rotation ROM in the dominant injured extremity means the physical therapist must include interventions that specifically address the loss of IR.[40-42] Finally, the findings of focal posterior rotator cuff weakness indicate the need for specific exercise interventions to improve strength and endurance of key stabilizing muscles to improve humeral head control and optimize shoulder function.

A functional outcome measure for an overhead athlete may include an activity-specific rating scale such as the Kerlan-Jobe Orthopaedic Clinic Shoulder and Elbow Score, which has been designed for overhead athletes with upper extremity (shoulder and elbow) injury.[43-45] Other functional rating scales (*e.g.*, American

Table 1-1 PASSIVE SHOULDER RANGE OF MOTION IN ELITE JUNIOR TENNIS PLAYER		
Movement	Left	Right
External rotation (ER) at 90° abduction	90°	95°
Internal rotation (IR) at 90° abduction	55°	30°
Total rotation	145°	125°
Horizontal cross-arm adduction	45°	28°

Shoulder and Elbow Surgeons Standardized Shoulder Assessment Form, University of Washington's Simple Shoulder Test)[46,47] often do not adequately assess the demands for overhead function because they focus more on activities of daily living (ADLs) and lower-level functional demands. While these assessments may not be the best choice for this patient, they can still be applied based on their predominance in the shoulder literature.

Plan of Care and Interventions

The prognosis for this overuse shoulder injury is good, given the patient's young age, good fitness level, and strong motivation to improve. Outcomes following nonoperative rotator cuff rehabilitation have been reported.[48,49] Morrison et al.[49] profiled 616 patients with GH impingement and found that more than two-thirds of these patients reported success (as measured by reduction of pain and return to function) with physical therapy and nonsteroidal anti-inflammatory medication. While the current patient did *not* demonstrate signs of impingement, her rotator cuff injury was likely secondary to subtle underlying GH joint instability[21] and scapular pathology,[50,51] rather than the classically described external outlet type of GH impingement.[52] Nevertheless, nonoperative rotator cuff rehabilitation interventions are likely still applicable and her prognosis is very good for a complete recovery.

To address the patient's scapular dysfunction, the physical therapist initiated specific exercise progressions aimed at producing high levels of scapular muscle activation to improve strength. Van de Velde et al.[38] and De Mey et al.[39] have shown that a 6-week program of scapular exercises using upper extremity movement patterns such as sidelying shoulder ER, prone extension, prone horizontal abduction with humeral ER, and sidelying shoulder flexion can improve scapular activation and increase muscular strength. Kibler et al.[36] published a series of scapular exercises that can be used early in the rehabilitation process such as the robbery, low row, and lawnmower exercises (Figs. 1-7 through 1-9). Scapular stabilization exercises are progressed to include ER with retraction (Fig. 1-10), an exercise that utilizes the important position of scapular retraction and has been shown to recruit the lower trapezius at a rate 3.3 times greater than the upper trapezius.[53] During this early stage of rehabilitation, multiple exercises were used to strengthen the lower trapezius and other scapular stabilizers, including multiple seated rowing variations, scapular protraction/retraction exercises (with manual resistance provided by the therapist with hand placements directly on the scapula), and the 90° abducted ER exercise in prone (Fig. 1-11).[37]

Uhl et al.[54] have demonstrated the effects of increased weightbearing and of successive decreases in the number of weightbearing limbs on muscle activation of the rotator cuff and scapular musculature. Their work has provided guidance regarding closed-chain exercise progression in the upper extremity. The "plus" position (characterized by maximal scapular protraction in quadruped) has been recommended for its ability to maximally activate the serratus anterior during

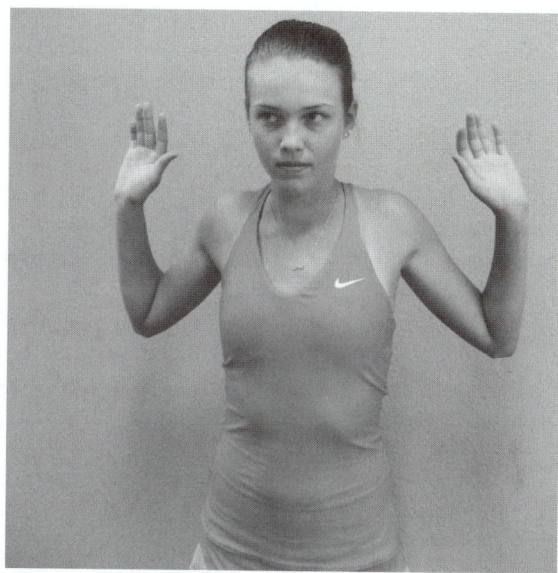

Figure 1-7. "Robbery" scapular exercise.

scapular protraction.[35,55] For the current patient, closed-chain step-ups performed with the upper extremities, quadruped position rhythmic stabilization, and variations of the pointer position (quadruped with extension of one arm and ipsilateral leg) were all used in endurance-oriented formats (timed sets of ≥30 seconds) to enhance scapular stabilization.

In the earlier phase of rehabilitation (after 2-3 weeks of therapy), the physical therapist progressed the athlete to exercises performed in 90° of abduction in the scapular plane to simulate the throwing and overhead patterning inherent in the tennis serve. Initially, the scapular plane position (30° anterior to the coronal plane of the body) only up to 90° of shoulder elevation was chosen as an optimal position for exercises because this is the position of optimal bony congruency between the humeral head and the glenoid[56] at which the rotator cuff is best able to maintain GH stability.[57] Basset et al.[58] have also shown the importance of training muscles in functional positions based on the change in muscular moment arms and subsequent function in the 90°/90° position. An example of an early shoulder elevation exercise performed with therapist guidance is rhythmic stabilization against a therapy ball (Fig. 1-12).

Two principles guided the prescription of rotator cuff strengthening exercises for this patient. First, the therapist selected exercises that placed the shoulder in positions that were well tolerated by patients with rotator cuff and scapular dysfunction. Second, exercise progression was based on research highlighting high levels of electromyographic (EMG) activity of the posterior rotator cuff musculature.[59-62] Sidelying ER and prone extension with the shoulder in an externally rotated (thumb out) position were utilized first. When the patient demonstrated

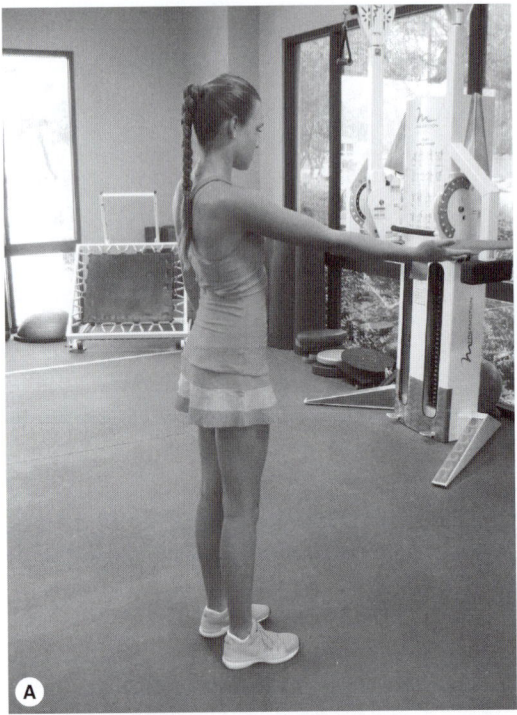

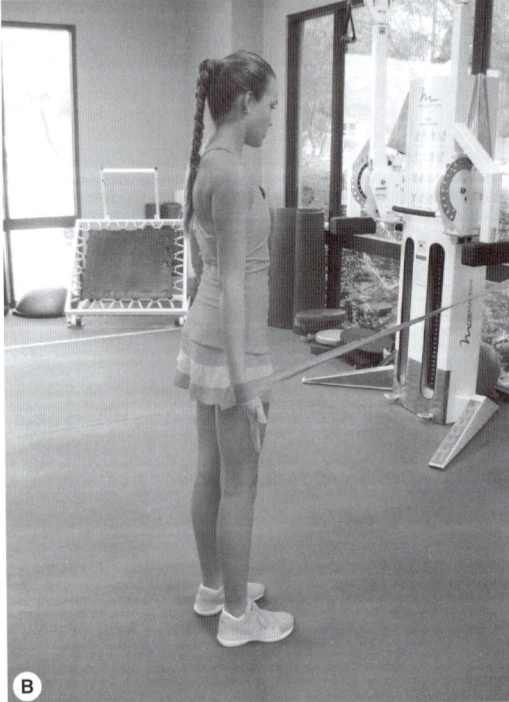

Figure 1-8. Low row exercise. **A.** Patient starts with arm elevated slightly less than 90°. **B.** Patient pulls arm down toward side.

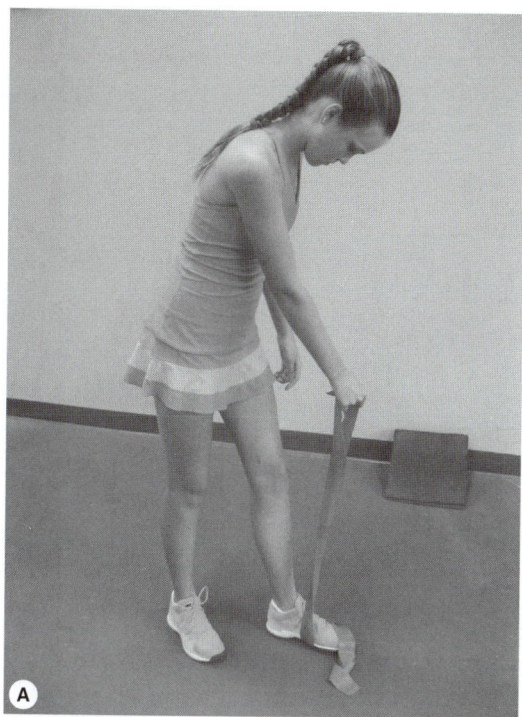

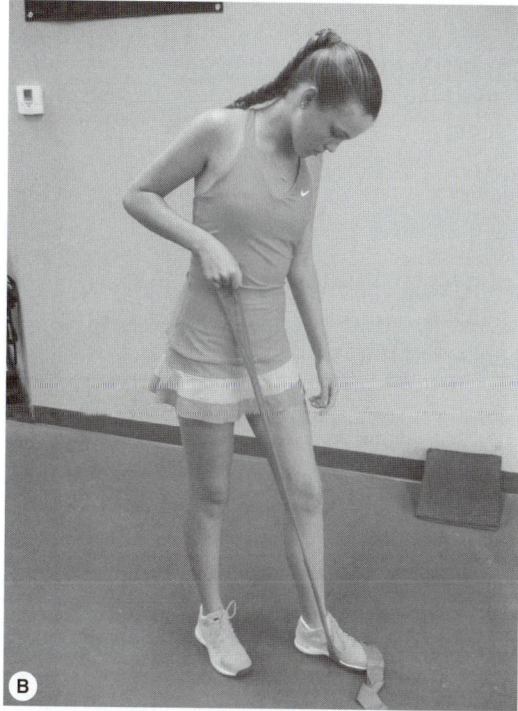

Figure 1-9. Lawnmower scapular exercise. **A.** Patient starts with slacked resistance band under left foot. **B.** Patient pulls right arm up against the resistance of the band, in simulated motion of starting a lawn mower.

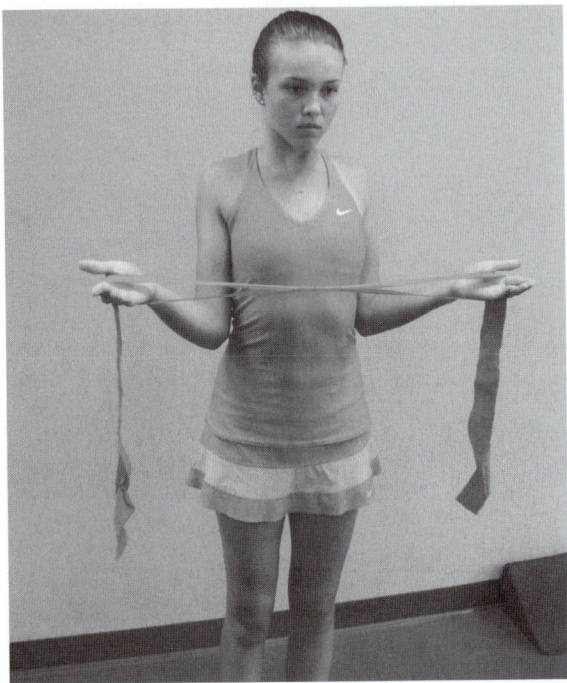

Figure 1-10. External rotation with scapular retraction.

pain-free tolerance to these initial 2 exercises, the therapist progressed her to prone horizontal abduction and prone ER with scapular retraction. The prone horizontal abduction position minimizes subacromial impingement[63] and creates high levels of supraspinatus activation.[60,61,64] This position is a superior alternative to the widely used empty can exercise, which may cause impingement because the shoulder is elevated through the combined movements of IR and elevation.[65] Three sets of 15 to 20 repetitions are recommended to create a fatigue response and improve muscular endurance.[66] Moncrief et al.[67] have shown 8% to 10% increases in isokinetic IR and ER strength in healthy subjects after a 4-week training program. These exercises have also produced improvements in strength and muscular endurance in tennis players and overhead athletes.[68-70] Training of the rotator cuff and scapular musculature modifies and improves the ER to IR ratio, improves strength and endurance of the rotator cuff, and enhances performance.[68,70,71]

All exercises for ER strengthening in standing and sidelying were performed with a small towel roll in the axilla to position the shoulder in 20° to 30° of abduction (Fig. 1-13). In addition to controlling unwanted movements, use of the towel roll increases activity in the infraspinatus muscle by 10% when compared with identical exercises performed without the towel placement.[60] Another theoretical advantage is that this position prevents the "wringing out" phenomenon shown in cadaver research investigating shoulder microvascularity.[72] In an MRI study of 12 healthy adults, Graichen et al.[73] positioned uninjured shoulders at 30°, 60°, 90°, 120°, and 150° of abduction with a towel roll or pillow under the axilla between the

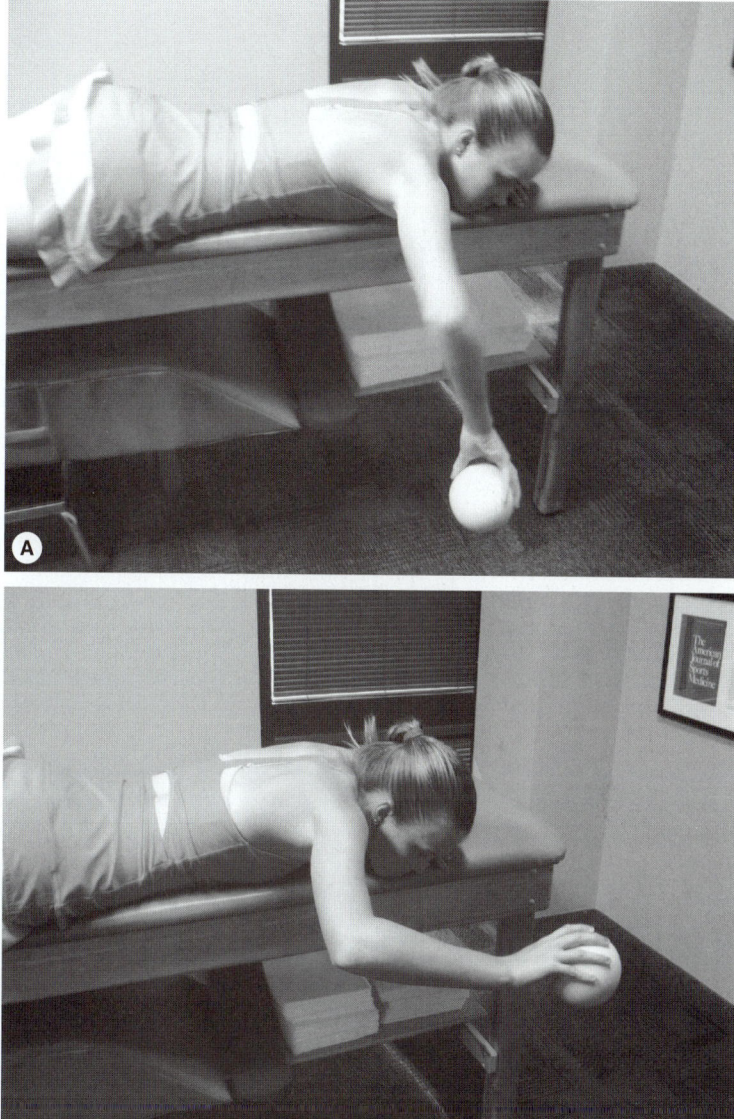

Figure 1-11. Prone external rotation exercise at 90° shoulder abduction. **A.** Patient grasps weighted ball in hand (or dumbbell), and **B.** slowly brings the ball up inline with the body by externally rotating the shoulder.

humerus and the torso. During a humeral rotational training exercise, an isometric abduction or adduction contraction of a 15-Newton force was produced. During the adduction isometric contraction, a significant increase in the subacromial space occurred in all positions of GH joint abduction. The clinical application from this study implies that use of the towel roll facilitates an adduction isometric contraction

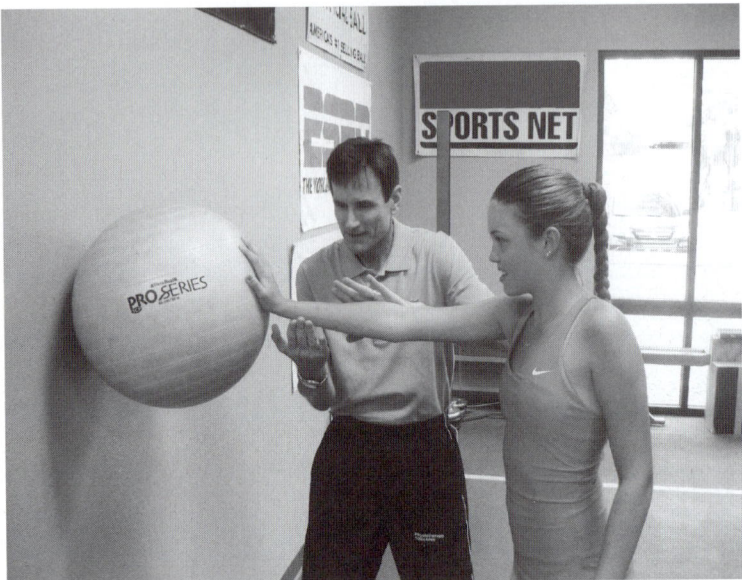

Figure 1-12. Rhythmic stabilization performed with an exercise ball at 90° of elevation in the scapular plane. Therapist provides perturbations to the proximal and distal aspects of the upper extremity.

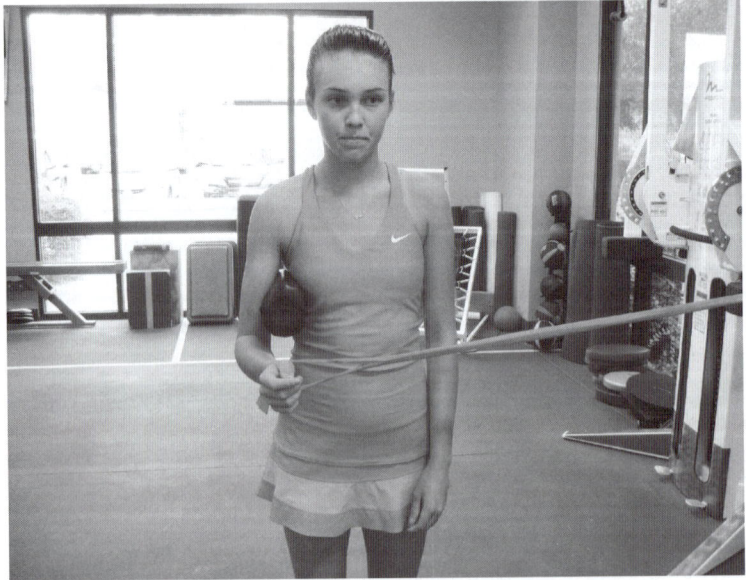

Figure 1-13. Shoulder external rotation performed in standing with elastic resistance showing a towel roll placed under the shoulder for optimal positioning.

in patients who may need enhanced shoulder positioning due to impingement during humeral rotation exercise.[73] To optimize activation of the rotator cuff and to de-emphasize activation from the deltoid and other prime movers of the shoulder, the physical therapist used lower-intensity strengthening exercises. Bitter et al.[74] have measured EMG activity of the infraspinatus and middle and posterior deltoid during ER exercises performed at 10%, 40%, and 70% of maximal contraction in healthy subjects. When resistance was 40% of maximal effort, there was increased relative infraspinatus activity and less compensatory activation of the deltoid as compared to activations at 70%.

To simulate the functional position during serving in tennis[75] or throwing in baseball,[76] the external oscillation or "Statue of Liberty" exercise (Fig. 1-14) and the Impulse Trainer (Impulse Training System, Newnan, Georgia) were used to provide ER eccentric overload training in a position of 90° of elevation in the scapular plane and 90° of ER. The importance of ER fatigue resistance training has ramifications for the proper biomechanical function of the entire upper extremity kinetic chain. Tsai et al.[77] demonstrated significant decreases in posterior scapular tilting and scapular ER following fatigue of the GH external rotators. In a similar study, Ebaugh et al.[78] used an ER fatigue protocol to fatigue the posterior rotator cuff muscles of normal adults with no history of shoulder pathology. Following fatigue of the external rotators, subjects demonstrated less posterior tilting during subsequent arm elevation, indicating scapular compensations and abnormal movement patterns. These studies provide a rationale for the use of ER-based training for the athlete with shoulder dysfunction to potentially avoid compensations that occur with fatigue of the external rotators.

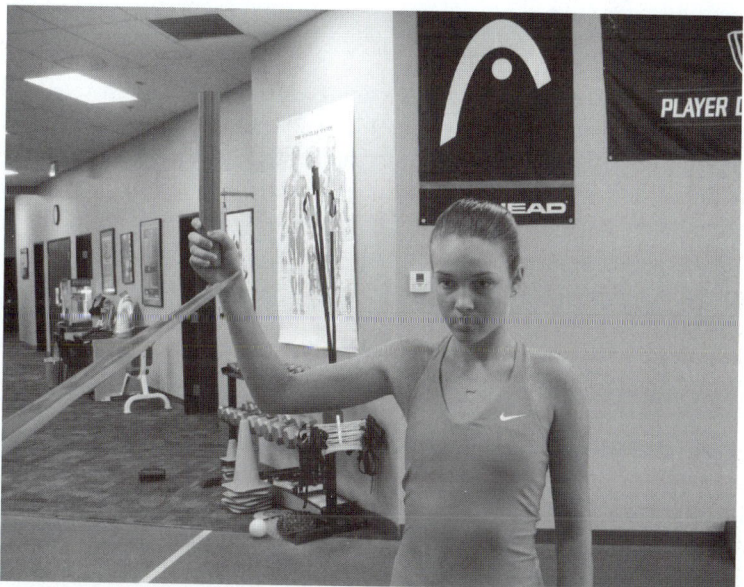

Figure 1-14. Statue of Liberty exercise. The patient externally rotates the shoulder against the applied resistance of the elastic band. Once in the 90/90 position of shoulder abduction and external rotation, the patient performs oscillations with the FlexBar by flexing and extending the wrist.

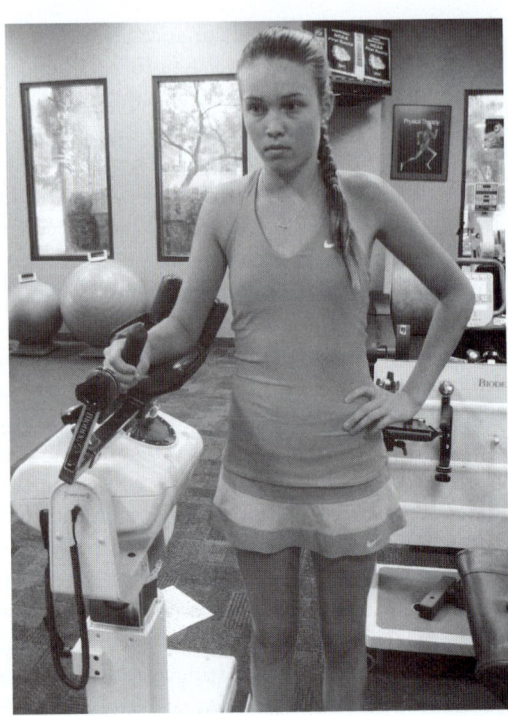

Figure 1-15. Isokinetic shoulder internal/external rotation "modified base" position for testing and training.

Once the patient tolerated isotonic exercise with 2 to 3 lb and could perform rotational training using elastic resistance without pain, the therapist initiated isokinetic rotational exercise in the "modified base" position in which the base of the dynamometer is tilted 30° relative to the horizontal plane, which places the GH joint in 30° of flexion and 30° of abduction (Fig. 1-15). This well-tolerated position allows the patient to progress from submaximal levels of resistance at velocities ranging from 120° to 210° per second for nonathletic patients to 210° to 360° per second during later stages of rehabilitation in athletic patients. Use of the isokinetic dynamometer is important to objectively measure strength, especially the balance between the internal and external rotators.[25] Isokinetic training should focus primarily on shoulder IR/ER patterning. Quincy et al.[79] showed that IR/ER training for a period of 6 weeks not only produced significant gains in IR and ER strength, but also improved strength in shoulder extension/flexion and abduction/adduction. In contrast, training in the patterns of flexion/extension and abduction/adduction over the same 6 weeks only produced strength gains specific to the direction of training. Therefore, emphasis on IR/ER produces an overflow of training, allowing more time-efficient and effective focus in the clinic during isokinetic training.

The **ER/IR strength ratio** provides objective information for the clinician to determine whether there is an appropriate strength balance between anterior and posterior dynamic shoulder stabilizers. Ratios in normal, healthy shoulders have been reported at 66%,[25,80] meaning that external rotators are 66% as strong as the internal rotators. However, pathologic shoulders typically have abnormal ER/IR strength ratios with the shoulder external rotators significantly weaker on the involved side. Emphasis on strength development of the external rotators (posterior rotator cuff) in rehabilitation for a patient with an anterior instability has led to the concept of a "posterior dominant" shoulder (*i.e.*, a shoulder that essentially has a unilateral strength ratio > 66%) with a goal of attaining a ratio of 75% to 80% to improve shoulder dynamic stabilization. The posterior dominant shoulder theoretically provides greater humeral head control and is recommended as a key goal in shoulder rehabilitation. Careful assessment with a dynamometer allows the therapist to objectively measure strength gains and focus the rehabilitation program to promote the return of muscular balance.

During the final stage of rotator cuff rehabilitation (in this case after approximately 4-6 weeks), individuals returning to overhead activities and sports are candidates for advanced isokinetic training using functionally specific rotational training. After 6 weeks of isokinetic training at 90° of GH joint abduction in the scapular plane, athletes have reported increases in rotator cuff strength and functional overhead sport enhancement.[68,81] Plyometric exercise progressions should also be initiated. A functional eccentric pre-stretch followed by a powerful concentric muscular contraction that occurs during plyometric exercises closely parallels many upper extremity sport activities and serves as an excellent exercise modality for transitioning the active patient to interval return-to-sport programs. After an 8-week training program of **plyometric upper extremity exercise and ER strengthening** with elastic resistance, Carter et al.[71] found increased eccentric ER strength, concentric IR strength, and improved throwing velocity in collegiate baseball players. Ellenbecker et al.[82] published a descriptive EMG study of 2 commonly recommended plyometric exercises used in end-stage shoulder rehabilitation. These exercises include a prone 90/90 drop exercise (Fig. 1-16) and reverse catch exercise (Fig. 1-17). High

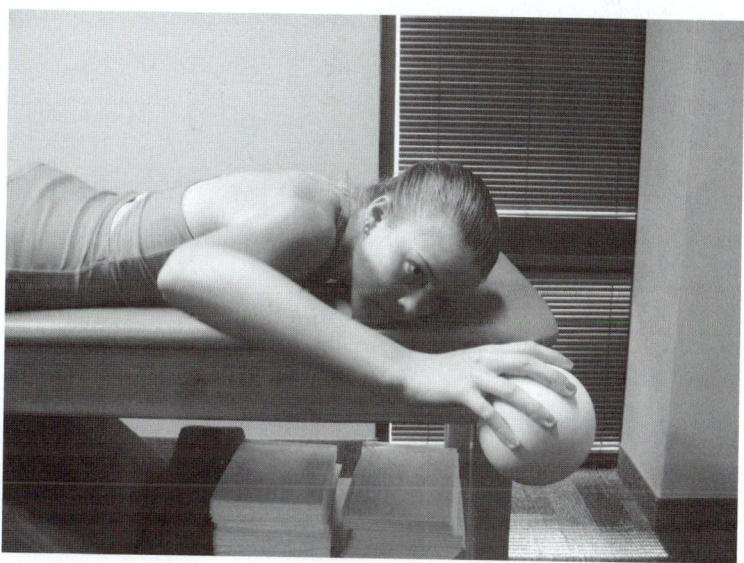

Figure 1-16. The 90/90 plyometric drop exercise. With the shoulder at 90° of abduction and the elbow at 90° of flexion, the patient drops the ball and quickly internally rotates the shoulder to catch it. The shoulder is externally rotated to return the upper extremity to the start position.

levels of lower trapezius and infraspinatus activation were measured using a 0.5- and 1.0-kg medicine ball during the performance of these exercises.[82]

Specific interventions to address loss of shoulder IR must be initiated. Because this patient has underlying anterior instability of the GH joint, the decision to proceed with interventions to increase IR strength must be seriously considered.

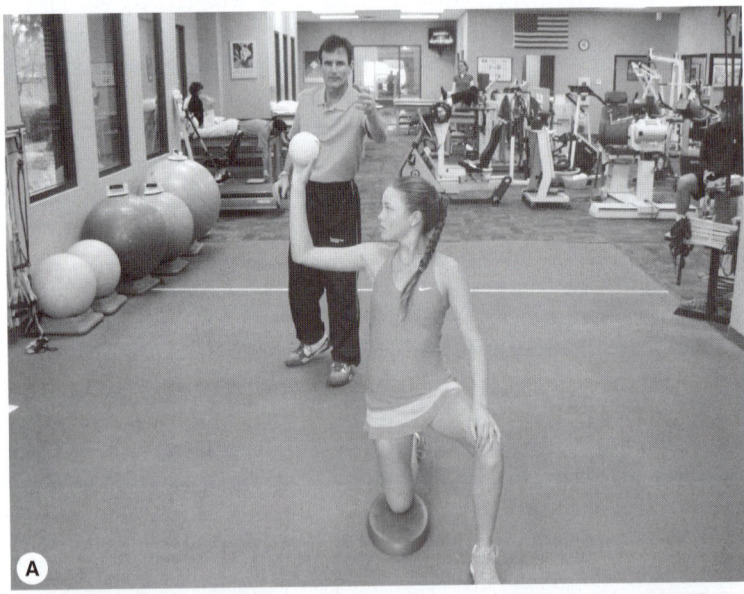

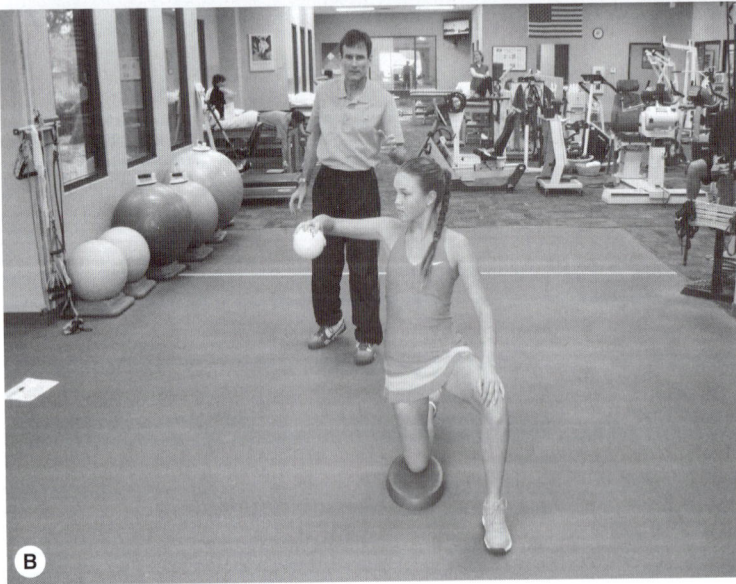

Figure 1-17. The 90/90 reverse catch plyometric exercise. **A.** The therapist lobs a Plyoball over the patient's upper extremity. **B.** The patient catches the Plyoball, decelerating it as the shoulder internally rotates.

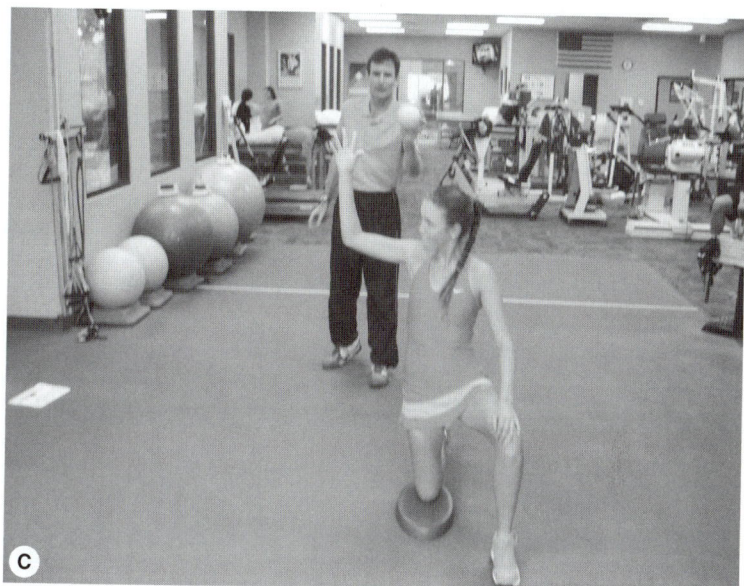

Figure 1-17. *(Continued)* The 90/90 reverse catch plyometric exercise. **C.** The patient quickly reverses the motion by externally rotating the shoulder to throw the ball back to the therapist.

The last thing any therapist wishes to do is to inappropriately increase rotational ROM, which would accentuate GH joint instability. This patient presented with a loss of both isolated dominant arm IR (25°) as well as a loss of total rotation (20°). Therefore, this indicates the need for interventions geared at increasing IR because the threshold widely accepted for rotational ROM loss without increasing injury lies in the window of 5° to 10° of total ROM compared to the contralateral extremity in overhead athletes.[28,29] Because this patient has an IR loss *and* a total rotation loss, she is an ideal candidate for specific interventions to improve IR. Prior to performing interventions to increase ROM, a review of the patient's initial examination findings is indicated. The physical therapist evaluated both physiologic ROM (IR, ER, TROM) and accessory ROM (anterior, posterior, and caudal glides). At the time of evaluation, there were no decrements noted in accessory mobility, only deficiencies in physiologic motion (i.e., IR). Therefore, specific interventions to address IR using physiologic mobilization were indicated. The use of posterior glides or other accessory glides would *not* be indicated due to the patient's underlying hypermobility.

Several studies have been performed to guide clinical decision making on which **specific IR ROM interventions** to utilize.[40,42,83] Figures 1-18 and 1-19 demonstrate versions of shoulder IR stretching positions that utilize the scapular plane position and can be performed in various positions of GH joint elevation. Each stretching position requires an anterior hand placement to provide posterior pressure to minimize scapular compensation and to limit anterior humeral head translation during the IR stretch (due to the effects of obligate translation). In cadaveric studies, Izumi et al.[83] determined which shoulder position placed optimal stress on the

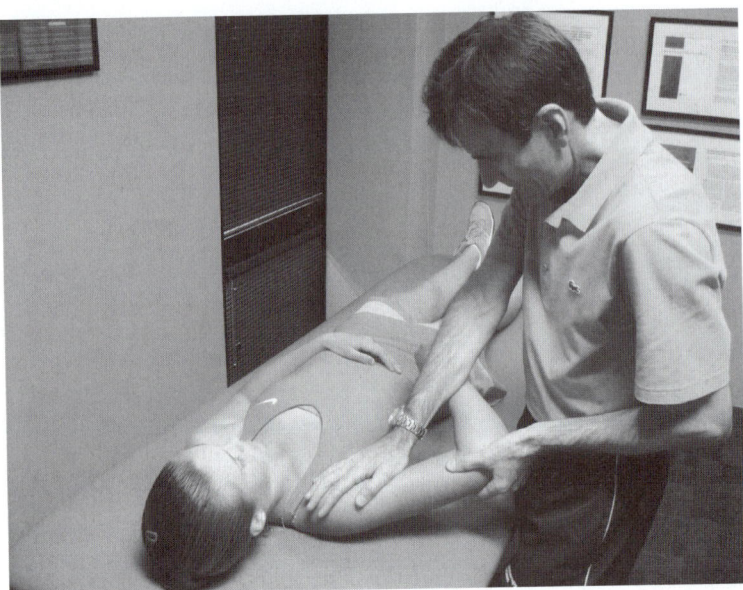

Figure 1-18. Figure 4 internal rotation stretch in the scapular plane. Therapist uses one hand to stabilize the scapula, whereas the other hand grasps the upper extremity at the elbow to perform an internal rotation stretch at the shoulder.

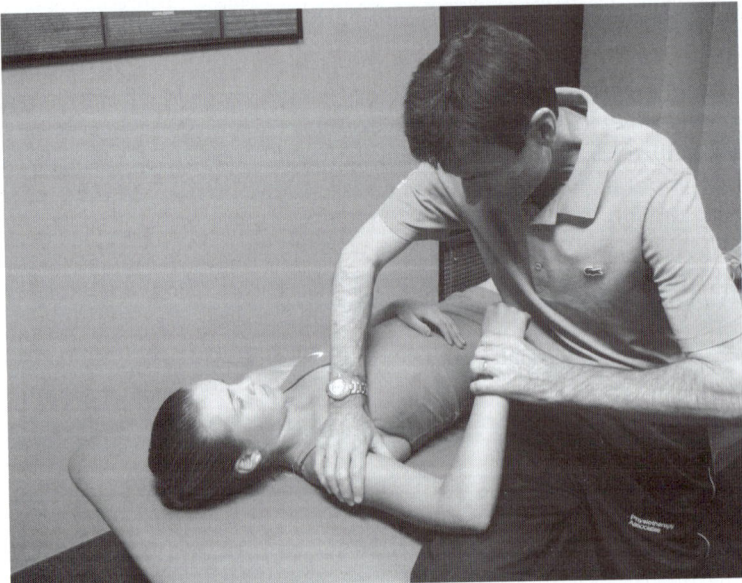

Figure 1-19. Internal rotation stretch modification in scapular plane. Therapist stabilizes scapula with one hand and grasps the wrist with his other hand. The therapist internally rotates the shoulder to create the stretch.

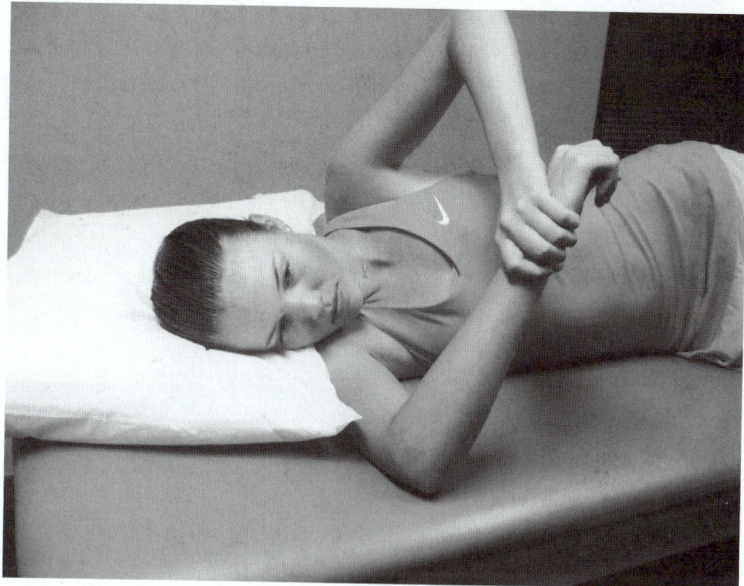

Figure 1-20. Traditional sleeper stretch. The patient grasps her affected arm at the wrist applying a gentle force to internally rotate the shoulder.

posterior capsule. They found that large strains in the posterior capsule occurred during a stretching position of 30° of elevation in the scapular plane with IR. They concluded that this position produced acceptable levels of posterior capsular strain and would be very effective for clinical use. These stretches for the posterior capsule and muscle tendon unit can also be used in a proprioceptive neuromuscular facilitation (PNF) contract-relax format following a low-load prolonged stretch-type paradigm to facilitate the increase in ROM. The sleeper stretch and cross-arm adduction stretch are examples of home stretches given to patients to address IR ROM deficiency (Figs. 1-20 and 1-21). The physical therapist must ensure that the patient maintains scapular stabilization during these stretches. In the sleeper stretch, the patient's body weight on the lateral border of the scapula stabilizes the scapula; in the cross-arm stretch, a wall or supportive object prevents scapular protraction. In a population of recreational athletes (some with significant IR ROM deficiency), McClure et al.[42] compared the effects of the cross-arm stretch versus the sleeper stretch. Four weeks of stretching produced significantly greater IR gains in the group performing the cross-body stretch compared to the sleeper stretch. Despite the results of the aforementioned study, the use of the sleeper stretch is still advocated. However, instead of the full sidelying position that can cause anterior shoulder discomfort, a semi-sidelying position is often recommended (Fig. 1-22). This semi-sidelying position is characterized by the body being rotated backward one-third from true sidelying, still producing scapular stabilization, but decreasing the amount of anterior compression and the induced shoulder pain often inherent with the traditional sleeper stretch. Laudner et al.[84] found an acute increase of 3.3° of IR following three 30-second sleeper stretches. Further research is needed to

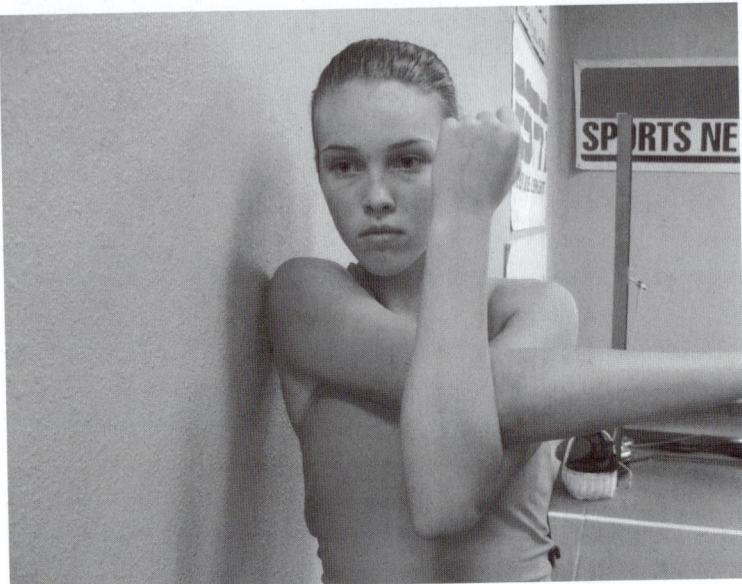

Figure 1-21. Cross-arm adduction stretch with scapular stabilization applied to the lateral scapular border against the wall.

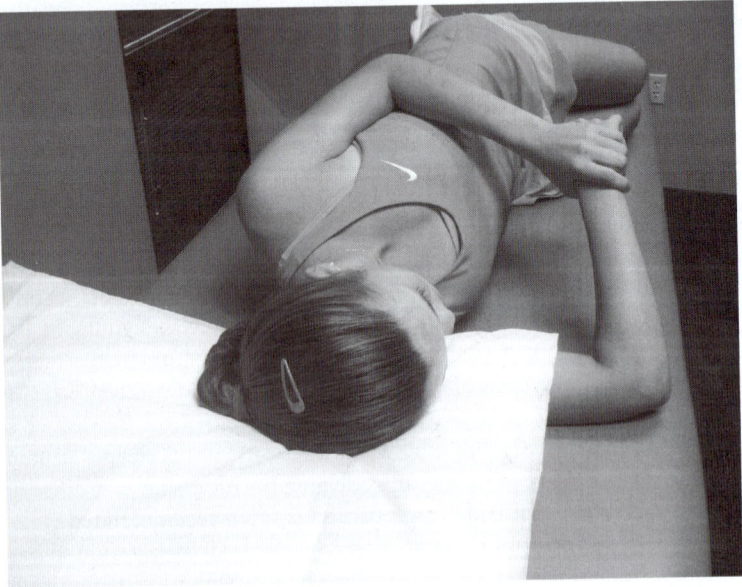

Figure 1-22. Sleeper stretch in one-third rolled-back position (semi-sidelying position). The patient uses her left arm to internally rotate the right shoulder.

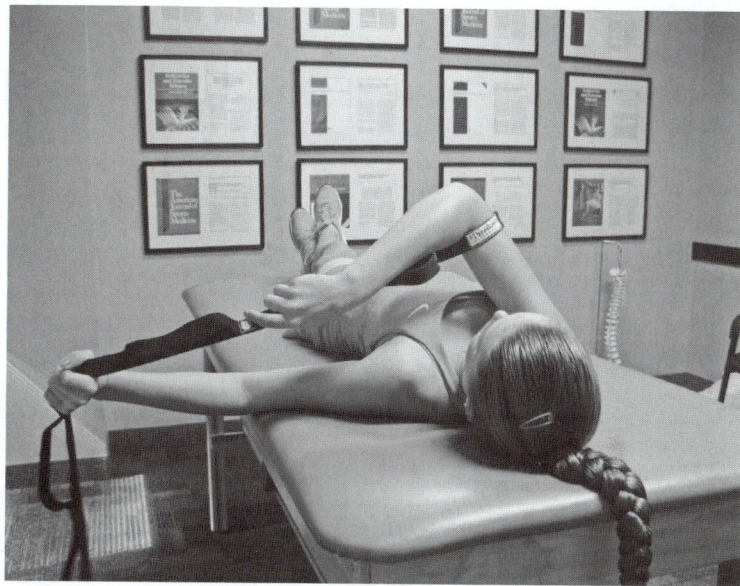

Figure 1-23. Contract-relax cross-arm adduction stretch in supine using a stretch strap.

better define the optimal application of these stretches; however, studies have supported improved IR ROM with a home stretching program.[42]

Additional methods of cross-arm adduction can be used to stress the posterior shoulder structures and improve GH joint IR.[40,41,85] Moore et al.[40] found significantly greater immediate ROM improvements following a cross-arm adduction contract-relax stretch in IR ROM, compared to a contract-relax stretch in the direction of IR. Ellenbecker et al.[85] found an acute increase of 8.4° in IR after 3 patient-directed 30-second contract-relax stretches using an elastic stretch strap in the direction of cross-arm adduction (Fig. 1-23). Another method to improve IR ROM using cross-arm adduction is shown in Fig. 1-24. These stretches use ample scapular stabilization by the therapist and overpressure in the movement of cross-arm adduction to influence posterior shoulder tissue elongation.

Several precautions should be taken during the rehabilitation process. The physical therapist must educate the patient to minimize stress to the rotator cuff, specifically cautioning her to avoid overhead positions (>90° elevation) with resistance exercises and ADLs. In addition, traditional upper extremity weightlifting movement patterns that recruit the prime movers (deltoid, latissimus dorsi, upper trapezius, pectoralis major) should be avoided in an attempt to promote muscular balance. End-range stretching into ER and movement patterns and positions that create stress on the anterior capsule should also be avoided due to her underlying hypermobility.

Psychosocial factors have a significant impact on the rehabilitation of the young athlete. Based on her reported history, the patient exhibits high achievement

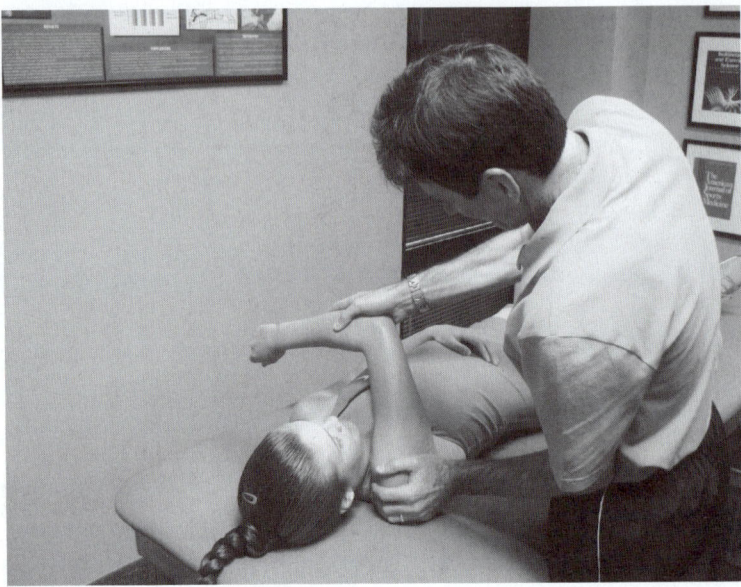

Figure 1-24. Cross-arm adduction stretch performed by the physical therapist with scapular stabilization. The therapist grasps the patient's forearm and horizontally adducts the upper extremity across the chest.

motivation, which can lead to overtraining and overuse.[86] At age 14, elite players are often doing a significant amount of both off-court and on-court training. However, they usually do not understand or have the discipline to consistently execute routines that prepare them for physical exertion or for optimal recovery. With the onset of injury, there is uncertainty about the future that creates anxiety and negative effects on self-confidence, self-esteem, and sense of identity.[87] This player has not been injured before and that may increase her anxiety including the potential of struggling with fears of losing tennis or at least the ability to play at a previous level of proficiency. How the player appraises her ability to cope with the injury and how it affects her tennis goals will influence the rehabilitation process.[88] Furthermore, the player has scheduled tournaments in a month, so there will be pressure to return to play and play well. Often, athletes push to come back sooner to training than they should.

Anxiety and stress related to injury and rehabilitation increase the chance of negative cognition about the rehabilitation process, which can affect commitment and create excessive muscular tension. Feeling connected to the physical therapist can help adherence to the treatment plan, including the home exercise program. Being mindful of the athlete's desire to get back to training and playing, the therapist should remind the young athlete to be patient and make good decisions for the long-term health of her shoulder. In addition, belief in the plan and optimism that the shoulder will regain full strength and function can enhance commitment to the plan of care. Setting short-term and process-focused goals allows the patient to feel success in the rehabilitation journey, thus enhancing motivation. The therapist should also encourage the patient to use positive self-talk to encourage herself to stick to the training and remind herself that she will return healthy and eventually to greater levels of performance. Use of visualization of playing tennis with power and execution can also enhance her readiness to return to play.

Because the physical therapy referral initially came from an orthopaedic surgeon who specializes in shoulder and upper extremity injuries, no additional medical referral is indicated at this time. However, in the event that this patient does not progress with her treatment program and symptoms continue, a referral back to the orthopaedic surgeon for additional imaging and evaluation would be indicated. It is important that the physical therapist work very closely with the player's coach who can provide valuable insight on the player's stroke mechanics, ensuring that proper biomechanical analysis is done on the court to optimize performance and prevent further injury. A key area for the physical therapist to direct the coach to focus on for serving mechanics is proper toss location to minimize impingement forces.

One of the major differences between the values of the patient and clinician lie in the relative importance of returning to play. The clinician has the responsibility to ensure the safe return of the player to tennis without jeopardizing health and well-being, while the player values time on the court and continued competition to achieve pre-set goals within her sport. Clearly communicating the player's status and return-to-sport criteria to the player, coach, and parents is imperative to ensure that improper return to sport timing is encountered.

The professional obligation of the therapist is to couple evidence-based interventions with objective return-to-play guidelines to ensure a comprehensive and complete plan of care from the initial evaluation to discharge. In this case, return-to-play guidelines have been set at returning ER strength equal to the contralateral side, and ER/IR unilateral strength ratios greater than 66% on the dominant injured side.[25] Restoration of total rotation ROM to within 10° of the contralateral side and addressing the GIRD on the dominant side are required to minimize re-injury and return to full activity.[32,89]

Evidence-Based Clinical Recommendations

SORT: Strength of Recommendation Taxonomy
A: Consistent, good-quality patient-oriented evidence
B: Inconsistent or limited-quality patient-oriented evidence
C: Consensus, disease-oriented evidence, usual practice, expert opinion, or case series

1. To optimize dynamic stabilization of the shoulder, the strength of the shoulder external rotators should be at least 66% of the strength of the shoulder internal rotators. **Grade B**
2. The inclusion of plyometric exercises for the shoulder increases eccentric external rotation strength and concentric internal rotation strength in athletes. **Grade B**
3. The sleeper stretch or the cross-arm stretch increase shoulder internal rotation passive range of motion. **Grade B**

COMPREHENSION QUESTIONS

1.1 Which of the following is *not* considered a risk factor for overuse shoulder injury in an elite level overhead athlete?
   A. Scapular pathology
   B. External rotation weakness
   C. Increased internal rotation range of motion
   D. Decreased internal rotation range of motion (GIRD)

1.2 Which factors should be applied in an optimal exercise progression to increase rotator cuff strength?
   A. Low-load, high-repetition formats with exercise intensity for external rotation at 40% or less of maximal levels with movement patterns less than 90° of elevation to minimize impingement
   B. High-load, low-repetition formats with exercise intensity for external rotation at 80% of one's 1 repetition maximum
   C. Maximal effort overhead lifting
   D. Exercises emphasizing shoulder internal rotation strengthening

1.3 Several important clinical characteristics should be evaluated before an overhead athlete returns to play. Which of the following would *not* be one of those factors?
   A. ER/IR ratio between 66% and 75%
   B. Ability to bench press 120% of body weight
   C. No pain with external rotation MMT in 90° of abduction
   D. Pain-free range of motion in 90° of external rotation and 90° of abduction

ANSWERS

1.1 **C.**

1.2 **A.**

1.3 **B.**

REFERENCES

1. Beighton P, Horan F. Orthopaedic aspects of the Ehlers-Danlos syndrome. *J Bone Joint Surg Br.* 1969;51:444-453.
2. Kovacs M, Ellenbecker T. An 8-stage model for evaluating the tennis serve: implications for performance enhancement and injury prevention. *Sports Health.* 2011;3:504-513.
3. Ryu RK, McCormick J, Jobe FW, Moynes DR, Antonell DJ. An electromyographic analysis of shoulder function in tennis players. *Am J Sports Med.* 1988;16:481-485.
4. Roetert EP, Groppel JL. Mastering the kinetic chain. In: Roetert EP, Groppel JL, eds. *World Class Tennis Technique.* Champaign, IL: Human Kinetics; 2001:99-113.
5. Ellenbecker TS. *Clinical Examination of the Shoulder.* St Louis, MO: Elsevier Saunders; 2004.

6. Burkart SS, Morgan CD, Kibler WB. The disabled throwing shoulder: spectrum of pathology. Part I: pathoanatomy and biomechanics. *Arthroscopy*. 2003;19:404-420.
7. Kibler WB, Kuhn JE, Wilk K, et al. The disabled throwing shoulder: spectrum of pathology-10-year update. *Arthroscopy*. 2013;29:141-161.
8. Ellenbecker TS. Rehabilitation of shoulder and elbow injuries in tennis players. *Clin Sports Med*. 1995;14:87-110.
9. Kovacs M, Ellenbecker TS, Kibler WB, Roetert EP, Lubbers P. Injury trends in American competitive junior tennis players. *J Sci Med Tennis*. 2014; 19:19-24.
10. Jayanthi N, Feller E, Smith A. Junior competitive tennis: ideal tournament and training recommendations. *J Med Sci Tennis*. 2013;18:50-58.
11. Tate AR, McClure P, Kareha S, Irwin D, Barbe MF. A clinical method for identifying scapular dyskinesis, part 2: validity. *J Athl Train*. 2009;44:165-173.
12. McClure P, Tate AR, Kareha S, Irwin D, Zlupko E. A clinical method for identifying scapular dyskinesis, part 1: reliability. *J Athl Train*. 2009;44:160-164.
13. Ellenbecker TS, Kibler WB, Bailie DS, Caplinger R, Davies GJ, Riemann BL. Reliability of scapular classification in examination of professional baseball players. *Clin Orthop Rel Res*. 2012; 470:1540-1544.
14. Kibler WB, Uhl TL, Maddux JW, Brooks PV, Zeller B, McMullen J. Qualitative clinical evaluation of scapular dysfunction: a reliability study. *J Shoulder Elbow Surg*. 2002;11:550-556.
15. Priest JD, Nagel DA. Tennis shoulder. *Am J Sports Med*. 1976;4:28-42.
16. Romeo AA, Rotenberg DD, Bach BR Jr. Suprascapular neuropathy. *J Am Acad Orthop Surg*. 1999; 7:358-367.
17. Kibler WB, Uhl TL, Cunningham TJ. The effect of the scapular assistance test on scapular kinematics in the clinical exam. *J Orthop Sports Phys Ther*. 2009;39:A12.
18. Rabin A, Irrgang JJ, Fitzgerald GK, Eubanks A. The intertester reliability of the Scapular Assistance Test. *J Orthop Sports Phys Ther*. 2006;36:653-660.
19. Manske R, Ellenbecker T. Current concepts in shoulder examination of the overhead athlete. *Int J Sports Phys Ther*. 2013;8:554-578.
20. O'Brien SJ, Pagnani MJ, Fealy S, McGlynn SR, Wilson JB. The active compression test: a new and effective test for diagnosing labral tears and acromioclavicular joint abnormality. *Am J Sports Med*. 1998;26:610-613.
21. Jobe FW, Bradley JP. The diagnosis and nonoperative treatment of shoulder injuries in athletes. *Clin Sports Med*. 1989;8:419-437.
22. Hamner DL, Pink MM, Jobe FW. A modification of the relocation test: arthroscopic findings associated with a positive test. *J Shoulder Elbow Surg*. 2000;9:263-267.
23. Kelley MJ, Kane TE, Leggin BG. Spinal accessory nerve palsy: associated signs and symptoms. *J Orthop Sports Phys Ther*. 2008;38:78-86.
24. Riemann BL, Davies GJ, Ludwig L, Gardenhour H. Hand-held dynamometer testing of the internal and external rotator musculature based on selected positions to establish normative data and unilateral ratios. *J Shoulder Elbow Surg*. 2010;19:1175-1183.
25. Ellenbecker TS, Davies GJ. The application of isokinetics in testing and rehabilitation of the shoulder complex. *J Athl Train*. 2000;35:338-350.
26. Wilk KE, Reinold MM, Macrina LC, et al. Glenohumeral internal rotation measurements differ depending on stabilization techniques. *Sports Health*. 2009;1:131-136.
27. Awan R, Smith J, Boon AJ. Measuring shoulder internal rotation range of motion: a comparison of 3 techniques. *Arch Phys Med Rehabil*. 2002;83:1229-1234.
28. Wilk KE, Macrina LC, Fleisig GS, et al. Correlation of glenohumeral internal rotation deficit and total rotational motion to shoulder injuries in professional baseball pitchers. *Am J Sports Med*. 2011;39:329-335.

29. Shanley E, Rauh MJ, Michener LA, Ellenbecker TS, Garrison JC, Thigpen CA. Shoulder range of motion measures as risk factors for shoulder and elbow injuries in high school softball and baseball players. *Am J Sports Med*. 2011;39:1997-2006.
30. Ellenbecker TS, Roetert EP, Bailie DS, Davies GJ, Brown SW. Glenohumeral joint total rotation range of motion in elite tennis players and baseball pitchers. *Med Sci Sports Exerc*. 2002;34:2052-2056.
31. Chandler TJ, Kibler WB, Uhl TL, Wooten B, Kiser A, Stone E. Flexibility comparisons of elite junior tennis players to other athletes. *Am J Sports Med*. 1990;18:134-136.
32. Ellenbecker T, Roetert EP. Age-specific isokinetic glenohumeral internal and external rotation strength in elite junior tennis players. *J Sci Med Sport*. 2003;6:63-70.
33. Laudner KG, Moline MT, Meister K. The relationship between forward scapular posture and posterior shoulder tightness among baseball players. *Am J Sports Med*. 2010;38:2106-2112.
34. Ellenbecker TS, Kovacs M. Bilateral comparison of shoulder horizontal adduction range of motion in elite tennis players. *J Orthop Sports Phys Ther*. 2013;43:A51-A52.
35. Moseley JB Jr, Jobe FW, Pink M, Perry J, Tibone J. EMG analysis of the scapular muscles during a shoulder rehabilitation program. *Am J Sports Med*. 1992;20:128-134.
36. Kibler WB, Sciascia AD, Uhl TL, Tambay N, Cunningham T. Electromyographic analysis of specific exercises for scapular control in the early phases of shoulder rehabilitation. *Am J Sports Med*. 2008;39:1789-1798.
37. Ekstrom RA, Donatelli RA, Soderberg GL. Surface electromyographic analysis of exercises for the trapezius and serratus anterior muscles. *J Orthop Sports Phys Ther*. 2003;33:247-258.
38. Van de Velde A, De Mey K, Maenhout A, Calders P, Cools AM. Scapular muscle performance: two training programs in adolescent swimmers. *J Athletic Train*. 2011;46:160-167.
39. De Mey K, Danneels L, Cagnie B, Cools AM. Scapular muscle rehabilitation exercises in overhead athletes with impingement symptoms: effect of a 6-week training program on muscle recruitment and functional outcome. *Am J Sports Med*. 2012;40:1906-1915.
40. Moore SD, Laudner KG, McLoda TA, Shaffer MA. The immediate effects of muscle energy technique on posterior shoulder tightness: a randomized controlled trial. *J Orthop Sports Phys Ther*. 2011;41:400-407.
41. Manske RC, Meschke M, Porter A, Smith B, Reiman M. A randomized controlled single-blinded comparison of stretching versus stretching and joint mobilization for posterior shoulder tightness measured by internal rotation motion loss. *Sports Health*. 2010;2:94-100.
42. McClure P, Balaicuis J, Heiland D, Broersma ME, Thorndike CK, Wood A. A randomized controlled comparison of stretching procedures in recreational athletes with posterior shoulder tightness. *J Orthop Sports Phys Ther*. 2005;35:A5.
43. Kraeutler MJ, Ciccotti MG, Dodson CC, Frederick RW, Cammarota B, Cohen SB. Kerlan-Jobe Orthopaedic Clinic overhead athlete scores in asymptomatic professional baseball pitchers. *J Shoulder Elbow Surgery*. 2013;22:329-332.
44. Domb GB, Davis JT, Alberta FG, et al. Clinical follow-up of professional baseball players undergoing ulnar collateral ligament reconstruction using the new Kerlan-Jobe Orthopaedic Clinic overhead athlete shoulder and elbow score (KJOC score). *Am J Sports Med*. 2010;38:1558-1563.
45. Alberta FG, ElAttrache NS, Bissell S, et al. The development and validation of a functional assessment tool for the upper extremity in the overhead athlete. *Am J Sports Med*. 2010;38:903-911.
46. Matsen FA III, Artnz CT. Subacromial impingement. In: Rockwood CA Jr, Matsen FA III, eds. *The Shoulder*. Philadelphia, PA: WB Saunders; 1990.
47. Richards RR, An KN, Bigliani LU, et al. A standardized method for the assessment of shoulder function. *J Shoulder Elbow Surg*. 1994;3:347-352.
48. Kuhn JE, Dunn WR, Sanders R, et al. Effectiveness of physical therapy in treating atraumatic full-thickness rotator cuff tears: a multicenter prospective cohort study. *J Shoulder Elbow Surg*. 2013;22:1371-1379.

49. Morrison DS, Frogameni AD, Woodworth P. Non-operative treatment of subacromial impingement syndrome. *J Bone Joint Surg Am*. 1997;79:732-737.
50. Kibler WB. Role of the scapula in the overhead throwing motion. *Cont Orthop*. 1998;22:525-532.
51. Kibler WB. The role of the scapula in athletic shoulder function. *Am J Sports Med*. 1998;26:325-337.
52. Neer CS. Impingement lesions. *Clin Orthop Relat Res*. 1983;173:70-77.
53. McCabe RA, Orishimo KF, McHugh MP, Nicholas SJ. Surface electromyographic analysis of the lower trapezius muscle during exercises performed below ninety degrees of shoulder elevation in healthy subject. *N Am J Sports Phys Ther*. 2007;2:34-43.
54. Uhl TL, Carver TJ, Mattacola CG, Mair SD, Nitz AJ. Shoulder musculature activation during upper extremity weight-bearing exercise. *J Orthop Sports Phys Ther*. 2003;33:109-117.
55. Decker MJ, Hintermeister RA, Faber KJ, Hawkins RJ. Serratus anterior muscle activity during selected rehabilitation exercises. *Am J Sports Med*. 1999;27:784-791.
56. Saha AK. The classic. Mechanism of shoulder movements and a plea for the recognition of "zero position" of the glenohumeral joint. *Clin Orthop Relat Res*. 1983;173:3-10.
57. Happee R, Van der Helm FC. The control of shoulder muscles during goal directed movements, an inverse dynamic analysis. *J Biomech*. 1995;28:1179-1191.
58. Bassett RW, Browne AO, Morrey BF, An KN. Glenohumeral muscle force and moment mechanics in a position of shoulder instability. *J Biomech*. 1994;23:405-415.
59. Townsend H, Jobe FW, Pink M, Perry J. Electromyographic analysis of the glenohumeral muscles during a baseball rehabilitation program. *Am J Sports Med*. 1991;19:264-272.
60. Reinhold MM, Wilk KE, Fleisig GS, et al. Electromyographic analysis of the rotator cuff and deltoid musculature during common shoulder external rotation exercises. *J Orthop Sports Phys Ther*. 2004;34:385-394.
61. Blackburn TA, McLeod WD, White B, Wofford L. EMG analysis of posterior rotator cuff exercises. *Athl Train*. 1990;25:40-45.
62. Ballantyne BT, O'Hare SJ, Paschall JL, et al. Electromyographic activity of selected shoulder muscles in commonly used therapeutic exercises. *Phys Ther*. 1993;73:668-682.
63. Wuelker N, Plitz W, Roetman B. Biomechanical data concerning the shoulder impingement syndrome. *Clin Orthop Relat Res*. 1994;303:242-249.
64. Malanga GA, Jenp YN, Growney E, An K. EMG analysis of shoulder positioning in testing and strengthening the supraspinatus. *Med Sci Sports Exerc*. 1996;28:661-664.
65. Thigpen CA, Padua DA, Morgan N, Kreps C, Karas SG. Scapular kinematics during supraspinatus rehabilitation exercise: a comparison of full-can versus empty-can techniques. *Am J Sports Med*. 2006;34:644-652.
66. Fleck SJ, Kraemer WJ. *Designing Resistance Training Programs*. Champaign IL: Human Kinetics Publishers; 1987.
67. Moncrief SA, Lau JD, Gale JR, Scott SA. Effect of rotator cuff exercise on humeral rotation torque in healthy individuals. *J Strength Cond Res*. 2002;16:262-270.
68. Ellenbecker TS, Davies GJ, Rowinski MJ. Concentric versus eccentric isokinetic strengthening of the rotator cuff: objective data versus functional test. *Am J Sports Med*. 1988;16:64-69.
69. Treiber FA, Lott J, Duncan J, Slavens G, Davis H. Effects of Theraband and lightweight dumbbell training on shoulder rotation torque and serve performance in college tennis players. *Am J Sports Med*. 1998;26:510-515.
70. Niederbracht Y, Shim AL, Sloniger MA, Paternostro-Bayles M, Short TH. Effects of a shoulder injury prevention strength training program on eccentric external rotator muscle strength and glenohumeral joint imbalance in female overhead activity athletes. *J Strength Cond Res*. 2008;22:140-145.
71. Carter AB, Kaminski TW, Douex AT Jr, Knight CA, Richards JG. Effects of high volume upper extremity plyometric training on throwing velocity and functional strength ratios of the shoulder rotators in collegiate baseball players. *J Strength Cond Res*. 2007;21:208-215.

72. Rathburn JB, Macnab I. The microvascular pattern of the rotator cuff. *J Bone Joint Surg Br.* 1970;52:540-553.
73. Graichen H, Hinterwimmer S, von Eisenhart-Rothe R, Vogl T, Englmeier KH, Eckstein F. Effect of abducting and adducting muscle activity on glenohumeral translation, scapular kinematics and subacromial space width in vivo. *J Biomech.* 2005;38:755-760.
74. Bitter NL, Clisby EF, Jones MA, Magarey ME, Jaberzadeh S, Sandow MJ. Relative contributions of infraspinatus and deltoid during external rotation in healthy shoulders. *J Shoulder Elbow Surg.* 2007;16:563-568.
75. Elliott B, Marsh T, Blanksby B. A three dimensional cinematographic analysis of the tennis serve. *Int J Sports Biomech.* 1986;2:260-271.
76. Fleisig GS, Andrews JR, Dillman CJ, Escamilla RF. Kinetics of baseball pitching with implications about injury mechanisms. *Am J Sports Med.* 1995;23:233-239.
77. Tsai NT, McClure PW, Karduna AR. Effects of muscle fatigue on 3-dimensional scapular kinematics. *Arch Phys Med Rehabil.* 2003;84:1000-1005.
78. Ebaugh DD, McClure PW, Karduna AR. Scapulothoracic and glenohumeral kinematics following an external rotation fatigue protocol. *J Orthop Sports Phys Ther.* 2006;36:557-571.
79. Quincy RI, Davies GJ, Kolbeck KJ, Szymanski JL. Isokinetic exercise: the effects of training specificity on shoulder strength development. *J Athl Train.* 2000;35:S64.
80. Byram IR, Bushnell BD, Dugger K, Charron K, Harrell FE Jr, Noonan TJ. Preseason shoulder strength measurements in professional baseball pitchers: identifying players at risk for injury. *Am J Sports Med.* 2010;38:1375-1382.
81. Mont MA, Cohen DB, Campbell KR, Gravare K, Mathur SK. Isokinetic concentric versus eccentric training of the shoulder rotators with functional evaluation of performance enhancement in elite tennis players. *Am J Sports Med.* 1994;22:513-517.
82. Ellenbecker TS, Sueyoshi T, Bailie DS. Muscular activity during plyometric exercises in 90° of glenohumeral joint abduction. *Sports Health.* 2015;7:75-79.
83. Izumi T, Aoki M, Muraki T, Hidaka E, Miyamoto S. Stretching positions for the posterior capsule of the glenohumeral joint: strain measurement using cadaveric specimens. *Am J Sports Med.* 2008;36:2014-2022.
84. Laudner KG, Sipes RC, Wilson JT. The acute effects of sleeper stretch on shoulder range of motion. *J Athl Train.* 2008;43:359-363.
85. Ellenbecker TS, Manske R, Sueyoshi T, Bailie DS. The acute effect of a contract-relax horizontal cross body adduction stretch on shoulder internal rotation using a thera-band stretch strap. Proceedings of Thera-Band Research Advisory Meeting (Moscow, Russia). 2013. http://www.thera-bandacademy.com/elements/clients/docs/TRAC2013Proceedings__635126902900036533.pdf. Accessed March 1, 2015.
86. Peterson K. Overtraining: balancing practice and performance. In: Murphy S, ed. *The Sport Psych Handbook.* Champaign, IL: Human Kinetics; 2004.
87. Brown C. Injuries: the psychology of recovery and rehab. In: Murphy S, ed. *The Sport Psych Handbook.* Champaign, IL: Human Kinetics; 2004.
88. Brewer BW. The role of psychological factors in sport injury rehabilitation outcomes. *Int Rev Sport Exerc Psychol.* 2010;3:40-61.
89. Manske R, Wilk KE, Davies G, Ellenbecker T, Reinold M. Glenohumeral motion deficits: friend or foe? *Int J Sports Phys Ther.* 2013;8:537-553.

Acute Anterior First-Time Shoulder Dislocation

Robert C. Manske
Daniel Quillin
B.J. Lehecka

CASE 2

A 16-year-old male football player is referred to an outpatient physical therapy clinic following a first-time anterior glenohumeral dislocation of his dominant right shoulder one week ago when he reached out to tackle a running back.

- Based on the patient's diagnosis, what is the best method of glenohumeral immobilization?
- How long should glenohumeral immobilization occur in a younger athletic population?
- What are the more common physical therapy subjective outcome measures that can be obtained following this injury?
- What are the most appropriate physical therapy interventions for an anterior shoulder dislocation?
- Are there possible complications that could interfere with physical therapy following this injury?

KEY DEFINITIONS

DYNAMIC STABILIZATION: Use of strengthening or stabilization exercises to help maintain joint congruency

GLENOHUMERAL INSTABILITY: Excessive translation of the humeral head on the glenoid fossa, associated with pain and loss of shoulder function; classified according to many factors such as direction, degree, mechanism, and frequency

JOINT HYPERMOBILITY: Condition in which joints can move beyond the normal range of motion (ROM)

NEUROMUSCULAR CONTROL: Training the neuromuscular system to maintain dynamic stability of the body

PLYOMETRIC EXERCISES: Advanced exercises that train muscles in short, timed intervals; designed to increase the velocity of muscle contraction, which results in increased muscular power

TUBS: Acronym describing glenohumeral instability that is created by a one-time traumatic event in which T = traumatic; U = unilateral extremity; B = Bankart tear; S = surgery that is usually required to repair a torn labrum

Objectives

1. Describe causes of anterior glenohumeral dislocation.
2. Describe the proper treatment following a first-time anterior dislocation.
3. Understand concerns during rehabilitation following an anterior dislocation.
4. Describe exercises designed to obtain dynamic glenohumeral stability.
5. Utilize subjective outcome measurement tools that can be used to track progress.

Physical Therapy Considerations

PT considerations during management of the young athlete following glenohumeral dislocation:

- **General physical therapy plan of care/goals:** Decrease pain; gradually increase ROM and flexibility; increase dynamic glenohumeral control; maintain dynamic scapular stability and return to prior functional level

- **Physical therapy interventions:** Progressive passive and active assisted ROM and gradual progression of strengthening of shoulder and arm (starting with gentle submaximal isometrics and progressing to maximal isotonic exercises); once ROM and strength are regained, slow and gradual return-to-sport progressions; modalities to decrease effusion and edema, as needed

- **Precautions during physical therapy:** Glenohumeral immobilizer is typically worn during the early rehabilitation period to ensure sufficient stabilization to protect healing soft tissue or bony structures; immobilizer typically discontinued in approximately 3 weeks to allow progression of exercises

▶ **Complications interfering with physical therapy:** Persistent pain and swelling; loss of ROM; soft tissue re-rupture (uncommon with appropriate rehabilitation)

Understanding the Health Condition

There is frequently confusion when making the distinction between glenohumeral laxity and instability because these 2 terms are often used interchangeably. Laxity is a constitutional trait that involves the asymptomatic, normal passive translation of the humeral head on the glenoid and may be beneficial to athletic performance.[1] In contrast, glenohumeral instability (the condition discussed in the present case) is a pathologic condition characterized by symptoms of pain and apprehension, which occur with abnormal translations of the humeral head.[1] The total contact surface area of the humeral head with the glenoid is typically about 30%, which means that the joint has limited osseous constraints so that stability is primarily provided by soft tissue components.[2] In the young athletic individual with a loose capsule and a relatively large humeral head in comparison to a shallow and small glenoid fossa, the glenohumeral joint is predisposed to anterior instability. These factors make this joint extremely susceptible to anterior dislocation.[3] When a dislocation occurs, it usually results in a detachment of the anterior inferior labrum from the glenoid fossa, known as a Bankart lesion. **Bankart lesions** occur in 87% to 100% of first-time dislocations.[4-6]

The glenohumeral joint is the most commonly dislocated joint in the human body representing 1.7% of all dislocations occurring each year.[7] Approximately 96% of all shoulder dislocations are acute and anterior in direction.[8,9] Younger athletic individuals usually suffer a dislocation from sporting or recreational activities, whereas older adults may suffer the same injury because of falling on an outstretched hand.[7] Forced abduction and external rotation of the shoulder generally cause anterior dislocation with resulting instability.[10] Dislocation recurrence rates have historically been reported to be as high as 94%.[7,11-16] This is especially problematic for younger athletes who continue to participate in high-risk activities, such as football, rugby, hockey, and wrestling. This case involves a 16-year-old male football player who dislocated his right dominant shoulder while tackling a player on the opposing team.

Risk factors for recurrent anterior glenohumeral instability include young age, participation in high-demand contact sports, previous history of ipsilateral traumatic glenohumeral dislocation, the presence of a Hill-Sachs lesion, presence of an osseous or soft tissue Bankart lesion, ipsilateral rotator cuff or deltoid muscle insufficiency, and any underlying ligamentous laxity issues that have gone undetected.[17-20]

Physical Therapy Patient/Client Management

Following a first-time anterior glenohumeral dislocation, **nonoperative conservative rehabilitation** is attempted prior to surgery. However, the reported success of nonoperative care (as measured by lack of recurrent dislocation) varies widely from

4% to 75%.[11,21] Given the high rate of recurrent instability, there is controversy regarding the best management of first-time dislocation in the young athletic population. Arciero et al.[17] were one of the first groups to examine operative versus nonoperative treatment in this population. Thirty-six military cadets (average age 20 years) were divided into either a conservatively treated group with shoulder immobilization for 1 month followed by rehabilitation or a group who underwent arthroscopic Bankart repair. Twelve of the 15 (80%) conservatively treated athletes developed recurrent instability and 7 of the 12 required open Bankart repair. In contrast, only 3 of 21 (14%) athletes who underwent initial surgical repair developed recurrent instability. This study demonstrated the value of early arthroscopic surgery to reduce the incidence of recurrence in young athletes.[17] A recent systematic review reported that 5 randomized controlled trials consisting of 288 patients supported the use of early operative management in a focused population of young adults.[22] These patients were mostly active males who came from several populations including emergency departments, general hospitals, and active duty military. However, no long-term data (beyond ~3 years postsurgery) are available to determine the effects of surgical intervention on the development of arthritis. Because the young athlete in this case incurred his injury during the end of the football season, the decision was made to initially attempt a nonoperative course of treatment, and if needed, he could have surgical stabilization following the end of the season. With this decision, the athlete and his family must be aware that the attempt at nonoperative care could result in further structural damage such as recurrent dislocations, increased size of Hill-Sachs lesion, and ultimately anterior glenoid bone loss and arthritis.

Examination, Evaluation, and Diagnosis

Examination of the athlete with a first-time anterior shoulder dislocation should consist of a **systematic approach** to direct the examination process for assessing glenohumeral stability. Assessment of active and passive ROM plays a critical role in examining an athlete with glenohumeral instability. Active motion of the shoulder allows the physical therapist to observe the quality and quantity of motion that the athlete is willing to move through. This is especially true when the athlete attempts motions of abduction and external rotation. The therapist asks the athlete to move through the cardinal planes of flexion/extension, internal/external rotation, abduction/adduction, and horizontal abduction/adduction. The therapist asks the athlete to move the shoulder as far as he can and then asks if his shoulder feels as though it would slip, or pop out of place near the end of each motion. If the patient reports a sensation of "giving way," it is important to note where in the range this occurs. It is in this range that the therapist should be careful when assessing passive ROM. Due to the patient's apprehension, passive ROM is usually performed in a relaxed, supine position.

There are several physical examination special tests that can be used specifically to assess for glenohumeral dislocations in athletic individuals.[23] Testing for general ligamentous laxity can be done with the sulcus sign and anterior load and shift test. A dislocation can be assessed with the apprehension test.

The sulcus sign is not necessarily used to determine if an athlete has dislocated his shoulder, but rather is performed to give the examiner an idea of the overall laxity of the glenohumeral joint. While this test can be performed with the patient standing, it is recommended that it be performed with the patient in a seated position because this position allows for more precise control of shoulder position and limits muscle guarding in the apprehensive patient.[24] When performed with the patient seated and the shoulder in a neutrally adducted position, this test primarily assesses the laxity of the superior glenohumeral and coracohumeral ligaments, which are the main passive stabilizing structures of the arm in this position.[25,26] The patient sits with his arm relaxed in his lap so the shoulder is neutrally rotated and adducted. In this position, the patient's elbow is flexed approximately 60° to 80° with the forearm in neutral. Sitting beside the patient, the therapist uses the thumb and fingers of one hand to grasp the acromion. With the other hand, the therapist grasps the athlete's distal humerus and provides a brief downward pull while observing for any separation between the humeral head and the acromion (Fig. 2-1). A positive sulcus sign is a tethering or dimple in the skin between the lateral edge of the acromion and the humerus during the downward pull. This dimple is caused by a widening of the subacromial space due to an increase in inferior humeral translation. A positive sulcus sign is graded by the amount of inferior humeral translation. Grade I is less than 1.0 cm, grade II is 1.0 to 1.5 cm of translation, and grade III is 1.5 cm or greater.[27] In our clinic, we usually determine grades I to III based on the corresponding number of fingerbreadths of the actual sulcus. Therefore, a grade I sulcus would be indicated by one fingerbreadth in sulcus width. In the present case, the athlete exhibited only a trace sulcus sign bilaterally (less than a single fingerbreadth). Because the sulcus sign was minimal and

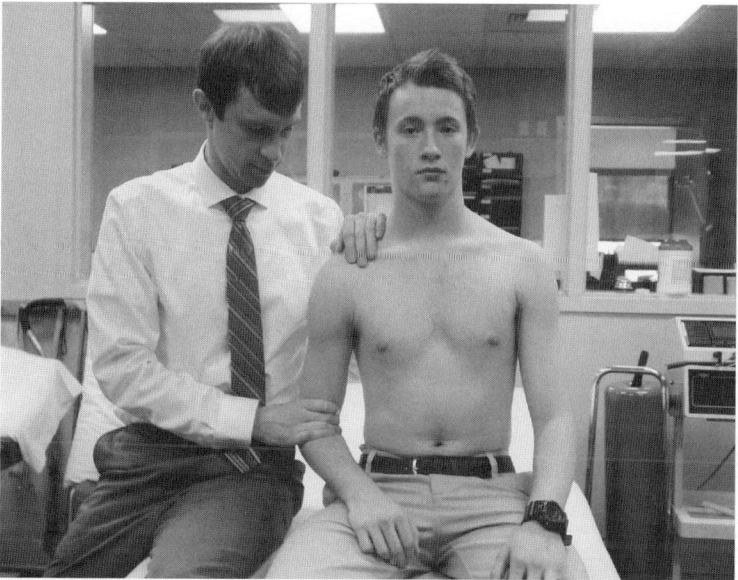

Figure 2-1. Sulcus sign.

bilaterally equal, it was determined that this was likely not the result of a unilateral injury but rather just a slight degree of bilateral congenital laxity.

The anterior load and shift test can be performed to assess the amount of anteroposterior (AP) humeral head laxity. Similar to the sulcus sign, this test is performed with the patient in the sitting position with the glenohumeral joint in the neutral adducted position. This test can also be performed with the patient in the supine position, which allows various degrees of abduction to be assessed. With the arm in adduction with neutral rotation, this test primarily assesses the integrity of the superior glenohumeral ligament of the anterior capsule; however, as the humerus is moved into more abduction, the therapist can assess the integrity or laxity of the middle glenohumeral ligament. Because changing humeral position and testing passive mobility is more difficult in the seated position, the supine position is recommended if the therapist wants to assess the middle glenohumeral ligament. The athlete's hand can be placed in his lap to facilitate relaxation. The patient should be tested in an upright, optimal posture because sitting in a slumped forward shoulder position may lead to a false sense of *less* translation due to the positioning of the humeral head in this posture. The therapist's hand is placed over the patient's shoulder so that the index, second, and third fingers can palpate across the clavicle to the humeral head and coracoid process of the scapula. This hand is therefore used to stabilize the scapula, but also to appreciate any anterior translation of the humeral head from the resting neutral position. With the second hand, the thumb is placed posteriorly and the fingers anteriorly along the proximal humerus. A gentle load can be placed to center the humeral head into the glenoid fossa. Using the thumb on the posterior shoulder to provide the moving force, the therapist attempts to shift the humerus in an anteromedial direction (Fig. 2-2). This anteromedial shift

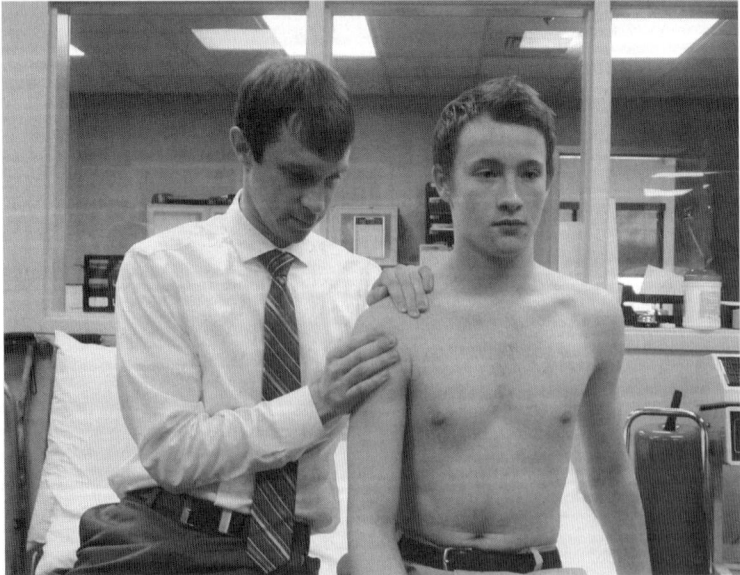

Figure 2-2. Anterior load and shift test.

moves the humeral head along the face of the glenoid, which is oriented at 30° relative to the sagittal plane. Incorrectly performing the shifting movement in a straight sagittal plane will result in tightening of the capsule sooner. This could result in a false-negative result in which it appears that the capsule is tighter than it actually is. A positive anterior load and shift test indicating capsular insufficiency is a unilateral increase in translation compared to the noninvolved extremity. Grading the amount of humeral head translation has been described by Altchek and Dines.[28] In their categorization, a grade I translation indicates that the humeral head translates within the confines of the glenoid rim; a grade II translation occurs when the head translates up and over the glenoid rim with a spontaneous reduction on removal of the anteromedial load; a grade III translation occurs when the head moves up and over the glenoid rim, but does not spontaneously reduce upon removal of the load. In a grade III translation, the humerus must be manually placed back within the area of the glenoid fossa. While there is a large variation in the degree of AP humeral head laxity, grade I and II translations are more common. Several pearls can be offered for therapists inexperienced at performing the anterior load and shift technique. First, care should be taken to avoid pinching with the fingers that are placed over the patient's shoulder because the long head of the biceps lies directly underneath and it is typically a very sensitive area in those with shoulder pain. Second, the grasp must be wide enough to contain the entire humeral head and not just subcutaneous tissue and deltoid muscle that overlie the humeral head. Last, the direction of the translation force must be parallel to the joint surface of the glenoid fossa. This means that the shift should be in the anteromedial direction rather than along the direct sagittal plane. In the current case, the patient had guarded motion and was not able to relax enough during the anterior load and shift test to enable an accurate assessment of laxity in this direction, which may suggest the presence of a labral tear. Because of the pain and guarding that he exhibited as the therapist moved the humeral head near the point of dislocation, the results of this test were inconclusive.

The apprehension test is done to determine whether an individual has had a recent dislocation. This test involves placing the patient in a position similar to that in which he originally dislocated his shoulder. With the athlete relaxed in the supine position, the therapist places the athlete's involved shoulder in one of the more vulnerable positions following a dislocation: abduction, external rotation, and horizontal abduction. The therapist stands on the side of the shoulder being tested to allow a clear view of the athlete's facial expressions during the test. The therapist brings the athlete's shoulder into 90° of abduction, external rotation, and horizontal abduction. Next, the therapist brings the extremity to the end range of the combined motion and provides slight overpressure (Fig. 2-3). If no response is noted, the therapist can provide an anteriorly directed force with one hand placed on the posterior aspect of the humerus. This strategy subjects a greater anterior stress to the humerus, in an attempt to provoke the athlete's symptoms. It must be stressed that this test only evaluates the patient's apprehension—not the amount of anterior translation or pain experienced. A positive test is the patient's apprehensive response to the anteriorly directed force, indicating a lack of glenohumeral joint stability most likely due to a previous glenohumeral dislocation. The apprehension

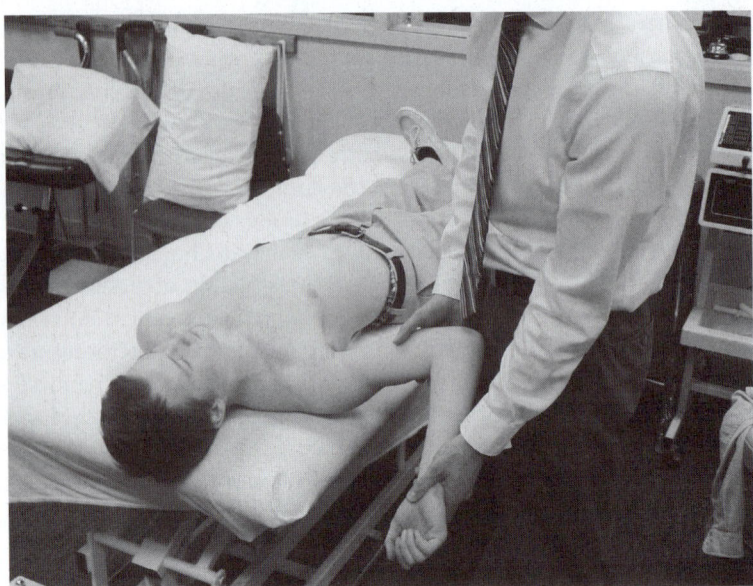

Figure 2-3. Apprehension test.

test may be a fairly good test to rule in the likelihood of a glenohumeral joint dislocation because its reported specificity ranges from moderate to high (63%-99%). However, its sensitivity is quite low (30%-50%).[29,30] Furthermore, the inter-rater reliability of this test is poor [ICC (intraclass correlation coefficient) = 0.47].[31] The athlete in this case demonstrated slight apprehension in the 90/90 position with some overpressure. He stated that it "felt like it was about to slip." The test did not cause another dislocation; however, it was considered a positive apprehension test due to his sensation of an impending dislocation or subluxation.

An acutely dislocated shoulder is readily detectable. However, many times a glenohumeral joint may dislocate and spontaneously relocate, making the diagnosis somewhat more difficult. Following the acute dislocation, the athlete in this case was unable to independently reduce his shoulder. With help from the athletic trainer, his shoulder was reduced on the sideline while at the game. The following day, this athlete was taken to his primary care physician where radiographs were taken to ensure adequate reduction had occurred and that no bony lesion was present. Initial radiographs confirmed adequate reduction and absence of any fractures.

The American College of Radiology recommends that an AP radiograph and an axillary or scapular Y radiograph be performed as the initial imaging for all trauma cases to rule out fracture or dislocation.[32] A standard AP projection is done with the arm at the side and the shoulder slightly externally rotated in anatomical position. This radiograph should demonstrate the proximal third of the humerus, lateral two-thirds of the clavicle, the acromioclavicular joint, and the upper and lateral portions of the scapula. The axillary view, performed supine or prone, is done to help determine the exact relationship of the humeral head to the glenoid fossa in the evaluation of dislocations. The scapular Y view is taken with the athlete in sidelying with the upper extremity in neutral at the patient's side. This view is named for the appearance of the scapula seen in this position, in which it looks like the letter "Y." If there is doubt regarding the extent of the injury and if any labral or rotator cuff damage is suspected, a magnetic resonance imaging sequence can be taken with or without gadolinium. If a bony Bankart detachment from the inferior glenoid is suspected or if there is concern regarding other potential osseous defects such as a Hill-Sachs lesion, a regular or 3-dimensional computed tomography (CT) scan can be performed. Although transient axillary nerve palsy is common following glenohumeral dislocations, many nerves within the brachial plexus can be damaged. Any persistent neurologic deficits should be thoroughly assessed through the use of a nerve conduction study.

Plan of Care and Interventions

The athlete described in this case study is a 16-year-old high school student who dislocated his dominant right shoulder while reaching to tackle a player in a football game. The rehabilitation program used following this injury was a 3-phase program described in Table 2-1.

At times, exercises within these phases may overlap depending on the progress of the individual athlete. There are several factors used to consider the length of rehabilitation. These include the degree of shoulder instability and laxity following the dislocation, shoulder strength and ROM, and the athlete's performance and activity demands. Phases I and II require some degree of caution to ensure that undue stress on the anterior joint capsule is avoided while dynamic joint stability is restored through strengthening of the active stabilizers. The focus of phase II is on progressive isotonic exercises in preparation for returning to prior activity level.

During the first 3 weeks after the acute injury, the athlete is placed in a shoulder sling (Fig. 2-4) and immobilizer. Early on, a cold compressive dressing can be used intermittently to decrease pain and edema. During the acute phase (phase I), electrical stimulation and cryotherapy may be used to help reduce pain and swelling and facilitate the athlete's progress to higher-level activity and demands.

ROM is performed passively, actively, or actively assisted, as tolerated (creating minimal to no pain or apprehension; Figs. 2-5 and 2-6). To avoid overstressing the anterior joint capsule, shoulder abduction and external rotation should be performed in the scapular plane (~20°-30°) anterior to the frontal plane. Shoulder hyperextension should be avoided because this position also places excessive strain on the anterior capsule, which has been injured following an anterior glenohumeral dislocation.

In rare cases, joint mobilization of the posterior shoulder capsule may be needed due to obligate glenohumeral translation from an overly tight capsule. Because an obligate translation occurs opposite the direction of the tight capsule, forward movements of the shoulder with a tight posterior capsule would create an obligate anterior translation, which may cause further pain and exacerbate the already irritable shoulder.

Table 2-1 CONSERVATIVE REHABILITATION FOLLOWING FIRST-TIME GLENOHUMERAL DISLOCATION

Phase	Days-Weeks	Goals	Restrictions	Treatment	Clinical Milestones
Phase I: Immediate postinjury phase	Day 1–Week 4	Decrease pain and inflammation Prevent negative effects of immobilization Restore normal glenohumeral arthrokinematics Prevent primary/secondary hypomobility Promote dynamic stability Prevent reflex inhibition and secondary muscle atrophy	Sling × 3 weeks	Weeks 1-2 AROM/PROM of shoulder as tolerated Wrist/elbow AROM/PROM Shoulder isometrics (no ER) Elbow isometrics Scapular isometric exercises Scapular isotonic exercises Weeks 3-4 Isotonic exercises: Full can (scapular plane shoulder elevation with thumb up) Lateral raises (shoulder abduction) Biceps/triceps exercises ER/IR exercises (light)	No elbow pain No effusion No instability 4/5 shoulder, elbow, and forearm strength
Phase II: Intermediate phase	Weeks 4-8	Progressively restore ROM (full by weeks 6-8) Maintain glenohumeral stability Progressively restore motion, strength, and balance	Avoid activities that provoke pain Do not push motion into ER, ABD, horizontal ABD	Continue to progress AROM/PROM, if full ROM not achieved yet Progress previous UE strengthening exercises by altering intensity and speed Begin light exercises with 1-2 lb. weights Wrist curls Pronation/supination isotonic exercises	Full glenohumeral motion (by week 8) No pain No swelling 4+/5 shoulder, elbow, and forearm strength

Phase IIIA: Return to activity phase	Weeks 8-14+	Full and pain-free AROM/PROM Restoration of muscle strength, power, and endurance No pain or tenderness Gradual initiation of functional activities	Avoid activities that provoke pain Initiate progressive strengthening	Maintain full ROM Increase intensity and decrease repetitions of standard exercises Sidelying ER Two-handed plyometric exercises such as chest pass and wood chopper Wrist flips Wrist slams (with forearm resting on thigh, patient throws 2-lb ball forcefully to ground)	Full symmetrical AROM/PROM No pain or swelling 5/5 shoulder, elbow, forearm, wrist, hand, and scapular muscle strength
Phase IIIB: Return to full activity phase	Weeks 14-21+	Maintain muscle strength, power, and endurance Maintain elbow motion Progress functional activities Return to unrestricted sports activity	None	Continue previous exercises Initiate more advanced double- and single-arm exercises Advance sport-specific training Progress interval sports Plyometric exercises: Single-arm dribble Single-arm IR throws Single-arm ER catches Prone 90/90 drops (see Fig. 1-16)	Return to activity and/or sport

Abbreviations: ABD, abduction; AROM, active range of motion; ER, external rotation; IR, internal rotation; PO, postoperative; PROM, passive range of motion; ROM, range of motion; UE, upper extremity.

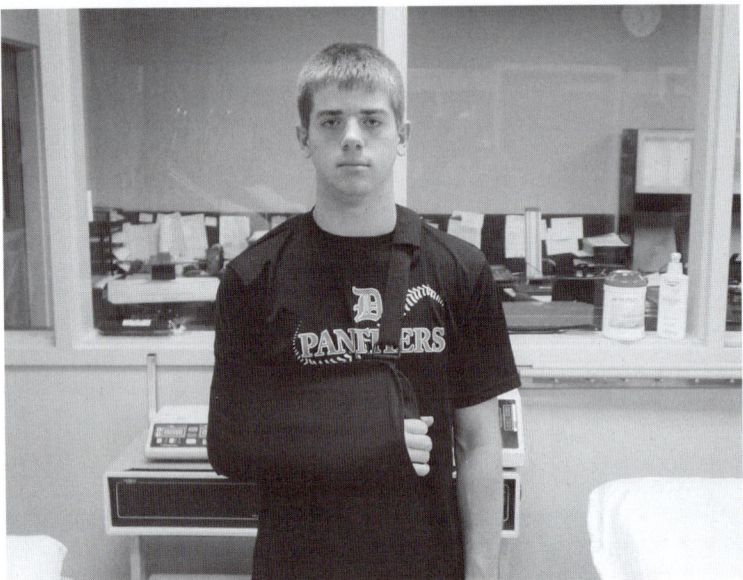

Figure 2-4. Postoperative shoulder sling.

To initiate exercises after an anterior dislocation, arm position should be at the athlete's side with elbow flexed 90°. Strengthening of internal and external glenohumeral rotators begins with isometric exercises and is followed by isotonic exercises as tolerated with light weights or resistive tubing (Figs. 2-7 and 2-8). To avoid stress to the anterior capsule, the amount of external rotation should be no greater than

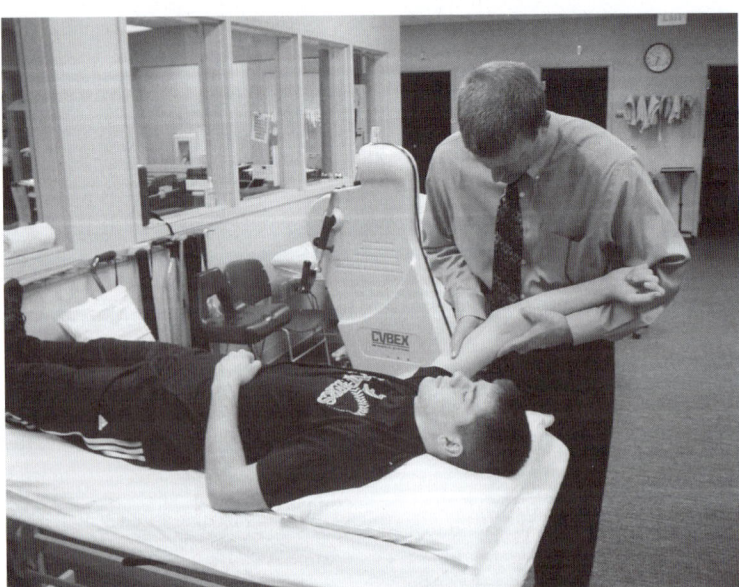

Figure 2-5. PROM: shoulder flexion.

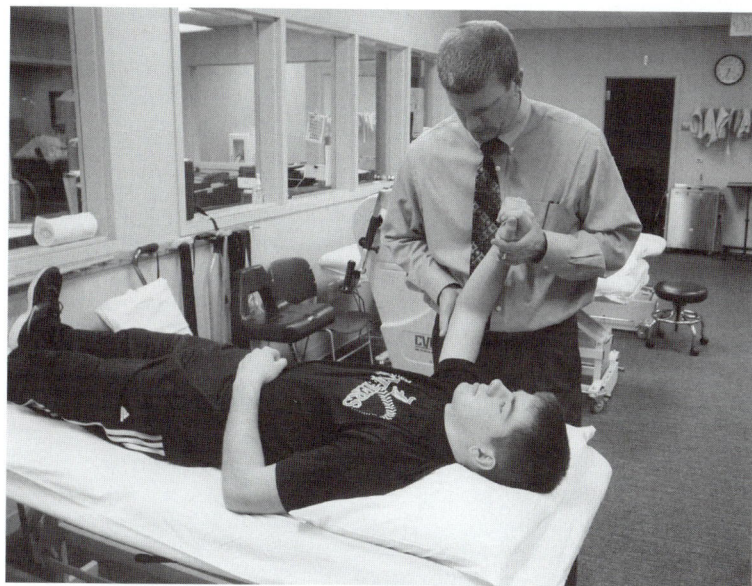

Figure 2-6. PROM: shoulder internal and external rotation.

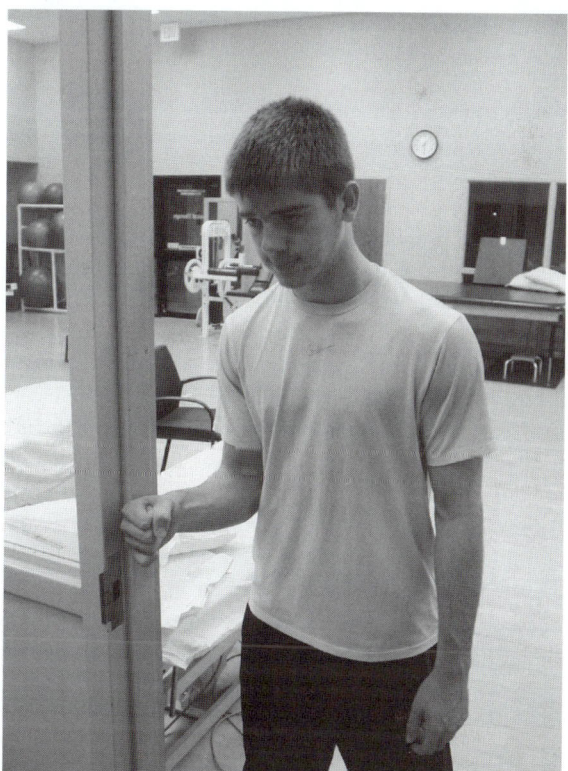

Figure 2-7. Isometric shoulder external rotation exercise.

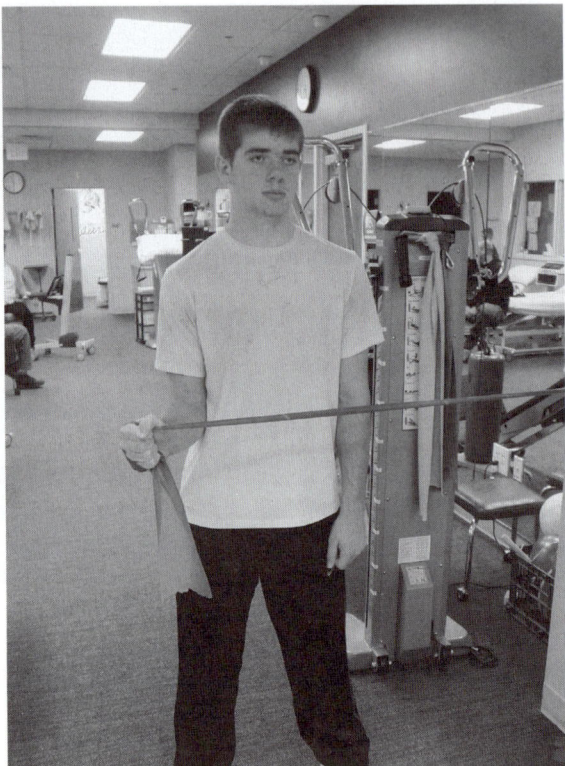

Figure 2-8. Shoulder external rotation with resistive band.

30° to 45°, or as tolerated. Once the athlete is able to tolerate exercises to strengthen the supraspinatus (*e.g.,* full can, lateral raises; Fig. 2-9), he can begin movement in the scapular plane if adequate ROM (up to 90°) is tolerated. Isotonic shoulder flexion exercises can also commence. Prone or standing shoulder extension exercises should be performed with limited extension to the midline of the body. Forearm, wrist, and hand strengthening exercises can be performed as tolerated.

During phase II exercises, posterior cuff/capsule stretching and mobilizations continue, as needed. Strengthening can progress by either increasing resistance or repetitions of each exercise. During phase II, an increased emphasis is placed upon eccentric training of the rotator cuff muscles to better assist with dynamic control of the shoulder. More traditional exercises can begin in phase II, though modifications should be made. For example, push-ups should not be performed in the traditional method in the prone plank position. Instead, the therapist should instruct the athlete to initiate push-ups by performing standing wall push-ups. In addition, to prevent undue stress on the anterior capsule, the shoulder should not horizontally extend past the midline of the body, or the body should not be lowered below the elbows during push-ups. As strength improves, the athlete can move to a modified push-up on the floor by performing the motion on his knees and then progressing to a traditional full push-up from the feet. To protect the anterior

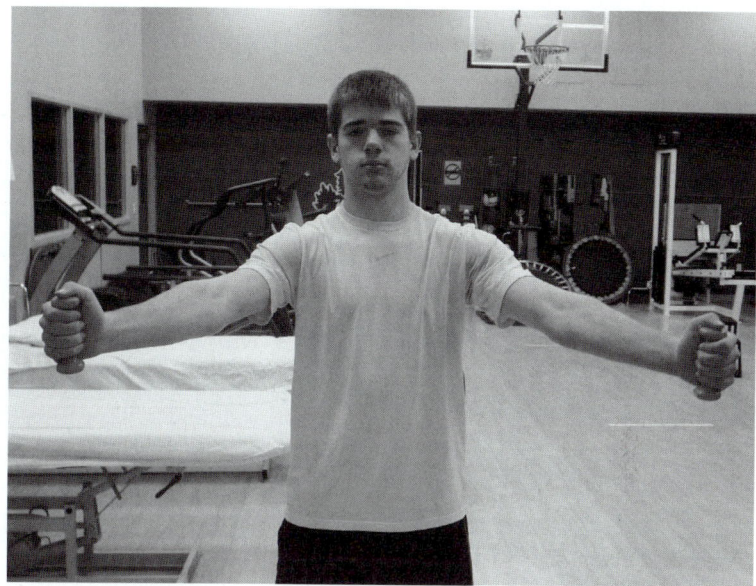

Figure 2-9. Shoulder elevation in scapular plane.

capsule, shoulder presses and latissimus dorsi pull-down exercises should be performed with the bar pulled down in front of the head, and not behind the head.

Phase III exercises progress to higher levels of shoulder elevation. Glenohumeral internal and external rotation exercises are performed in positions that gradually stress the anterior capsule. This is accomplished by progressively positioning the upper extremity at 45°, 80°, and 90° of abduction. These rotator cuff strengthening exercises should be progressed to positions that are specific to the athlete's sporting demands.

It is in phase III that the athlete attempts to return to play. The athlete may begin a return-to-sport program once he has full control of the glenohumeral joint without incidences of subluxation or feelings of instability. Manual muscle testing of the scapula and rotator cuff should not reveal any deficits. Because the current patient is a football player, once these conditions are met he would be able to begin light drills. It is preferred to gradually increase tolerance to practice situations and provide a slow return to full contact and game situations for several weeks. In this manner, the athlete is able to return to full activity in a slow and controlled manner.

In some contact sports, athletes may be prescribed a shoulder brace in an attempt to prevent recurrent anterior instability of the glenohumeral joint. Because of the inherent mobility of the glenohumeral joint and the exacerbated nature of this mobility in individuals with glenohumeral instability, it is very difficult to completely immobilize a shoulder and still maintain acceptable ROM. Most braces limit motion at the glenohumeral joint to 90° of abduction and 70° to 90° of external rotation, which is typically acceptable for a football player. However, for a basketball player's dominant shooting arm or a baseball player's dominant throwing arm (activities that require overhead motion), this type of brace may be unacceptable.

Evidence-Based Clinical Recommendations

SORT: Strength of Recommendation Taxonomy
A: Consistent, good-quality patient-oriented evidence
B: Inconsistent or limited-quality patient-oriented evidence
C: Consensus, disease-oriented evidence, usual practice, expert opinion, or case series

1. Physical therapists should consider the potential of a Bankart tear any time an athlete incurs an anterior shoulder dislocation. **Grade A**
2. Recurrent glenohumeral dislocations are common despite completion of supervised nonoperative treatment for glenohumeral instability. **Grade A**
3. Examination of the athlete with a first-time anterior shoulder dislocation should consist of a systematic approach to direct the examination process for assessing glenohumeral stability. **Grade C**

COMPREHENSION QUESTIONS

2.1 What is the typical length of time that an athlete is immobilized in a shoulder sling following a first-time anterior glenohumeral dislocation?
  A. 1 week
  B. 2 weeks
  C. 3 weeks
  D. 4 weeks

2.2 A positive apprehension test would be indicative of which pathology?
  A. Posterior glenohumeral dislocation
  B. Nontraumatic anterior laxity
  C. Chronic glenohumeral subluxation
  D. Acute traumatic anterior glenohumeral dislocation

ANSWERS

2.1 **C.**

2.2 **D.**

REFERENCES

1. Murray IR, Ahmed I, White NJ, Robinson CM. Traumatic anterior shoulder instability in the athlete. *Scan J Med Sci Sports*. 2013;23:387-405.
2. Bigliani LU, Keldar R, Flatow EL, Pollack RG, Mow VC. Glenohumeral stability. Biomechanical properties of passive and active stabilizers. *Clin Orthop Relat Res*. 1996;330:13-30.

3. Calliet R. Shoulder pain. In: Rowe CR, ed. *The Shoulder.* New York, NY: Churchill Livingstone; 1988.

4. Taylor DC, Arciero RA. Pathologic changes associated with shoulder dislocations. Arthroscopic and physical examination findings in first-time shoulder dislocations. *Am J Sports Med.* 1997;25:306-311.

5. Baker CL, Uribe JW, Whitman C. Arthroscopic evaluation of acute initial anterior shoulder dislocations. *Am J Sports Med.* 1990;18:25-28.

6. Norlin R. Intraarticular pathology in acute, first-time anterior shoulder dislocations: an arthroscopic study. *Arthroscopy.* 1993;9:546-549.

7. Hovelius L. Incidence of shoulder dislocation in Sweden. *Clin Orthop Rel Res.* 1982;166:127-131.

8. Kazar B, Relovszky E. Prognosis of primary dislocation of the shoulder. *Acta Orthop Scand.* 1969;40:216-224.

9. Wintzell G, Haglund-Akerlind Y, Nowak J, Larsson S. Arthroscopic lavage compared with nonoperative treatment for traumatic primary anterior shoulder dislocation: a 2-year follow-up of a prospective randomized study. *J Shoulder Elbow Surg.* 1999;8:399-402.

10. Kaplan LD, Flanigan DC, Norwig J, Jost P, Bradley J. Prevalence and variance of shoulder injuries in elite collegiate football players. *Am J Sports Med.* 2005;33:1142-1146.

11. Aronen JG, Regan K. Decreasing the incidence of recurrence of first time anterior shoulder dislocations with rehabilitation. *Am J Sports Med.* 1984;12:283-291.

12. Hill HA, Sachs MD. The grooved defect of the humeral head: a frequently unrecognized complication of dislocations of the shoulder joint. *Radiology.* 1940;3:690-700.

13. Hovelius L, Olofsson A, Sandstrom B, et al. Nonoperative treatment of primary anterior shoulder dislocation in patients forty years of age and younger: a prospective twenty-five year follow-up. *J Bone Joint Surg Am.* 2008;5:945-952.

14. McLintock LH, Cavallaro WU. Primary anterior dislocation of the shoulder. *Am J Surg.* 1950;80:615-621.

15. Rowe CR, Sakellarides HT. Factors related to recurrences of anterior dislocations of the shoulder. *Clin Orthop Rel Res.* 1961;20:40-48.

16. Simonet WT, Cofield RH. Prognosis in anterior shoulder dislocation. *Am J Sports Med.* 1984;12:19-24.

17. Arciero RA, Wheeler JH, Ryan JB, McBride JT. Arthroscopic Bankart repair versus nonoperative treatment for acute, initial anterior shoulder dislocations. *Am J Sports Med.* 1994;22:589-594.

18. Burkhart SS, De Beer JF. Traumatic glenohumeral bone defects and their relationship to failure of arthroscopic Bankart repairs. Significance of the inverted-pear glenoid and the humeral engating Hill-Sachs lesion. *Arthroscopy.* 2000;16:677-694.

19. Hovelius L, Augustini BG, Fredin H, Johansson O, Norlin R, Throrling J. Primary anterior dislocation of the shoulder in young patients. A ten year prospective study. *J Bone Joint Surg Am.* 1996;78:1677-1684.

20. Robinson CM, Kelly M, Wakefield AE. Redislocation of the shoulder during the first six weeks after a primary anterior dislocation: risk factors and results of treatment. *J Bone Joint Surg Am.* 2002;84A:1522-1559.

21. Hovelius L. Anterior dislocation of the shoulder in teenagers and young adults. Five-year prognosis. *J Bone Joint Surg Am.* 1987;69:393-399.

22. Godin J, Sekiya JK. Systematic review of rehabilitation versus operative stabilization for the treatment of first-time anterior shoulder dislocation. *Sports Health.* 2010;2:156-165.

23. Manske RC, Ellenbecker TS. Current concepts in shoulder examination of the overhead athlete. *Int J Sports Phys Ther.* 2013;8:554-578.

24. McFarland EG, Campbell G, McDowell J. Posterior shoulder laxity in asymptomatic adolescent athletes. *Am J Sports Med.* 1996;24:468-471.

25. Pagnani MJ, Warren RF. Stabilizers of the glenohumeral joint. *J Shoulder Elbow Surg.* 1994;3:73-90.
26. O'Brien SJ, Neves MC, Arnoczky SJ, et al. The anatomy and histology of the inferior glenohumeral ligament complex of the shoulder. *Am J Sports Med.* 1990;18:449-456.
27. Mallon WJ, Speer KP. Multidirectional instability: current concepts. *J Shoulder Elbow Surg.* 1995;4:54-64.
28. Altchek DW, Dines DW. The surgical treatment of anterior instability: selective capsular repair. *Op Tech Sports Med.* 1993;1:285-292.
29. Guanche CA, Jones DC. Clinical testing for tears of the glenoid labrum. *Arthroscopy.* 2003;19:517-523.
30. Lo IK, Nonweiler B, Woolfrey M, Litchfield R, Kirkley A. An evaluation of the apprehension, relocation and surprise tests for anterior shoulder instability. *Am J Sports Med.* 2004;32:301-307.
31. Tzannes A, Paxinos A, Callanan M, Murrell GA. An assessment of the interexaminer reliability of tests for anterior instability. *J Shoulder Elbow Surg.* 2004;13:24-29.
32. American College of Radiology. Appropriateness criteria for shoulder trauma. https://acsearch.acr.org/docs/69433/Narrative/. Accessed March 15, 2015.

Glenohumeral Joint Dislocation: Postsurgical Management

Christopher Seagrave

CASE 3

A 17-year-old high school football running back was tackled during a routine play and sustained a left (non-dominant) shoulder dislocation. Following the incident, the athlete removed himself from the game and presented to the team's athletic trainer and orthopaedic physician with an obvious, gross deformation of the left shoulder. Upon examination, it was determined that the athlete had sustained a first-time anteroinferior dislocation of his glenohumeral joint which was relocated within 20 minutes of the incident by the team orthopaedic physician. Follow-up examination included radiographs that confirmed the dislocation (and presence of a Hill-Sachs lesion) and physical findings suggestive of a Bankart tear. The decision to proceed with surgery was made, and the athlete underwent an arthroscopically assisted anterior shoulder stabilization procedure. Postoperatively, he was placed in a sling with a bolster that protected his shoulder in approximately 20° of abduction in the scapular plane. The patient was initially seen in the outpatient physical therapy clinic 5 days after surgery for a single visit of postoperative wound care and instruction in passive range of motion (PROM) activities to be performed for the first 4 weeks after surgery. Two weeks later, the patient returned to the physical therapist to progress rehabilitation following a set of predetermined postoperative guidelines.

- What factors contributed to the decision to progress to operative intervention with this athlete?
- What are the examination priorities of this patient 4 weeks after shoulder stabilization surgery?
- What precautions should be taken during physical therapy?
- Given the diagnosis and surgery, what are the most appropriate physical therapy interventions?
- What is his rehabilitation prognosis?

KEY DEFINITIONS

BANKART REPAIR: Surgical procedure used to repair recurrent shoulder dislocations that can be performed arthroscopically or with an open procedure

BICEPS TENODESIS: Surgical procedure involving relocation of the proximal attachment of the biceps tendon on the glenoid

HILL-SACHS LESION: Cortical depression in the posterolateral aspect of the humeral head, resulting from forceful impaction of the humerus against the anteroinferior glenoid rim when the shoulder is dislocated anteriorly

SHOULDER INSTABILITY: Clinical condition in which the humeral head is unable to maintain articulation within the glenoid because of excessive translatory movements leading to subluxation or dislocation of the joint; may be a primary problem or a secondary result of another concurrent pathology, and may result in singular or multidirectional instability

Objectives

1. Understand the decision-making criteria for treating anterior shoulder instability conservatively versus surgically.
2. Identify appropriate physical therapy interventions within a 5-phase rehabilitation protocol.
3. Implement initial precautions following surgical stabilization of anterior shoulder instability.
4. Understand the criteria for making a functional return-to-play decision.

Physical Therapy Considerations

PT considerations following surgical stabilization of a dislocating shoulder:

- **General physical therapy plan of care/goals:** Decrease pain; increase muscular flexibility; increase muscular strength; protect the surgical repair by guiding the athlete through the rehabilitative progression
- **Physical therapy interventions:** Patient education regarding postoperative precautions and immobilization requirements to protect the repair; graded progression of exercises from PROM to active assisted range of motion (AAROM) to active range of motion (AROM) and strengthening; manual therapy interventions to the thoracic spine, scapulothoracic articulation, glenohumeral joint, elbow, wrist, and hand to optimize the arthrokinematic movement patterns of the entire kinetic chain; restoration of functional neuromuscular movement patterns to return the athlete to activity

▶ **Precautions during physical therapy:** Postoperative precautions including ROM limitations and active movement limitations to allow for appropriate healing of the surgical repair; monitor for early signs of infection, arthrofibrosis, and compliance with home exercise program

▶ **Complications interfering with physical therapy:** Psychological effects of injury occurrence and subsequent influence on the athlete's return-to-sport attitude and future performance; secondary adhesive capsulitis resulting from inappropriate or mistimed therapeutic interventions

Understanding the Health Condition

Shoulder instability is a common clinical diagnosis encountered in a sports physical therapy practice. Classifications of shoulder instability include considerations for the degree of instability (subluxation or dislocation), the nature (voluntary or involuntary), and the chronology (acute, chronic, recurrent).[1,2] The concept of instability has been described as a progressive continuum ranging from atraumatic to traumatic. The acronyms "AMBRI" and "TUBS" have been proposed to help describe the specifics of the ends of the pathology continuum and assist the clinician in formulating an appropriate treatment approach. AMBRI stands for *atraumatic, multidirectional,* frequently *bilateral,* responsive to *rehabilitation,* and in cases where rehabilitation fails, an *inferior capsular shift* may be considered. The "AMBRI" shoulder is generally related to an individual who is considered "born loose," whereas the "TUBS" shoulder is related to an individual with an injury that is "torn loose."[3,4] The first line of treatment for an individual with an AMBRI shoulder should be rehabilitation. If conservative rehabilitation fails, surgical intervention may be considered in the form of an inferior capsular shifting procedure. TUBS refers to a *traumatic unilateral* lesion (e.g., dislocation) resulting in a *Bankart* lesion that usually requires *surgery*[5] (Figs. 3-1 and 3-2). The treatment priority is surgical stabilization using an anterior labral reconstruction procedure. A common finding following traumatic dislocation is a Hill-Sachs lesion, which is a cortical depression of the humeral head occurring when it makes contact with the glenoid labrum during dislocation or relocation. Essentially, this results in a "dent"

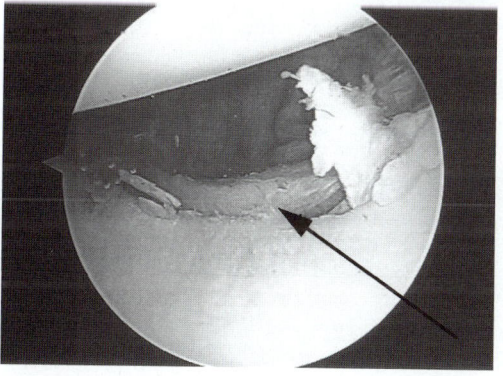

Figure 3-1. Arthroscopic view of an anterosuperior glenoid labrum injury known as a Bankart lesion that often results from traumatic shoulder dislocation. The arrow is pointing to the tear in the glenoid labrum.

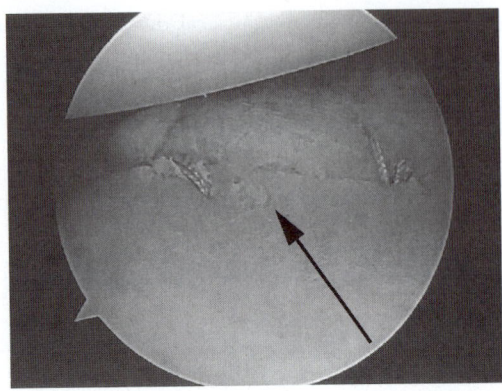

Figure 3-2. Arthroscopic view of a repaired Bankart lesion. The arrow is pointing to the repaired glenoid labrum.

to the humeral head, which is readily seen on radiographs and during arthroscopic exploration (Fig. 3-3). The **presence of a Hills-Sachs lesion** does not significantly influence the treatment options; however, it assists in confirming the history of an episode of subluxation/dislocation in the absence of radiographic confirmation.[6] The "SLAP" lesion refers to a *superior labral tear* occurring in an *anterior* to *posterior* direction. This type of injury is often associated with tensile overload forces frequently seen in the overhead-throwing athlete, but it may also occur because of biceps load during a shoulder dislocation.

The annual incidence of shoulder joint dislocation is estimated to be 17 dislocations out of every 100,000 shoulders. Ninety-six percent of dislocations are believed to be anterior in nature and most commonly occur in young men involved in contact-related sports and in elderly women as a result of falls.[7,8] In 1956, Rowe reported an 83% recurrence rate in 107 subjects younger than 20 years.[9] More recently, recurrence rates have been reported to be nearly 100% for skeletally immature individuals and as high as 96% for adolescents and adults younger than 30 years.[10]

The decision regarding when to surgically repair a first-time shoulder dislocation and when to attempt conservative immobilization has been controversial.[4,5,11,12]

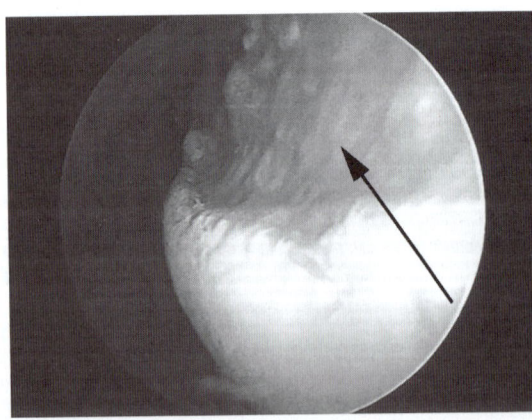

Figure 3-3. Arthroscopic example of a Hills-Sachs lesion. The arrow is pointing to a cortical depression within the humeral head.

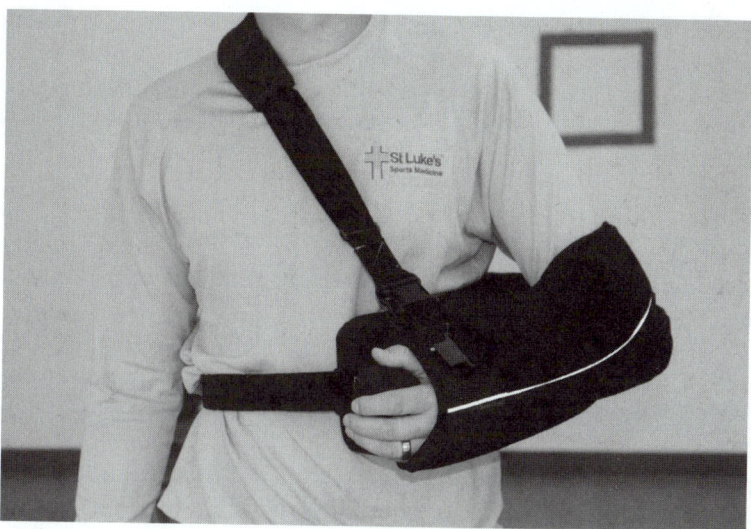

Figure 3-4. Postoperative sling with a bolster to protect shoulder in approximately 20° of abduction in the scapular plane.

Given the high incidence of recurring dislocations in adults younger than 30 years, there is a shifting trend from conservative shoulder immobilization for 4 to 6 weeks in various anatomical positions to **early surgical capsulolabral repair** (Fig. 3-4).[4,13,14] Open surgical procedures have been replaced by arthroscopic techniques with comparable outcomes involving functional return to sport.[14,15] Advances in arthroscopic surgical techniques combined with evidence showing decreased recurrence rates following surgery is likely contributing to this trend.[5,16] Despite the changes from conservative to surgical management, physical therapy management has remained somewhat consistent with a focus on restoring glenohumeral compression-based stability, scapulohumeral motion synchrony, and proprioceptive mechanisms.[16]

Physical Therapy Patient/Client Management

Individuals with shoulder instability presenting to physical therapy following surgical stabilization are often managed based on a 5-phase rehabilitation protocol approach.[16] The first 4 weeks postsurgery is phase 1, which is designed for maximum protection of the repair. Phase 2 (4-6 weeks postsurgery) includes progressive stretching and active motion progression. Phase 3 (6-10 weeks postsurgery) is a minimal protection phase to assure full range of motion (ROM) and improve muscle strength. Phase 4 (8-16 weeks postsurgery) is an advanced strengthening phase that leads to the final return-to-sport phase occurring between 4 and 9 months. Specific interventions within each phase are dictated by the individual's presentation and functional status. Typical interventions include ROM exercises, neuromuscular re-education and strengthening exercises, manual therapy, and modalities (to decrease pain). The decision to progress from one phase of rehabilitation to the next is based on the stage of healing and a collaborative interaction between the orthopaedic surgeon and the physical therapist. It is also important to consider the needs of the patient from a sports psychology perspective.[17] The injury, subsequent surgery, and rehabilitation process can affect recovery and future athletic performance. The athlete's social support and coping strategies are key indicators of recovery success.[18] Although not a mental health expert, the physical therapist can positively influence the patient's attitude about the rehabilitation process, which is invaluable during the recovery.[19]

Examination, Evaluation, and Diagnosis

The patient initially presents to physical therapy 5 to 7 days after a surgical stabilization procedure with a shoulder brace and bolster in place (Fig. 3-4). Examination begins with a thorough history to determine the athlete's prior level of function and to establish the goals of the therapeutic interventions. Objective examination includes inspection of the incision to ensure that the wound margins are well approximated and there are no signs/symptoms of infection. Although active ROM is avoided during the first 4 weeks after surgery, the therapist should assess and perform passive ROM, within the limits outlined by the surgeon. Most protocols suggest ROM limits around 90° of flexion, 0° external rotation (ER), and approximately 45° of internal rotation (IR) in the scapular plane (as occurs when the arm is held across the abdomen) for the first 4 weeks to specifically protect the repaired subscapularis muscle. The therapist should assess the neurovascular status of the patient's involved upper extremity including distal radial pulse, grip/pinch, and dermatome sensation.

Serial measurements of shoulder ROM and strength will be ongoing throughout the duration of rehabilitation. The collaborative nature of the medical and athletic team is important to assure a unified approach to returning the athlete to sport. In the event of complications such as infection, excessive stiffening, or a failure to maintain compliance with postoperative precautions, collaboration within the medical team may become more frequent for the good of the athlete.

As rehabilitation progresses, special testing includes sport-specific proprioceptive evaluation of the glenohumeral and scapulothoracic articulations. Any remaining dyskinesis in the overhead-throwing athlete may delay progression to the return-to-sport phase of recovery. The therapist's assessment of the athlete's coordination and neuromuscular control as well as his cognitive ability to understand and coordinate movement patterns contribute to the needs of the athlete's treatment plan. Biomechanical analysis of the athlete's specific sport will be critical to understand to assure a safe return to competitive status.[20,21] In this case, the specific considerations for a football running back may include assessment of the athlete's ability to assume his stance position, receive the ball either as a pass or handoff, and cradle and protect the ball while moving in various dynamic planes of motion.

Plan of Care and Interventions

The ultimate goal of postoperative management of the Bankart repair is to return the athlete to normal functional levels to allow for a successful return to sport. Progression through a sequential 5-phase rehabilitation protocol[22] occurs in a collaborative manner with the patient, physician, and physical therapist. The rate of progression is based on many factors including the quality of the repair and the rate of healing, which depends on the individual's age and the complexity of the repair. Table 3-1 outlines physical therapy goals, interventions, and activities allowed after anterior stabilization with a Bankart repair.

This patient is starting the first phase of rehabilitation (postoperative weeks 1-4), which focuses on maximum protection of the repair. The surgical repair of the Bankart lesion includes a re-attachment of the labrum and rotator cuff to the glenoid rim. Initial ROM restrictions (such as avoiding ER beyond 0°) protect the re-attachment from tensile forces that could disrupt the repair. During the first week, the patient's glenohumeral joint is kept completely immobilized using a sling and bolster 24 hours/day, which protects the shoulder in approximately 20° of abduction in the scapular plane (Fig. 3-4). Ice should be used frequently (e.g., for 20 minutes every 1-2 hours) to reduce pain and inflammation. During the first postsurgical week, wrist and hand motion is started, as the patient tolerates. Between postoperative weeks 1 and 2, modalities for pain and inflammation are utilized. Passive shoulder ROM is allowed within the following limits: flexion up to 90°, abduction to 45°, IR to the patient's belly within the scapular plane (45°), and ER to 0°. During the second week, wrist and hand active movement may progress to gentle strengthening and manually resisted scapular elevation and retraction are permitted (Fig. 3-5). Weeks 2 through 4 allow for increased shoulder PROM, progressing flexion up to 130°, abduction to 90°, and ER to 30° with the arm at the side of the body and to 50° with the shoulder at 45° of abduction. Internal rotation is gradually restored based on the patient's tolerance. Wrist/hand movement continues and elbow AROM is added. In the presence of an associated biceps tenodesis, elbow extension is avoided in order to limit unnecessary tensile forces at the repair that would result from stretching the long head of the biceps tendon. Submaximal shoulder isometrics (ER, IR, abduction, adduction, flexion, and extension) begin between weeks 2 and 4.

Phase 2 of the postoperative Bankart repair protocol (4-6 weeks postsurgery) includes progressive stretching and an active movement phase. Between weeks 4 and 5, shoulder PROM is gradually increased in all planes of motion to patient tolerance. While restoration of full ROM is desired at 10 to 12 weeks postsurgery, it should not be achieved before then to reduce the risk of a "stretched out" repair. However, there may be additional considerations regarding how quickly emphasis is placed on restoring ROM. Although not specifically supported by current evidence, some physicians adjust ROM demands based on the age of the patient. In individuals older than 35 years, early emphasis is often placed on shoulder ROM because they tend to lose mobility quicker than younger patients. In general, active shoulder ROM is begun approximately 6 weeks after surgery in patients younger

Table 3-1 PHYSICAL THERAPY GUIDELINES AFTER ANTERIOR STABILIZATION WITH BANKART REPAIR

Phase (Time After Surgery)	Goals	Interventions	Activities Allowed/Not Allowed
Phase 1 (0-4 weeks) • Week 0-1	Reduce pain and inflammation	Modalities (*e.g.*, ice) Complete immobilization of GHJ (wear sling 24 h/day) Begin AROM wrist and hand Passive elbow flexion (if biceps tenodesis)	No active shoulder ROM throughout all of Phase 1
• Week 1-2	Reduce pain and inflammation Initiate shoulder PROM Initiate wrist, hand, and scapular strengthening	Modalities (*e.g.*, ice) Shoulder PROM exercises: • Flexion to 90° • ER to 0° • IR to belly in scapular plane (45°) • Abduction to 45° Resisted manual scapular elevation and retraction Wrist and hand strengthening exercises	Return to computer activities at 10 days
• Weeks 2-4	Progress shoulder ROM Initiate shoulder isometric strengthening	Shoulder PROM exercises: • Flexion to 130° • ER to 30° with arm at side; 50° at 45° abduction • IR to patient's tolerance • Abduction to 90° Continue passive elbow flexion (if biceps tenodesis) Begin submaximal isometric exercises (ER, IR, abduction, adduction, flexion, extension)	

Phase 2 (4-6 weeks)	Initiate shoulder AROM Gradually achieve ROM goals at (but not before) 10-12 weeks (earlier if patient is a thrower)		Active shoulder ROM allowed
• Week 4-5		Begin shoulder AROM exercises for patients ≥ 35 years old Progressive AROM exercises to achieve: • Flexion to 140° • ER to 70° at 45° abduction; 60° at 90° abduction • Abduction to 90°	
• Week 5-6	Progressive rotator cuff strengthening, if meeting ROM goals	Begin shoulder AROM exercises for patients ≤ 35 years old Resisted tubing exercises for rotator cuff Biceps and triceps strengthening exercises Proprioception drills emphasizing neuromuscular control	
Phase 3 (6-8 weeks)	Strengthening	Shoulder AROM exercises Rotator cuff and scapular strengthening/stabilization exercises Proprioception drills emphasizing neuromuscular control	Return to running at 7-8 weeks

(continued)

Table 3-1 PHYSICAL THERAPY GUIDELINES AFTER ANTERIOR STABILIZATION WITH BANKART REPAIR (CONTINUED)

Phase (Time After Surgery)	Goals	Interventions	Activities Allowed/Not Allowed
Phase 4 (8-16 weeks)	Advanced strengthening Plyometrics Shoulder AROM goals at 10-12 weeks (comparisons are to uninvolved side): • 5° shy of full flexion • 5° shy of ER • 10° shy of IR at 90° abduction • 90° of ER at 90° abduction By end of Phase 4: Full functional shoulder AROM, with strength 90% of uninvolved side	Initiate closed kinetic chain strengthening exercises in protective range (*i.e.*, do not cross midline of body): • Wall push-up progression • Seated serratus push-up Initiate plyometric exercises: • Plyoball wall drills • One-arm rebounder drills	At week 12, patient may begin gym strengthening 3-4 times/week: • Seated rows • Front latissimus pull-downs • Dumbbell chest press and flys (on ground to avoid crossing midline of body) Return to: Golf chipping and putting at 8-10 weeks Road biking at 10-12 weeks Full golf activities at 12-14 weeks
Phase 5 (4+ months)	Gradual progression to return to unrestricted participation in sport Maintain motion, stability, and strength Follow-up with surgeon	Initiate interval throwing program (as directed by surgeon) Progressive gym strengthening	In gym exercises, patient should always see the back of his/her hands. Avoid wide grip push-ups, deep flies, military press, and latissimus pull-downs behind the head. Return to mountain biking at 4 months and full contact sports, per surgeon approval

Abbreviations: AROM, active range of motion; ER, external rotation; GHJ, glenohumeral joint; IR, internal rotation; PROM, passive range of motion; ROM, range of motion.

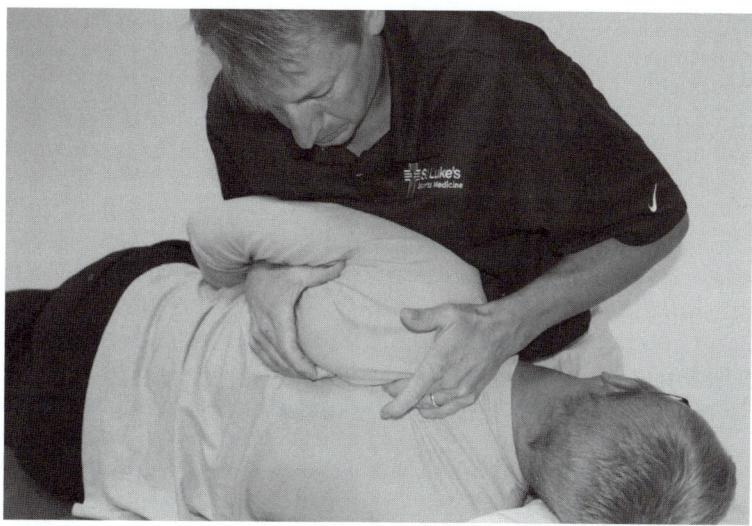

Figure 3-5. Therapist providing manual resistance to scapular retraction.

than 35 years old (and earlier in older patients). Shoulder AROM goals during phase 2 are abduction to 90°, ER to 70° at 45° of abduction, and 60° at 90° of abduction. Between weeks 5 and 6, if the patient is meeting shoulder ROM goals, the physical therapist introduces gentle progressive resistance exercises for the rotator cuff. Progression into rotator cuff specific movements is based on ensuring that scapulothoracic control is maintained to avoid compensatory scapular elevation movement patterns. Biceps and triceps strengthening may be prescribed as well as proprioception drills emphasizing neuromuscular control between weeks 5 and 6. An example of a proprioceptive drill at this stage is rhythmic stabilization of the arm in various planes while the patient is in supine.

Phase 3 begins at postoperative week 6 and continues through postoperative week 10. This is considered the strengthening phase of the rehabilitation protocol. The physical therapist must closely monitor the patient for compensatory movement patterns. It has been shown that **early, uncontrolled compensatory scapulothoracic substitution patterns** delay the ability to generate forces through the rotator cuff, resulting in delayed strengthening and probable delayed return to sport.[16] By weeks 10 and 12, shoulder AROM is gradually increased to normal end-range goals. Rotator cuff and scapular strengthening exercises are advanced within biomechanically correct movement patterns. Proprioception and closed kinetic chain (CKC) neuromuscular control drills are progressed according to the patient's abilities and continually advanced as ROM is restored.

While the third and fourth phases of rehabilitation have some inherent overlaps in goals and interventions, activity progression is dependent on how the athlete progresses. The fourth phase (postoperative weeks 8-16) involves advanced strengthening and plyometric activities in addition to continuation of the previously prescribed parascapular and rotator cuff specific strengthening. Strengthening exercises typically include CKC activities within a protected ROM. For example, to avoid compression forces to the anterolateral joint surfaces that could aggravate the repair, the therapist encourages the athlete to avoid midline crossover movements. CKC activities may include wall push-up progressions, seated serratus press-ups with strict control of biomechanically correct movements. The most common compensatory movement pattern involves early scapular elevation concurrent with glenohumeral flexion or abduction resulting in a "shrugging" type movement pattern. Plyometric and advanced CKC exercises are initiated such as Plyoball wall drills and 1-arm rebounder drills (Fig. 3-6).

Between 10 and 12 weeks postsurgery, shoulder ROM goals should be focused on achieving 5° short of full flexion and ER as compared to uninvolved shoulder. External rotation (at 90° abduction) should be limited to 90° and not overstretched. Internal rotation (at 90° abduction) should be approximately 10° shy of the uninvolved shoulder. Because stretching will continue to occur over time, it is desirable to leave the Bankart-repaired shoulder just short of full end-range movement during rehabilitation. At week 12, the athlete may begin gym-based strengthening 3 to 4 times per week. Typical exercises include seated rowing, front latissimus pull-downs, and biceps and triceps strengthening. Dumbbell chest press and flys may be performed with the patient sitting on the ground and avoiding crossing the midline of the body.

The final rehabilitation phase, known as the return to activity phase, begins 4 months following an anterior stabilization procedure. The criterion to progress into the final phase is based on obtaining full shoulder active and passive ROM and strength equivalent to 90% of the contralateral side.[1,16] The goals of this phase are to gradually progress sports activities to unrestricted participation. It is during this phase that interval-based programs are prescribed and increased intensity with gym-based programs occurs. The decision for full, unrestricted clearance to sport is based on performance of functional testing such as the upper extremity stability

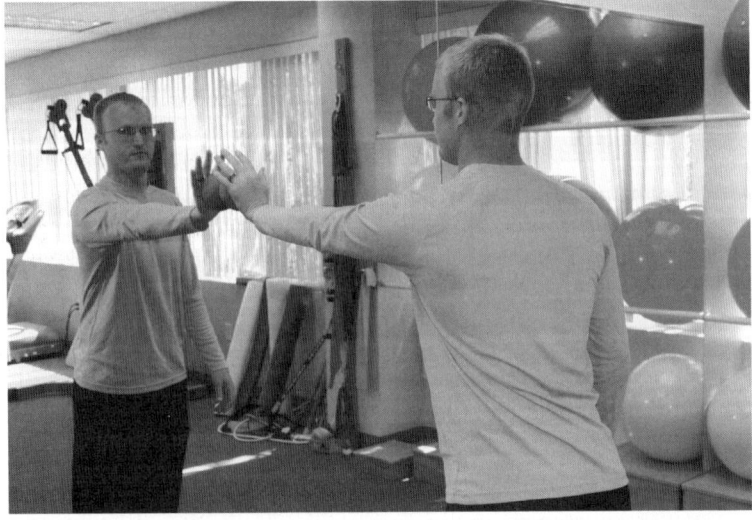

Figure 3-6. Patient performing closed kinetic chain (CKC) shoulder exercises.

test as well as collaborative understanding between the patient, physical therapist, physician, and coach.[23-25]

Evidence-Based Clinical Recommendations

SORT: Strength of Recommendation Taxonomy
A: Consistent, good-quality patient-oriented evidence
B: Inconsistent or limited-quality patient-oriented evidence
C: Consensus, disease-oriented evidence, usual practice, expert opinion, or case series

1. The presence of a Hills-Sachs lesion does not significantly influence the decision-making process for treatment options for anterior shoulder instability. **Grade C**
2. Because of the high recurrence rate of anterior shoulder dislocations, primary operative intervention following first-time dislocation in young active adults (<30 years old) is the recommended treatment choice. **Grade A**
3. Rotator cuff strengthening exercises in the presence of poor neuromuscular scapulothoracic control will significantly prolong the athlete's appropriate recovery and return to play timeline. **Grade B**

COMPREHENSION QUESTIONS

3.1 Which lesion involves detachment of the anterior labrum as a result of traumatic anterior instability?
   A. Hill-Sachs lesion
   B. SLAP lesion
   C. Bankart lesion
   D. Osteochondral lesion

3.2 During phases 1 to 2 of the rehabilitation progression after shoulder stabilization surgery, avoidance of active internal rotation or passive external rotation beyond neutral protects which anatomical structure?
   A. Supraspinatus
   B. Infraspinatus
   C. Teres minor
   D. Subscapularis

3.3 The final stage of rehabilitation after shoulder stabilization surgery of an athlete should focus on which of the following?
   A. Interval return-to-sport programs
   B. Submaximal isometrics
   C. Scapular stabilization focused exercises
   D. Shoulder range of motion gains

ANSWERS

3.1 **C.** In 1923, Bankart described anterior labral detachment as the essential lesion in traumatic anterior instability.[5,15]

3.2 **D.** The subscapularis muscle serves as the prime internal rotator of the shoulder and is frequently re-attached during a Bankart repair. Avoidance of passive ER that could stretch the subscapularis and active IR that may contract against the repair are important considerations.

3.3 **A.** Sport-specific interval programs are used to simulate the demands placed upon the athlete within his sport. Interval programs are frequently used to prepare the athlete in the final stages of rehabilitation prior to returning to sport. Submaximal isometrics are performed during phase 1 (option B). Full shoulder ROM should have already been achieved during phase 4 (option D), and scapular stabilization exercises are integrated and progressed between phases 1 and 4 (option C).

REFERENCES

1. Andrews JR, Wilk KE. *The Athlete's Shoulder*. London: Churchill Livingstone Inc.;1994.
2. Provencher MT, LeClere LE, King S, et al. Posterior instablity of the shoulder: diagnosis and management. *Am J Sports Med*. 2011;39:874-886.
3. Matsen FA, Thomas SC, Rockwood CA, Wirth MA. Glenohumeral instability. *The Shoulder*. Philadelphia, PA: Saunders; 2004:633-639.
4. Wang RY, Arciero RA, Mazzocca AD. The recognition and treatment of first-time shoulder dislocation in active individuals. *J Orthop Sports Phys Ther*. 2009;39:118-123.
5. Bankart ASB. Pathology and treatment of recurrent dislocation of shoulder-joint. *Br J Surg*. 1938;26:23-29.
6. Bhatia S, Ghodadra NS, Romeo AA, et al. The importance of the recognition and treatment of glenoid bone loss in an athletic population. *Sports Health*. 2011;3:435-440.
7. Godin J, Sekiya JK. Systematic review of rehabilitation versus operative stabilization for the treatment of first-time anterior shoulder dislocations. *Sports*. 2010;2:156-165.
8. Hovilius L. Incidence of shoulder dislocation in Sweeden. *Clin Orthop Relat Res*. 1982;166:127-131.
9. Rowe CR. Prognosis in dislocations of the shoulder. *J Bone Joint Surg Am*. 1956;38(A):957-977.
10. Deitch J, Mehlman CT, Foad SL, Obbehat A, Mallory M. Traumatic anterior shoulder dislocation in adolescents. *Am J Sports Med*. 2003;31:758-763.
11. DeBerardino TM, Arciero RA, Taylor DC, Uhorchak JM. Prospective evaluation of arthroscopic stabilization of acute, initial anterior shoulder dislocations in young athletes. Two- to five-year follow-up. *Am J Sports Med*. 2001;29:586-592.
12. Roach CJ, Cameron KL, Westrick RB, Posner MA, Owens BD. Rotator cuff weakness is not a risk factor for first-time anterior glenohumeral instability. *Orth J Sports Med*. 2013;1:1-6.
13. Scheibel M, Kuke A, Nikulka C, Magosch P, Ziesler O, Schroeder RJ. How long should acute anterior dislocations of the shoulder be immobilized in external rotation? *Am J Sports Med*. 2009;37:1309-1316.
14. Mazzocca AD, Brown FM, Carreira DS, Hayden J, Romeo AA. Arthroscopic anterior shoulder stabilization of collision and contact athletes. *Am J Sports Med*. 2005;33:52-60.
15. Karlsson J, Magnusson L, Ejerhed L, Hultenheim I, Lundin O, Kartus J. Comparison of open and arthroscopic stabilization for recurrent shoulder dislocation in patients with a Bankart lesion. *Am J Sports Med*. 2001;29:538-542.

16. Hayes K, Callanan M, Walton J, Paxinos A, Murrell GA. Shoulder instability: management and rehabilitation. *J Orthop Sports Phys Ther*. 2002;32:497-509.
17. Sharp L. Sport psychology consulting effectiveness: the sport psychology consultant's perspective. *J Appl Sports Psychology*. 2011;23:360-376.
18. Junge A. The influence of psychological factors on sports injuries. Review of the literature. *Am J Sports Med*. 2000;28:S10-S15.
19. Kraemer W, Denegar C, Flanagan S. Recovery from injury in sport: considerations in the transition from medical care to performance care. *Sports Health*. 2009;1:392-395.
20. Reinold MM, Gill TJ. Current concepts in the evaluation and treatment of the shoulder in overhead-throwing athletes, part 1: physical characteristics and clinical examination. *Sports Health*. 2009;2:39-50.
21. Shin SJ, Yun YH, Kim DJ, Yoo JD. Treatment of traumatic anterior shoulder dislocation in patients older than 60 years. *Am J Sports Med*. 2012;40:822-827.
22. St. Luke's Sports Medicine-Intermountain Orthopaedics: Post-operative Bankart Repair Protocol. Boise, Idaho; 2013.
23. Negrete RJ, Hanney WJ, Kolber MJ, et al. Reliability, minimal detectable change and normative values for tests of upper extremity function and power. *J Strength Cond Res*. 2010;24:3318-3325.
24. Negrete RJ, Hanney WJ, Kolber MJ, Davies GJ, Riemann B. Can upper extremity functional tests predict the softball throw for distance: a predictive validity investigation. *Int J Sports Phys Ther*. 2011;6:104-111.
25. Baumgarten KM, Vidal AF, Wright RW. Rotator cuff repair rehabilitation: a Level I and II systematic review. *Sports Health*. 2009;1:125-130.

Rehabilitation and Return to Sport After a SLAP Repair in a College Baseball Player

Craig Garrison
Joseph Hannon

CASE 4

A 20-year-old collegiate baseball pitcher presents to the physical therapy clinic 3 days after an arthroscopic repair and debridement of the posterior labrum with a subacromial decompression. The patient's initial injury and diagnosis of a superior labrum anterior to posterior (SLAP) tear was due to the repetitive and excessive stresses brought on by pitching competitively since he was 7 years old. One month ago, the patient noted that he started to experience pain in the back of his right shoulder every time he pitched. His pain was brought on by throwing, especially during the late cocking phase. The patient underwent conservative care (ice and electrical stimulation) from his athletic trainer for 1 month while continuing to pitch; however, his symptoms did not improve. The patient was referred to a board-certified and fellowship-trained orthopaedic surgeon who specialized in the treatment of overhead athletes. Magnetic resonance imaging (MRI) with contrast revealed a posterior-superior and posterior labral tear in addition to synovitis and a thickening of the subacromial bursa. The patient underwent an arthroscopic posterior labral repair with debridement and subacromial decompression. The patient was given immediate postoperative instructions on donning and doffing his sling and pendulum exercises. The patient presents to the physical therapy clinic 3 days following surgery with a referral to "evaluate and treat." The patient presents with his right shoulder immobilized in a sling with an axillary pillow that places his arm into approximately 20° of abduction. He has no complaints of radicular symptoms; he rates his current pain 2/10 at rest and 5/10 with moving his arm during dressing. The patient's medical history is unremarkable.

▶ How would this individual's contextual factors influence or change your patient/client management?
▶ Based on the patient's diagnosis, what are potential contributing factors that may have predisposed him to this injury and eventual surgical intervention?
▶ What is his rehabilitation prognosis following surgery?
▶ What are some baseball-specific considerations for his eventual return to play?

KEY DEFINITIONS

INSTABILITY: Increased mobility or excessive shifting of the humeral head on the glenoid that occurs when the baseball player's shoulder is in the position of abduction and maximal external rotation (ER) during either the late cocking or acceleration phases of the throwing motion

INTERNAL IMPINGEMENT: Pinching of the posterior-superior portion of the labrum and/or joint capsule as the shoulder moves into a position of abduction and maximum ER during the late cocking phase of the throwing motion

LABRUM: Projection of cartilage on the glenoid fossa that provides stability to the glenohumeral joint (GHJ)

PAINT LESION: Acronym for partial thickness articular surface intratendinous tear that involves a superficial undersurface tear of the posterior supraspinatus and anterior infraspinatus tendons; this injury may occur during the throwing motion and is due to high tensile stresses.

PASTA LESION: Acronym for partial thickness articular surface tendon avulsion that involves a superficial undersurface tear of the distal supraspinatus or infraspinatus tendons; this injury may occur during the throwing motion and is due to high tensile stresses.

SUBACROMIAL DECOMPRESSION: Arthroscopic surgical procedure used to open up the space or clean the area under the acromion that may be abutting against adjacent structures such as a fibrotic bursa sac or frayed rotator cuff

Objectives

1. Understand the pathology involved in a glenohumeral labral injury and the potential mechanisms of this injury.
2. Identify and provide the rationale for the postoperative precautions associated with a SLAP repair and subacromial decompression surgery.
3. Describe appropriate rehabilitation interventions in the early phase after SLAP repair with subacromial decompression.
4. Identify objective criteria required for returning to throwing and playing baseball after SLAP repair with subacromial decompression.

Physical Therapy Considerations

PT considerations during management of the baseball player after SLAP surgical repair with subacromial decompression:

- ▶ **General physical therapy plan of care/goals:** Increase active and passive shoulder range of motion (ROM); decrease pain; increase scapular stability and rotator cuff strength; maintain or improve lower extremity ROM, strength, and balance; return athlete to throwing with proper mechanics

- **Physical therapy interventions:** Patient education regarding functional anatomy and injury pathomechanics and general precautions regarding protection of healing tissue; modalities and manual therapy to decrease pain; mobilization and passive stretching to improve joint mobility and minimize/prevent capsular restriction; submaximal resistance exercises to increase muscular strength and endurance of the rotator cuff and scapular stabilizers; lower extremity strength and balance exercises; normalize or re-establish neurodynamics of the upper extremity; home exercise program
- **Precautions during physical therapy:** Monitor neural tension signs and symptoms; address precautions or contraindications for exercise based on patient's recent surgery
- **Complications interfering with physical therapy:** Location and extent of repair; tissue quality; athlete's eagerness to return to sport too quickly; common psychological traits of a pitcher such as fear of re-injury and inability to pitch with the same velocity or control

Understanding the Health Condition

The glenoid labrum is a fibrocartilagenous ring that sits on the glenoid and deepens the glenoid fossa by up to 50%, which adds stability to an otherwise unstable bony articulation.[1] In addition to increasing the overall articulation of the humerus on the glenoid, the labrum also acts to provide a suction-cup effect, which further increases stability. The GHJ is surrounded by the capsule that blends with 3 glenohumeral ligaments (GHLs): the superior GHL, middle GHL, and inferior GHL complex. Together, the labrum, capsular ligaments, and rotator cuff musculature all act to stabilize the GHJ.[1]

The etiology of labral pathologies in the throwing athlete is multifaceted and distinct from that of the non-throwing athlete. Acute/traumatic shoulder dislocations or subluxations that can occur from a fall on an outstretched arm have the potential to cause different labral pathologies (and potential corresponding humeral pathologies) depending on the direction and extent of the dislocation. These types of labral tears are treated differently than the chronic or "adaptive" tears that typically develop in throwers.[2-4] During the throwing motion, the shoulder is maximally abducted and externally rotated during the late cocking phase, requiring the labrum, GHJ ligaments, and rotator cuff to provide stability for the humeral head within the glenoid labrum in this very unstable position.[5,6] Over time, micro-instability may occur.[3,7,8] Micro-instability is not the same as true "shoulder instability." Shoulder instability refers to gross GHJ instability of greater than 1 cm as tested with the sulcus sign or apprehension testing. In contrast, micro-instability refers to small shifts of the humeral head on the glenoid through only *millimeters* of motion. Ultimately, this small shift can cause abutting of the humeral head against the posterior superior labrum and the undersurface (articular side) of the rotator cuff.[7,8] The result is internal impingement, which is not the same as subacromial impingement.[9] In subacromial impingement, the structures that pass under the acromion (supraspinatus tendon and subacromial bursa) become impinged by the greater tuberosity. With internal impingement, the orientation of the GHL changes as the arm is brought into maximal abduction and ER (*e.g.*, in late cocking phase), resulting in the inferior GHL complex sliding into an anterior/inferior position. This new position pushes the humeral head posteriorly and superiorly.[3,10] This shifted position can shear the labrum, and eventually cause a posterior-sided labral tear and/or an articular-sided rotator cuff tear (PASTA or PAINT lesion).[10]

Other factors predispose the overhead athlete to labral pathologies, including glenohumeral internal rotation deficit (GIRD), scapular dyskinesis, and poor throwing mechanics.[9,11] GIRD is a common phenomenon in athletes subject to repetitive throwing (see Case 1).[9,12] As the athlete's dominant throwing arm begins to lose internal rotation (IR) motion, the shoulder subsequently tends to increase ER in an attempt to maintain total rotational motion. GIRD has been identified in throwing athletes from pre-teenagers to professionals and predisposes these athletes to shoulder and/or elbow injuries.[13-16] GIRD can be caused by soft tissue changes (*e.g.*, tight posterior capsule, specifically the inferior GHL complex or posterior musculature) or a bony abnormality (*e.g.*, humeral retrotorsion).[12] Often, both soft tissue changes and bony abnormalities are present.[12] Precisely why GIRD increases injury risk is not completely understood; however, if the humerus cannot internally rotate to allow a more fluid deceleration, the forces may transfer up the arm to the shoulder and/or elbow.[17] From a rehabilitation standpoint, GIRD improves with directed therapeutic interventions.[18-21]

While the role of scapular dyskinesis in shoulder pathologies is less understood, most clinicians and researchers agree that if scapular dyskinesis is present, addressing this deficit with physical therapy is warranted.[19,22,23] With an already complex joint that is mobile by nature, a dyskinetic scapula increases the chances of this mobility becoming pathologic. As the arm is moved overhead, the glenoid and humeral head must remain in contact and the scapula should elevate, upwardly rotate, and posteriorly tilt on the thorax.[24] If one of these motions does not occur, ideal alignment of the glenoid and humeral head is not achieved. This can alter the arthrokinematics of the joint and place increased stress on structures that normally should not be stressed in this position.

Last, throwing mechanics play an important role in shoulder and elbow pathologies.[5,6,25] Correct arm and trunk position are important. Lower extremity balance,[26] hip ROM,[27,28] and coordination may also play a role. It has been hypothesized that a breakdown in the lower extremity kinetic chain potentially increases the forces at the shoulder and elbow, thus creating an environment that is detrimental to the upper extremity.[29] In general, addressing these issues in the throwing athlete independently can be difficult; therefore, it may be beneficial for the physical therapist to work in conjunction with a pitching coach in order to identify possible deficiencies that could contribute to shoulder dysfunction.

Arthroscopic repair of SLAP tears is common in overhead athletes.[30,31] In a retrospective review of 30 overhead athletes with SLAP tears, the overall satisfaction rate was 93.3% and the mean time to return to sport was 11.7 months.[30] However, while overhead athletes who were throwers reported improvements in daily activities, their return-to-sport functional outcome scores were slightly *lower* than those who were not throwers. Similarly, in a systematic review of return to play after SLAP repairs in athletes, overhead athletes demonstrated a lower return-to-play percentage than those participating in non-throwing sports.[31] There are likely many reasons for lower rates of return to play in overhead athletes after SLAP repair, including concomitant pathologies such as rotator cuff tears and shoulder instability.

Physical Therapy Patient/Client Management

Patients presenting for physical therapy following arthroscopic labral repair can benefit from interventions consisting of manual therapy and submaximal therapeutic exercise to restore shoulder ROM, muscular strength, and shoulder function. Information regarding tissue quality, potential stresses to the tissue during movement, and the location of injury following labral repair helps the physical therapist to optimize the initial ROM of the shoulder without jeopardizing tissue healing. Access to the surgery report following the SLAP repair is essential for understanding the procedures and the surgeon's assessment of the situation. It is also important for the physical therapist to develop a good line of communication with the orthopaedic surgeon in order to discuss any precautions or special considerations for the rehabilitation process.

Examination, Evaluation, and Diagnosis

Highlights of the examination for an athlete 3 days after SLAP repair include ROM assessment within the precautions for the surgery and scapular resting alignment and positional control. At this time, the athlete's shoulder is typically immobilized in a sling. Shoulder ROM should be passively assessed in a supine position. At this point following surgery, active ROM is *avoided* because activation of the muscles could potentially increase stress across the surgical site, increasing pain and possibly damaging the repair. It is important to recognize that IR of the humerus will cause a posterior glide of the humeral head on the glenoid, which could compromise the tissue by causing a shear force across the recently repaired labrum. Therefore, the safest way to assess passive shoulder IR is with the arm at the patient's side at 0° of abduction to limit the overall available ROM. External rotation, flexion, and abduction should theoretically not stress the repaired site because these motions will cause the humeral head to glide anteriorly, thus avoiding the posterior portion of the labrum that was repaired. Because the patient may be apprehensive or complain of pain during assessment of passive ROM (PROM), the physical therapist should proceed with caution when assessing these motions. In the clinical experience of the authors, it is important to gradually progress these ranges of motions within a pain level of 4 or less (on numerical pain rating scale [NPRS] of 0-10).

Scapular position and neuromuscular control of the scapula can be examined with the patient in sitting or standing. Assessment of the resting alignment of the scapula is done by visual inspection and palpation on the patient's scapulae, comparing the involved to the uninvolved side. To appreciate the patient's normal posture, the therapist evaluates for excessive scapular protraction, elevation, or depression.[32] Baseball players, especially pitchers, often present with the scapula of the throwing arm in a depressed and protracted resting position when compared to the non-throwing arm. Next, the physical therapist asks the patient to actively elevate, depress, protract, and retract his involved scapula with his arm relaxed at his side. This allows the therapist to assess the patient's scapular control without active engagement of the GHJ. When the patient is cleared for active shoulder ROM (~4-6 weeks after surgery), the physical therapist can perform the scapular dyskinesis test, which is a more accurate assessment of scapular control.[33] In addition to upper extremity examination, it is important to assess lower extremity strength, mobility, and overall neuromuscular control.[27-29,34] This can help the physical therapist identify (and correct) any deficiencies that might decrease the baseball player's ability to efficiently transfer forces through the kinetic chain.

Plan of Care and Interventions

Initial postsurgical rehabilitation focuses on increasing shoulder ROM to prevent capsular adhesions while protecting the surgically repaired tissues.[35,36] Some rehabilitation protocols specify shoulder ROM limitations during the first 4 to 6 weeks after surgery, including flexion to 90° and with the arm at the side, IR to neutral (0°), and ER to 30°.[30,31] Several studies have provided rationale for the GHJ movements that allow joint excursion and capsular lengthening, yet provide safe and protective inherent tensions produced across the labrum.[37-39]

Scapular positioning exercises should be initiated immediately.[23] These exercises are designed to promote kinesthetic awareness and are not necessarily designed to be strengthening exercises. Following surgery, proprioception may be altered secondary to scope incisions, swelling, and pain. Early implementation of exercises to regain proprioceptive awareness of the shoulder complex can be beneficial and provide a base on which to advance the therapeutic exercises.

For the athlete presented in this case, glenohumeral IR will be the most limited motion secondary to the arthrokinematics of the GHJ. During IR, the humeral head posteriorly translates, which may result in shearing of the repaired tissue, especially at 90° of abduction. Initial IR ROM can be implemented with the arm in 0° of abduction. Approximately 4 to 6 weeks after surgery, passive abduction of the arm to 45° and gentle passive IR ROM can be initiated in the scapular plane. Shoulder flexion and abduction should be limited to 90° for the first 6 weeks.[30] However, the physical therapist should use his/her clinical judgment to determine if shoulder mobility is returning with proper arthrokinematics. If the patient is having difficulty achieving 90° of shoulder flexion/abduction, more time may be spent stretching and mobilizing in these planes. As a common clinical guideline, shoulder mobilizations and/or stretching during this timeframe should typically be pain-free up to 90° of flexion and abduction (Fig. 4-1). During this initial phase, gentle grade 1 and 2 GHJ mobilizations inferiorly may be used to help achieve the desired ROM and assist with pain control.[35] Anterior to posterior mobilizations should be avoided to minimize stress across the posterior labrum. If the

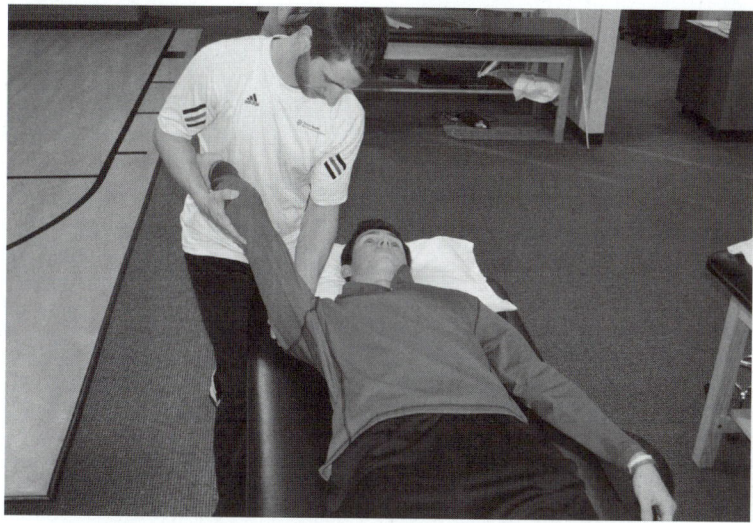

Figure 4-1. Initial shoulder mobilizations. The patient is supine with the therapist at the head of the table and on the side to be treated. The therapist passively moves the patient's arm into flexion and abduction while simultaneously applying an inferior glenohumeral glide.

patient can easily achieve the desired ROM, care must be taken to avoid pushing the shoulder too far too early because this could result in poor healing of the labral tissue.

At 6 weeks after surgery, active assisted range of motion (AAROM) and active range of motion (AROM) may be initiated at the discretion of the surgeon and therapist. At this time, achieving full ROM becomes the priority. However, a gradual progression is needed. Passive stretching with and without scapular stabilization, GHJ mobilizations, and active motions are used to help achieve and maintain shoulder ROM.[35,36] If the patient can tolerate low-intensity IR stretching in 90° of abduction with no to moderate discomfort (0-4 on the NRPS), this can be initiated (Fig. 4-2). Active movements include unweighted or weighted shoulder flexion, scaption, and abduction.[23,34] With these motions, it is important that the physical therapist identify and attempt corrections of any compensatory movement patterns such as excessive scapular elevation during shoulder flexion. In addition, assessment of neural tension in the involved upper extremity is warranted because it is common in the overhead athlete.[40] If increased tension is noted, upper limb neural tension gliding (Fig. 4-3) can be used as part of the treatment approach.[41] Use of inferior GHJ mobilizations in supine, sitting, or with active motion may be beneficial. Verbal and manual feedback may be used to help the patient regain proper movement patterns.

More aggressive scapular strengthening and control exercises may be initiated at 6 weeks after surgery. **Exercises that promote scapular retraction and activation of the rotator cuff, middle and lower trapezius, and the serratus muscles are beneficial.**[22,23,42] These exercises should be progressed from basic movements that require

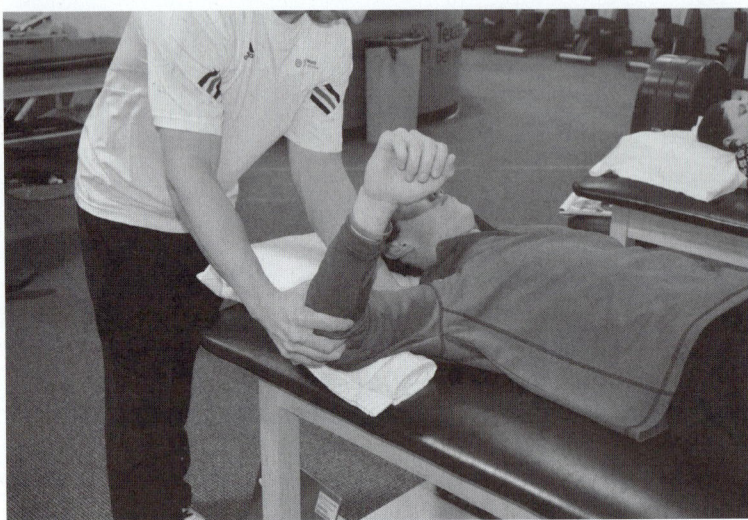

Figure 4-2. Manual internal rotation stretching with mobilization. The patient is supine with the therapist at the head of the table and on the side to be treated. The patient's upper extremity is positioned into 90° shoulder abduction and 90° elbow flexion. The therapist depresses the scapula from superior to inferior and passively moves the flexed arm into internal rotation until movement is felt at the scapula.

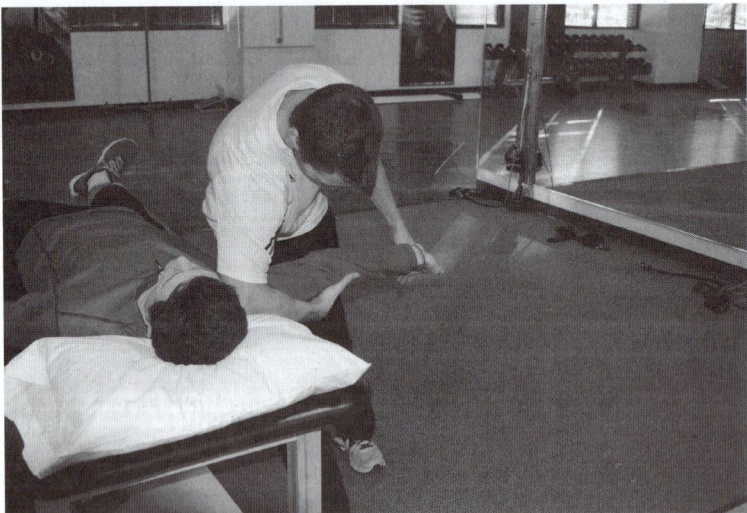

Figure 4-3. Upper limb neural tension gliding (median nerve). The patient is supine with the therapist on the side to be treated. The patient's upper extremity is positioned into 90° of abduction at the shoulder with the elbow and wrist fully extended. The therapist depresses the patient's shoulder using his elbow while using his opposite hand to move the patient's wrist and fingers into extension in order to apply tension to the median nerve.

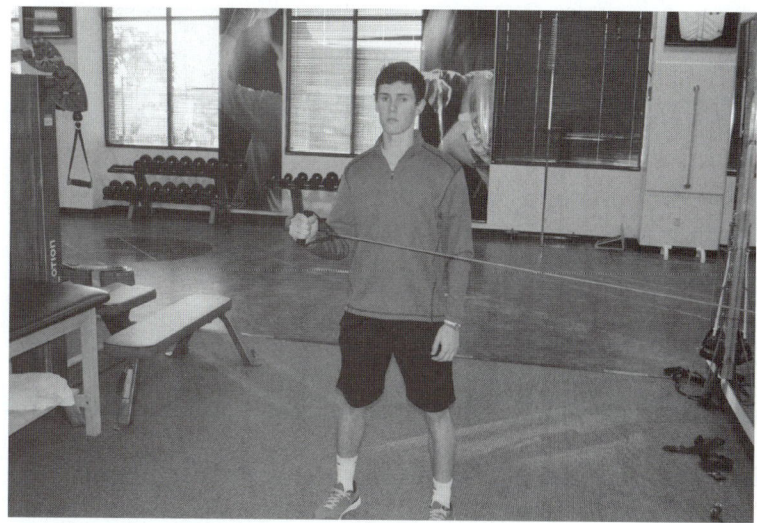

Figure 4-4. Resisted external rotation walkout. The patient stands with the involved upper extremity flexed to 90° at the elbow while grasping the resistance cord. The upper extremity should be held to the side of the body (neutral position). The patient is instructed to retract the scapula (pulling involved shoulder posteriorly) and maintain this position while stepping away from the resistance (1-2 steps) and then slowly returning without losing scapular retraction or elbow flexion.

little shoulder motions and elicit low levels of electromyographic (EMG) activity in the scapular muscles[43] (*e.g.*, resisted ER walkout; Fig. 4-4) to more advanced motions (*e.g.*, the lawnmower; Fig. 4-5) that require full body movements and produce higher EMG activation in muscles such as the lower trapezius.[23] The therapist should have the patient initiate these exercises with the involved arm at the side of the body and progress to overhead motions with emphasis placed on driving off of the contralateral lower extremity to activate the involved shoulder to promote sequential muscle activation[44] (Fig. 4-6).

At approximately 3 months after SLAP repair, the athlete should demonstrate good scapular control and the physical therapist can initiate more aggressive strengthening. **More closed chain exercises to compress the joint and promote stability should be implemented.**[44] These exercises can be initiated in the standing position and gradually progressed to a baseball-specific functional position. Once the athlete has achieved adequate control and stability with the arm in the overhead position, gentle plyometric activities can be initiated. These may include "wall ball" exercises (Fig. 4-7), eccentric catches, and Bodyblade exercises that promote baseball-specific movements. The athlete can begin an interval throwing program when several criteria are met. These include total shoulder ROM (passive combined motions of internal and ER measured at 90° of abduction) less than or equal to within 5° of the opposite side,[13] 75% ratio of ER to IR rotator cuff strength,[36] normalized lower extremity balance (>94% Y Balance Test Composite Score),[26]

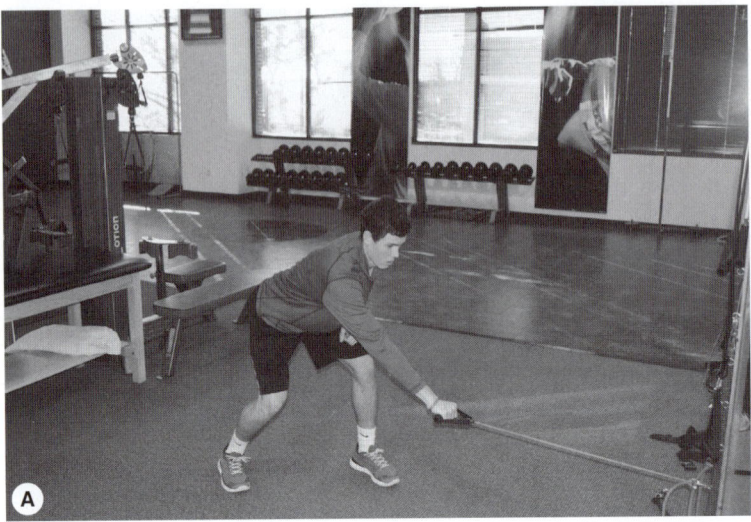

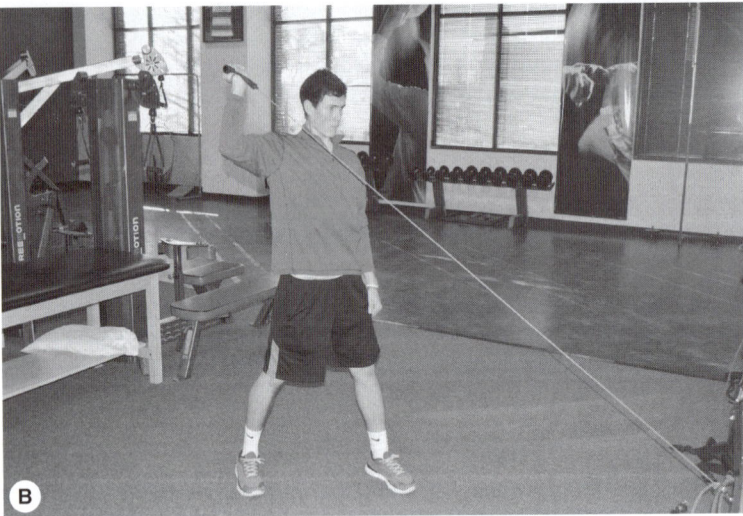

Figure 4-5. Double-leg lawnmower. **A.** The patient begins in a squatted position with the trunk and knees flexed and the involved upper extremity fully extended at the elbow while grasping the resistance cord. The patient is instructed to move from a squatted to a standing position by driving from the lower limbs while simultaneously pulling the resistance band with the involved upper extremity. **B.** The patient should finish the movement with the involved upper extremity abducted to 90° at the shoulder and elbow (*i.e.*, position of throwing).

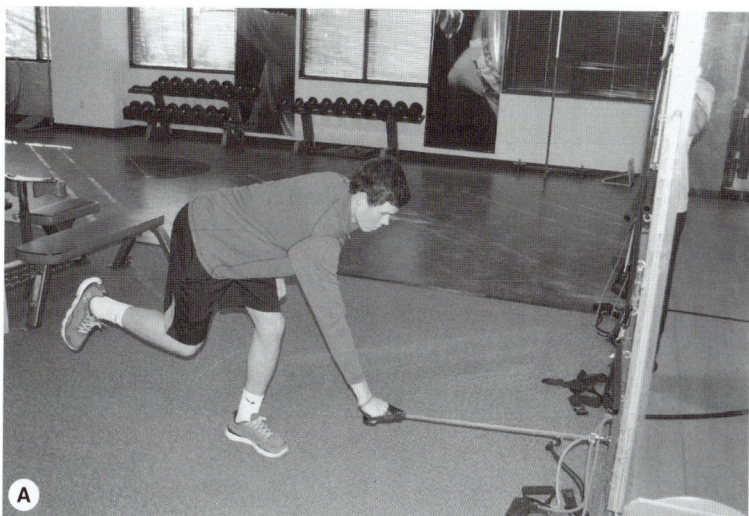

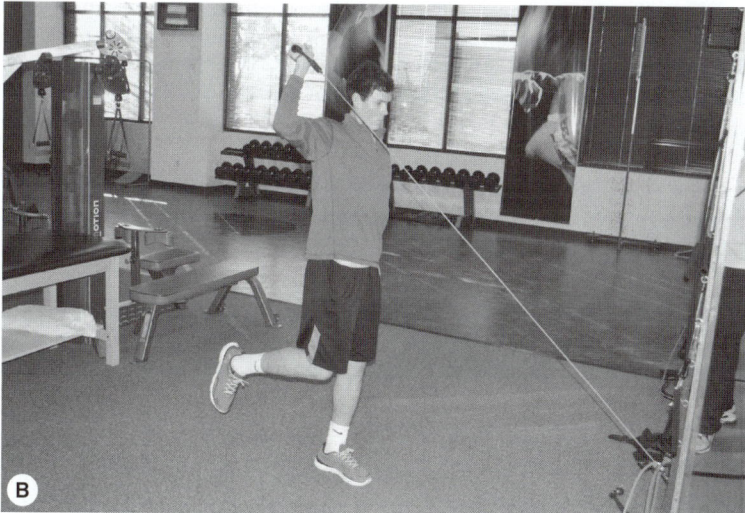

Figure 4-6. Single-leg lawnmower. **A.** The patient begins by standing on the limb contralateral to the throwing arm in a squatted position with the trunk and knees flexed. The patient grasps the resistance cord with the involved upper extremity fully extended at the elbow. The patient is instructed to initiate moving to a standing position from the lower extremity, while simultaneously pulling the resistance band with the involved upper extremity. **B.** The patient should finish the movement with the involved upper extremity abducted to 90° at the shoulder and elbow (*i.e.*, position of throwing).

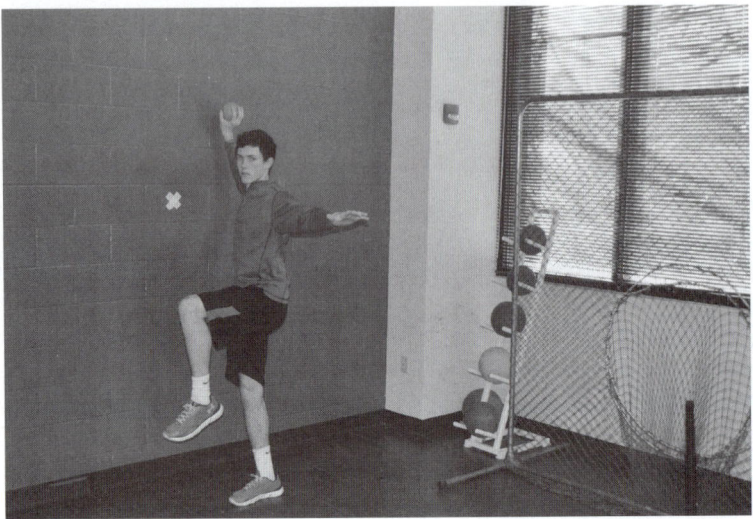

Figure 4-7. Wall ball dribbles. The patient begins by standing on ipsilateral limb of the involved throwing arm with the knee slightly flexed and the contralateral limb raised off the ground with the hip and knee flexed (~90°). The throwing upper extremity is abducted to 90° at the shoulder and the elbow is flexed while holding a 2-lb plyometric ball. The patient is instructed to maintain his balance on the stance limb while dribbling the plyometric ball off the wall in order to replicate the beginning of the throwing motion.

and normal scapular neuromuscular control. This milestone usually occurs around 4 months postsurgery,[30,36] but may be pushed back to 5 months depending upon the individual progression of the patient.

Evidence-Based Clinical Recommendations

SORT: Strength of Recommendation Taxonomy
A: Consistent, good-quality patient-oriented evidence
B: Inconsistent or limited-quality patient-oriented evidence
C: Consensus, disease-oriented evidence, usual practice, expert opinion, or case series

1. Altered throwing mechanics in the overhead athlete may contribute to labral injury of the shoulder. **Grade B**
2. Restoration of normal scapular mechanics is important in the rehabilitation of the overhead athlete following labral repair and debridement. **Grade B**
3. The use of closed-chain sport-specific therapeutic exercise helps retrain proper movement patterns and neuromuscular control in overhead athletes. **Grade C**

COMPREHENSION QUESTIONS

4.1 A sports physical therapist evaluates a baseball player with a diagnosis of posterior labral tear of his throwing shoulder. The patient reports pain in his shoulder during the throwing motion. The phase of throwing *most* likely to contribute to this type of pain in an overhead athlete is:
   A. Early cocking phase
   B. Late cocking phase
   C. Acceleration phase
   D. Deceleration phase

4.2 After the first 6 weeks following shoulder labral repair and debridement in a baseball player, use of a therapeutic strengthening exercise such as the "lawn-mower" elicits high EMG activity in which of the following muscles?
   A. Upper trapezius
   B. Middle trapezius
   C. Posterior deltoid
   D. Lower trapezius

4.3 Which of the following is *not* a component of the objective criteria used to determine when a baseball player is ready to begin an interval throwing program?
   A. Good rotator cuff strength (75% ratio)
   B. Total shoulder range of motion equal to 180°
   C. Normalized lower extremity balance
   D. Proper neuromuscular control of the scapula

ANSWERS

4.1 **B.** During the late cocking phase of the throwing motion, the shoulder is in a position of abduction and maximal external rotation. In this position, the humeral head is rotating posteriorly and gliding anteriorly. If the posterior portion of the joint capsule (specifically the posterior portion of the inferior GHL complex) is tight or restricted, the humeral head will be displaced in a posterior and superior direction causing a shear force and impingement on the posterior portion of the labrum.

4.2 **D.** The movements of the "lawnmower" exercise elicit higher EMG activity in the lower trapezius than other muscles such as the upper or middle trapezius and posterior deltoid because the scapula is pulled into retraction and posterior tilting toward the end of the movement.

4.3 **B.** Total shoulder range of motion should be less than or equal to 5° of the uninvolved side. This is one of the objective criteria used when determining whether a baseball player is ready to begin an interval throwing program. Option A is not correct because 75% ratio of rotator cuff strength (external to internal) is an objective criterion for determining whether or not a baseball player is ready to begin an interval throwing program. Options C and D are good criteria for the athlete to meet, but they are not objective outcome measures.

REFERENCES

1. Terry GC, Chopp TM. Functional anatomy of the shoulder. *J Athl Train*. 2000;35:248-255.
2. Provencher MT, Frank RM, LeClere LE, et al. The Hill-Sachs Lesion: diagnosis, classification, and management. *J Am Acad Orthop Surg*. 2012;20:242-252.
3. Drakos MC, Rudzki JR, Allen AA, Potter HG, Altcheck DW. Internal impingement of the shoulder in the overhead athlete. *J Bone Joint Surg Am*. 2009;91:2719-2728.
4. Knesek M, Skendzel JG, Dines JS, Altcheck DW, Allen AA, Bedi A. Diagnosis and management of superior labral anterior posterior tears in throwing athletes. *Am J Sports Med*. 2013;41:444-460.
5. Fortenbaugh D, Fleisig GS, Andrews JR. Baseball pitching biomechanics in relation to injury risk and performance. *Sports Health*. 2009;1:314-320.
6. Seroyer ST, Nho SJ, Bach BR, Bush-Joseph CA, Nicholson GP, Romeo AA. The kinetic chain in overhand pitching: its potential role for performance enhancement and injury prevention. *Sports Health*. 2010;2:135-146.
7. Reinold MM, Curtis AS. Microinstability of the shoulder in the overhead athlete. *Int J Sports Phys Ther*. 2013;8:601-616.
8. Chambers L, Altcheck DW. Microinstability and internal impingement in overhead athletes. *Clin Sports Med*. 2013;32:697-707.
9. Burkhart SS, Morgan CD, Kibler WB. The disabled throwing shoulder: spectrum of pathology Part I: pathoanatomy and biomechanics. *Arthroscopy*. 2003;19:404-420.
10. Conway JE. Arthroscopic repair of partial-thickness rotator cuff tears and SLAP lesions in professional baseball players. *Orthop Clin North Am*. 2001;32:443-456.
11. Burkhart SS, Morgan CD, Kibler WB. The disabled throwing shoulder: spectrum of pathology Part III: the SICK scapula, scapular dyskinesis, the kinetic chain, and rehabilitation. *Arthroscopy*. 2003;19:641-661.
12. Tokish JM, Curtin MS, Kim YK, Hawkins RJ, Torry MR. Glenohumeral internal rotation deficit in the asymptomatic professional pitcher and its relationship to humeral retroversion. *J Sport Sci Med*. 2008;7:78-83.
13. Wilk KE, Macrina LC, Fleisig GS, et al. Correlation of glenohumeral internal rotation deficit and total rotational motion to shoulder injuries in professional baseball pitchers. *Am J Sports Med*. 2011;39:329-335.
14. Garrison JC, Cole MA, Conway JE, Macko MJ, Thigpen C, Shanley E. Shoulder range of motion deficits in baseball players with an ulnar collateral ligament tear. *Am J Sports Med*. 2012;40:2597-2603.
15. Dines JS, Frank JB, Akerman M, Yocum LA. Glenohumeral internal rotation deficits in baseball players with ulnar collateral ligament insufficiency. *Am J Sports Med*. 2009;37:566-570.
16. Shanley E, Rauh MJ, Michener LA, Ellenbecker TS, Garrison JC, Thigpen C. Shoulder range of motion measures as risk factors for shoulder and elbow injuries in high school softball and baseball players. *Am J Sports Med*. 2011;39:1997-2006.

17. Putnam CA. Sequential motions of body segments in striking and throwing skills: descriptions and explanations. *J Biomechanics*. 1993;26:125-135.
18. Tyler TF, Nicholas SJ, Lee SJ, Mullaney M, McHugh MP. Correction of posterior shoulder tightness is associated with symptom resolution in patients with internal impingement. *Am J Sports Med*. 2010;38:114-119.
19. Braun S, Kokmeyer D, Millet PJ. Shoulder injuries in the throwing athlete. *J Bone Joint Surg Am*. 2009;91:966-978.
20. Laudner KG, Sipes RC, Wilson JT. The acute effects of sleeper stretches on shoulder range of motion. *J Athl Train*. 2008;43:359-363.
21. McClure P, Balaicuis J, Heilland D, Broersma ME, Thorndike CK, Wood A. A randomized controlled comparison of stretching procedures for posterior shoulder tightness. *J Orthop Sports Phys Ther*. 2007;37:108-114.
22. De Mey K, Danneels L, Cagnie B, Cools AM. Scapular muscle rehabilitation exercises in overhead athletes with impingement symptoms. Effect of a 6-week training program on muscle recruitment and functional outcome. *Am J Sports Med*. 2012;40:1906-1915.
23. Kibler WB, Sciascia A, Uhl T, Tambay N, Cunningham T. Electromyographic analysis of specific exercises for scapular control in early phases of shoulder rehabilitation. *Am J Sports Med*. 2008;36:1789-1798.
24. Ludewig PM, Reynolds JF. The association of scapular kinematics and glenohumeral joint pathologies. *J Orthop Sports Phys Ther*. 2009;39:90-104.
25. Davis JT, Limpisvasti O, Fluhme D, et al. The effect of pitching biomechanics on the upper extremity in youth and adolescent baseball pitchers. *Am J Sports Med*. 2009;37:1484-1491.
26. Garrison JC, Arnold A, Macko MJ, Conway JE. Baseball players diagnosed with ulnar collateral ligament tears demonstrate decreased balance compared to healthy controls. *J Orthop Sports Phys Ther*. 2013;43:752-758.
27. Robb AJ, Fleisig GS, Wilk KE, Macrina LC, Bolt B, Pajaczkowski J. Passive ranges of motion of the hips and their relationship with pitching biomechanics and ball velocity in professional baseball pitchers. *Am J Sports Med*. 2010;38:2487-2493.
28. Scher S, Anderson K, Weber N, Bajorek J, Rand K, Bey MJ. Associations among hip and shoulder range of motion and shoulder injury in professional baseball players. *J Athl Train*. 2010;45:191-197.
29. Kibler WB, Sciascia A. Kinetic chain contributions to elbow function and dysfunction in sports. *Clin Sports Med*. 2004;23:545-552.
30. Neuman BJ, Boisvert CB, Reiter B, Lawson K, Ciccotti MG, Cohen SB. Results of arthroscopic repair of Type II superior labral anterior posterior lesions in overhead athletes. *Am J Sports Med*. 2011;39:1883-1888.
31. Sayde WM, Cohen SB, Ciccotti MG, Dodson CC. Return to play after Type II superior labral anterior-posterior lesion repairs in athletes. *Clin Orthop Relat Res*. 2012;470:1595-1600.
32. Thigpen CA, Padua DA, Michener LA, et al. Head and shoulder posture affect scapular mechanics and muscle activity in overhead tasks. *J Electromyogr Kinesiol*. 2010;20:701-709.
33. McClure P, Tate AR, Kareha S, Irwin D, Zlupko E. A clinical method for identifying scapular dyskinesis, Part 1: reliability. *J Athl Train*. 2009;44:160-164.
34. Sciascia A, Cromwell R. Kinetic chain rehabilitation: a theoretical framework. *Rehabil Res Pract*. 2012;2012:853037. doi: 10.1155/2012/853037.
35. Reinold MM, Gill TJ, Wilk KE, Andrews JR. Current concepts in the evaluation and treatment of the shoulder in overhead throwing athletes, part 2: injury prevention and treatment. *Sports Health*. 2010;2:101-115.
36. Wilk KE, Meister K, Andrews JR. Current concepts in the rehabilitation of the overhead throwing athlete. *Am J Sports Med*. 2002;30:136-15.

37. Zhang S, Li H, Tao H, et al. Delayed early passive motion is harmless to shoulder rotator cuff healing in a rabbit model. *Am J Sports Med.* 2013;41:1885-1893.
38. Koo SS, Parsley BK, Burkhart SS, Schoolfield JD. Reduction of postoperative stiffness after arthroscopic rotator cuff repair: results of a customized physical therapy regimen based on risk factors for stiffness. *Arthroscopy.* 2011;27:155-160.
39. Cuff DJ, Pupello DR. Prospective randomized study of arthroscopic rotator cuff repair using an early versus delayed postoperative physical therapy protocol. *J Shoulder Elbow Surg.* 2012;21:1450-1455.
40. Esposito MD, Arrington JA, Blackshear MN, Murtagh FR, Silbiger ML. Thoracic outlet syndrome in a throwing athlete diagnosed with MRI and MRA. *J Magn Reson Imaging.* 1997;7:598-599.
41. Walsh MT. Upper limb neural tension testing and mobilization. Fact, fiction, and a practical approach. *J Hand Ther.* 2005;18:241-258.
42. Kibler WB, Kuhn JE, Wilk KE, et al. The disabled throwing shoulder: spectrum of pathology-10-year update. *Arthroscopy.* 2013;29:141-161.
43. Reinold MM, Escamilla R, Wilk KE. Current concepts in the scientific and clinical rationale behind exercises for glenohumeral and scapulothoracic musculature. *J Orthop Sports Phys Ther.* 2009;39:105-117.
44. McMullen J, Uhl T. A kinetic chain approach for shoulder rehabilitation. *J Athl Train.* 2000;35:329-337.

Ulnar Collateral Ligament Reconstruction

Robert C. Manske
B.J. Lehecka

CASE 5

A 28-year-old professional baseball player is referred to physical therapy following ulnar collateral ligament (UCL) reconstruction of his dominant right elbow. The original injury occurred 1 month earlier during a bout of repetitive throwing. He remembers the exact pitch that caused his symptoms. He felt an extreme cramping sensation in his proximal forearm, but he did not report feeling a popping sensation. Prior to surgery, he reported the ability to throw, but his velocity had decreased and he felt as though he continued to have cramping in his forearm that limited his ability to increase velocity or maintain control over his pitching. The physical therapist is evaluating him 7 days after right UCL reconstruction using his hamstring tendon as a graft source.

- Based on the patient's diagnosis, what do you anticipate may be contributing factors to his condition?
- What are the most appropriate physical therapy interventions for this condition?
- Are there possible complications that could interfere with physical therapy?

KEY DEFINITIONS

DYNAMIC STABILIZATION: Stabilization of the elbow joint via active muscle contractions

ELBOW EXTENSION LAG: Loss of active or passive elbow extension compared to uninvolved elbow or age- and activity-appropriate norms

THROWING PROGRESSION: Gradual, graded, and progressive increase in both throwing distance and number of repetitions used to gain shoulder endurance in a manner conducive to returning to throwing with minimal risk of overuse

Objectives

1. Describe UCL injury and its potential causes.
2. Describe postoperative treatment following UCL reconstruction.
3. Understand postoperative concerns regarding soft tissue healing timeframes (*e.g.*, avoidance of fast elbow movement, stretching out graft, or bone tunnel incorporation).
4. Describe exercises utilized to obtain dynamic elbow stability.

Physical Therapy Considerations

PT considerations during management of the baseball player following UCL reconstruction:

- **General physical therapy plan of care/goals:** Decrease pain; gradually increase elbow and shoulder range of motion (ROM) and flexibility; increase dynamic elbow control; maintain dynamic shoulder stability; return to throwing
- **Physical therapy interventions:** Modalities to decrease edema and effusion; progressive passive and active assisted ROM; gradual strengthening progression for elbow and shoulder muscles (*i.e.*, beginning with gentle submaximal isometrics and progressing to maximal isotonic exercises and ultimately plyometrics); return to throwing progression
- **Precautions during physical therapy:** Postoperative brace with ROM stops (typically worn during first 6 weeks after surgery) to ensure gradual return of ROM and protect the healing graft
- **Complications that can interfere with physical therapy:** Persistent postoperative pain and swelling, loss of motion, ligament re-rupture, ulnar nerve palsy or irritation

Understanding the Health Condition

The elbow joint consists of 3 articulations: the humeroulnar, humeroradial, and superior radioulnar. Most of the stability to the elbow is provided by the humeroulnar joint. This joint occurs at the convex portion of the trochlea of the distal humerus and the concave trochlear notch of the proximal ulna. The humeroulnar joint is considered a diarthrodial modified hinge joint because the ulna also has a slight axial rotation and slight side-to-side motion during flexion and extension. The humeroradial joint is the articulation between the convex capitulum of the humerus and the concave fovea of the radial head. Because this is considered a sellar joint, it provides minimal joint stability. The superior radioulnar joint is a diarthrodial joint formed by the concave radial notch and the annular ligament and the convex radial head.

The UCL stabilizes the medial side of the elbow. The UCL is composed of 3 bands: anterior, posterior, and oblique. The anterior band is the strongest and provides the majority of resistance to a valgus force placed on the medial elbow. The fibers run from the anterior aspect of the medial epicondyle and insert on the medial portion of the coronoid process; these fibers are taut at full extension and provide stability throughout the entire ROM. The posterior band attaches to the posterior part of the medial epicondyle and inserts on the medial side of the olecranon process. These fibers become taut in extreme elbow flexion. The oblique band attaches to both the anterior and posterior bands and provides little stability. Like all ligaments, the UCL contains receptors that normally provide proprioception and detect safe limits of tension in surrounding structures.

Using MRI scans from a sample of 16 asymptomatic professional baseball players, Kooima and colleagues[1] found that 87% had abnormalities in their dominant elbows indicative of chronic UCL injury and 81% demonstrated posteromedial osteochondral injury. In asymptomatic major league baseball pitchers, increased medial laxity on valgus stress is not uncommon.[2,3] Insufficiency of the UCL means a loss of ligament competency due to a sprain. UCL injuries are graded based on severity of ligamentous injury. A grade I injury causes little loss of function. There is a slight disruption of ligament tissue that may cause mild pain and swelling and discomfort when the ligament is stressed. Despite the damage to the ligament, it is not severe enough to cause instability with a valgus stress test. However, a grade II injury causes moderate instability with a valgus stress test. Moderate swelling and discoloration occur; ROM is likely limited due to swelling. A grade III sprain can cause severe swelling, pain, and definite functional limitations. Throwing will cause pain due to the inherent instability this injury causes. While the player may be able to function with a mild grade I UCL sprain, grade II and III injuries generally cause some degree of impairment. Because of the high prevalence of medial elbow laxity and evidence of UCL injury in competitive throwing or hitting athletes, **insufficiency of the UCL should always be considered as a differential or concomitant diagnosis in an overhead athlete with pain on the medial side of the elbow.**

Damage to the UCL can occur because of an acute injury. However, more often, UCL injuries occur because of chronic, repetitive low-level stresses during overhead activity that lead to microtearing of the UCL. These injuries can occur in any of the grades I to III. Most of these medial elbow injuries occur during the acceleration phase of throwing when valgus forces reach as high as 64 N·m.[4] Motion recording and analysis allows high-speed actions to be slowed down, which enables therapists to examine the kinetics and kinematics involved in the throwing motion. During overhead pitching, the elbow experiences significant valgus stress; approximately 300 N of shear force is experienced by the medial elbow.[4] This valgus torque is concentrated at the medial elbow, primarily at the anterior bundle of the UCL.[5,6]

Several authors have described 5 phases of throwing.[7,8] These phases include: (1) wind-up, (2) cocking, (3) acceleration, (4) release and deceleration, and (5) follow-through. The *wind-up phase* prepares the athlete to throw. It occurs when the athlete shifts the throwing shoulder away from the direction of the pitch with the opposite leg cocked high and the ball is removed from the glove. Because the shoulder is moved posteriorly in preparation for throwing, the elbow has minimal muscular activity to provide dynamic support during the wind-up phase. *Cocking* starts when the lead foot touches the ground and continues until the shoulder is abducted approximately 90° and externally rotated 90° or greater with some horizontal abduction, while the elbow is flexed about 85°.[9] At the point of maximal shoulder external rotation, a varus torque is produced to resist the valgus stress placed on the elbow during throwing. Just before maximum external shoulder rotation is achieved, the varus torque reaches approximately 85 N·m because the elbow is flexed to roughly 95°.[10] Morrey and An[11] have reported that at this point in the pitching motion, the UCL is contributing 54% of the resistance to the valgus load. This implies that during cocking, a strain of 45 N·m (54% of 85 N·m) is applied to the UCL, which is near the maximum load capacity for failure of the ligament.[12] *Acceleration* begins at the point of maximum shoulder external rotation and ends at ball release. *Release and deceleration* occur as the ball is released and the arm begins to decelerate. Last, the *follow-through* phase begins as the body moves forward with the arm and creates a distraction force on the shoulder and elbow.

The ability of an overhead athlete to return to sport after nonsurgical treatment of a UCL sprain is only about 42%.[13] Thus, for many of these athletes, surgical repair is required to successfully return to sport. Surgical choices include direct repair or reconstruction. Direct repair involves re-approximation of the torn fibers of the UCL. Reconstruction is distinct from repair. Reconstruction attempts to restore the static stabilizing function of the anterior band of the UCL by using a graft. Common graft sources are the semitendinosus tendon, gracilis tendon, or the palmaris longus tendon. These grafts are passed in a figure-8 pattern through drill holes placed in the sublime tubercle of the distal ulna and medial epicondyle. While direct repair of the UCL results in higher return to play than nonsurgical treatment (50%-63% vs. 42%, respectively),[14,15] **reconstruction of the UCL using a graft source has the highest rate of return to play for overhead athletes at 80% to 92%.**[16,17]

Physical Therapy Patient/Client Management

Postsurgical protocols after UCL reconstruction vary based on many factors including the surgical technique, graft source used, whether the ulnar nerve was transposed, and the surgeon's preference for immobilization versus immediate motion. Generally, a short period (4-6 weeks) of controlled motion is utilized to prevent excessive stress on reconstructed soft tissue. This controlled motion is provided by a splint or brace. During the first week, a posterior splint that holds the elbow in 90° of flexion may be used (Fig. 5-1). After this, the patient progresses to a motion controlled hinge brace that has motion stops allowing only a given ROM for the elbow, while allowing free motion for the forearm, wrist, and hand. A graduated progression of increased ROM at dedicated timeframes

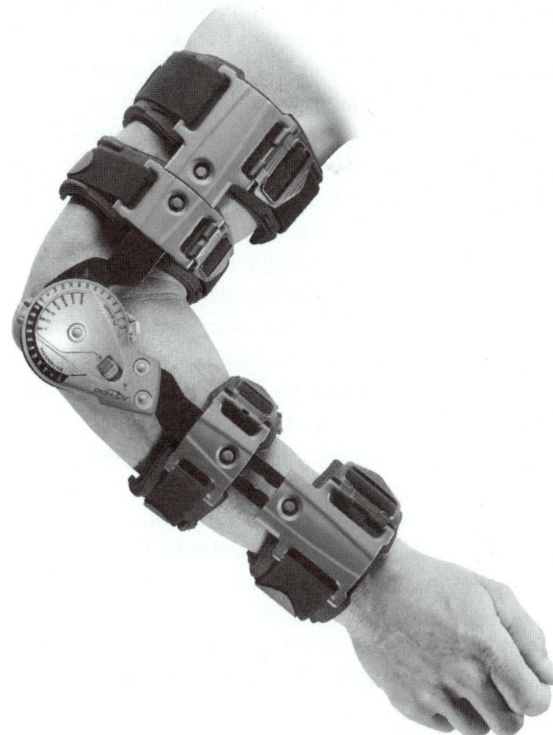

Figure 5-1. Hinged brace to provide varus and valgus elbow stability. (Reproduced with permission from http://www.djoglobal.com/products/donjoy/x-act-rom-elbow. Accessed July 28, 2015.)

typically results in full ROM and discontinuation of the protected brace around 6 weeks after surgery. The first physical therapy session may be 2 to 3 days or up to a week following surgery, pending surgeon preference. Prior to the initial physical therapy evaluation, a clinician at the surgeon's office should have shown the patient how to move the wrist and forearm in a pain-free ROM to decrease stiffness in the forearm and hand. There should be a short time of relative rest between surgery and initiation of formal physical therapy sessions to allow initial soft tissue healing to occur.

Examination, Evaluation, and Diagnosis

The UCL can either be injured from an acute rupture or from repetitive microtrauma over months of dysfunctional and painful throwing. Although some athletes are able to continue throwing through chronic microtrauma, many find it too painful following an acutely ruptured UCL. Those with chronic injury who are able to continue throwing usually describe a loss of control, an inability to throw at the same speed, or a cramping sensation in the medial elbow and forearm. Once the ligament ruptures, the athlete is usually able to recall the specific event that created sudden and sharp medial elbow pain. Tenderness at the medial elbow is expected; at times, a general joint effusion can be present.

A physical therapy evaluation of the individual after UCL reconstruction is typically performed several days to 1 week after surgery; timing varies pending surgeon and therapist preference. Following surgery, active and passive elbow and forearm ROM are generally limited due to pain and edema and/or effusion. Key motions that are tested include elbow flexion and extension and forearm supination and pronation. The therapist should be aware that pitchers who have spent years throwing often have an asymmetrical elbow extension lag (*i.e.*, loss of full elbow extension) on the dominant arm. When assessing an individual who has opted for conservative (nonsurgical) treatment of a UCL injury, manual muscle testing may reveal weakness of elbow flexor and extensor muscles and forearm pronator and supinator muscles mostly due to pain inhibition rather than actual loss of muscle strength. In the athlete post-UCL reconstruction, the therapist observes active ROM to determine strength against gravity. Further strength assessment is not performed immediately following surgery and can be assessed later during progressive rehabilitation (~3 weeks after surgery).

For any individual with suspected injury to the UCL, the therapist should perform ligament integrity tests. These physical examination tests are not performed immediately following UCL reconstruction. They are reserved for initial examination of the athlete with a nonsurgical UCL injury and may be used 6 to 12 weeks after UCL reconstruction to examine the integrity of the surgical reconstruction. There are 3 classic clinical tests for the structural integrity of the UCL. These tests are usually performed to assess the degree of medial laxity when the joint is stressed. A positive response to any of these tests is an abnormal end feel to the applied valgus stress, medial joint opening, and/or pain.

The valgus instability test is performed with the patient in the seated or standing position. The elbow is tested near full extension (Fig. 5-2A) and at 25° to 30° of flexion (Fig. 5-2B). The examiner stabilizes the patient's arm with one hand at the elbow and the other hand placed above the patient's wrist on the mid-forearm. The therapist applies an abduction or valgus force at the distal forearm to stress the UCL while palpating the UCL with the hand stabilizing the elbow.[18] With the fingers over the UCL, the therapist assesses the extent of opening or gapping as well as the end feel. Prior to testing, it is helpful to externally rotate the patient's shoulder to prevent the upper extremity from further rotation that may lead the examiner to falsely perceive increased medial elbow joint laxity. Excessive gapping, a soft end feel, or localized medial pain can each indicate a UCL injury.[19]

In the milking maneuver, the athlete sits or stands with the elbow flexed at 90° or greater and the forearm supinated. The therapist grasps the athlete's thumb and pulls it laterally, imparting a valgus stress to the elbow (Fig. 5-3). Reproduction of symptoms indicates a positive test and suggests a partial tear of the medial collateral ligament.[18,20] To date, there have been no studies evaluating the sensitivity or specificity of either the valgus instability test or the milking maneuver.

The last test is the moving valgus stress test, which has been shown to be 100% sensitive and 75% specific for detecting a partial UCL tear.[21] This test can also be performed with the athlete supine or standing with the arm abducted (Fig. 5-4). With the patient's elbow fully flexed, the examiner quickly extends the elbow while providing a valgus stress. Reproduction of the athlete's medial elbow pain between 120° and 70° indicates a positive test and a partial tear of the UCL.[18,20,21]

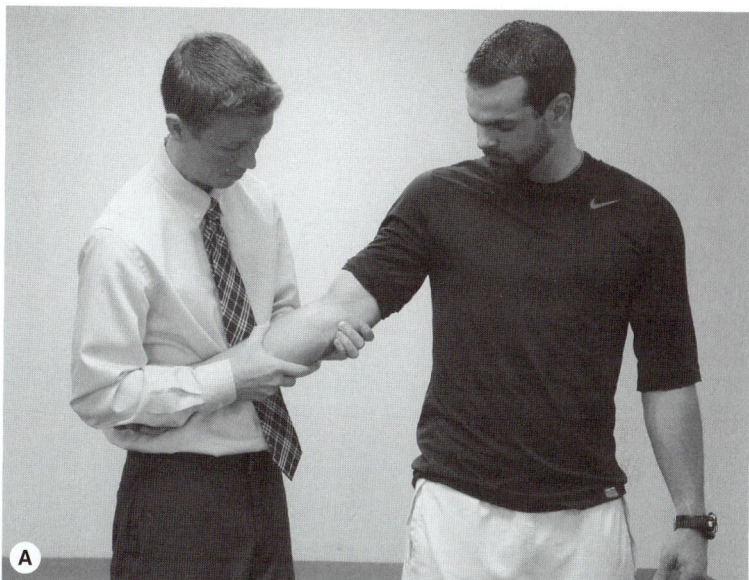

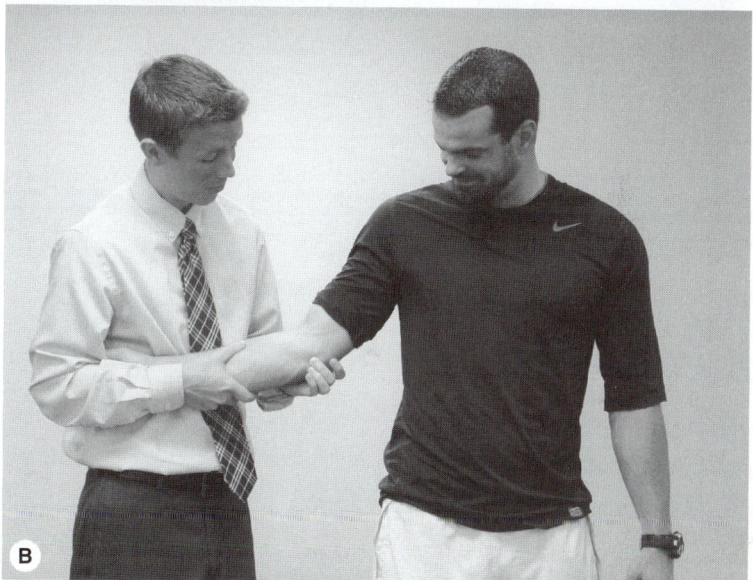

Figure 5-2. Valgus stress test with the elbow (**A**) near full extension and (**B**) at 25° to 30° flexion.

Plan of Care and Interventions

The athlete in this case study is a 28-year-old professional baseball pitcher who injured his UCL about 1 month ago and underwent UCL reconstruction with a gracilis tendon autograft 1 week ago. Table 5-1 shows the rehabilitation program following autologous reconstruction of the UCL. During the first postoperative

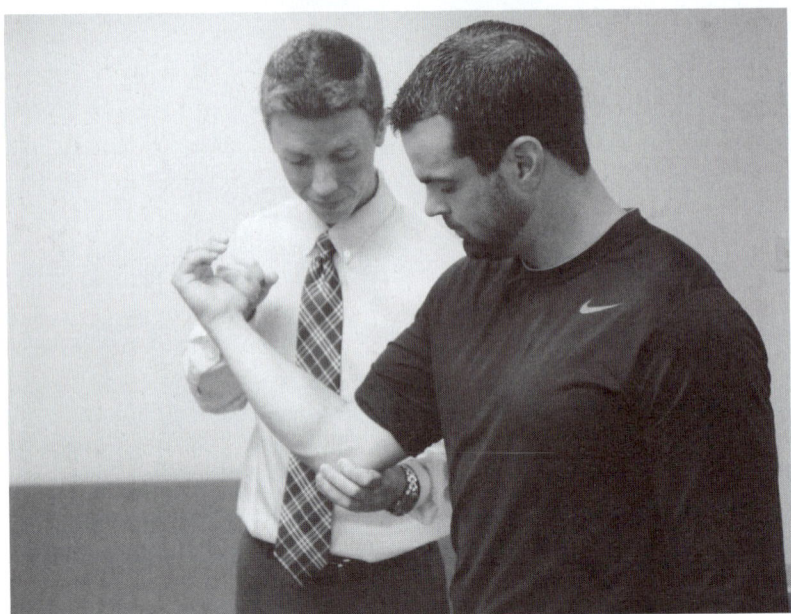

Figure 5-3. Milking maneuver for elbow ulnar collateral ligament (UCL) instability.

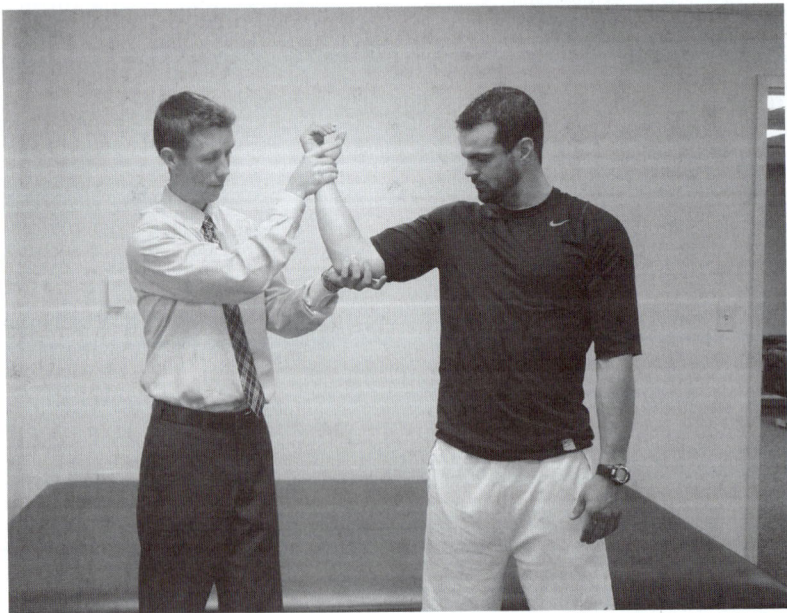

Figure 5-4. Midpoint during the moving valgus stress test for elbow ulnar collateral ligament (UCL) instability.

Table 5-1 POSTOPERATIVE REHABILITATION AFTER UCL RECONSTRUCTION USING AUTOLOGOUS GRAFT (GRACILIS)

Phase	Postoperative Days—Weeks	Goals	Restrictions	Treatment	Clinical Milestones
Phase I—Immediate postoperative	Day 1 to week 4	Protect surgical repair Decrease pain and inflammation Prevent negative effects of immobilization Restore normal elbow arthrokinematics Prevent primary/secondary hypomobility Promote dynamic stability Prevent reflex inhibition and secondary muscle atrophy	Brace: *Week 1:* locked in 90° elbow flexion *Week 2:* opened as tolerated, with goal of 15°-105° *Week 3:* opened, with goal of 5°-120°	*Weeks 1-2:* *ROM* Elbow: AROM/PROM (brace unlocked during therapy sessions) Shoulder AROM (no ER) Wrist: AROM/PROM *Strengthening* Shoulder isometrics (no IR/ER) Elbow isometrics Scapular isometrics Scapular isotonic exercises *Weeks 3-4:* Full can: shoulder elevation with thumbs pointing up Lateral raises: shoulder elevation to 0° with wrist and forearm in neutral Scapular plane elevation Biceps/triceps isotonic exercises ER/IR light isotonic exercises	No elbow pain No effusion No instability 4/5 shoulder, elbow, and forearm strength

(continued)

Table 5-1 POSTOPERATIVE REHABILITATION AFTER UCL RECONSTRUCTION USING AUTOLOGOUS GRAFT (GRACILIS) (CONTINUED)

Phase	Postoperative Days—Weeks	Goals	Restrictions	Treatment	Clinical Milestones
Phase II—Intermediate	Weeks 4-7	Progressively restore elbow ROM (full by weeks 6-8) Maintain repair Progressively restore motion, strength, and muscular balance	Discontinue brace at 6 weeks (per surgeon approval) Avoid pain-provoking activities Begin isotonic strengthening exercises	Continue to progress elbow AROM/PROM (full by weeks 6-8) Progress previous UE strengthening exercises by altering intensity and speed Begin light exercises with 1-2 lb weights Wrist curls Pronation/supination isotonic exercises	Full elbow flexion and extension (by weeks 6-8) No pain No swelling 4/5 shoulder, elbow, and forearm strength
Phase III—Advanced strengthening	Weeks 8-14	Full pain-free elbow AROM/PROM Restoration of muscle strength, power, and endurance No pain or tenderness Gradual initiation of functional activities	Avoid pain-provoking activities Initiate progressive strengthening exercises	Maintain full ROM Increase intensity and decrease repetitions of standard exercises Sidelying shoulder ER Two-handed plyometric exercises (e.g., chest pass and wood chopper) Wrist flips and wrist slams: throwing 2-lb ball to floor with emphasis on wrist flexion action	Full symmetrical elbow AROM/PROM No pain No swelling 5/5 elbow, forearm, wrist, and hand strength 5/5 scapular muscle strength

Phase IV—Return to full activity	Weeks 14-21+	Maintain muscle strength, power, and endurance Maintain elbow motion Progress functional activities Return to unrestricted sports activity	None	Continue previous exercises Initiate more advanced double- and single-arm exercises Advanced sport-specific training Progress interval sports programs Plyometric exercises: Single-arm dribble Single-arm IR throws Single-arm ER catches Prone 90/90 drops: prone on table with shoulder and elbow in 90/90 position, with quick release and catching of 2-lb ball	Return to activity and/or sport

Abbreviations: AROM, active range of motion; ER, external rotation; IR, internal rotation; PROM, passive range of motion; ROM, range of motion; UCL, ulnar collateral ligament; UE, upper extremity.

week, the athlete was placed in a posterior splint at 90° of elbow flexion; a compressive dressing with cryotherapy is often used to decrease edema, joint effusion, and pain. Gripping and active wrist motion exercises for flexion and extension are prescribed with dosing based on a number of factors including the athlete's pain tolerance, age, and postoperative strength. On the athlete's initial visit, his uninvolved active elbow ROM was 3° of hyperextension to 140° of flexion. His right active elbow ROM was limited to a 30° to 90°arc of motion. Forearm supination and pronation on the uninvolved side were 80° each; these motions on the involved side were 40° each. After the first week, the posterior splint was replaced with the motion-controlled hinged brace. The motion-controlled hinged brace not only controls motion, but also provides varus and valgus stability to the elbow during activities. The brace can be unlocked to allow elbow ROM as tolerated during therapy sessions and while performing home exercises. After the first few physical therapy sessions, the therapist noted that the athlete could tolerate elbow and forearm ROM exercises with little to no pain, so biceps and shoulder isometrics were prescribed. At this time (and until 4-6 weeks after surgery), the only motion that should be restricted to protect graft integrity is external rotation due to the stress that this motion places on the UCL. Modalities such as cryotherapy and interferential electrical stimulation (*e.g.*, 90-120 pulses per second for 15 minutes) can be utilized to decrease pain and reduce edema.

Between the first and second postsurgical weeks, all previous exercises are continued and progressed within the athlete's tolerance. Gentle elbow extensor isometric exercises are initiated. Elbow motion is generally allowed to progress by 10° of extension and 20° of flexion per week until full active ROM is achieved. In this fashion, full elbow ROM (0°-145°) should be achieved by the end of week 6. Between the second and third postsurgical weeks, shoulder AROM exercises and scapular strengthening exercises are initiated. By the end of week 3 and the start of week 4, the athlete's elbow active ROM had increased to 130° of flexion to 11° shy of full extension. At this time, manual muscle testing was performed for the first time and graded 4$^-$/5 for the biceps, triceps, wrist flexors and extensors, supinators, and pronators. At the end of the sixth postsurgical week, the physical therapist and the surgeon decided that the athlete could discontinue use of the hinged elbow brace.

After UCL reconstruction, some individuals have difficulty achieving full elbow ROM, especially extension. In this case, the athlete's active elbow ROM was 8° to 135°. Because he was a professional pitcher, he did not exhibit full symmetrical extension on his pitching arm prior to surgery; thus, he was very near his presurgical elbow extension. To try to gain the last few degrees of extension, joint mobilization (Fig. 5-5) and low-load, long-duration stretching into elbow extension was initiated (Fig. 5-6). At week 6, light isotonic exercises for the shoulder, elbow (Fig. 5-7), wrist, and hand were also initiated using light weights and band resistance. The emphasis for strengthening exercises should be on the flexor and pronator muscle groups of the elbow and wrist because they lie over the medial elbow and provide the required dynamic support and resistance to valgus stress and overload. In particular, the flexor carpi ulnaris and flexor digitorum superficialis, which lie over the top of the UCL, are extremely important for dynamic stabilization of the medial elbow. At week 8, light sport-specific exercises were allowed.

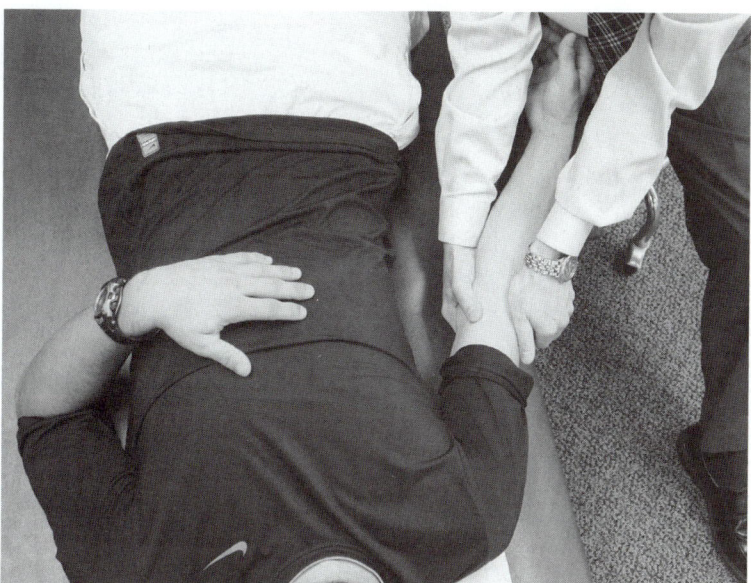

Figure 5-5. Manual therapy joint mobilizations to increase elbow extension.

Postsurgical weeks 9 to 16 are used to advance exercises to higher levels. Eccentric training and plyometric exercises are incorporated to start simulating functional activities. At this time, the athlete should be able to tolerate light plyometric exercises with both hands, progressing to single hand (at ~14 weeks), and start similar activities (*e.g.*, throwing, tennis forehand and backhand, swimming). By

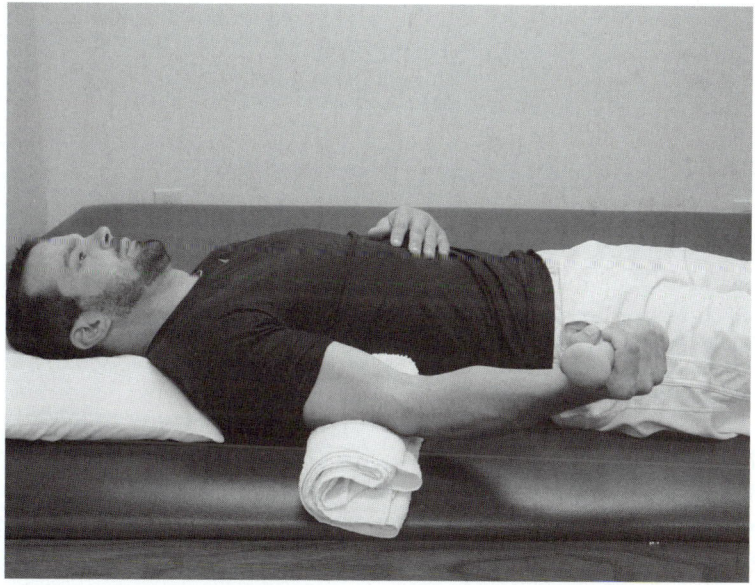

Figure 5-6. Low-load, long-duration stretching to increase elbow extension.

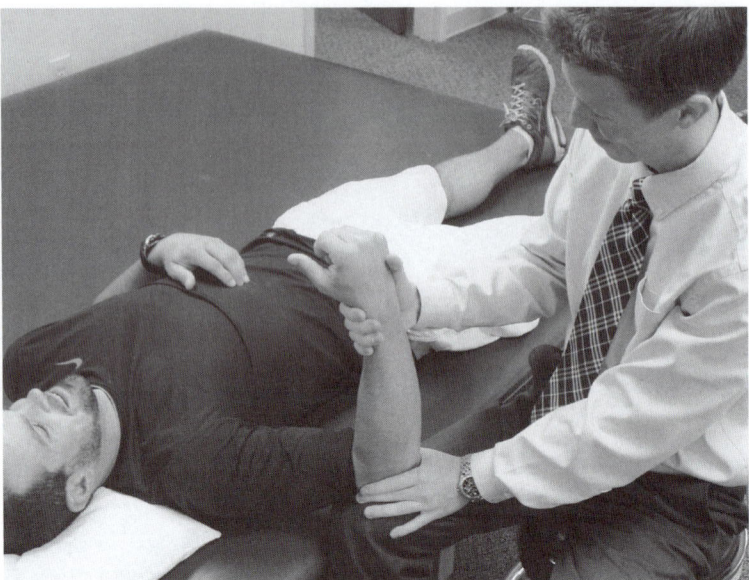

Figure 5-7. Therapist providing manual resistance to biceps and triceps for submaximal pain-free isometrics.

week 16, the athlete's elbow active ROM was 5° to 145°. He still exhibited a slight extensor lag; however, this represented a return to his normal asymmetry. Manual muscle testing was 5/5 for all shoulder, elbow, forearm, wrist, and hand muscles. Four months after surgery, an interval throwing progression is allowed; in most instances, throwing from the mound is progressed within 4 to 8 weeks after initiation of the interval throwing program. The surgeon typically allows a return to competitive pitching 9-12 months or more after surgery.

Evidence-Based Clinical Recommendations

SORT: Strength of Recommendation Taxonomy
A: Consistent, good-quality patient-oriented evidence
B: Inconsistent or limited-quality patient-oriented evidence
C: Consensus, disease-oriented evidence, usual practice, expert opinion, or case series

1. Physical therapists should consider UCL injury when a pitcher complains of medial elbow pain with a valgus stress to the humeroulnar joint. **Grade B**
2. Ulnar collateral ligament reconstruction for UCL insufficiency allows the majority of overhead athletes to return to pre-injury level. **Grade A**
3. Examination of the individual with suspected injury to the UCL should include ligament integrity tests with good diagnostic accuracy. **Grade C**

COMPREHENSION QUESTIONS

5.1 During progressive rehabilitation of a competitive collegiate pitcher's elbow, which feature would be *most* anticipated regarding elbow range of motion?
   A. Symmetrical motion bilaterally
   B. More hyperextension on the throwing side
   C. Slight loss of extension on throwing side
   D. Symmetrical extension and loss of flexion throwing side

5.2 Which of the following is uncommon in a pitcher that continues to throw following a chronic ulnar collateral ligament injury?
   A. Loss of control
   B. Loss of speed
   C. Cramping sensations
   D. Burning

ANSWERS

5.1 **C.** Slight loss of extension on the dominant throwing side is common after years of throwing.

5.2 **D.** Loss of control and speed as well as cramping sensations are common following chronic UCL injury in pitchers. Burning is not a common symptom of UCL injury.

REFERENCES

1. Kooima CL, Anderson K, Craig JF, Teeter DM, van Holsbeeck M. Evidence of subclinical medial collateral ligament injury and posteromedial impingement in professional baseball players. *Am J Sports Med*. 2004;32:1602-1606.
2. Nazarian LN, McShane JM, Ciccotti MG, O'Kane PL, Harwood MI. Dynamic US of the anterior band of the ulnar collateral ligament of the elbow in asymptomatic major league baseball pitchers. *Radiology*. 2003;227:149-154.
3. Ellenbecker TS, Mattalino HA, Elam EA, Caplinger RA. Medial elbow joint laxity in professional baseball pitchers. A bilateral comparison using stress radiography. *Am J Sports Med*. 1998;26:420-424.
4. Fleisig GS, Andrews JR, Dillman CJ, Escamilla RF. Kinetics of baseball pitching with implications about injury mechanisms. *Am J Sports Med*. 1995;23:233-239.
5. Davidson PA, Pink M, Perry J, Jobe FW. Functional anatomy of the flexor pronator muscle group in relation to the medial collateral ligament of the elbow. *Am J Sports Med*. 1995;23:245-250.
6. Glousman RE, Barron J, Jobe FW, Perry J, Pink M. An electromyographiuc analysis of the elbow in normal and injured pitchers with medial collateral ligament insufficiency. *Am J Sports Med*. 1992;20:311-317.
7. McCleod WD. The pitching mechanism: In: Zarins B, Andrews JR, Carson WG, eds. *Injuries to the Throwing Arm*. Philadelphia, PA: Saunders; 1985:22-29.

8. Fleisig GS, Dillman CJ, Andrews JR. Biomechanics of the shoulder during throwing. In: Andrews JR, Wilk KE, eds. *The Athlete's Shoulder*. New York, NY: Churchill Livingstone; 1997:355-368.
9. Werner SL, Fleisig GS, Dillman CJ, Andrews JR. Biomechanics of the elbow during baseball pitching. *J Orthop Sports Phys Ther*. 1993;17:274-278.
10. Dun S, Kingsley D, Fleisig GS, Loftice J, Andrews JR. Biomechanical comparison of fastball from wind-up and the fastball from stretch in professional baseball pitchers. *Am J Sports Med*. 2008;36:137-141.
11. Morrey BF, An KN. Articular and ligamentous contributions to the stability of the elbow joint. *Am J Sports Med*. 1983;11:315-319.
12. Fleisig GS, Barrentine SW. Biomechanical aspects of the elbow in sports. *Sports Med Arthrosc Rev*. 1995;3:149-159.
13. Rettig AC, Sherrill C, Snead DS, Mendler JC, Meiling P. Nonoperative treatment of ulnar collateral ligament injuries in throwing athletes. *Am J Sports Med*. 2001;29:15-17.
14. Conway JE, Jobe FW, Glousman RE, Pink M. Medial instability of the elbow in throwing athletes. Treatment by repair or reconstruction of the ulnar collateral ligament. *J Bone Joint Surg Am*. 1992;74:67-83.
15. Azar FM, Andrews JR, Wilk KE, Groh D. Operative treatment of ulnar collateral ligament injuries of the elbow in athletes. *Am J Sports Med*. 2000;28:16-23.
16. Thompson WH, Jobe FW, Yocum LA, Pink MM. Ulnar collateral ligament reconstruction in athletes: muscle-splitting approach without transposition of the ulnar nerve. *J Shoulder Elbow Surg*. 2001;10:152-157.
17. Rohrbough JT, Altchek DW, Hyman J, Williams RJ 3rd, Botts JD. Medial collateral ligament reconstruction of the elbow using the docking technique. *Am J Sports Med*. 2002;30:541-548.
18. Magee DJ. *Orthopedic Physical Assessment*. 6th ed. St. Louis, MO: Elsevier; 2014.
19. Andrews JR, Whiteside JA. Common elbow problems in the athlete. *J Orthop Sports Phys Ther*. 1993;17:289-295.
20. O'Driscoll SW. Acute, recurrent and chronic elbow instabilities. In: Norris TR, ed. *Orthopedic Knowledge Update 2: Shoulder and Elbow*. Rosemount, IL: American Academy of Orthopedic Surgeons; 2002.
21. O'Driscoll SW, Lawton RM, Smith AM. The "moving valgus stress test" for medial collateral ligament tears of the elbow. *Am J Sports Med*. 2005;33:231-239.

Spondylolysis in a Gymnast

Kaan Celebi
Airelle O. Hunter-Giordano

CASE 6

A 14-year-old female gymnast was referred to physical therapy after a fall sustained during gymnastics practice 2 weeks ago. While performing a flight series on the balance beam, she missed the beam with her hands, forcing her into spinal hyperextension prior to falling onto the mat. When she was first evaluated 2 weeks after the incident by a sports physical therapist, the patient presented with a positive lumbopelvic screen, tenderness to palpation along L5/S1 vertebrae, significant pain with lumbar extension, and hypermobility at L3/4 and L4/5. At that time, the physical therapist recommended that the gymnast rest (*i.e.*, not participate in gym practice) for 2 weeks. However, the gymnast continued practicing and competing because she had a good chance to qualify for Nationals in 2 months because she ranked in the top 10 and finished as a junior national finalist. The gymnast was taking over-the-counter nonsteroidal anti-inflammatories; physical therapy interventions focused primarily on pain management (electrical stimulation, ice, soft tissue mobilization) in order to get the athlete through her competitive season. During the past few months, the patient has continued to complain of intermittent low back pain. Following her initial physical therapy evaluation more than 2 months ago, her back pain still had not decreased from 4/10 (on the 0-10 numeric pain rating scale). Based upon the athlete's mechanism of injury, gross physical examination findings, and the nature of the athlete's sport, the physical therapist suspected that the underlying cause of her pain could be due to spondylolysis.

▶ What signs may be associated with the diagnosis of a spondylolysis?
▶ What are the examination priorities?
▶ Based on the patient's suspected diagnosis, what do you anticipate may be the contributing factors to her condition?
▶ What are the most appropriate physical therapy interventions?
▶ What is her rehabilitation and return-to-sport prognosis?

KEY DEFINITIONS

SPONDYLOLISTHESIS: Translation of one vertebra over another due to a congenital defect or fracture in the pars interarticularis

SPONDYLOLYSIS: Degeneration or defect of a portion of the vertebra; commonly involves the pars interarticularis of the neural arch; 5 types of spondylolysis have been described

SPONDYLOSIS: Age-related degeneration of the spine, either in the vertebrae, facet joints, or intervertebral discs, which may be diagnosed through conventional radiographs; hallmark signs include decreased joint spaces and sclerotic formations

STRESS FRACTURE: Next stage in bony injury following a stress reaction and the first sign of an actual break in a bone; occurs if the stress reaction continues without being noticed or if the athlete continues the aggravating activity

STRESS REACTION: Initial form of a bony injury that occurs when stresses affecting the bone occur at a greater rate than the rate of the bone rebuilding; initially presents as localized bony tenderness

Objectives

1. Define spondylolysis and identify risk factors associated with this condition.
2. Identify an appropriate medical referral and diagnostic imaging that should be completed to rule in or rule out spondylolysis.
3. Describe the most appropriate physical therapy interventions for an individual with a spondylolysis.
4. Describe the prognosis for a young athlete with a spondylolysis.

Physical Therapy Considerations

PT considerations during management of the teenage gymnast with a suspected diagnosis of a spondylolysis:

- **General physical therapy plan of care/goals:** Decrease pain; increase pain-free range of motion (ROM) and muscular flexibility; increase spine and lower-quadrant strength, endurance, and motor control of the trunk; maintain aerobic fitness capacity while avoiding extension-based movements

- **Physical therapy interventions:** Patient education regarding functional anatomy and injury pathomechanics; instruct patient in avoiding symptomatic positions and maneuvers; referral for radiographs; if radiographs confirm diagnosis of spondylolysis, begin to immobilize in brace; therapeutic exercises for spinal stabilization (in "neutral spine" position); stretch and/or mobilize inflexible areas (i.e., muscles and spinal segments that contribute to increased lordosis)

▶ **Precautions during physical therapy:** Avoid lumbar extension; if the injury is a stress reaction, progression back to sport can begin as long as activities are pain-free; if stress fracture is present, participation in gymnastics must cease to allow proper rest and healing

▶ **Complications interfering with physical therapy:** Symptomatic nonunion of fracture sites; progression into spondylolisthesis; noncompliance with avoidance of painful lumbar extension ranges

Understanding the Health Condition

Spondylolysis is defined as a defect in the pars interarticularis of the neural arch.[1] It occurs in about 6% of the general population and is often asymptomatic.[1,2] In young athletes, however, the incidence is much higher. It has been reported that 47% of young athletes who report low back pain were diagnosed with a spondylolysis.[2,3] Within the elite gymnast population, 15% to 20% have this diagnosis and they are often very symptomatic.[2,3]

The pathogenesis of spondylolysis has been suggested to be acute and repetitive microtrauma to the spinal unit.[4] Mechanical stresses to the spine can be caused by isolated hyperextension movements as well as hyperextension combined with rotational movements.[4] Flexion movements may also produce shear forces, particularly on the pars, which can cause a fatigue type stress and/or fracture.[4,5] Although any spinal level may be affected, 71% to 95% of all spondylolytic defects occur at L5/S1 and 5% to 25% occur at L4/L5.[1,2,6-8] Table 6-1 outlines the classification scheme originally developed by Wiltse et al.[9] to describe 5 main types of spondylolysis.

Many factors can contribute to the development of a spondylolytic defect. These include severe scoliosis, spina bifida occulta, and participation in sports that require repetitive extension movements (*e.g.*, gymnastics, ballet, figure skating, soccer, volleyball).[2,9] An increased lordosis or factors that contribute to increased lordosis (iliopsoas tightness, thoracolumbar fascia tightness, abdominal weakness, thoracic

Table 6-1	CLASSIFICATION SCHEME OF SPONDYLOLYSIS	
Type 1	Dysplastic	Genetic dysplasia of the neural arch of L5 or upper sacrum such that the body of L5 may sublux anteriorly on the body of S1. This may occur in the presence of an elongated and intact pars, or a pars that has physically divided into 2 separate pieces.
Type 2	Isthmic	A lesion of the pars of 1 of 3 types: 1. Lytic: true separation in the pars resulting from a fatigue fracture 2. Elongation: elongation of the pars without separation 3. Acute fracture: always secondary to severe trauma
Type 3	Degenerative	Secondary to longstanding intersegmental instability with associated remodeling of the articular process
Type 4	Traumatic	Secondary to acute trauma that fractures a part of the arch other than the pars
Type 5	Pathologic	Generalized or focal bone disease that results in interruption of the neural arch

kyphosis) can also contribute to the development of spondylolysis.[10] In the adolescent, the spine is still undergoing growth and osseous remodeling; full skeletal maturation does not occur until the mid-20s.[10] This puts the younger individual at higher risk of sustaining repetitive stress injuries secondary to numerous points of weakness in the non-mature bone.[10]

Early diagnosis is essential to enhance healing of a stress reaction or stress fracture in the spine. If pars defects in the immature spine are detected at an early stage, higher rates of healing have been documented.[5,11] However, the mean time between onset of symptoms and time of diagnosis is 3 years for L5/S1 defects and up to 11 years for L4/L5 or higher-level defects.[5,11] If a particular defect in the spine is not diagnosed early and properly treated, a spondylolisthesis (anterior translation of the vertebrae) can develop. In the current patient case, the gymnast's acute injury caused by her fall from the beam is presumed to have caused macrotrauma superimposed upon the multiple chronic stress reactions induced by the repetitive spinal extension motion in the sport of gymnastics.

Physical Therapy Patient/Client Management

If there is a concern for a spondylolysis based upon patient history and physical examination, the physical therapist should educate the patient on functional anatomy and injury pathomechanics and refer her for diagnostic imaging. The role of imaging is to aid in diagnosis, guide therapeutic decision making, develop a prognosis, and determine whether the athlete can be cleared to return to sport. If a spondylolysis is confirmed by imaging, the physical therapist must attempt to determine if the anatomical defect is the primary source of her pain or merely an incidental finding. The primary goal for most injured individuals is to return to pain-free activity as quickly and as safely as possible in a manner that does not overload the healing structures.

Examination, Evaluation, and Diagnosis

Patients with symptomatic spondylolysis often present with insidious onset of localized low back pain. Pain can range from "low level" to "severe" and may radiate into the buttocks or posterior thighs. Some patients may report a single traumatic event that led to the onset of pain; however, most complain of a gradual worsening of pain. Pain associated with spondylolysis typically worsens with activity and improves with rest. When a patient presents primarily with low back pain and no prior history of symptoms in that region, the physical therapist may overlook spondylolysis as a potential cause. Instead, the therapist may focus interventions directed to address the patient's symptoms and the findings from the musculoskeletal examination. In most cases, this would be an appropriate plan of care. However, when insidious onset of low back pain occurs in athletes participating in sports with repetitive lumbar extension movements, the therapist should consider spondylolysis as part of the differential diagnosis. Failure to suspect a spondylolysis can delay early diagnosis and lead to further progression of the current stress reaction and potentially lead to a spondylolisthesis. In younger patients, specifically athletes known to experience repetitive extension stresses to the lumbar spine, the physical therapist must keep in mind the potential for this defect during examination of the low back.

During palpation, **patients with spondylolysis commonly experience** localized lumbosacral tenderness and muscle spasm, which can often be one-sided and may resemble symptoms produced by a scoliotic curve.[12] **Other key findings** may include a hyperlordotic posture and pain reproduced with lumbar hyperextension. In most cases, the patient is asymptomatic in spinal flexion and the neurologic examination (e.g., reflexes, dermatomal and myotomal screens) is negative. In this patient case, hallmark findings from the spinal musculoskeletal examination included decreased and painful active right side bending and left rotation; other gross active spinal ROM was normal to excessive in all directions. On closer visual assessment and lumbar mobility testing, the physical therapist noted that the gymnast's spinal motion occurred primarily at the L3/L4 spinal segment and above, with no notable extension ROM occurring below. Major muscle imbalances were evident with tightness in bilateral iliopsoas (measured with the Thomas test) and lengthened hamstrings (measured with passive straight leg raise, >90°).

Imaging is essential to confirm the suspected diagnosis of spondylolysis or spondylolisthesis. Initially, a physician orders a set of plain radiographs; the recommended films are in the posteroanterior, standing lateral, and oblique views.[13] Plain radiographs may reveal the pars lesion of a spondylolysis, overall spinal alignment (e.g., scoliosis), and/or the presence of other bony lesions. In individuals with lumbar spondylolysis or spondylolisthesis, the posteroanterior view often shows findings of a lateral deviation of the spinous process and/or sclerosis of the contralateral pedicle.[14,15] The lateral view is ideal for detection of any pars lesions as well as a possible spondylolisthesis. The oblique view can highlight the "neck of the scotty dog" lesion. Single-photon emission computed tomography (SPECT) of the spine is indicated for those patients with inconclusive radiographs, but whose history and clinical examination suggest a presence of spondylolysis.[12,16,17] Positive findings on a SPECT examination include increased uptake in the pars, adjunct lamina, or pedicle; these are suggestive of a stress reaction, stress fracture, or symptomatic spondylolytic defect. Following a SPECT examination, computed axial tomography (CT) can be used to examine the area of increased uptake. CT has been shown to be the best imaging modality to define the bony morphology of spondylolysis.[12] A CT scan is also the best modality for identifying *chronic* lesions, in which the pars defect appears sclerotic in nature.[7] Magnetic resonance imaging (MRI) is most frequently ordered for patients with a suspected spondylolysis when neurologic symptoms are present in conjunction with back pain. Some researchers suggest it may be a useful diagnostic test for early diagnosis of active spondylolysis when missed on traditional radiographs.[12,18,19]

Plan of Care and Interventions

Diagnosing spondylolysis can be difficult and may even be overlooked by sports medicine clinicians; however, it must be suspected when examining athletes who perform repetitive extension-based movements in their sport. Although there is no agreed upon best treatment protocol in the literature for athletes with spondylolysis, most agree that **treatment should include a period of rest** to allow for healing. d'Hemecourt et al.[10,20] suggest athletes diagnosed with spondylolysis should be

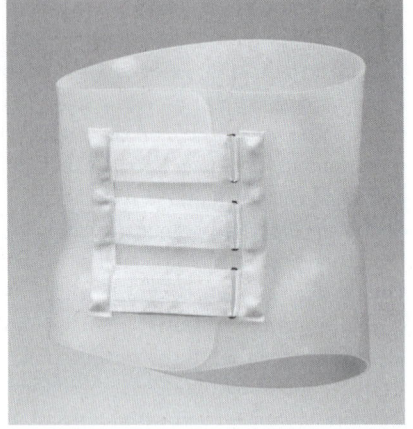

Figure 6-1. Boston overlap brace (www.boston-brace.com). Initially, typical wearing schedule is 24 hours per day. Brace may be taken off for short periods for personal hygiene. Duration of wear is based on degree of symptoms and compliance with prescribed activity restriction. (Reproduced with permission from Boston Brace. www.boston-brace.com.)

removed from sporting activities and be immobilized in 0° of lumbosacral extension in a **Boston overlapping brace** (Fig. 6-1) to be worn up to 24 hours per day. Upon diagnosis of a spondylolysis, physical therapy interventions may be initiated and should focus on **pain control, restoring the balance between anterior and posterior pelvic muscles, and antilordotic strengthening**. Lumber extension should be avoided in all interventions. Table 6-2 includes examples of recommended exercises for the young athlete with a spondylolysis or spondylolisthesis in the early rehabilitation phase when large lumbar movements are not permitted. The goals of these exercises are to strengthen muscles that promote lumbar stabilization (with primary emphasis on transversus abdominis and multifidi) and to stretch or mobilize those structures that promote lumbar extension, especially the hip flexors.

In addition to traditional spinal stability and strengthening exercises, neuromuscular electrical stimulation (NMES) to the lumbar paraspinals can be used to promote proper muscle recruitment and stability in the lumbar region.[21] The patient is positioned in prone in neutral or slight lumbar flexion (facilitated by placing 2-3 pillows under the abdomen/hip region) with her pelvis strapped to the treatment table to prevent anterior tilt during electrical stimulation (Fig. 6-2).[21] Electrical stimulation typically is performed for 15 minutes per physical therapy session, with an on:off ratio of 10 sec:50 sec. The goal is to achieve a total of only 15 contractions with ample rest time to avoid muscle fatigue.

In 4 to 6 weeks, the athlete may return to sporting events while wearing a brace.[10,15] However, this decision must be made based on the individual and should only include a return to sports that are *not* extension biased (*e.g.*, soccer, field hockey, softball, baseball). By 4 months, if there is evidence of bony healing on the CT scan or a pain-free nonunion (*i.e.*, individual does not have pain with any spinal motion, even though there is no radiographic evidence of healing), weaning off the brace can begin.[10,15] For sports such as gymnastics in which use of a brace is not feasible, **a pain-free gradual return-to-sport progression** should be implemented with sport-specific drills and return to sporting activities. Prognosis is patient specific. Rehabilitation guidelines have not been consistent within the literature, although return to play is typically based on pain-free progressions. Anatomic outcomes of

Table 6-2 RECOMMENDED THERAPEUTIC EXERCISES FOR THE ATHLETE WITH SPONDYLOLYSIS

Stretching/Mobilization	Strengthening
Perform each exercise in this category 1-2 times/day. Mobilizations: 30 repetitions Stretches: 3 repetitions, holding each repetition for 30 sec	Perform 30 repetitions of each basic exercise 1-2 times/day. Perform 10 repetitions of each dynamic core stabilization exercise 1-2 times/day. Initiate program with basic exercises utilizing a TA contraction. Once patient can perform isometric TA contraction, dynamic core stabilization exercises may be added.
"Cat/camel" mobilization (alternating lumbar spine position from neutral to kyphotic position via anterior and posterior pelvic tilts)	TA contraction in hooklying with 5-sec hold
Supine pelvic tilt (posteriorly tilting pelvis from neutral spine position)	TA contraction in hooklying with single heel slide
Half-kneeling hip flexor stretch	TA contraction in hooklying with single-leg extension
	TA contraction in hooklying with double-leg extension
	Front (Fig. 6-3) and side planks (Fig. 6-4) with 10-sec holds, 10 repetitions (first with knees bent and progressing to straight knees). Increase from 10- to 60-sec holds before progressing to next exercise.
	"Bird dog" exercise: begin with single LE extension; progress to UE and contralateral LE extension in kneeling position (Fig. 6-5) and then in push-up position (Fig. 6-6).
	Once plank exercises are mastered, progress to arms extended (Fig. 6-7). Increase from 10-sec to 60-sec holds.
	Side planks with hip abduction (Fig. 6-8): Initiate hip abduction with 10-sec holds. Increase in increments of 10 sec, finishing at 60-sec holds.

Abbreviations: LE, lower extremity; TA, transversus abdominis; UE, upper extremity.

spondylolysis include 1 of 3 scenarios: complete bony healing, healing with fibrous tissue, or nonunion. The case of nonunion is only problematical if the athlete continues to have pain. For example, athletes can have positive signs of spondylolysis on imaging but continue to be pain-free and partake in their sports.[2,22]

In determining when it is safe for a gymnast to return to sport, the physical therapist not only has to think about her injury, but also must consider how that injury impacts each of the 4 apparatuses she needs to perform (vault, uneven bars, balance beam, floor exercise). When a gymnast has a spondylolysis, the restriction on uncontrolled and/or forced extension needs to be slowly eased. She must be progressed back into the rehabilitation program in a pain-free manner in order to prevent further injury and pathology. In this case, the gymnast could start returning to the gym with swinging on the uneven bars while limiting extremes in spinal ROM, followed by the acceptance of force and shock with small leaps and jumps on the floor exercise and balance beam. Dance throws and leap throws can also be done on the balance beam and the floor exercise in order to keep cardiovascular fitness. After performing these activities pain-free, the gymnast should be able to run

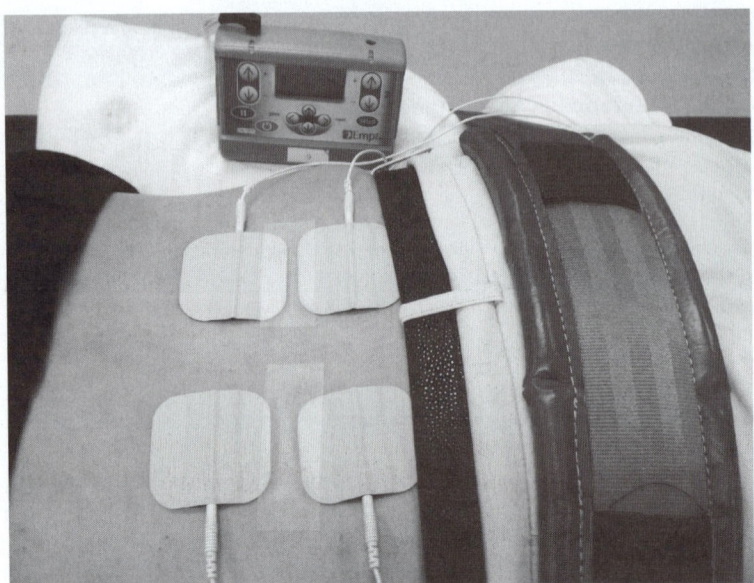

Figure 6-2. Neuromuscular electrical stimulation (NMES) to the lumbar paraspinal muscles in a patient with lumbar spondylolysis. Note 4-electrode placement with 1 pair on either side of the symptomatic spinal level (L3-L5). Mode is set at isometric and intensity should be maximal tolerable with visible contraction causing a tetanic contraction and extension of the spine against the restraints.

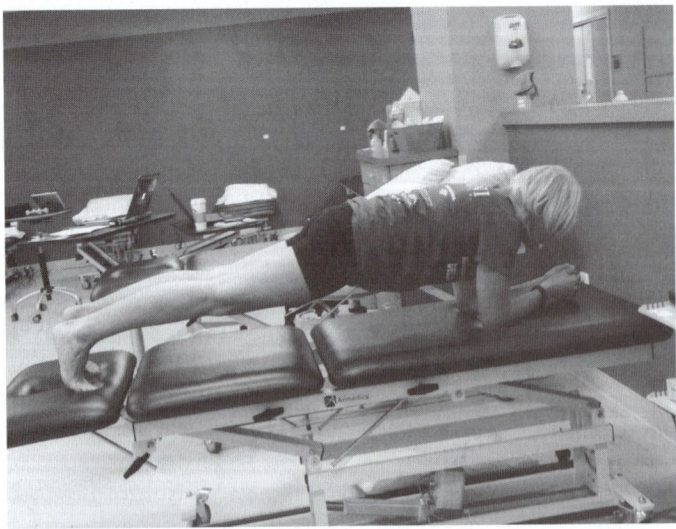

Figure 6-3. Front plank exercise on forearms.

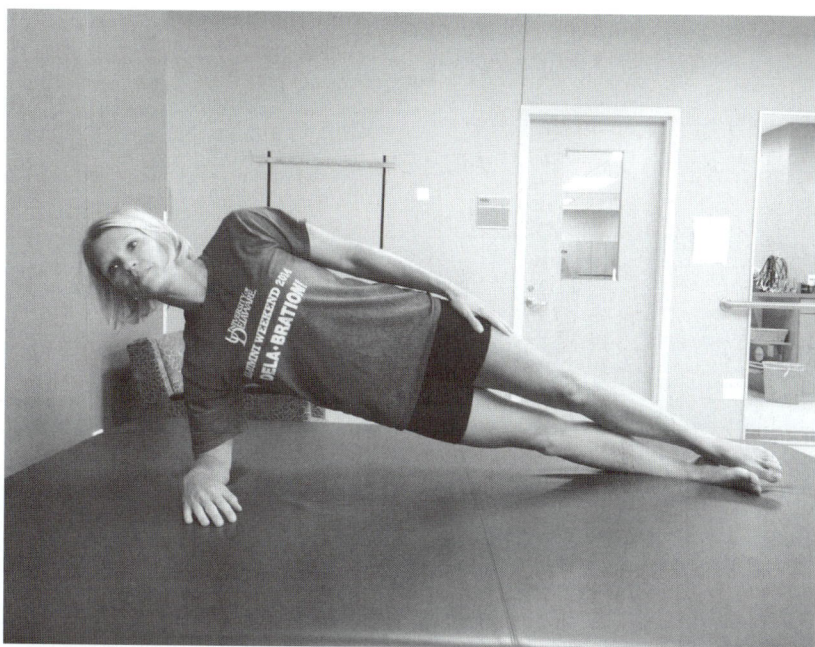

Figure 6-4. Side plank exercise.

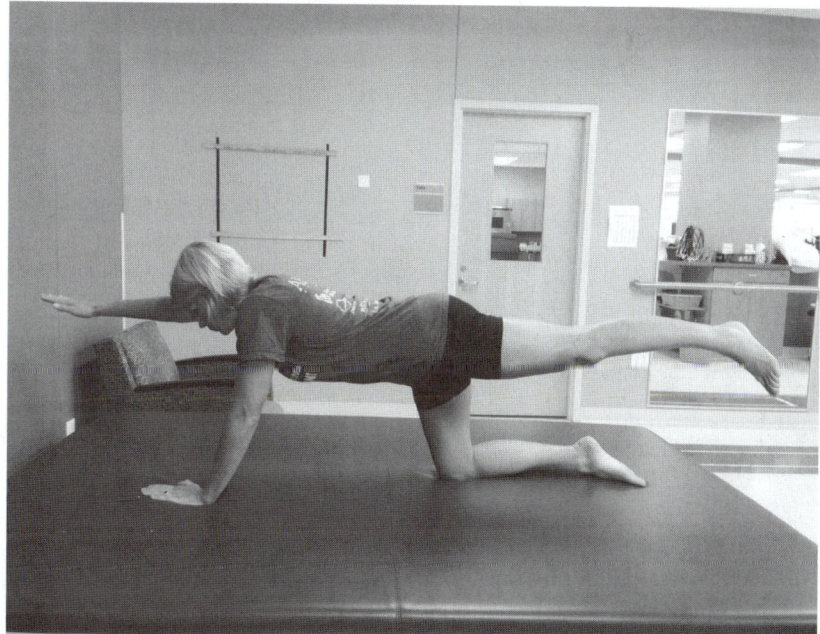

Figure 6-5. Bird dog exercise.

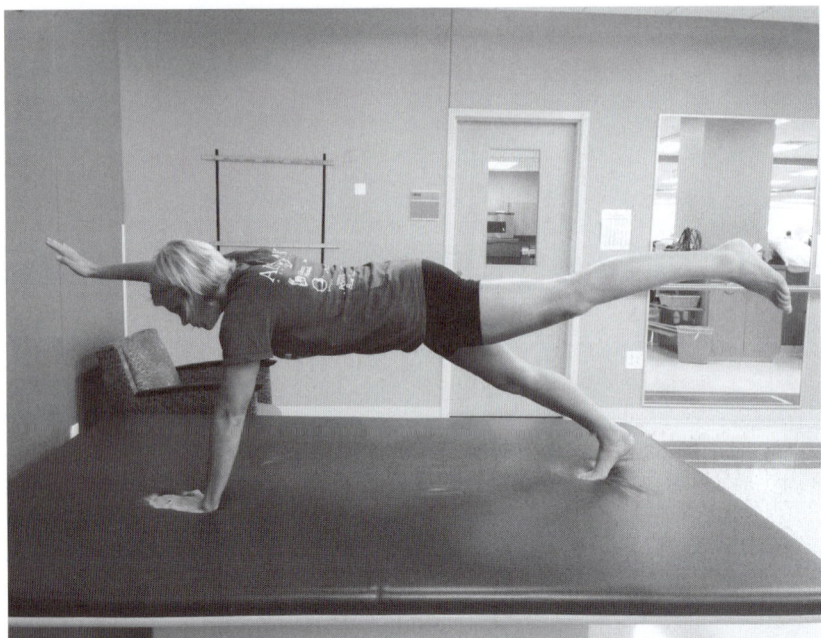

Figure 6-6. Bird dog with opposite arm and leg in push-up position.

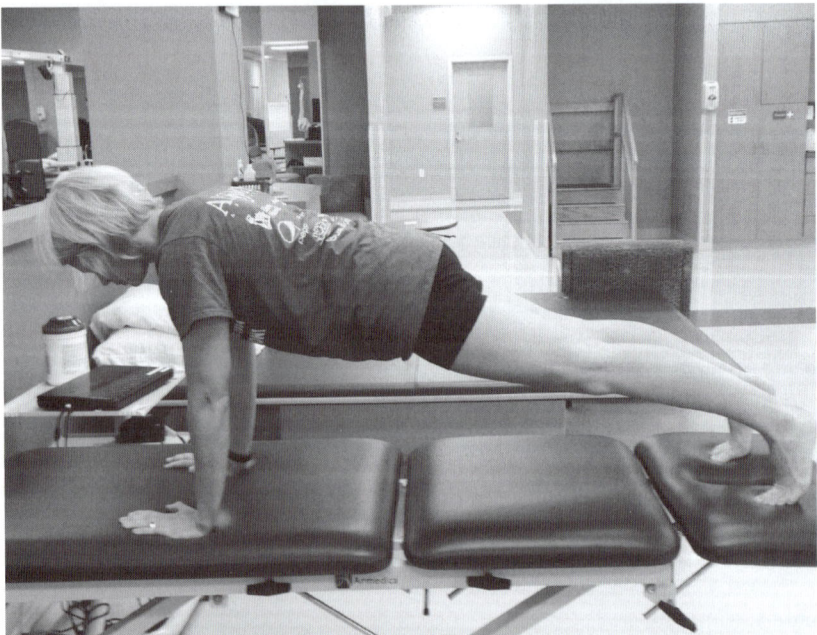

Figure 6-7. Front plank exercise with elbows extended.

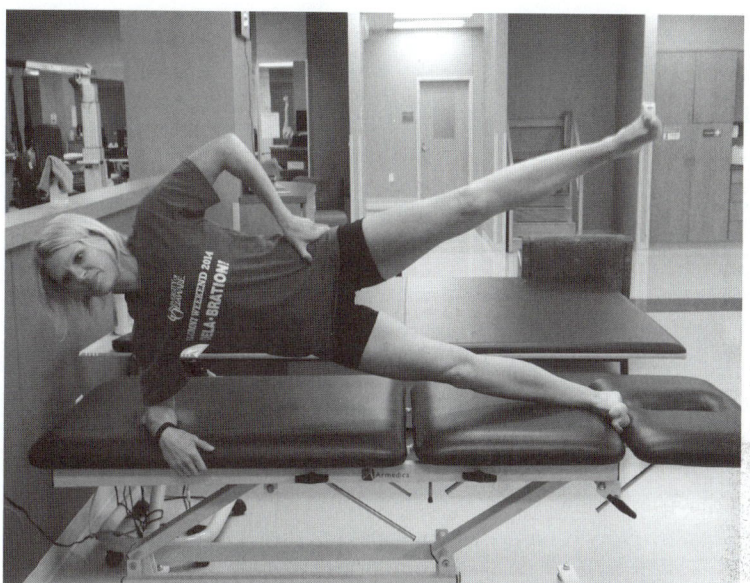

Figure 6-8. Side plank exercise with hip abduction.

and complete less challenging compulsory vaults in which landings are most likely to be on both feet or in a roll-through fashion with no unexpected hard landings. Next, completion of back bends should be tried because this type of extension can be controlled. More dynamic activities can be added such as back handsprings and leaps and jumps with spinal extension. First, elements with isolated lumbar extension should be introduced, followed by more complex movements including lumbar extension with hip extension activities. In addition, incorporation of release moves on the uneven parallel bars and flight series and tumbling can be added back in slowly. Each individual move should be assessed separately to ensure that the gymnast has a pain-free response. Increase in repetitions in future sessions occurs if the patient continues to be asymptomatic with the activity. The physical therapist should also ensure that the athlete performs flexibility exercises and certain gymnastic moves correctly. For example, if the gymnast turns out her hip when performing splits or leaps in the split position, instead of performing true hip extension, she will "take up the slack" in her lumbar spine. This places excess stress in this area. Ideally, the coach and the sports physical therapist should assess each maneuver that is reintroduced to the athlete to ensure proper form and pain-free movement and landing.

Evidence-Based Clinical Recommendations

SORT: Strength of Recommendation Taxonomy
A: Consistent, good-quality patient-oriented evidence
B: Inconsistent or limited-quality patient-oriented evidence
C: Consensus, disease-oriented evidence, usually practice, expert opinion, or case series

1. Physical examination of individuals with a spondylolysis typically reveals localized lumbosacral tenderness and muscle spasm, hyperlordosis, and pain reproduced with lumbar hyperextension. **Grade C**
2. When history and physical examination findings are concerning for spondylolysis, particularly in those involved with repetitive extension sports—radiography should include posteroanterior, standing lateral, and bilateral oblique views of the lumbar spine to identify any pars defects. **Grade B**
3. Treatment for athletes with spondylolysis includes initial rest from the aggravating activity with lumbar brace support, lumbar stabilization program, and progressive pain-free reintroduction to sport. **Grade B**

COMPREHENSION QUESTIONS

6.1 A physical therapist is evaluating a 13-year-old right-handed pitcher presenting with a 6-week history of right-sided low back pain. Initial onset was insidious; however, after 7 innings of pitching the previous day, the patient complained of severe right-sided low back pain extending into the buttocks and posterior thigh. Physical examination reveals localized tenderness and muscle spasms through the lower paraspinals and quadratus lumborum, along with severely limited lumbar extension and right side bending motions secondary to pain. Which of the following would be the *best* radiographic imaging view to assess for a defect in the pars articularis?
  A. Oblique
  B. Posteroanterior
  C. Prone ¾
  D. Standing lateral

6.2 Which of the following is the *best* indicator to advance an athlete to the next stage of return-to-sport progression following diagnosis of a spondylolysis?
  A. Pain-free response with current activities
  B. Proper technique and movement with exercise
  C. Time
  D. Upcoming game/competition

ANSWERS

6.1 **A.** Although the standard recommended radiographic views for assessing the lumbar spine are posteroanterior, standing lateral, and oblique views (options A, B, D), the best imaging technique to assess the pars articularis is the oblique view.

6.2 **A.** Although there will be many factors and indicators one may follow in order to advance an athlete through the stages of return-to-play progression, the best indicator in the aforementioned case would be a pain-free response with current activities.

REFERENCES

1. Iwamoto J, Takeda T, Wakano K. Returning athletes with severe low back pain and spondylolysis to original sporting activities with conservative treatment. *Scand J Med Sci Sports.* 2004;14:346-351.
2. McCleary MD, Congeni JA. Current concepts in the diagnosis and treatment of spondylolysis in young athletes. *Curr Sports Med Rep.* 2007;6:62-66.
3. Micheli LJ, Wood R. Back pain in young athletes. Significant differences from adults in causes and patterns. *Arch Pediatr Adolesc Med.* 1995;149:15-18.
4. Hu SS, Tribus CB, Diab M, Ghanayem AJ. Spondylolisthesis and spondylolysis. *J Bone Joint Surg Am.* 2008;90:656-671.
5. Sundell CG, Jonsson H, Ådin L, Larsén KH. Clinical examination, spondylolysis and adolescent athletes. *Int J Sports Med.* 2013;34:263-267.
6. Congeni J, McCulloch J, Swanson K. Lumbar spondylolysis. A study of natural progression in athletes. *Am J Sports Med.* 1997;25:248-253.
7. Morita T, Ikata T, Katoh S, Miyake R. Lumbar spondylolysis in children and adolescents. *J Bone Joint Surg Br.* 1995;77:620-625.
8. Amato M, Totty WG, Gilula LA. Spondylolysis of the lumbar spine: demonstration of defects and laminal fragmentation. *Radiology.* 1984;153:627-629.
9. Wiltse LL. The etiology of spondylolisthesis. *J Bone Joint Surg Am.* 1962;44-A:539-560.
10. d'Hemecourt PA, Gerbino PG 2nd, Micheli LJ. Back Injuries in the young athlete. *Clin Sports Med.* 2000;19:663-679.
11. Saraste H. Symptoms in relation to the level of spondylolysis. *Int Orthop.* 1986;10:183-185.
12. Herman MJ, Pizzutillo PD. Spondylolysis and spondylolisthesis in the child and adolescent: a new classification. *Clin Orthop Relat Res.* 2005;434:46-54.
13. McKinnis LN. *Fundamentals of Musculoskeletal Imaging.* 4th ed. Philadelphia, PA: FA Davis Company; 2014.
14. Harvey CJ, Richenberg JL, Saifuddin A, Wolman RL. The radiological investigation of lumbar spondylolysis. *Clin Radiol.* 1998;53:723-728.
15. McTimoney CA, Micheli LJ. Current evaluation and management of spondylolysis and spondylolisthesis. *Curr Sports Med Rep.* 2003;2:41-46.
16. Bellah RD, Summerville DA, Treves ST, Micheli LJ. Low-back pain in adolescent athletes: detection of stress injury to the pars interarticularis with SPECT. *Radiology.* 1991;180:509-512.
17. Lusins JO, Elting JJ, Cicoria AD, Goldsmith SJ. SPECT evaluation of lumbar spondylolysis and spondylolisthesis. *Spine.* 1994;19:608-612.

18. Saifuddin A, Burnett SJ. The value of lumbar spine MRI in the assessment of the pars interarticularis. *Clin Radiol*. 1997;52:666-671.
19. Kobayashi A, Kobayashi T, Kato K, Higuchi H, Takagishi K. Diagnosis of radiographically occult lumbar spondylolysis in young athletes by magnetic resonance imaging. *Am J Sports Med*. 2013;41:169-176.
20. d'Hemecourt PA, Zurakowski D, Kriemler S, Micheli LJ. Spondylolysis: returning the athlete to sports participation with brace treatment. *Orthopedics*. 2002;25:653-657.
21. Coghlan S, Crowe L, McCarthypersson U, Minogue C, Caulfield B. Neuromuscular electrical stimulation training results in enhanced activation of spinal stabilizing muscles during spinal loading and improvements in pain ratings. *Conf Proc IEEE Eng Med Biol Soc*. 2011;2011:7622-7625.
22. Shipley JA, Beukes CA. The nature of the spondylolytic defect. Demonstration of a communicating synovial pseudoarthrosis in the pars interarticularis. *J Bone Joint Surg Br*. 1998;80:662-664.

Acute Low Back Pain: Spinal Manipulation and Manual Therapy Intervention

Jaynie Bjornaraa

CASE 7

A 22-year-old female athlete is referred to physical therapy following a soccer injury that occurred 3 days ago. The patient's injury occurred during a slide tackle in which she landed forcefully on her right hip and buttock. She tried to continue playing, but could not due to increasing low back pain (LBP) that extended into her gluteal area. That evening, she experienced pain while rolling in bed, transferring from sitting to standing, and standing on 1 leg while she was dressing. The patient indicates that she has had several falls on her right side while playing soccer, but has not experienced back pain of this intensity before. Because her pain continued the next day, she consulted her doctor who then referred her to physical therapy. No imaging was performed at this time. As the patient walked into the outpatient therapy clinic, the therapist noted that she displayed a wide-based gait. She rates her LBP as 7/10 (using the visual analog scale) during pain provoking movements like walking and 4/10 at rest. She describes her pain as mostly limited to her right low back and gluteal area; however, she also has some hamstring and groin pain at times. The patient's medical history is otherwise unremarkable. The patient's mechanism of injury, signs, and symptoms are consistent with sacroiliac joint (SIJ) pathology.

▶ What examination signs may be associated with this diagnosis?
▶ What are the most appropriate examination tests?
▶ What are the most appropriate physical therapy interventions?
▶ Describe a physical therapy plan of care based on each stage of the health condition.

KEY DEFINITIONS

CENTRALIZATION: Phenomenon whereby the performance of certain repeated movements or postures causes radiating pain to move proximally to the midline of the spine

CLINICAL PREDICTION RULE: Structured decision-making tools that contain selected patient-specific prognostic variables to assist in making a diagnosis, establishing a prognosis, or determining a patient management strategy

FAMILIAR SYMPTOMS: Pain or other symptoms (*e.g.*, aching, burning, or numbness) produced by a special or diagnostic test and previously identified on the patient's pain drawing, and verified by the patient as the reason for seeking care; these symptoms must be distinguished from other symptoms that are produced by the special or diagnostic test

FORCE CLOSURE: Stability of the SIJ that results from the surrounding musculature and soft tissues primarily through dynamic activation

FORM CLOSURE: Stability of the SIJ that results from the bony structure of the sacrum and ilium that allows the SIJ to be stable and resistant to shearing forces

NEGATIVE PROVOCATION SIJ TEST: A provocation SIJ test that does *not* produce or increase familiar symptoms

PERIPHERALIZATION: Phenomenon whereby the performance of certain repeated movements or postures causes symptoms to move distally

POSITIVE PROVOCATION SIJ TEST: A provocation SIJ test that produces or increases familiar symptoms

RED FLAGS: Signs and symptoms that require immediate evaluation and referral to a primary healthcare provider due to their potential indication of a serious health problem outside the scope of physical therapy practice

SACROILIAC JOINT PATHOLOGY: Term used to indicate that the SIJ structures are the pain-generating tissues

Objectives

1. Describe and apply appropriate examination tests that provide confidence in a SIJ dysfunction diagnosis.
2. Describe how the clinical prediction rule (CPR) for spinal manipulation can be applied to the athlete with acute LBP.
3. Identify evidence-based physical therapy interventions for acute LBP.
4. Describe a physical therapy plan of care based on stage of recovery from LBP.

Physical Therapy Considerations

PT considerations during management of acute LBP in a young adult athlete using spinal manipulation and other manual interventions:

- **General physical therapy plan of care/goals:** Decrease pain; restore asymmetrical pelvic and sacral positions; increase active spinal range of motion (ROM); promote spinal and sacral stability; return to sport
- **Physical therapy interventions:** Patient education on pertinent lumbar and sacral anatomy, biomechanics, and pathomechanics relating to her injury (*e.g.*, body mechanics and movements to reduce risk of re-injury); soft tissue mobilization (STM) and manual therapy to reduce pain and optimize healing; spinal manipulation for pain relief and improved mechanics; exercises to increase spinal stability, strength, and endurance; home exercise instruction
- **Precautions during physical therapy:** Monitor signs and symptoms, especially neurologic complaints; avoid movements and unilateral positions that stress symptomatic SIJ
- **Complications interfering with physical therapy:** Noncompliance with exercise and patient education; inaccurate assessment of pain-generating tissues, which may interfere with optimal treatment effectiveness

Understanding the Health Condition

Low back pain (LBP) is a very common health problem and creates an extensive personal burden financially, physically, and emotionally. Most people experience LBP at some point in their life. The first episode typically occurs between 20 and 40 years of age. Most cases resolve with little or no intervention.[1] However, approximately one-third of individuals experiencing their first bout of acute LBP will not fully recover to their original state of health within 6 months.[2] Estimates of the 1-year incidence of first-ever LBP range between 6.3% and 15.4%, whereas the 1-year incidence of any episode of LBP ranges between 1.5% and 36%.[3] According to clinic- or health facility-based studies, episode remission rates at 1 year range from 54% to 90%; however, these results need to be considered with caution due to lack of clarity of what defined the "episode" of LBP. Despite this, most people who experience back pain that limits their activities go on to have back pain again. Estimates of recurrence at 1 year range from 24% to 80%.[3] A more recent study estimated the global point prevalence of LBP that limits activity at roughly 12% and the 1-month prevalence at roughly 23%.[4] The clinical challenge of treating LBP is determining the origin of the pain and symptoms so that the plan of care can address these structures. Most of the structures and tissues in the low back, hip, and pelvis can produce pain in the back, gluteal region, groin, and lower extremity.[5-7] The SIJ and associated ligaments, zygapophyseal joints, lumbar discs, nerve roots, and other structures can also be nociceptive sources of LBP.[8] Using specific tests to determine whether the source of the LBP is limited to the lumbar spine or SIJ is important for establishing a plan of care that will be most effective and efficient.

Acute LBP is defined as pain lasting up to 12 weeks.[1] After 12 weeks, the pain can be classified as chronic. LBP may present between the costal angles and gluteal folds and may radiate into one or both legs. LBP is often defined as nonspecific because it cannot be attributed to a definite cause.[1] However, a differential diagnosis for the etiology of acute back pain over other potentially more serious causes is imperative. Possible uncommon causes of acute LBP include infection, tumor, osteoporosis, fracture, and inflammatory arthritis.[1,8] Differential diagnosis depends on history, examination, and recognition of red flags. Red flag conditions include cancer, cauda equina syndrome, fracture, and infection. It is critical to question patients about constitutional signs and symptoms such as unexplained weight loss, night pain, fever, and debilitating fatigue. Presence of these signs and symptoms may indicate a systemic disease such as cancer. Complaints of bilateral leg weakness and sensory loss, and bladder and/or bowel incontinence may indicate a more serious condition such as cauda equina syndrome.[1,8] Prolonged use of systemic glucocorticoids (e.g., prednisone), history of osteoporosis, and/or trauma with vertebral tenderness and limited motion may indicate fracture. Severe pain with history of surgery with fever, presence of wound, vertebral tenderness, and/or limited spinal ROM may indicate infection. All these situations require immediate referral.[1,8] According to a 2009 study,[9] some red flags are more important than others and overall they are poor at ruling *in* more serious causes of back pain. The authors found that patients seeking care in the primary care setting for back pain tend to have at least 1 red flag, yet rarely have a serious condition.[9] However, for physical therapists, vigilance in red flag assessment, differential diagnosis, and referral cannot be over-emphasized. Table 7-1 presents the differential diagnosis of acute LBP.[1,8]

Diagnostic imaging is typically not indicated for patients with acute LBP. Clinical outcomes are not improved in patients unless signs and symptoms indicating the likelihood of a serious pathology are noted.[10-13] If a serious condition is suspected, magnetic resonance imaging (MRI) is likely the best option because radiography has little diagnostic value due to its low sensitivity and specificity for the cause of acute LBP.[11] Laboratory tests, such as blood counts, may be beneficial if infection or malignancy is suspected.

Physical Therapy Patient/Client Management

Physical therapists offer several treatment options for patients with acute LBP. Clinical decision making regarding the use of manual therapy interventions can be based on a combination of biomechanical principles of normal and abnormal spinal movement and evaluation of criteria in CPRs. Spinal manipulation and mobilization are common interventions for patients with acute LBP.[1,14,15] Other beneficial treatment techniques include manual therapy techniques such as STM, muscle energy techniques (METs), trunk stabilization exercises, aerobic activity, and patient education.[1,16-30]

Table 7-1 DIFFERENTIAL DIAGNOSIS OF ACUTE LOW BACK PAIN WITH KEY CLINICAL FINDINGS

Diagnosis	Key Clinical Findings
Musculoskeletal System	
Compression fracture	History of trauma or osteoporosis, point tenderness, pain increases with spinal flexion and movement from supine to sit to stand
Herniated lumbar disc	Radiating leg pain worse than back pain, positive neurologic findings (motor, sensory, reflexes), worsens with sitting
Spinal stenosis	Pain in one or both lower extremities that worsens with ambulation and standing and is relieved with rest and spinal flexion; clumsiness with gait
Spondylolisthesis or spondylolysis	Pain with spinal extension and activity, "step-off" with palpation
Degenerative disc disease (DDD) or facet joint arthropathy	Generalized back pain with or without gluteal pain; for DDD, pain worsens with spinal flexion; for facet joint problems, pain worsens with spinal extension
Lumbar strain or sprain	Generalized back pain with or without gluteal pain, pain increases with movement and is relieved with rest
Sacroiliac dysfunction	Back pain that is localized to PSIS, S2 region and below, may refer to groin, gluteals, hamstrings, or entire leg; unilateral
Other systems	
Abdominal aortic aneurysm	Abdominal discomfort, visual, and/or palpable (wider than expected) abdominal pulse
Gastrointestinal (GI) conditions	GI signs and symptoms, back pain associated with eating, positive abdominal palpation findings
Pelvic conditions	Lower abdominal, pelvis, or hip pain or discomfort
Renal conditions	Costovertebral angle pain, urinary symptoms and signs, possible fever
Herpes zoster	Unilateral dermatomal pain and hypersensitivity, rash
Systemic	
Cancer	Constitutional symptoms in addition to back pain; tender spine
Ankylosing spondylitis	Morning pain and stiffness in lower back, pain after inactivity, problems with eyes or bowels
Osteomyelitis or discitis	Constant pain, spinous process tenderness, possible fever, recent surgery
Autoimmune diseases or related conditions (e.g., fibromyalgia)	Multiple joint arthralgias, fever, weight loss, fatigue

Examination, Evaluation, and Diagnosis

Optimizing treatments may minimize the development of chronic pain, which accounts for most of the healthcare costs related to LBP.[31] Key aspects of the examination include a thorough subjective history followed by examination techniques to determine whether the patient's history, subjective report, and examination results predict whether or not she will benefit from spinal manipulation as an intervention for her acute back pain.[14] In 2002, Flynn et al.[14] developed a CPR for one manipulation technique that had historically been used for patients with probable sacroiliac (SI) dysfunction. Seventy-one patients with acute LBP who met specific subjective and objective inclusion and exclusion criteria were enrolled in this CPR derivation study. The following self-report measures were captured: pain diagram, pain rating using a visual analog scale, Fear-Avoidance Beliefs Questionnaire (FABQ), and the Oswestry Disability Questionnaire (ODQ). The FABQ was used to assess each subject's fear of pain and beliefs about activity. The authors used FABQW, the work subscale of the FABQ, to help determine which subjects would benefit from manipulation. A score of less than 19 suggested that the subject had a reduced likelihood of current and future work loss and disability and may be a good candidate for spinal manipulation. The authors performed neurologic screening (e.g., dermatome, myotome, and reflex testing) to determine the presence of findings that would contraindicate spinal manipulation. Positive or negative findings were established based on comparison to the opposite side. These exclusion criteria ensured that participants did not exhibit any contraindications to spinal manipulation. The authors assessed prone hip ROM and supine straight leg raise and performed spring testing of the lumbar spine to assess for pain and hyper-, hypo-, or normal segmental mobility. Several special tests proposed to confirm SI dysfunction were also performed. The SIJ tests were divided into 3 categories: position (tests assessing symmetry of bony landmarks), provocation (tests to reproduce symptoms), and mobility (tests assessing symmetry of pelvic motion). Participants received up to 2 sessions of the spinal manipulation technique. Approximately 2 to 4 days after the spinal manipulation, subjects were assessed for improvement. Those who improved at least 50% on the ODQ were deemed "successfully" treated. Those who did not meet this threshold received another manipulation and were assessed for improvement 2 to 4 days later. Again, those meeting the 50% improvement threshold were considered successfully treated with the remaining subjects classified as having been treated without success. Using the results of several traditional SI region special tests, outcome assessments, and subjective and objective information, Flynn et al.[14] used a logistic regression analysis to predict which factors influenced whether manipulation was successful for treating LBP. They concluded that the **presence of 5 criteria could identify patients with acute LBP who would likely benefit from spinal manipulation**: (1) FABQW score of less than 19 points (i.e., low fear-avoidance beliefs about work activities); (2) duration of current episode less than 16 days; (3) no symptoms extending distal to the knee; (4) at least 1 hypomobile lumbar spine segment; and (5) at least 1 hip with greater than 35° of internal rotation ROM.

Observation and palpation are the initial components of the spinal examination. The current patient demonstrated a wide-based gait as she ambulated to the treatment room. In standing, the physical therapist noted that the patient had a mild forward head and shoulder posture and a normal lordotic curve. Bony landmark palpation of bilateral posterior superior iliac spine (PSIS), iliac crest (IC), and anterior superior iliac spine (ASIS) indicated the following asymmetry in standing: higher right ASIS, lower right PSIS, and slightly higher left IC. This asymmetry suggests right innominate upslip and posterior rotation, meaning that the right innominate bone was sheared superiorly on the sacrum and also rotated in a posterior direction on the sacrum in the sagittal plane. The therapist palpated soft tissue to assess the tone of the lumbar and pelvic musculature; the patient demonstrated tenderness and spasm on the right side within the following musculature: lumbar paraspinals, gluteals, piriformis, quadratus lumborum, and iliopsoas. The muscle tone of the same muscles on the left side was increased, but not to the same extent.

Next, neurologic screening, ROM, and spinal mobility activities were assessed. The patient had normal lower extremity reflexes and sensation to sharp/dull, and had no myotomal weakness. The therapist asked the patient to perform single and repeated spinal ROM. Repeated spinal movements can identify centralization or peripheralization of symptoms that may indicate discogenic pain; this pain behavior can help distinguish between lumbar and sacral pathology, allowing for a more specific treatment.[32] Single repetition active ROM of the lumbar spine was limited in flexion with pain and apprehension (limited 70%), extension (limited 25%), and side bending right and left (limited 25% and 50%, respectively). No centralization or peripheralization was noted with any repetitive lumbar ROM activities. Prone passive hip rotation demonstrated limited internal rotation on the right side (20°) relative to the left (33°). She had normal mobility of the lumbar spine as noted with spring testing.

Spinal examination often includes special tests to determine if pathology or biomechanical dysfunction of the SIJ is the source of the patient's LBP. These tests are also the basis for various therapeutic interventions, including manipulation and METs. Although several SIJ pain provocation tests have been advocated as capable of determining SIJ dysfunction, evidence suggests that the results of *individual* tests are not as accurate as a positive diagnostic injection.[33-35] A positive diagnostic injection is when the injection of solutions into the SIJ provokes the patient's familiar pain and injecting a local anesthetic (*e.g.*, lidocaine) reduces it by 80% or more for the duration of the anesthetic. Current evidence shows that using a *combination* of SIJ pain provocation tests can more accurately determine SIJ dysfunction. **A composite of 3 positive provocation SIJ tests in the absence of centralization during lumbar ROM testing** has clinically meaningful sensitivity, specificity, and positive likelihood ratios for the diagnosis of SIJ dysfunction.[32,36-38] According to Laslett et al.,[38] the type and order of SI provocation tests are also important. Laslett et al.[38] chose 5 provocation tests based on their acceptable inter-rater reliability: SI distraction, SI compression, thigh thrust, sacral thrust, and Gaenslen's test. In a blinded gold-standard related design (*i.e.*, local anesthetic injection into the SIJ) with 48 patients, they found that the SI distraction test had the highest single positive predictive value. The thigh thrust, SI compression, and sacral thrust tests added positively to the overall diagnostic accuracy for SIJ pathology, whereas Gaenslen's did not improve the diagnostic ability. The authors concluded that the optimal strategy is to perform SI distraction first, followed by thigh thrust, SI compression, and sacral thrust tests and to stop when 2 of these are positive because adding 1 more test only minimally increased the specificity.[38] However, the physical therapist treating the current patient decided to perform a third test after 2 SI tests were positive for 2 reasons. First, van der Wurff et al.[36] reported that the likelihood that pain is related to SIJ dysfunction is between 65% and 93% when 3 or more provocation tests were positive. Second, closer examination of the data from Laslett et al.[38] confirms that improved diagnostic accuracy was achieved with 3 or more positive tests. Therefore, the physical therapist performed the SI distraction test first. With the patient in a supine position, the therapist applied pressure on bilateral ASISs down and outward to "spread apart" the ASISs. A positive test occurs when pain is felt in the gluteal or posterior leg of the affected side.[39] This patient felt her familiar pain in the right gluteal region. Next, the physical therapist performed the thigh thrust SIJ provocation test. With the patient still in supine, the therapist flexed the patient's right hip and knee to 90°. After placing her hand under the patient's sacrum, the therapist applied a posterior shear force to the SIJ through the long axis of the femur.[39] The patient complained of familiar pain in the right SIJ with this test, which was considered positive. Third, the therapist completed the SI compression test. Standing behind the sidelying patient, the therapist applied a downward force on the anterior aspect of the ilium down toward the table to spread the SIJ.[39] This test was also positive, reproducing pain on the patient's right side. Given the 3 positive tests which suggested that the source of the patient's pain was the right SIJ, the therapist determined that no further provocation testing was necessary.

To assess the SI region further, the physical therapist performed 3 active mobility tests. The Gillet test assesses for SI dysfunction by noting movement of the PSIS with respect to S2. A positive test occurs when the PSIS *fails* to move posterior and inferior relative to S2 as the patient flexes her hip in standing.[39] This test was positive on the right side for this patient. Next, the standing flexion test was performed. After the therapist palpates the PSIS levels, the standing patient flexes at her trunk as far as she can. A test is considered positive when one PSIS moves more superior and faster relative to the other PSIS.[39] The standing flexion test was negative for this patient. Last, the therapist asked the patient to perform an active straight leg raise (ASLR) in which the patient compares the difficulty of raising her leg off the table with and without an external compressive force through the SI joints. This patient noted improved ability to actively raise her leg 5 cm with a manual compressive force applied through bilateral ilia, indicating augmentation of force closure of the SIJ.[40,41] The ASLR has been promoted as a reliable assessment of load transfer quality through the lumbopelvic region.[40] O'Sullivan et al.[41] proposed that when patients have difficulty performing the ASLR due to pain or apparent lack of ability, altered motor responses and neuromuscular system compensation are needed to load transfer due to form and/or force closure impairment.

To summarize the results of the examination, this patient presented with pelvic asymmetry (higher right ASIS, lower right PSIS, and slightly higher left IC) and decreased right hip passive internal rotation. She demonstrated reduced lumbar spine ROM with no centralization or peripheralization noted. She had soft tissue tenderness and increased tone in right-sided lumbar and pelvic musculature and posterior SI ligaments, suggesting guarding, inflammation, and/or irritation of these tissues. She also presented with findings consistent with SIJ pain and dysfunction. She had 3 positive right SIJ pain provocation tests (distraction, thigh thrust, and compression) and positive Gillet and ASLR tests on the right. Spring testing to the lumbar spine demonstrated normal mobility. According to the criteria of a CPR for spinal manipulation,[14] the current patient had the following positive findings: FABQW less than 19, duration of episode less than 16 days, and no symptoms extending distal to the knee. Given the presence of these findings, lack of positive neurologic signs, and absence of centralization or peripheralization, this patient's examination results supported trying spinal manipulation as an initial intervention.[14,15] In addition, the patient's bony anatomic landmark asymmetry findings and lumbar and hip motion test findings created a clinical picture consistent with low back and pelvis dysfunction. If the spinal manipulation intervention was unsuccessful, specific SIJ intervention implementation would be appropriate. This is based on the assumption that SIJ displacement does occur and is detectable,[42,43] which has been questioned.[5,14,34,38,43-45] However, radiographic and biomechanical evidence have demonstrated that definite but small degrees of relative displacement do occur at the SIJ.[46]

Plan of Care and Interventions

Based on the examination findings that were suggestive of SIJ pathology, initial rehabilitation included patient education, exercise, and spinal manipulation. Spinal manipulation has been advocated for individuals presenting with SIJ biomechanical dysfunction.[15] If 3 of the 5 prediction criteria as outlined by Flynn et al.[14] are met, the probability of post-treatment success (defined as ≥50% improvement in ODQ score) increases from a near coin-toss likelihood to 68%. If 4 of the Flynn et al.[14] criteria are met, the likelihood of manipulation being successful jumps to 95%.

In studies by Childs et al.[15] and Flynn et al.,[14] an audible click was required to consider the spinal manipulation successful. If the investigators did not hear a click with manipulation on the more symptomatic side after 2 attempts, the other side was manipulated. Since the development of the CPR, others have found that an audible click is not needed for a successful manipulation.[47] According to Cibulka et al.,[48] changes in pelvic position occur with manipulation to either side, so essentially the decision for which side to manipulate could be random.

The physical therapist considered these newer data, but followed the original protocols as outlined by Childs et al. and Flynn et al.[14,15] Prior to the manipulation intervention, the therapist administered several STM techniques to reduce soft tissue tightness and discomfort in the SIJ region. Often, surrounding musculature is tight in an attempt to guard and/or stabilize a symptomatic SIJ. The following bilateral STM techniques were utilized on this patient: bony contouring of pelvis, quadratus lumborum trigger point and myofascial releasing, piriformis release with contract-relax, gluteus medius trigger point release, and iliopsoas release.[16-19,49] Following STM, the physical therapist performed the lumbopelvic spine manipulation upon which the CPR was based. The more symptomatic right side was selected for manipulation to be consistent with the protocol in Flynn et al.[14] The patient was supine with the therapist on the opposite side to be treated. The therapist passively moved the patient into side bending toward her painful right side. With the patient's fingers interlocked behind her head, the therapist rotated her arms and

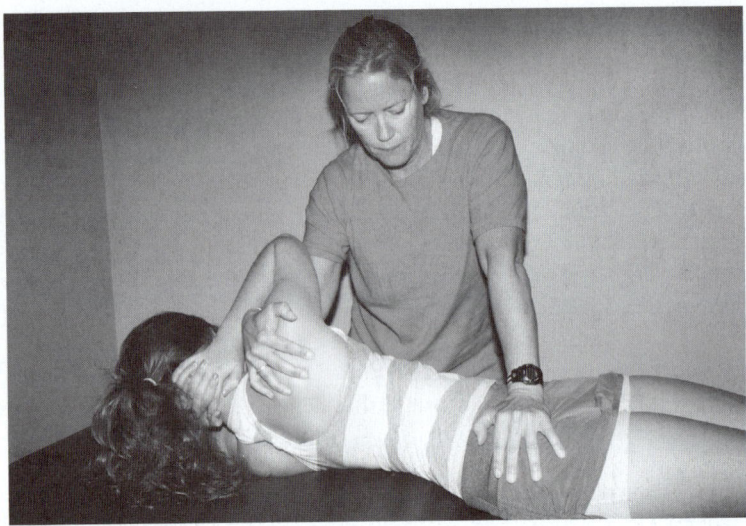

Figure 7-1. Supine lumbopelvic manipulation technique. The patient is supine with the therapist on the opposite side to be treated. The therapist passively moves the patient into side bending toward her painful right side. With the patient's fingers interlocked behind her head, the therapist rotates her arms and upper body opposite of the side of manipulation and applies a quick thrust to her right anterior superior iliac spine (ASIS) in a posterior and inferior direction.

upper body opposite of the side of manipulation and applied a quick thrust to her right ASIS in a posterior and inferior direction (Fig. 7-1). The therapist heard a click with the manipulation to this patient.

Immediately following the manipulation, the patient was instructed in lumbar stabilization exercises, including the drawing-in/bracing maneuver, bridging, supine rotations with knees at 90° and feet on the mat, prone alternating single-leg hip extension, and side plank from the knees. All exercises emphasized the drawing-in/bracing maneuver prior to movement. She was instructed to perform a set of 10 repetitions of each exercise 3 times daily. She was also instructed to remain as active as she could without increasing her pain.[1,20]

This patient returned for a follow-up appointment 3 days after the initial examination and first interventions. At this time, a pain rating and ODQ were reassessed. The patient rated her pain as slightly improved over her initial rating, with a decrease to 5/10 with movement and 3/10 at rest. However, her ODQ score decreased by only 25%—not enough to be considered successful.[14,15,50] Therefore, the therapist chose to perform a different spinal manipulation than was performed at the initial intervention. The therapist chose the alternate sidelying lumbar spine manipulation described by Cleland et al.[50] This method of manipulation is different than the one used in the article by Flynn et al.[14] (i.e., lumbopelvic spine manipulation) and targets the L4-L5 segment instead of the innominate bone of the pelvis. Because abundant research supports that manipulative techniques are nonspecific from a vertebral-level perspective,[47,51-56] the physical therapist was confident in trying the alternate method described by Cleland et al.[50] Research has also supported greater benefits of manual therapy directed at the lower lumbar spine versus

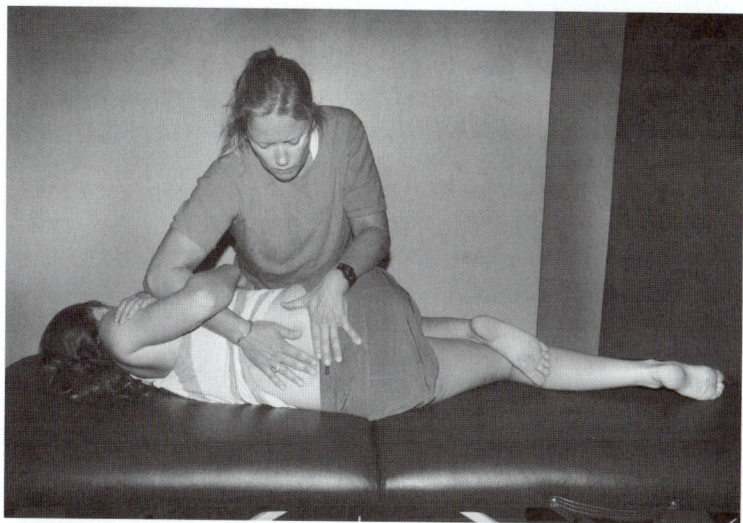

Figure 7-2. Alternative lumbar manipulation technique. The patient is positioned with the painful side up with the therapist standing in front of her. The patient's top leg is passively flexed until the therapist can palpate movement at the L4-L5 interspinous space. The therapist pulls the patient's lower shoulder and arm to side bend her toward the table while rotating her away until movement can be palpated at L4-L5 again. The therapist applies a high velocity, low amplitude thrust of the pelvis in the anterior direction.

the upper lumbar spine.[57] The patient was treated with her right side up with the therapist standing in front of her. The patient's top leg was flexed until the therapist could palpate movement at the L4-L5 interspinous space. The patient placed her foot into the popliteal fossa of her bottom leg. The therapist then pulled the patient's lower shoulder and arm to side bend her toward the table and rotate away from the table again until movement was noted at L4-L5 interspinous space. The therapist applied a high velocity, low-amplitude thrust of the pelvis in the anterior direction[50] (Fig. 7-2). Next, the therapist performed another lumbopelvic manipulation as was done on the first therapy session because a recent report suggests that a single session of SIJ and lumbar manipulation was more effective for improving functional disability than SIJ manipulation alone in patients with SIJ syndrome.[58] The therapist encouraged the patient to continue with the same lumbar stabilization home exercise program (HEP).

Three days later, the patient returned for her next scheduled therapy visit. Her pain and perceived disability had not substantially changed. Given this, the focus of therapy was modified to focus on restoration of biomechanical dysfunction utilizing METs. **MET can be effective for reducing LBP and improving function.**[21,22,59] The therapist performed STM as described previously prior to initiation of the MET. Bony palpation of symmetry was repeated (similar to examination procedures) and the same asymmetry was confirmed from the patient's initial examination: right ASIS higher, right PSIS lower, and IC slightly higher on the left. First, a "pubic clearing" was performed with the patient in supine with knees flexed to 90° and feet flat on the table with the patient resisting hip adduction to the therapist's forearm

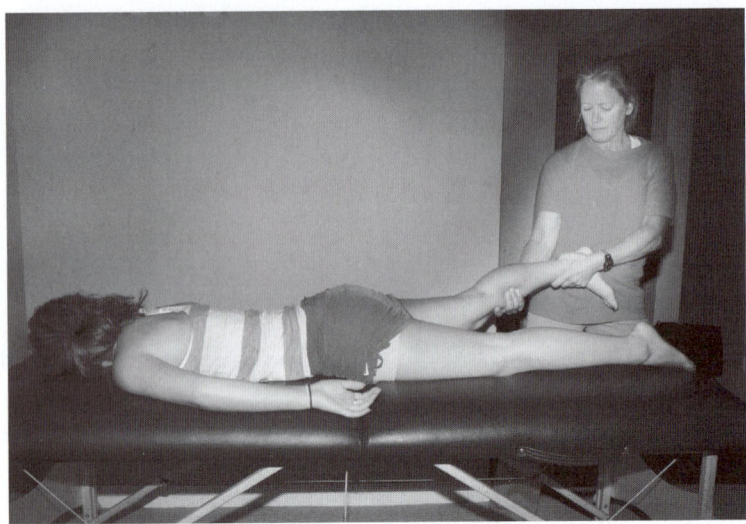

Figure 7-3. Long axis grade V thrust manipulation for right innominate upslip.

placed between her knees. This technique is often used prior to specific right- or left-sided techniques. Contraction of the adductor musculature can restore pubic tubercle position so they are even right to left. This suggests a movement of the innominate as well, which often causes an audible pop. An audible pop was noted with this maneuver suggesting position resolution. Next, the patient was asked to move into the prone position and the therapist performed a long axis grade V thrust to the right lower extremity to correct the right innominate upslip (Fig. 7-3). This technique resulted in a "clunk" perceived by both therapist and patient.

Following this maneuver, MET was performed to correct the posterior rotation of the right innominate (Fig. 7-4). To complete this technique, the therapist resisted hip flexion on the right while maintaining full posterior tilt on the left. The position was held for 5 seconds and repeated 5 times. The right hip was passively extended to take up the slack prior to each resistance phase (Fig. 7-4). Following the entire treatment, the therapist noted resolution of symmetry of ASIS, PSIS, and ICs. The patient also demonstrated increased active lumbar ROM with less pain. To improve lumbopelvic control and stability, the therapist also initiated resisted concentric and eccentric diagonal movements of the pelvis in all directions. The therapist did not alter the HEP at this stage.

The patient returned 2 days later. Pain rating and perceived disability were reduced substantially. She stated she was sore in her right gluteal region for only a day after the previous therapy session. Treatment during this session consisted of STM and the following exercises to improve lumbopelvic stability: manually resisted pelvic diagonal movements, resisted bridging in various planes, prone and reverse planks, side planks from the feet, and prone alternating arm and leg lifts. These exercises were added to her HEP and the drawing-in maneuver was removed, because she had mastered this activity. She was instructed to continue being active while still avoiding aggravating activities. She continued physical therapy for 4 more

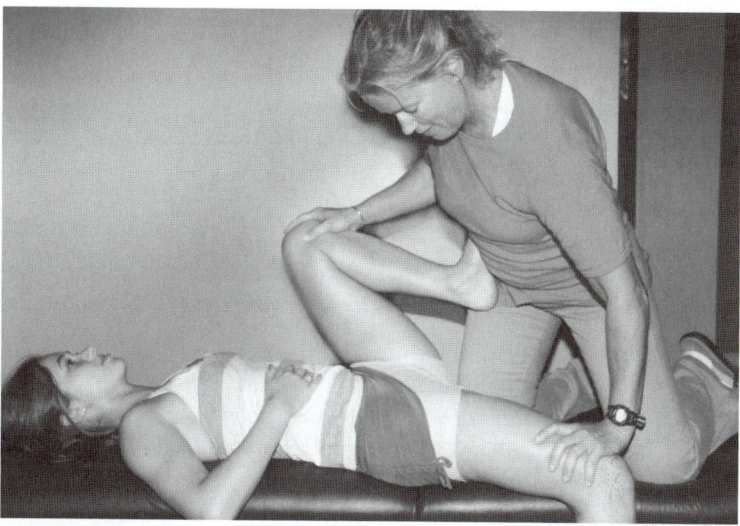

Figure 7-4. Muscle energy technique (MET) for right posterior rotation of innominate. With the patient's left hip flexed up and right leg hanging off the edge of the table, the therapist resists hip flexion on the right while maintaining full posterior tilt on the left. The position is held for 5 seconds and repeated 5 times. The right hip is passively extended to take up the slack prior to each resistance phase.

visits. These visits consisted of supervised exercise instruction for lumbopelvic stabilization and progression to athletic activity. Although most research has focused on the benefits of exercise for chronic LBP, the **addition of proper deep abdominal and segmental stabilization exercises to general exercise** is beneficial for pain relief, restoration of function, and prevention of further back pain.[23-29,60] The patient was also instructed in home MET techniques for self-treatment, if needed. These mimicked MET for a posterior rotation of the right innominate without therapist resistance. She also added swimming to her exercise regimen given the activation of the posterior musculature and its benefit for trunk strengthening and stabilization. At her eighth and final visit, the patient was pain-free and had returned to soccer.

A key component of rehabilitation for an episode of acute LBP requires clinical decision making that is based upon subjective history and examination that directs the clinician to the most effective treatment outcome. The CPR for spinal manipulation offers clinicians an efficient, evidence-based tool to initiate treatment for patients with LBP while optimizing outcomes.[61] Adding standing performance of repeated active lumbar flexion, extension, and side bending movements for assessment of pain and centralization or peripheralization of symptoms to rule in or out discogenic pain and further qualify patients for a specific treatment is also prudent. Capturing outcomes at *each* visit is another key component of effective patient management. If expected outcomes are not met, a thorough re-evaluation can provide guidance toward another intervention that may have more success. A CPR can encourage spinal manipulation as a treatment for those who meet criteria, but having other tools in the toolkit to allow for implementation of other potentially successful interventions is imperative. Exercise, education, and consideration of the patient's goals and lifestyle are important pieces of LBP management.[30] Future research will continue to reveal diagnostic tests and criteria to optimize treatment interventions for patients with acute and chronic LBP.

Evidence-Based Clinical Recommendations

SORT: Strength of Recommendation Taxonomy
A: Consistent, good-quality patient-oriented evidence
B: Inconsistent or limited-quality patient-oriented evidence
C: Consensus, disease-oriented evidence, usually practice, expert opinion, or case series

1. A trial of spinal manipulation for the treatment of acute low back pain is advocated when 3 or more of the following criteria are met: (1) FABQW score of less than 19 points; (2) duration of current episode less than 16 days; (3) no symptoms extending distal to the knee; (4) at least 1 hypomobile lumbar spine segment; and (5) at least 1 hip with greater than 35° of internal rotation ROM. **Grade B**
2. Three or more positive sacroiliac joint provocation tests improve the likelihood of a diagnosis of sacroiliac joint pain and dysfunction. **Grade B**
3. A rehabilitation program including METs may help restore sacroiliac joint biomechanical dysfunction and symmetry, reduce pain, and improve function. **Grade C**
4. The addition of deep abdominal and segmental stabilization ("core stabilization") exercises to a physical therapy treatment program is beneficial for pain relief, restoration of function, and prevention of further low back pain. **Grade B**

COMPREHENSION QUESTIONS

7.1 Which of the following contains criteria in the clinical prediction rule developed by Flynn et al. (2002) that predict when spinal manipulation is likely to benefit patients with acute low back pain?
   A. Fear-Avoidance Beliefs Questionnaire Work (FABQW) score less than 19 points, duration of current episode less than 12 weeks
   B. No symptoms distal to knee, at least 1 hip with greater than 35° of external rotation range of motion (ROM)
   C. At least 1 hypermobile lumbar segment, FABQW score less than 19
   D. No symptoms distal to knee, at least 1 hip with greater than 35° internal rotation ROM

7.2 Which of the following contains the tests with the highest sensitivity, specificity, and positive likelihood ratio for indication of sacroiliac joint (SIJ) pain and dysfunction?
   A. Patrick's test, compression test, sacral thrust
   B. Gillet test, distraction test, thigh thrust
   C. Distraction test, compression test, thigh thrust
   D. Gaenslen's test, sacral thrust, Patrick's test

ANSWERS

7.1 D. The 5 criteria in the clinical prediction rule developed by Flynn et al.[14] are listed below.

Criterion	Definition of Positive
Symptom location	No symptoms distal to knee
Duration of current episode	<16 days
FABQ work subscale	<19 points
Segmental mobility testing in a posteroanterior direction (spring testing)	At least 1 hypomobile segment in the lumbar spine
Hip internal rotation ROM	At least 1 hip with >35° of internal rotation

7.2 C. According to Laslett et al.,[32,38] performance of SIJ tests in a specific order (distraction, thigh thrust, compression, and sacral thrust tests) improves their overall diagnostic ability. When 2 tests are positive, there is satisfactory specificity, sensitivity, and positive likelihood ratio; diagnostic accuracy improves only slightly with an additional positive test.

REFERENCES

1. Casazza BA. Diagnosis and treatment of acute low back pain. *Am Fam Physician*. 2012;85:343-350.
2. Carey TS, Garrett J, Jackman A, McLaughlin C, Fryer J, Smucker DR. The outcomes and costs of care for acute low back pain among patients seen by primary care practitioners, chiropractors, and orthopedic surgeons. The North Carolina Back Pain Project. *N Engl J Med*. 1995;333:913-917.
3. Hoy D, Brooks P, Blyth F, Buchbinder R. The epidemiology of low back pain. *Best Pract Res Clin Rheumatol*. 2010;24:769-781.
4. Hoy D, Bain C, Williams G, et al. A systematic review of the global prevalence of low back pain. *Arthritis Rheum*. 2012;64:2028-2037.
5. Dreyfuss P, Michaelsen M, Pauza K, McLarty J, Bogduk N. The value of medical history and physical examination in diagnosing sacroiliac joint pain. *Spine*. 1996;21:2594-2602.
6. Fortin JD, Dwyer AP, West S, Pier J. Sacroiliac joint: pain referral maps upon applying a new injection/arthrography technique. Part I: Asymptomatic volunteers. *Spine*. 1994;19:1475-1482.
7. Fortin JD, Aprill CN, Ponthieux B, Pier J. Sacroiliac joint: pain referral maps upon applying a new injection/arthrography technique. Part II: Clinical evaluation. *Spine*. 1994;19:1483-1489.
8. Goodman CC, Snyder TEK. *Differential Diagnosis for Physical Therapists: Screening for Referral*, 5th ed. St. Louis, MO: Elsevier Saunders; 2013.
9. Henschke N, Maher CG, Refshauge KM, et al. Prevalence of and screening for serious spinal pathology in patients presenting to primary care settings with acute low back pain. *Arthritis Rheum*. 2009;60:3072-3080.
10. Chou R, Fu R, Carrino JA, Deyo RA. Imaging strategies for low back pain: systematic review and meta-analysis. *Lancet*. 2009;373:463-472.
11. Davis PC, Wippold FJ II, Cornelius RS, et al. Expert panel on neurologic imaging. ACR Appropriateness Criteria® low back pain. Reston, VA: American College of Radiology (ACR); 2011:8. http://www.guideline.gov/content.aspx?id=35145. Retrieved on July 30, 2013.
12. Webster BS, Cifuentes M. Relationship of early magnetic resonance imaging for work-related acute low back pain with disability and medical utilization outcomes. *J Occup Environ Med*. 2010;52:900-907.

13. Andersen JC. Is immediate imaging important in managing low back pain? *J Athl Train.* 2011;46:99-102.
14. Flynn T, Fritz J, Whitman J, et al. A clinical prediction rule for classifying patients with low back pain who demonstrate short-term improvement with spinal manipulation. *Spine.* 2002;27:2835-2843.
15. Childs JD, Fritz JM, Piva SR, Erhard RE. Clinical decision making in the identification of patients likely to benefit from spinal manipulation: a traditional versus an evidence-based approach. *J Orthop Sports Phys Ther.* 2003;33:259-272.
16. Tozzi P, Bongiorno D, Vitturini C. Fascial release effects on patients with non-specific cervical or lumbar pain. *J Bodyw Mov Ther.* 2011;15:405-416.
17. Ramsook RR, Malanga GA. Myofascial low back pain. *Curr Pain Headache Rep.* 2012;16:423-432.
18. Malanga GA, Cruz Colon EJ. Myofascial low back pain: a review. *Phys Med Rehabil Clin N Am.* 2010;21:711-724.
19. Lavelle ED, Lavelle W, Smith HS. Myofascial trigger points. *Med Clin North Am.* 2007;91:229-239.
20. Dahm KT, Brurberg KG, Jamtvedt G, Hagen KB. Advice to rest in bed versus advice to stay active for acute low-back pain and sciatica. *Cochrane Database Syst Rev.* 2010;(6):CD007612.
21. Wilson E, Payton O, Donegan-Shoaf L, Dec K. Muscle energy technique in patients with acute low back pain: a pilot clinical trial. *J Orthop Sports Phys Ther.* 2003;33:502-512.
22. Selkow NM, Grindstaff TL, Cross KM, Pugh K, Hertel J, Saliba S. Short-term effect of muscle energy technique on pain in individuals with non-specific lumbopelvic pain: a pilot study. *J Man Manip Ther.* 2009;17:E14-E18.
23. Wang XQ, Zheng JJ, Yu ZW, et al. A meta-analysis of core stability exercise versus general exercise for chronic low back pain. *PLoS One.* 2012;7:e52082.
24. Liddle SD, Gracey JH, Baxter GD. Advice for the management of low back pain: a systematic review of randomised controlled trials. *Man Ther.* 2007;12:310-327.
25. Hayden JA, van Tulder MW, Malmivaara AV, Koes BW. Meta-analysis: exercise therapy for nonspecific low back pain. *Ann Intern Med.* 2005;142:765-775.
26. Macedo LG, Maher CG, Latimer J, McAuley JH. Motor control exercise for persistent, nonspecific low back pain: a systematic review. *Phys Ther.* 2009;89:9-25.
27. van Middelkoop M, Rubinstein SM, Verhagen AP, Ostelo RW, Koes BW, van Tulder MW. Exercise therapy for chronic nonspecific low-back pain. *Best Pract Res Clin Rheumatol.* 2010;24:193-204.
28. Lizier DT, Perez MV, Sakata RK. Exercises for treatment of nonspecific low back pain. *Rev Bras Anestesiol.* 2012;62:838-846.
29. Inani SB, Selkar SP. Effect of core stabilization exercises versus conventional exercises on pain and functional status in patients with non-specific low back pain: a randomized clinical trial. *J Back Musculoskelet Rehabil.* 2013;26:37-43.
30. Wand BM, Bird C, McAuley JH, Doré CJ, MacDowell M, De Souza LH. Early intervention for the management of acute low back pain: a single-blind randomized controlled trial of biopsychosocial education, manual therapy, and exercise. *Spine.* 2004;29:2350-2356.
31. Becker A, Held H, Redaelli M, et al. Low back pain in primary care: costs of care and prediction of future health care utilization. *Spine.* 2010;35:1714-1720.
32. Laslett M, Young SB, Aprill CN, McDonald B. Diagnosing painful sacroiliac joints: A validity study of McKenzie evaluation and sacroiliac provocation tests. *Aust J Physiother.* 2003;49:89-97.
33. Dreyfuss PH, Dreyer SJ, NASS. Lumbar zygapophysial (facet) joint injections. *Spine J.* 2003;3 (3 suppl):50S-59S.
34. Maigne JY, Aivaliklis A, Pfefer F. Results of sacroiliac joint double block and value of sacroiliac pain provocation tests in 54 patients with low back pain. *Spine.* 1996;21:1889-1892.
35. Slipman CW, Sterenfeld EB, Chou LH, Herzog R, Vresilovic E. The predictive value of provocative sacroiliac joint stress maneuvers in the diagnosis of sacroiliac joint syndrome. *Arch Phys Med Rehabil.* 1998;79:288-292.

36. van der Wurff P, Buijs EJ, Groen GJ. A multitest regimen of pain provocation tests as an aid to reduce unnecessary minimally invasive sacroiliac joint procedures. *Arch Phys Med Rehabil.* 2006;87:10-14.

37. Robinson HS, Brox JI, Robinson R, Bjelland E, Solem S, Telje T. The reliability of selected motion- and pain provocation tests for the sacroiliac joint. *Man Ther.* 2007;12:72-79.

38. Laslett M, Aprill CN, McDonald B, Young SB. Diagnosis of sacroiliac joint pain: validity of individual provocation tests and composites of tests. *Man Ther.* 2005;10:207-218.

39. Magee DJ. *Orthopedic Physical Assessment.* 5th ed. St. Louis, MO: Elsevier Saunders; 2008.

40. Mens JM, Vleeming A, Snijders CJ, Stam HJ, Ginai AZ. The active straight leg raising test and mobility of the pelvic joints. *Eur Spine J.* 1999;8:468-473.

41. O'Sullivan PB, Beales DJ, Beetham JA, et al. Altered motor control strategies in subjects with sacroiliac joint pain during the active straight-leg-raise test. *Spine.* 2002;27:E1-E8.

42. Hungerford BA, Gilleard W, Moran M, Emmerson C. Evaluation of the ability of physical therapists to palpate intrapelvic motion with the Stork test on the support side. *Phys Ther.* 2007;87:879-887.

43. Haneline MT, Young M. A review of intraexaminer and interexaminer reliability of static spinal palpation: a literature synthesis. *J Manipulative Physiol Ther.* 2009;32:379-86.

44. O'Haire C, Gibbons P. Inter-examiner and intra-examiner agreement for assessing sacroiliac anatomical landmarks using palpation and observation: pilot study. *Man Ther.* 2000;5:13-20.

45. Kilby J, Heneghan NR, Maybury M. Manual palpation of lumbo-pelvic landmarks: a validity study. *Man Ther.* 2012;17:259-262.

46. Stovall BA, Kumar S. Reliability of bony anatomic landmark asymmetry assessment in the lumbopelvic region: application to osteopathic medical education. *J Am Osteopath Assoc.* 2010;110:667-674.

47. Flynn TW, Fritz JM, Wainner RS, Whitman JM. The audible pop is not necessary for successful spinal high-velocity thrust manipulation in individuals with low back pain. *Arch Phys Med Rehabil.* 2003;84:1057-1060.

48. Cibulka MT, Delitto A, Koldehoff RM. Changes in innominate tilt after manipulation of the sacroiliac joint in patients with low back pain. An experimental study. *Phys Ther.* 1988;68:1359-1363.

49. Montañez-Aguilera FJ, Valtueña-Gimeno N, Pecos-Martín D, Arnau-Masanet R, Barrios-Pitarque C, Bosch-Morell F. Changes in a patient with neck pain after application of ischemic compression as a trigger point therapy. *J Back Musculoskelet Rehabil.* 2010;23:101-1044.

50. Cleland JA, Fritz JM, Whitman JM, Childs JD, Palmer JA. The use of a lumbar spine manipulation technique by physical therapists in patients who satisfy a clinical prediction rule: a case series. *J Orthop Sports Phys Ther.* 2006;36:209-214.

51. de Oliveira RF, Liebano RE, Costa Lda C, Rissato LL, Costa LO. Immediate effects of region-specific and non-region-specific spinal manipulative therapy in patients with chronic low back pain: a randomized controlled trial. *Phys Ther.* 2013;93:748-756.

52. Ross JK, Bereznick DE, McGill SM. Determining cavitation location during lumbar and thoracic spinal manipulation: is spinal manipulation accurate and specific? *Spine.* 2004;29:1452-1457.

53. Beffa R, Mathews R. Does the adjustment cavitate the targeted joint? An investigation into the location of cavitation sounds. *J Manipulative Physiol Ther.* 2004;27:e2.

54. Dunning J, Mourad F, Barbero M, Leoni D, Cescon C, Butts R. Bilateral and multiple cavitation sounds during upper cervical thrust manipulation. *BMC Musculoskelet Disord.* 2013;14:24.

55. Cramer GD, Ross JK, Raju PK, et al. Distribution of cavitations as identified with accelerometry during lumbar spinal manipulation. *J Manipulative Physiol Ther.* 2011;34:572-583.

56. Flynn TW, Childs JD, Fritz JM. The audible pop from high-velocity thrust manipulation and outcome in individuals with low back pain. *J Manipulative Physiol Ther.* 2006;29:40-45.

57. Chiradejnant A, Maher CG, Latimer J, Stepkovitch N. Efficacy of "therapist-selected" versus "randomly selected" mobilisation techniques for the treatment of low back pain: a randomised controlled trial. *Aust J Physiother.* 2003;49:233-241.

58. Kamali F, Shokri E. The effect of two manipulative therapy techniques and their outcome in patients with sacroiliac joint syndrome. *J Bodyw Mov Ther*. 2012;16:29-35.
59. Day JM, Nitz AJ. The effect of muscle energy techniques on disability and pain scores in individuals with low back pain. *J Sport Rehabil*. 2012;21:194-198.
60. Haladay DE, Miller SJ, Challis J, Denegar CR. Quality of systematic reviews on specific spinal stabilization exercise for chronic low back pain. *J Orthop Sports Phys Ther*. 2013;43:242-250.
61. Kuczynski JJ, Schwieterman B, Columber K, Knupp D, Shaub L, Cook CE. Effectiveness of physical therapist administered spinal manipulation for the treatment of low back pain: a systematic review of the literature. *Int J Sports Phys Ther*. 2012;7:647-662.

Athletic Pubalgia

Christine Panagos
Emily Ohlin

CASE 8

A 23-year-old male professional soccer player with complaints of left anterior hip and groin pain was referred to physical therapy by his athletic trainer following his preseason physical with the medical staff. He first experienced symptoms 4 months ago at the end of the previous season. Symptoms are most notable when he performs cutting and jumping activities. Although the patient notes a reduction in pain with 2 to 3 days of rest, his symptoms return with resumption of training activities. He is concerned about his ability to maintain a daily training schedule with the team. His past medical history is significant for a left acetabular labral repair with osteoplasty 2 years ago, multiple ankle sprains, and right medial meniscal tear 1 year ago.

- ▶ Based on the subjective information, what clinical evaluation methods will you utilize to determine intra-articular versus extra-articular hip pathology?
- ▶ What examination signs may be associated with the suspected diagnosis?
- ▶ What are the most appropriate physical therapy interventions if a nonoperative treatment plan is implemented?
- ▶ What is his rehabilitation prognosis?
- ▶ What are the complications that may limit the effectiveness of physical therapy?

KEY DEFINITIONS

ATHLETIC PUBALGIA: Commonly known as a "sports hernia"; weakness of the posterior inguinal wall without a clinically palpable hernia; symptoms include severe lower abdominal, pubic, low back, or groin pain with exertion[1-3]

FABER TEST: Acronym for Flexion, ABduction, and External Rotation; clinical test used to assess hip or sacroiliac joint dysfunction when the hip is brought into this combined position; pain elicited in anterior hip indicates possible hip pathology, while pain produced in posterior aspect of the pelvic region may indicate sacroiliac joint pathology, pain elicited in lateral hip may indicate piriformis or iliotibial band syndrome

FADIR TEST: Acronym for Flexion, ADduction, and Internal Rotation; pain elicited in the anterior hip when the patient's hip is brought into this combined position may indicate femoral acetabular impingement

FEMORAL ACETABULAR IMPINGEMENT (FAI): Condition in which the femoral head and/or neck makes excessive contact with the acetabulum

OSTEITIS PUBIS: Inflammation of the pubic symphysis

Objectives

1. Describe the clinical presentation of an individual with athletic pubalgia.
2. Describe the risk factors associated with athletic pubalgia.
3. Describe the clinical examination used to assess intra-articular versus extra-articular hip dysfunction.
4. List the differential diagnoses for athletic pubalgia.
5. Create an appropriate nonoperative treatment program for the athlete with athletic pubalgia.
6. Identify when appropriate medical referral is indicated.

Physical Therapy Considerations

PT considerations during management of the individual with athletic pubalgia (sports hernia):

- **General physical therapy plan of care/goals:** Decrease pain, increase muscular flexibility and joint mobility, improve lumbopelvic stability, increase hip and lower abdominal strength, increase postural awareness, increase ability to return to sport, prevent or minimize loss of aerobic fitness

- **Physical therapy interventions:** Patient education regarding functional anatomy and injury pathomechanics; modalities and manual therapy to decrease pain; flexibility exercises to restore or maintain normal range of motion (ROM); resistance exercises to increase muscular strength, alignment, and endurance capacity through the trunk musculature; aerobic exercise program

- **Precautions during physical therapy:** Monitor vital signs; address precautions or contraindications for exercise, based on patient's pre-existing condition(s); management of training volume to optimize healing and reduce risk of re-injury
- **Complications interfering with physical therapy:** Heavy travel and training volumes; inconsistency with physical therapy appointments and/or adherence to home exercise program

Understanding the Health Condition

Athletic pubalgia is a weakening of the posterior abdominal wall of the inguinal canal. The weakened wall allows the transversalis fascia to dilate, causing a widening of a region of the abdominal wall known as the inguinal triangle. The rectus abdominis (RA), the inguinal canal, and the inferior epigastric vessels create the borders of the inguinal triangle. The insertion of the RA and the origin of the adductor (ADD) longus conjoin in an aponeurosis, uniting at the pubic symphysis.[4] The pubic symphysis unites the superior rami of the pubic bones and is separated by a fibrocartilaginous disc.[5] The pubic symphysis also serves as a busy intersection for numerous musculotendinous attachments that dynamically stabilize and align the anterior pelvis. The muscles attaching at the pubic symphysis include the anterolateral portion of the RA, transversus abdominis (TA), external and internal obliques (EO, IO), and hip adductors (pectineus, ADD longus, ADD brevis, and ADD magnus).[1] When the inguinal triangle widens with athletic pubalgia, the RA retracts cranially and medially. Athletes may describe a dull or burning pain that radiates into the lower abdomen, inner thigh, or scrotum. The pain may be due to the tension produced as the inguinal triangle widens, allowing the RA to bulge, which may in turn compress the cutaneous branches of the iliohypogastric nerve (sensation to the lower abdomen), ilioinguinal nerve (sensation to the groin), and genital branch of the genitofemoral nerve (sensation to the scrotum or labia).[6] Physical exertion and strain in this area may exacerbate the condition, causing groin and scrotal pain that prevents the athlete from further participation in their sport.[6]

Although varied presentations of athletic pubalgia have been described, the most common involves injuries to the musculotendinous and insertional regions of the RA and/or the ADD longus and their associated aponeuroses.[3] The most likely causative factor for weakening of the posterior abdominal wall is a strength imbalance between the weaker RA and stronger ADD longus and the shear forces created across the pubic symphysis.[7-9] Hammound et al.[10] hypothesized that the **high prevalence of concomitant athletic pubalgia and femoroacetabular impingement (FAI) symptoms noted in professional soccer players** may be due to the abnormal stresses placed on the sacroiliac joint, pubic symphysis, and lumbar spine secondary to ROM limitations at the hip. Restricted motion at the hip leads to compensatory movement at the pubic symphysis, sacroiliac joint, and lumbar spine. Excessive movement in these structures can increase strain to the surrounding abdominal and hip muscles because they attempt to stabilize against the excessive movement.

Athletic pubalgia occurs more frequently in male athletes who participate in activities that involve cutting, pivoting, rapid acceleration and deceleration, kicking, and twisting.[7,11] Sports with the highest prevalence are soccer, ice hockey, and rugby.[6-7,11,12] For male soccer players, the annual incidence of groin pain ranges from 10% to 18%.[12-14] Athletic pubalgia is often a diagnosis of exclusion, even though it is recognized as a common source of groin pain in the athlete that fails to respond to conservative treatment.[6] Physical examination alone can only raise suspicion of athletic pubalgia. Methods such as protocol-specific magnetic resonance imaging (MRI), dynamic ultrasound, and diagnostic injection with local anesthetic have shown some promise in making the diagnosis.[15] Differential diagnosis of chronic groin pain can be classified into 4 general categories: hip ADD dysfunction, osteitis pubis, hip intra-articular and extra-articular pathology, and athletic pubalgia. When performed by skilled physical therapists, sports medicine physicians, or surgeons, diagnostic tests correlate well with surgical findings.[15-18] However, no group of clinical tests or diagnostic imaging can accurately diagnose athletic pubalgia. **Definitive diagnosis** of athletic pubalgia can only be made through laparoscopic examination.

If 3 months of conservative treatment fails to relieve symptoms, laparoscopic techniques can be used to repair the separation of the RA fascia from the pubis and inguinal ligament. Concurrent procedures may include an ADD tendon release and/or resection of the ilioinguinal and/or genitofemoral nerves.[1,6-7]

Physical Therapy Patient/Client Management

Physical therapy examination of the patient with hip, groin, and/or lower abdominal pain is generally challenging due to the poor diagnostic utility of many special tests for impairments in these regions and specifically challenging due to the lack of special tests for athletic pubalgia. Regardless of the specific location of the impairment, the physical therapist initially attempts to treat the athlete with hip, groin, and/or lower abdominal pain with interventions addressing identified postural deficits, muscular weakness, and muscular inflexibility. **Addressing the strength-tension ratio between the hip ADDs, pelvic floor, gluteal, and lower abdominals** through a well-designed therapeutic exercise program can provide the athlete with the best chance at a successful outcome.[15] A period of therapeutic exercise intervention should be attempted for approximately 3 months prior to surgical consideration.[3,16] An athlete who does not respond to conservative management should be referred to an appropriate surgeon.[19] **Surgical intervention** offers the greatest amount of symptom control and usually allows for return to competition within 3 months.[3]

Examination, Evaluation, and Diagnosis

When evaluating the patient with anterior hip and groin pain, all potential hip pathologies must be considered. It is helpful to start with a subjective evaluation that concisely guides which objective tests and measures the physical therapist should prioritize. In this case, the athlete reported an insidious onset of dull, left groin pain with radiation into the anterior thigh and lower abdominal region. He stated that the pain worsens with training activities (changing from dull to sharp) and resolves with approximately 3 days of rest. Activities such as sprinting, cutting, and jumping exacerbate his pain. Although this description is consistent with athletic pubalgia, it is also consistent with the clinical presentation of several intra-articular or extra-articular hip pathologies.[3] The therapist must be aware that the athlete may have one or more of these pathologies concurrently.

The objective portion of the examination begins with observation of posture. No asymmetries were noted when viewing the patient from the front. The athlete's anterior superior iliac spines and iliac crests were level; his lower extremities were slightly externally rotated, presenting as a bilaterally toed-out stance. From a side view, the athlete presented with an anteriorly tilted pelvis, increased lumbar lordosis, and highly developed lumbar paraspinal musculature. With the patient supine on the treatment table, active and passive hip mobility were assessed. The athlete demonstrated full, pain-free active and passive hip ROM that was equal to the contralateral side. However, during passive left hip abduction, the patient described a tightness in his left groin, consistent with the area that he reported hip pain. To assess for intra-articular pathology,[20,21] the therapist performed the log roll, FABER, FADIR, and resisted straight leg raise (SLR) tests. Pain described as "pinching" in the anterior hip during these tests may indicate FAI with concomitant labral tear and/or osteoarthritis (*i.e.*, intra-articular hip pathology).[6,19] If the patient reports snapping in the anterior or lateral hip or pain in the lateral hip, gluteal, or groin region with these tests, this could indicate the presence of extra-articular hip pathology. Examples of extra-articular hip pathology include snapping hip, osteitis pubis, ADD strain, piriformis syndrome, greater trochanteric bursitis, and iliotibial band syndrome. The patient reported no symptoms during any of these tests.

Next, passive SLR and resisted SLR at 30° were performed. The patient demonstrated pain-free SLR to 70°, which assisted in ruling out lumbar nerve root involvement. The therapist lowered his limb to approximately 30° and provided a downward resistance just above the knee. Pain elicited during the resisted SLR test may indicate iliopsoas, lower abdominal, or sacroiliac joint pathology. The patient reported left lower abdominal and mild groin discomfort with the left resisted SLR at 30°. To help rule out the possibility of a proximal femoral neck fracture, which can also produce pain in the anterior hip, the therapist performed a patellar-pubic percussion (PPP) test. With the patient still in supine with his lower extremities flat against the treatment table, the bell of a stethoscope was placed on the pubic symphysis. The therapist applied a percussive force alternately on each patella while stabilizing the ipsilateral leg in a neutral position. The therapist compared the sounds for differences in pitch and volume. If there is a bony disruption, a duller, diminished sound will be auscultated compared to the uninvolved side.[21] A meta-analysis of 14 articles concluded that the PPP test has good reported specificity at 86% (95% CI 78%-92%) and excellent sensitivity at 95% (95% CI 92%-97%).[22] There was no detectable difference in the athlete's PPP test from side to side. Based on the athlete's normal hip ROM findings, negative results in the hip special tests, and negative PPP test, the physical therapist determined that his symptoms were likely not intra-articular in nature.

Manual muscle testing was performed to assess the strength of the hip muscles and trunk stabilizers, focusing on those that attach at the pubic ramus. Prone gluteus maximus assessment revealed bilateral weakness and aberrant firing patterns of the hip extensors. Specifically, the physical therapist noted that the athlete initiated hip extension with the hamstrings and lumbar extensors, instead of the gluteal musculature. Other significant findings during hip strength testing were weakness in the left hip abductors and flexors and pain and weakness in the left hip ADDs. The therapist assessed the strength of the trunk muscles (TA, RA, obliques). During an active left SLR, the therapist observed a delay in TA contraction. With palpation, the therapist noted that TA contraction occurred *after* the leg raise was initiated as opposed to prior to the leg lift. This delayed TA contraction has been associated with long-standing groin pain.[23,24] When testing RA strength (with a partial sit-up), the athlete had pain in the left lower abdominal and groin regions. While strength testing the obliques, manual resistance at the right shoulder during a partial sit-up exacerbated left lower abdominal symptoms. Palpation revealed tenderness at the left superficial inguinal ring, the pubic symphysis, and the ADD longus insertion.

At this point in the examination, the therapist suspects a diagnosis of athletic pubalgia in this high-level athlete with a prior history of FAI based on the following findings: pain with activity that diminishes at rest, full pain-free hip ROM, negative special tests for intra-articular hip pathology, reproduction of lower abdominal/groin symptom with strength testing, and tenderness to palpation through inguinal landmarks without palpation of superficial herniation.

Special tests that can assist in the differential diagnosis of athletic pubalgia are the ADD squeeze test (Fig. 8-1) and the Valsalva maneuver (*i.e.*, bearing down against a closed glottis). The ADD squeeze test is performed with the patient in a hooklying position actively contracting the hip ADDs. Reproduction of symptoms

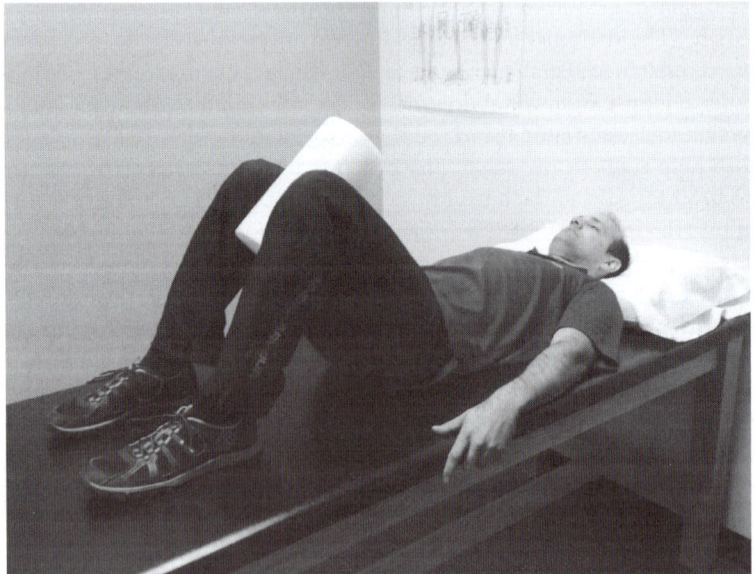

Figure 8-1. Adductor squeeze test. Position the patient in a supine hooklying position. Place an object approximately 6 inches wide between the knees and ask patient to squeeze the object. If the patient's symptoms are recreated, the adductor squeeze test is positive for adductor strain.

Table 8-1 DIFFERENTIAL DIAGNOSIS FOR HIP, GROIN, AND ABDOMINAL PAIN

Condition	Clinical Features	Diagnostic Test
FAI	Positive FABER test; pain with combined passive hip flexion, adduction, and internal rotation; decreased passive hip ROM compared to uninvolved side[23]	Radiograph: frog-leg view MRI[27]
Psoas major pathology	Painful active hip flexion; possibly decreased hip active and passive extension ROM; tenderness at iliospoas tendon[30]	Ultrasound, CT[28,29]
Intra-articular (e.g., osteoarthritis, labral tear)	Positive FABER test; positive scour test; possible decreased passive hip internal rotation ROM compared to uninvolved side[22]	MRI, MR arthrogram, injection[22]
Adductor strain/tendinopathy	Painful passive hip abduction; positive squeeze test; painful resisted hip adduction; tenderness at adductor tendon[18]	Ultrasound, MRI[4,27,31]
Femoral neck stress fracture	Positive heel percussion test; pain with impact activity[21]	MRI
Osteitis pubis	Tenderness at pubic symphysis; weakness and pain with resisted hip adduction; positive squeeze test[25]	MRI

Abbreviations: CT, computed tomography; FABER, Flexion, ABduction, and External Rotation; FAI, Femoroacetabular impingement; MRI, magnetic resonance imaging; ROM, range of motion.

in the ADD and pubic symphysis region indicates a positive test. Further research needs to be done to assess the clinical value of this test, but preliminary results show that the specificity of the bilateral ADD test ranges from 88% to 93%.[25] The Valsalva maneuver also reproduced pain (but no bulge) in the left lower abdominal region.[3,15]

Table 8-1 describes differential diagnoses and the clinical presentations for a patient presenting with anterior hip symptoms. With a provisional diagnosis of athletic pubalgia, the patient, physical therapist, and the medical team decided on conservative management of his impairments with physical therapy for a period of 8 to 12 weeks prior to pursuing further diagnostic testing. Conservative management, if successful, should allow the athlete to return to sport pain-free in 8 to 12 weeks.[26] If the patient is unable to return to training activity, further diagnostic testing is indicated. Non-contrast MRI, using a sports hernia protocol, is currently the imaging modality of choice.[27]

Plan of Care and Interventions

The first phase of the rehabilitation program should consist of interventions directed toward reducing pain and improving postural strength. Currently, this athlete did not present with any hip ROM deficits. However, 2 years ago, he had left hip ROM deficits that resolved with a femoral osteoplasty. Frequently, athletic pubalgia and FAI present concomitantly. In acute cases of athletic pubalgia, lumbar mobility, gluteal strength, active hip ROM, and timing of TA contraction may be adversely affected.[24] To address his identified deficits, an aquatic program of pain-free walking, hip strengthening, and bilateral squats with careful attention to pelvic alignment was initiated. The athlete progressed to the second phase when he was pain-free with normal activities of daily living.

The second phase of rehabilitation included lumbar stabilization exercises in supine, progressing to quadruped, kneeling, half-kneeling, and finally to standing. Exercises aimed at integrating strengthening of the TA, psoas major, the gluteals, and the obliques, through all planes of movement were chosen. The therapist instructed the athlete to perform clamshells (Fig. 8-2), supine dead bugs (Fig. 8-3), and opposite upper extremity (UE) and lower extremity (LE) lift in quadruped (Fig. 8-4). Bilateral bridging was progressed to bridging with marching, with cues to focus on lumbopelvic alignment in all planes. Clamshells are performed to address lateral hip weakness by specifically targeting the gluteus medius and hip external rotators. Supine dead bug exercises are used to improve the timing of TA contraction and promote lumbopelvic stabilization. The quadruped exercise involving lifting the opposing UE and LE (bird dog) promotes gluteal strength and rotational and lateral trunk stability. Bridging is also performed to increase gluteal strength; progression to bridging with marching helps isolate ipsilateral gluteal muscles and integrates the need for lumbopelvic

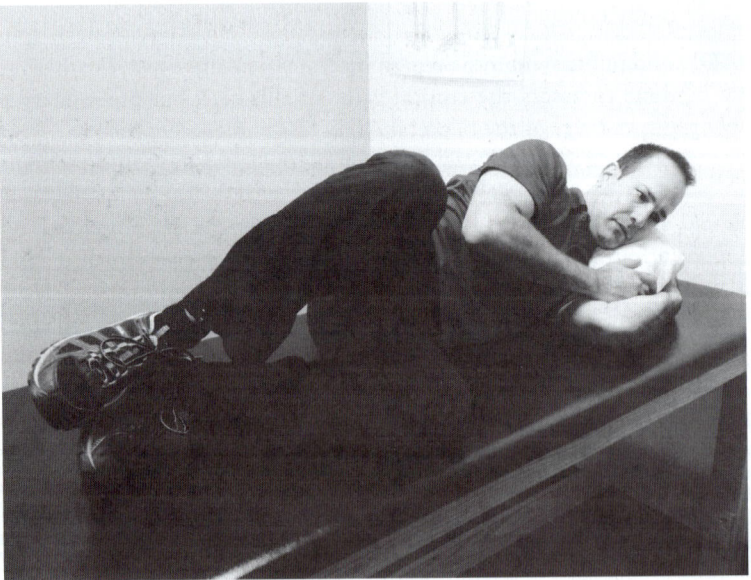

Figure 8-2. Clamshell exercise to strengthen gluteus medius and hip external rotators. The patient is positioned in a sidelying position with the pelvis rotated very slightly forward, knees and ankles together with knees flexed to 45°. The patient elevates the top knee upward, keeping the ankles together and preventing the pelvis from posteriorly rotating as the knee is elevated.

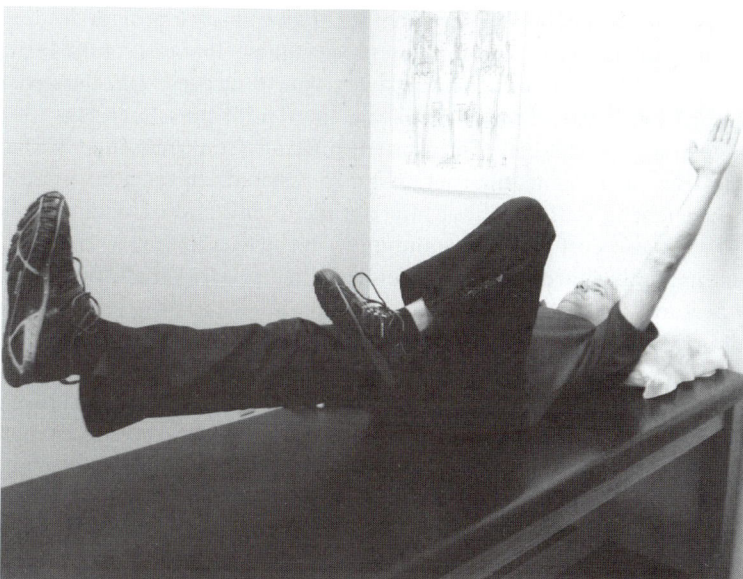

Figure 8-3. Supine dead bug exercise to improve timing of transversus abdominis (TA) contraction and promote lumbopelvic stabilization. The patient is positioned supine with arms at his side and knees and hips flexed to 90°. The patient extends the right leg while elevating the left upper extremity overhead and then alternates with left leg and right upper extremity. The patient may require cues to maintain a stable pelvis and trunk during performance.

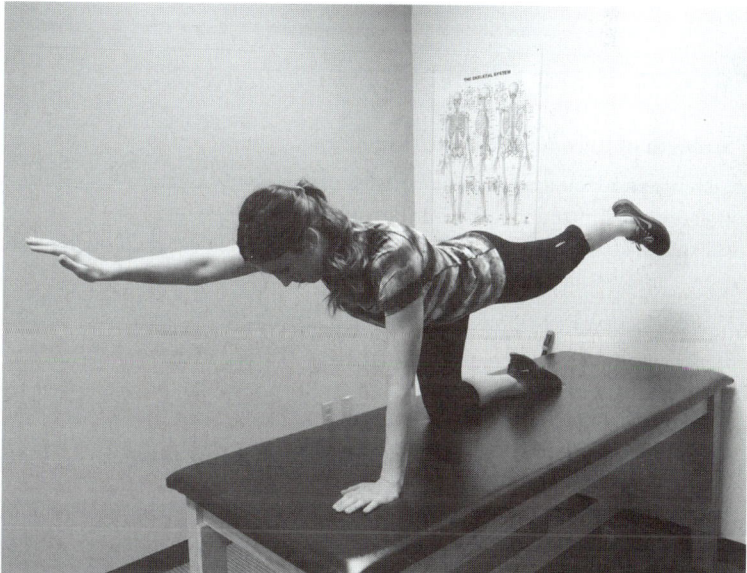

Figure 8-4. Bird dog exercise to increase gluteal strength and rotational and lateral trunk stability. Position the patient in quadruped. Instruct the patient to maintain a straight, flat trunk as he elevates the contralateral arm and leg up to body height. The therapist instructs the patient to lower the arm and leg down in a slow, controlled fashion and repeat the movement on the opposite side.

rotational stabilization. It is imperative for the therapist to provide feedback for the patient to avoid pelvic rotation, increased lumbar lordosis, trunk lean, and/or a hip drop. When the patient was able to perform these exercises correctly, the therapist progressed him to a tall-kneeling Pallof press (see Fig. 13-14) to challenge rotational stability. To promote hip and trunk muscular strength in a neutral pelvic alignment, the therapist also resisted UE motions in all planes with the patient in half-kneeling. Hip extension and abduction strengthening exercises were also performed in standing with the therapist providing feedback to lessen his lumbar lordosis and anteriorly tilted pelvis. When the patient was able to perform these exercises with internal and external perturbation while maintaining good lumbopelvic and hip control, plyometric exercises were introduced with gradual return to sport-specific drills.

It is recommended that athletes with symptoms of athletic pubalgia participate in a 12-week program of conservative treatment to address hip muscle strength and lumbopelvic stability. One case series study has shown that conservative management of athletic pubalgia provides successful return to sport within 6 to 8 weeks.[32] However, there are numerous case reports that support surgical repair; these studies report that up to 80% of those who underwent surgical repair returned to competition.[6] As the treating therapist, it is imperative to recognize patients who are not responding to conservative measures and refer them appropriately for further diagnostic testing and probable surgical intervention. Those who fail to respond to conservative treatment should be assessed for an accompanying FAI because it has been shown that stress from limited hip motion creates increased stresses to the pelvis and surrounding musculature, contributing to athletic pubalgia.[10]

Evidence-Based Clinical Recommendations

SORT: Strength of Recommendation Taxonomy

A: Consistent, good-quality patient-oriented evidence
B: Inconsistent or limited-quality patient-oriented evidence
C: Consensus, disease-oriented evidence, usual practice, expert opinion, or case series

1. The high prevalence of concomitant athletic pubalgia and femoroacetabular impingement (FAI) symptoms in high-performance athletes in sports such as soccer may be due to the abnormal stresses placed on the sacroiliac joint, pubic symphysis, and lumbar spine secondary to ROM limitations at the hip. **Grade C**
2. The diagnosis of athletic pubalgia is made through exclusion and can only be confirmed through surgical exploration. **Grade B**
3. Therapeutic exercises to address strength imbalances between the hip adductors, abductors, and lower abdominal musculature reduce symptoms in individuals with suspected athletic pubalgia. **Grade C**
4. Surgical correction of athletic pubalgia is effective for reducing pain and restoring individuals to their pre-existing level of performance. **Grade A**

COMPREHENSION QUESTIONS

8.1 What are 5 differential diagnostic tests and clinical signs utilized when evaluating a patient with suspected athletic pubalgia?

A. Resisted hip abduction, resisted hip adduction, tenderness at the iliopsoas tendon, pain with resisted sit-up, pain with Valsalva maneuver

B. Pain with resisted hip adduction, tenderness at pubic rami, pain with resisted sit-up, deep groin pain relieved with rest and exacerbated with sport, pain with Valsalva maneuver

C. Lower abdominal hip adductor pain, tenderness at pubic symphysis, loss of hip passive ROM, pain with resisted hip adduction, snapping hip

D. Tenderness at greater trochanter, tenderness at sacroiliac joint, pain with percussion testing, weakness in gluteus medius, pain with resisted hip abduction

8.2 Which of the following muscle groups typically require the prescription of therapeutic exercises to address musculoskeletal dysfunction in individuals with athletic pubalgia?

A. Obliques, hip adductors, back extensors
B. Transversus abdominis, obliques, multifidi, hip abductors
C. Hip internal rotators, hip abductors, quadriceps
D. Hip adductors, rectus abdominis, transversus abdominis

ANSWERS

8.1 **B.** Individuals with athletic pubalgia often have lower abdominal/groin pain that is exacerbated with sport and relieved with rest, pain with resisted hip adduction and resisted sit-up, tenderness at the pubic rami, and increased pain with cough/sneeze or the Valsalva maneuver. There is no change in passive hip ROM (option C) or resisted hip abduction (options A and D).

8.2 **B.** Muscle groups that affect lumbopelvic stability in the treatment for a sports hernia include but are not limited to transversus abdominis, obliques, hip abductors, and multifidii.

REFERENCES

1. Kachingwe AF, Grech S. Proposed algorithm for the management of athletes with athletic pubalgia (sports hernia): a case series. *J Orthop Sports Phys Ther*. 2000;38:768-781.

2. Ahumada LA, Ashruf S, Espinosa-de-los-Monteros A, et al. Athletic pubalgia: definition and surgical treatment. *Ann Plast Surg*. 2005;55:393-396.

3. Meyers WC, Foley DP, Garrett WE, Lohnes JH, Mandelbaum BR. Management of severe lower abdominal or inguinal pain in high-performance athletes. PAIN (Performing Athletes with Abdominal or Inguinal Neuromuscular Pain Study Group). *Am J Sports Med*. 2000;28:2-8.

4. Shortt CP, Zoga AC, Kavanaugh EC, Meyers WC. Anatomy, pathology, and MRI findings in the sports hernia. *Semin Musculoskelet Radiol.* 2008;12:54-61.
5. Gamble JG, Simmons SC, Freedman M. The symphysis pubis: anatomic and pathologic considerations. *Clin Orthop Relat Res.* 1986;203;361-372.
6. Minnich JM, Hanks JB, Muschaweck U, Brunt LM, Diduch DR. Sports hernia: diagnosis and treatment highlighting a minimal repair surgical technique. *Am J Sports Med.* 2011;39:1341-1349.
7. Anderson K, Strickland SM, Warren R. Hip and groin injuries in athletes. *Am J Sports Med.* 2001;29:521-533.
8. LeBlanc KE, LeBlanc KA. Groin pain in athletes. *Hernia.* 2003;7:68-71.
9. Morales-Conde S, Socas M, Barranco A. Sportsmen hernia: what do we know? *Hernia.* 2010;14:5-15.
10. Hammound S, Bedi A, Magennis E, Meyers WC, Kelly BT. High incidence of athletic pubalgia symptoms in professional athletes with symptomatic femoroacetabular impingement. *Arthroscopy.* 2012;28:1388-1395.
11. Gilmore J. Groin pain in the soccer athlete: fact, fiction, and treatment. *Clin Sports Med.* 1998;17:787-793.
12. Caudill P, Nyland J, Smith C, Yerasimides J, Lach J. Sports hernias: a systematic literature review. *Br J Sports Med.* 2008;42:954-964.
13. Taylor DC, Meyers WC, Moylan JA, Lohnes J, Bassett FH, Garrett E. Abdominal musculature abnormalities as a cause of groin pain in athletes: Inguinal hernias and pubalgia. *Am J Sports Med.* 1991;19:239-242.
14. Ekstrand J, Hilding J. The incidence and differential diagnosis of acute groin injuries in male soccer players. *Scand J Med Sci Sports.* 1999;9:98-103.
15. Farber AJ, Wilckens JH. Sports hernia: diagnosis and therapeutic approach. *J Am Acad Orthop Surg.* 2007;15:507-514.
16. Hackney RG. The sports hernia: a cause of chronic groin pain. *Br J Sports Med.* 1993;27:58-62.
17. Fricker PA. Management of groin pain in athletes. *Br J Sports Med.* 1997;31:97-101.
18. Orchard JW, Read JW, Neophyton J, Garlick D. Groin pain associated with ultrasound findings of inguinal canal posterior wall deficiency in Australian Rules footballers. *Br J Sports Med.* 1998;32:134-139.
19. Byrd JW. Evaluation of hip history and physical exam. *N Am J Sport Phys Ther.* 2007;2:231-240.
20. Muschaweck U, Berger LM. Sportsmen's groin-diagnostic approach with the minimal repair technique: a single center uncontrolled clinical review. *Sports Health.* 2010;2:216-221.
21. Martin RL, Irrgang JJ, Sekiya JK. The diagnosis accuracy of a clinical exam in determining intra-articular hip pain for potential hip scopes. *Arthoscopy.* 2008;24:1013-1018.
22. Reiman MP, Goode AP, Hegedus EJ, Cook CE, Wright AA. Diagnostic accuracy of clinical tests of the hip: a systematic review with meta-analysis. *Br J Sports Med.* 2013;47:893-902.
23. Cowan SM, Schache AG, Brinker P, et al. Delayed onset of transverse abdominals in long standing groin pain. *Med Sci Sports Exerc.* 2004;36:2040-2045.
24. Hemmingway AE, Herington L, Blower AL. Changes in muscle strength and pain in response to surgical repair of post abdominal wall disruption followed by rehab. *Br J Sports Med.* 2003;37:54-58.
25. Verrall GM, Slavotinek JP, Barnes PG, Fon GT. Description of pain provocation tests used for the diagnosis of sports-related chronic groin pain: relationship of tests to defined clinical (pain and tenderness) and MRI (pubic bone marrow oedema) criteria. *Scand J Med Sci Sports.* 2005;15:36-42.
26. Woodward JS, Parker A, MacDonald RM. Non-surgical treatment of a professional hockey player with signs and symptoms of sports hernia: a case report. *Int J Sports Phys Ther.* 2012;7:85-100.
27. Khan W, Zoga AC, Meyers WC. MRI of athletic pubalgia and the sports hernia: current understanding and practice. *Magn Reson Imaging Clin N Am.* 2013;21:97-110.

28. Kalebo P, Karlsson J, Sward L, Peterson L. Ultrasonography of chronic tendon injuries in the groin. *Am J Sports Med.* 1992;20:634-639.
29. Deslanders M, Guillin R, Hobden R, Burean NT. The snapping iliopsoas tendon: new mechanisms using dynamic sonography. *AJR Am J Roentgeol.* 2008:109:576-581.
30. Holmich P, Holmich LR, Bjerg AM. Clinical exam of athletes with groin pain: an intraobserver reliability study. *Br J Sports Med.* 2004;38:446-457.
31. Albers SL, Spritzer CE, Garrett WE, Meyers WC. MR findings in athletes with pubalgia. *Skeletal Radiol.* 2001;30:270-277.
32. Yuill EA, Pajaczkowshi JA, Howitt SD. Conservative care of sports hernias with in soccer players: a case series. *J Bodyw Mov Ther.* 2012;16:540-548.

Quadriceps Contusion

Jason Brumitt

CASE 9

A 22-year-old male Division II soccer player sustained an injury to his right thigh during today's game. He reports having been kicked in the anterior thigh by a defender from the opposing team during a corner kick. He was able to continue to play throughout the rest of the game; however, he sought care in the training room from the physical therapist after the match. After the game, he presented with pain, swelling, and stiffness. Examination of the right thigh reveals a hematoma and knee flexion active range of motion (ROM) limited by pain to 120°. He hopes to be able to play his next game in 10 days pain-free.

▶ Based on the patient's suspected diagnosis, what do you anticipate may be the contributing factors to his condition?
▶ What symptoms are associated with this diagnosis?
▶ What are the most appropriate examination tests?
▶ What are the most appropriate physical therapy interventions?

KEY DEFINITIONS

HEMATOMA: Collection of blood in the tissue resulting from damaged blood vessels

MYOSITIS OSSIFICANS (MO): Heterotopic ossification of bone within an injured muscle; exact pathogenesis is unknown; MO should be ruled out in athletes who have failed to recover after a thigh contusion.

QUAD SET: Isometric exercise for the quadriceps muscle. The standard quad set position is with the knee extended; however, this exercise can also be performed with the knee at any angle.

Objectives

1. Describe the signs and symptoms associated with a quadriceps contusion.
2. Describe the differential diagnosis for a quadriceps contusion.
3. Prescribe an evidence-based rehabilitation program for the athlete with a quadriceps contusion.

Physical Therapy Considerations

PT considerations during management of the college athlete with a quadriceps contusion:

- **General physical therapy plan of care/goals:** Decrease pain; increase muscular flexibility; increase active and/or passive ROM; increase lower-quadrant strength; prevent or minimize loss of aerobic fitness capacity
- **Physical therapy interventions:** Patient education regarding functional anatomy and injury pathomechanics; muscular flexibility exercises; resistance exercises to increase strength of the lower extremity; aerobic exercise program
- **Precautions during physical therapy:** Avoid prescribing manual therapy and aggressive strengthening exercises during early management of this condition; avoid subsequent contacts to same area during the immediate management phase
- **Complications interfering with physical therapy:** Development of a comorbidity associated with or resulting from the initial contusion injury; stress associated with pressure from coaching staff and teammates to return to play

Understanding the Health Condition

The quadriceps femoris muscle group, commonly referred to as the quadriceps or quads, is a collection of muscles that form the bulk of the anterior thigh. The 4 muscles that comprise the quadriceps are the rectus femoris, vastus medialis, vastus lateralis, and vastus intermedius. They originate from the pelvis or thigh and insert at the tibial tuberosity via the patellar tendon. Primary concentric muscular activation of the quadriceps extends the knee. Because of its origin at the anterior superior iliac spine, the rectus femoris also contributes to hip flexion.

A quadriceps contusion (also known as an anterior thigh contusion) results from a traumatic force to the musculature, typically a direct blow, such as a tackle to the thigh. These injuries are common, reported as the second most frequently experienced anterior thigh injury in sport.[1] Contusions to the anterior (or sometimes lateral) thigh have been reported in football, rugby, soccer, and martial arts.[2-8] A quadriceps contusion occurs when the muscle is compressed against the femur and the compressive force fails to disperse, which leads to damage in the impacted region's capillaries and myofibers.[9] The formation of a hematoma follows and may be accompanied by pain, swelling, a palpable mass, loss of strength, and loss of ROM.[1,3,6,10]

Contusion severity ranges from mild to severe with many athletes being able to continue practice or competition after injury. However, after a moderate or severe contusion, some athletes experience significant pain and loss of sport participation (average 45 days; range 2-180 days).[11] Usually, the athlete experiences pain in the presence of continued bleeding and increased swelling after a competition or practice.

Physical Therapy Patient/Client Management

The primary physical therapy interventions for an athlete with a quadriceps contusion include modalities, rest, and therapeutic exercises. Treatment should commence at the point that the athlete is no longer able to compete. Prior to initiating treatment, the physical therapist must perform a differential diagnosis to rule out other acute musculoskeletal conditions of the thigh. An athlete with signs and symptoms of an acute compartment syndrome injury (*e.g.*, paresthesia, pulselessness, excessive pain) should be referred to an emergency department for immediate treatment. An athlete who fails to achieve full, painless ROM within 4 weeks of injury onset requires referral to an orthopaedic physician to rule out heterotopic ossification.[4]

Examination, Evaluation, and Diagnosis

The athlete with a quadriceps contusion will be able to accurately recall the mechanism of injury during the practice or game as a traumatic impact (*e.g.*, tackle, kick to the thigh). An athlete who has sustained a contusion of the anterior thigh typically presents with one or more of the following: pain localized to the site of impact, a loss of ROM due to pain, discomfort with palpation to the injured region, hematoma, antalgic gait, and swelling or a palpable mass.[1,3,6,9] Circumferential girth measurements around the thigh can provide a measure of edema; however, this measure is not diagnostic and should only be used to help compare girth to the uninvolved side. Goniometric measurements of active ROM can help grade the severity of the injury. Jackson and Feagin[11] developed a classification system for quadriceps muscle contusions based on subsequent loss of flexion ROM (Table 9-1).[11]

Table 9-1 QUADRICEPS MUSCLE CONTUSION GRADING SYSTEM

Severity	Description
Mild	Knee flexion to at least 90°, hematoma, tenderness to palpation, no gait abnormalities
Moderate	Knee flexion to at least 90°, hematoma, swelling, tenderness to palpation, antalgic gait Inability to perform the following movements pain-free: deep squat, ascend stairs, stand from sitting position
Severe	Same as moderate, but with knee flexion less than 45°

Because athletes can experience several musculoskeletal injuries of the thigh, the physical therapist must perform a differential diagnosis for the athlete with a thigh contusion (Table 9-2). A muscular strain can typically be differentiated from a contusion based on its location and mechanism of injury. While muscular strains of the quadriceps can occur anywhere along the span of the muscle and/or tendon, they tend to occur primarily at the myotendinous junction.[10,12] The mechanism of injury for a quadriceps strain is usually eccentric contraction of the muscle,[13-15] such as occurs with sprinting and kicking (eccentric contraction of the rectus femoris). Similarly, a strain of the iliopsoas (psoas major and iliacus) is a

Table 9-2 DIFFERENTIAL DIAGNOSIS FOR INJURIES TO THE ANTERIOR THIGH

Diagnosis	Clinical Features
Quadriceps strain	Pain (minor to significant depending on severity) Pain associated with hip flexion and/or knee extension or pain with palpation of muscle at site of injury Palpation of a defect in the muscle Swelling (minimal to significant) Loss of strength (minimal to major depending on severity)
Iliopsoas strain	Pain and weakness associated with an injury to the psoas major and iliacus muscles Pain in anterior hip or groin region Injuries often result from sprinting or jumping
Coxa saltans ("snapping hip")	May have either intra- or extra-articular origins Audible snapping sound with or without pain during hip movement
Compartment syndrome	Excessive pain with thigh swelling Pain with passive quadriceps stretch May have paresthesia, paralysis, and/or pulselessness Elevated compartment pressure measurements
Osteomyelitis (bone infection)	May include loss of motion at adjacent joint(s), fever, fatigue, and signs/symptoms of inflammation (rubor, tumor, dolor, calor)
Myositis ossificans (heterotopic ossification in a muscle)	Persistent pain and loss of motion beyond the time period expected for recovery from a contusion May be a palpable mass

common acute injury experienced by athletes that can occur when these muscles are eccentrically activated.[3] In contrast, a contusion occurs in the location that has been impacted in a traumatic collision. Coxa saltans, also known as "snapping hip," is associated with pain in the anterior hip or groin region and the presence of an audible snapping sound that occurs with movement about the hip.[16,17] While a compartment syndrome of the thigh is rare, an athlete presenting with signs and symptoms of this condition should be taken immediately to an emergency department. A few cases of an acute thigh compartment syndrome developing subsequent to a quadriceps contusion have been reported.[18-22] This may occur because of the severity of the muscle damage or continued bleeding at the site of the injury.[18] The physical therapist should suspect compartment syndrome if the athlete presents with the 6 Ps: paresthesia, pulselessness, paralysis, pallor, pressure, and excessive pain.[18]

If the athlete fails to achieve full, painless ROM at the knee 4 weeks after injury, radiographs are indicated.[4] Bonsell et al.[4] reported a rare case of a high school football player who developed osteomyelitis that was discovered 5 months after a quadriceps contusion. In this case, the athlete returned to sport 2 months after the injury; however, he continued to experience pain and stiffness when playing football. The athlete sought care again 5 months post-injury due to residual pain and soreness associated with running. At this point, the physician questioned the patient if he had experienced symptoms associated with an infection (e.g., fever, chills) during the previous 5 months. The patient denied experiencing these systemic signs. The physician ordered a radiograph that revealed osteomyelitis. Additional tests performed subsequent to the radiograph included a magnetic resonance imaging (MRI) scan, erythrocyte sedimentation rate, and C-reactive protein test to confirm the osteomyelitis diagnosis.[4] Surgical procedures and intravenous medication over the course of 6 weeks were necessary to cure the infection. Bonsell et al.[4] hypothesized that the onset of osteomyelitis could have been pre-existing or occurred subsequent to the contusion injury. For the athlete who continues to have pain and loss of ROM beyond what would be expected for a recovery from a quadriceps contusion, the therapist should suspect myositis ossificans (MO), or the formation of abnormal bone in a muscle at the site of trauma.[23,24] An athlete with a moderate or severe quadriceps contusion has a greater likelihood of developing MO.[10,11] The athlete may also present with a palpable mass.[23,24] If the therapist suspects that an athlete has MO, therapeutic treatments should be deferred until after assessment by an orthopaedic physician.

Plan of Care and Interventions

A treatment program for an athlete with a quadriceps contusion should include rest, modalities, and therapeutic exercises.[1,25] As previously mentioned, some athletes may not immediately seek care after injury onset. An athlete who does not seek immediate care and is able to compete the duration of the event will likely seek medical attention after the event in response to increasing pain and loss of motion. The athlete should have his thigh and knee immobilized with an elastic wrap with the knee positioned in 120° of flexion (or to the point of pain tolerance in an athlete with a severe contusion).[25] Once immobilized, the athlete should be assisted to the training room by one or more individuals from the sports medicine team. In the training room, the elastic wrap is replaced by a **knee immobilizer with the flexion angle maintained at 120°** (or as close as possible).[25] For the next 24 hours, the athlete should wear the brace to avoid any weightbearing on the involved limb and ambulate with crutches. If the team physician is present, the athlete may be prescribed nonsteroidal anti-inflammatory drugs for 2 to 3 days.[25] The following day, the physical therapist can remove the brace and initiate therapeutic exercises (Table 9-3).[25] The athlete must continue ambulating with crutches (weightbearing as tolerated) until full pain-free lower extremity ROM has been restored. The use of cryotherapy (20 minutes per session, every hour or every other hour) is now indicated to help reduce pain and swelling.[9,25] Table 9-3 summarizes the treatment protocol that should result in an athlete being able to return to sport in 2 to 5 days.[25] The athlete will be able to return to sport when full knee ROM is restored, and he can perform sport-specific movements without pain. As a precaution, an athlete should wear a **thigh pad** to protect the region and avoid recurrence.[25]

Aronen et al.[25] utilized the treatment program described in Table 9-3 with 47 midshipmen who had sustained a quadriceps contusion. Twenty-four hours after injury, all the midshipmen had 120° of pain-free active ROM at the knee and 75% were able to initiate quad sets and a straight leg raise exercise without pain. All subjects had restored pain-free ROM equal to that of the uninvolved side. In 3.5 days (range 2-5 days), the midshipmen were able to return back to activity and sport without limitations, though they were required to wear a thigh pad to protect the region. This treatment protocol may also have reduced the incidence of MO in this sample. At 3 and 6 months after injury, radiographs performed on 23 of the 47 individuals showed that only 1 individual developed MO. **The overall incidence of MO in the midshipmen population was 4%,**[25] which is lower than the 9% to 17% incidence reported in the literature.[8,11,24,26-29]

Table 9-3 QUADRICEPS CONTUSION REHABILITATION PROTOCOL	
Injury Stage	**Treatment**
Sideline management for an acute injury	Knee immobilized in 120° flexion using elastic wrap. Athlete is assisted from the field to the on-site training room (sometimes referred to as the athletic training room)
Immediate management in on-site training room	Elastic wrap replaced by a knee immobilizer with flexion maintained at 120°. Athlete is instructed to wear brace for the next 24 hours and to ambulate with the use of crutches.
One day (24 hours) after injury	Brace is removed. Athlete is allowed to begin pain-free quadriceps stretching and quad sets (Fig. 9-1). Ambulation with crutches is continued until athlete has full, pain-free active ROM at the knee and hip and has restored strength of the involved quadriceps.

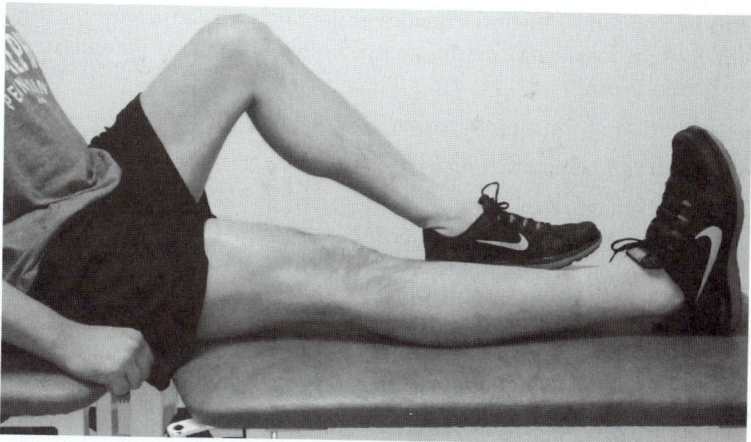

Figure 9-1. Quad set exercise.

Evidence-Based Clinical Recommendations

SORT: Strength of Recommendation Taxonomy
A: Consistent, good-quality patient oriented evidence
B: Inconsistent or limited-quality patient-oriented evidence
C: Consensus, disease-oriented evidence, usual practice, expert opinion, or case series

1. Immediate treatment for an athlete with a quadriceps contusion consists of knee immobilization at 120° of knee flexion and non-weightbearing ambulation with crutches. **Grade B**

2. After a quadriceps contusion, an athlete should wear a thigh pad to protect the region and reduce the risk of further injury. **Grade C**

3. Treating an individual with quadriceps contusion rehabilitation protocol outlined by Aronen et al. may reduce the formation of myositis ossificans. **Grade B**

COMPREHENSION QUESTIONS

9.1 A high school football player experiences a tackle to the right thigh near the end of the first half. He was unable to continue play due to pain. At halftime, the physical therapist examined the injured region. Visual observation of the thigh revealed a hematoma. The thigh was painful to palpation, and the athlete complained of loss of sensation in the thigh. The physical therapist was unable to detect pedal pulses on the right. Which of the following conditions should be immediately ruled out?
   A. Myositis ossificans
   B. Quadriceps strain
   C. Compartment syndrome
   D. Osteomyelitis

9.2 A quadriceps contusion and a quadriceps strain both cause anterior thigh pain. Which of the following examination techniques can help differentiate between the 2 conditions?
   A. Palpation of the injured region
   B. History of traumatic impact
   C. Loss of range of motion
   D. Pain with manual muscle testing

ANSWERS

9.1 **C.** Compartment syndrome is a potential complication associated with a quadriceps contusion. Hallmark features of compartment syndrome include excessive pain with swelling in the thigh, paralysis, pulselessness, and paresthesia. An athlete suspected of having a compartment syndrome of the thigh should be immediately referred to an emergency department.

9.2 **B.** A quadriceps contusion is because of a collision (*e.g.*, kick to the thigh, helmet to the thigh during a tackle), whereas a strain is usually because of eccentric overload of the quadriceps. Options A, C, and D would not be correct because both strains and contusions would likely result in pain during palpation and strength testing and loss of range of motion.

REFERENCES

1. Beiner JM, Jokl P. Muscle contusion injuries: current treatment options. *J Am Acad Orthop Surg*. 2001;9:227-237.
2. Alonso A, Hekeik P, Adams R. Predicting a recovery time from the initial assessment of a quadriceps contusion injury. *Aust J Physiother*. 2000;46:167-177.
3. Anderson K, Strickland SM, Warren R. Hip and groin injuries in athletes. *Am J Sports Med*. 2001;29:521-533.
4. Bonsell S, Freudigman PT, Moore HA. Quadriceps muscle contusion resulting in osteomyelitis of the femur in a high school football player. A case report. *Am J Sports Med*. 2001;29:818-820.
5. Chomiak J, Junge A, Peterson L, Dvorak J. Severe injuries in football players. Influencing factors. *Am J Sports Med*. 2000;28:S58-S68.
6. Diaz JA, Fischer DA, Rettig AC, Davis TJ, Shelbourne KD. Severe quadriceps muscle contusions in athletes. A report of three cases. *Am J Sports Med*. 2003;31:289-293.
7. Kary JM. Diagnosis and management of quadriceps strains and contusions. *Curr Rev Musculoskeletal Med*. 2010;3:26-31.
8. Ryan JB, Wheeler JH, Hopkinson WJ, Arciero RA, Kolakowski KR. Quadriceps contusions. West Point update. *Am J Sports Med*. 1991;19:299-304.
9. Trojian TH. Muscle contusion (thigh). *Clin Sports Med*. 2013;32:317-324.
10. Armfield DR, Kim DH, Towers JD, Bradley JP, Robertson DD. Sports-related muscle injury in the lower extremity. *Clin Sports Med*. 2006;25:803-842.
11. Jackson DW, Feagin JA. Quadriceps contusions in young athletes. Relation of severity of injury to treatment and prognosis. *J Bone Joint Surg Am*. 1973;55:95-105.

12. Pescasio M, Browning BB, Pedowitz RA. Clinical management of muscle strains and tears. *J Musculoskelet Med.* 2008;25:526-532.
13. Burns BJ, Sproule J, Smyth H. Acute compartment syndrome of the anterior thigh following quadriceps strain in a footballer. *Br J Sports Med.* 2004;38:218-220.
14. Zakaria AA, Housner JA. Managing quadriceps strains for early return to play. *J Musculoskeletal Med.* 2011;28:257-262.
15. Mendiguchia J, Alentorn-Geli E, Idoate F, Myer GD. Rectus femoris muscle injuries in football: a clinically relevant review of mechanisms of injury, risk factors and preventive strategies. *Br J Sports Med.* 2013;47:359-366.
16. Hoskins JS, Burd TA, Allen WC. Surgical correction of internal coxa saltans: a 20-year consecutive study. *Am J Sports Med.* 2004;32:998-1001.
17. Lewis CL. Extra-articular snapping hip: a literature review. *Sports Health.* 2010;2:186-190.
18. Joglekar SB, Rehman S. Delayed onset thigh compartment syndrome secondary to contusion. *Orthopedics.* 2009;32.
19. Mithofer K, Lhowe DW, Vrahas MS, Altman DT, Altman GT. Clinical spectrum of acute compartment syndrome of the thigh and its relation to associated injuries. *Clin Orthop Relat Res.* 2004;425:223-229.
20. Robinson D, On E, Halperin N. Anterior compartment syndrome of the thigh in athletes – indications for conservative treatment. *J Trauma.* 1992;32:183-186.
21. Rooser B. Quadriceps contusion with compartment syndrome. Evacuation of hematoma in 2 cases. *Acta Orthop Scand.* 1987;58:170-172.
22. Rooser B, Bengtson S, Hagglund G. Acute compartment syndrome from anterior thigh muscle contusion: a report of eight cases. *J Orthop Trauma.* 1991;5:57-59.
23. Beiner JM, Jokl P. Muscle contusion injury and myositis ossificans traumatica. *Clin Orthop Relat Res.* 2002;(403 suppl):S110-S119.
24. King JB. Post-traumatic ectopic calcification in the muscles of athletes: a review. *Br J Sports Med.* 1998;32:287-290.
25. Aronen JG, Garrick JG, Chronister RD, McDevitt ER. Quadriceps contusions: clinical results of immediate immobilization in 120 degrees of knee flexion. *Clin J Sport Med.* 2006;16:383-387.
26. Nalley J, Jay MS, Durant RH. Myositis ossificans in an adolescent following sports injury. *J Adolesc Health Care.* 1985;6:460-462.
27. Webner D, Huffman GR, Sennett BJ. Myositis ossificans traumatica in a recreational marathon runner. *Curr Sports Med Rep.* 2007;6:351-353.
28. Ryan JM. Myositis ossificans: a serious complication of a minor injury. *CJEM.* 1999;1:198.
29. Rothwell AG. Quadriceps hematoma. A prospective clinical study. *Clin Orthop Relat Res.* 1982;171:97-103.

Acute Hamstring Strain

Marc Sherry
Amanda Gallow
Bryan Heiderscheit

CASE 10

A 17-year-old male with an acute thigh injury was referred to physical therapy. Three days prior, the athlete was competing in a 200-m race, and upon sprinting through the turn, he felt a small pop and a sharp pain in the posterior aspect of his right thigh. He was unable to complete the race. When he was evaluated by the physical therapist, the patient presented with an antalgic gait pattern with decreased stride length and increased knee flexion on the involved side. The patient did not have any ecchymosis, but had significant pain to palpation 7 cm distal to the ischial tuberosity and a reproduction of this pain with strength and flexibility testing. The active popliteal angle was 40° on the uninvolved side and 56° on the involved side. Isometric knee flexion strength on the involved side was 5/5 at 90° of flexion and $4^+/5$ at 15° of flexion. When tested at 15° of knee flexion with varying tibial rotation, isometric knee flexion strength was 4/5 with external tibial rotation and $4^+/5$ with internal tibial rotation. Based on the history and physical examination findings, the physical therapist was concerned that the athlete presented with an acute hamstring strain.

▶ What additional patient-reported information is needed to establish a hypothesis-based differential diagnosis?
▶ What are the most appropriate examination tests?
▶ What are the most appropriate physical therapy interventions?
▶ What is his rehabilitation prognosis?

KEY DEFINITIONS

ACUTE HAMSTRING STRAIN: Disruption to the musculotendinous junction of one or more of the hamstring muscles with underlying hemorrhage and inflammatory reaction occurring within the previous 10 days

ANGLE OF PEAK TORQUE: Joint angle at which the greatest amount of torque production is observed. Individuals with a history of hamstring strain injuries often display a greater knee flexion angle of peak torque (~40°) in the injured limb compared to the uninjured limb (~30°).[1,2] Repetitive eccentric strengthening can alter this relationship so that peak torque is produced in a more extended joint position (*i.e.*, longer muscle length).

ECCENTRIC CONTRACTION: Muscle force production occurring when the muscle tendon unit is actively lengthening because it is opposing a force that is greater than the force it is generating. This type of muscle contraction has the potential to lead to elongation beyond the normal limits of the myofilament complex, creating fiber damage and tearing within the muscle.

RETURN-TO-SPORT TIME: Time to return to prior level of performance,[3] competition,[4] or practice.[5] For this case, it is defined as the time from injury to release for full athletic activity.[6] This may be the time of discharge from physical therapy,[7] although evidence has supported the need for continued rehabilitation even upon full release to activity.[7,8]

Objectives

1. Describe the most appropriate examination tests and likely findings in an individual following an acute hamstring injury and how the results relate to rehabilitation planning, prognosis, and return to sport.
2. Describe evidence-based rehabilitation interventions and treatment progressions following an acute hamstring injury.
3. Implement strategies to minimize the likelihood of re-injury when returning an athlete to his/her pre-injury level of performance.

Physical Therapy Considerations

PT considerations during management of the young sprinter with an acute hamstring strain injury:

- ▶ **General physical therapy plan of care/goals:** Normalize gait; restore pain-free and full range of motion (ROM) and strength; restore neuromuscular control during sport-specific movements; return to maximal speed during sport-specific movements without pain, stiffness, or apprehension
- ▶ **Physical therapy interventions:** Patient education regarding functional anatomy and injury pathomechanics and general precautions regarding protection of

healing muscle-tendon unit; cryotherapy for inflammation and pain management; exercises to increase neuromuscular control of lumbopelvic region; eccentric strengthening of hamstrings with emphasis on elongated positions

▶ **Precautions during physical therapy:** Avoidance of hamstring tissue over-stretching during early stages of rehabilitation; specific and graduated return to activity

▶ **Complications interfering with physical therapy:** Psychosocial factors including fear and apprehension of re-injury; injury location adjacent to the ischial tuberosity; injuries involving greater cross-sectional area or length; previous injury to the same hamstring muscle; lack of adherence to rehabilitation program

Understanding the Health Condition

An acute hamstring strain is a complex musculoskeletal condition often leading to a high re-injury rate, prolonged symptoms, and time lost from sport. In the athletic population, acute hamstring injuries occur during high-speed running that is common in football, track and rugby, or during activities that require a combination of excessive hip flexion and knee extension, such as dance or kicking sports.[9,10] The etiology of hamstring strains is multifactorial and can lead clinicians and patients down a challenging rehabilitation course. Successful rehabilitation and return to sport for an athlete following an acute hamstring strain relies on the clinician's understanding of hamstring anatomy, prognostic factors, mechanism of injury, and the role of eccentric strengthening and lumbopelvic neuromuscular control exercises to address deficits and prevent injury recurrence.

In a 10-year study of one National Football League team (1998-2007), hamstring strains were the second most common injury (behind knee sprains), with time lost from sport ranging from 8 to 25 days.[9] Hamstring strains in running backs, defensive backs/safeties, and wide receivers accounted for 22%, 14%, and 12% of all injuries in these groups, respectively.[9] When analyzing 51 professional European soccer teams over an 8-year period (2001-2009), 37% of muscle injuries involved the hamstrings with time lost from sport ranging from 1 to 128 days and a subsequent re-injury rate of 16%.[9,11] In a study of Australian footballers, injury recurrence following return to sport was the highest within the first 2 weeks.[10] The collective re-injury risk was 30.6% during the entire 22-week season. The high incidence of hamstring strain re-injuries following return to sport suggests that the rehabilitation programs utilized may be ineffective at targeting causative factors associated with hamstring injury and recurrence.

The hamstring muscle complex includes the long and short heads of the biceps femoris, the semitendinosus, and the semimembranosus. With the exception of the biceps femoris short head, the complex is biarticular, crossing both the hip and knee joints. A concentric contraction of the complex produces hip extension and knee flexion, whereas an eccentric contraction controls hip flexion and knee extension.[12] During many sport activities, the hamstrings produce high levels of force eccentrically for proper stabilization across the hip and knee joints. The inability to produce sufficient force in a lengthened position increases the muscle's susceptibility to injury. Following a hamstring injury, there is a shift in peak knee flexion torque development to a shorter musculotendon length (greater knee flexion angle).[1,2] Injury recurrence has been linked to this shift in the torque-angle relationship, because force development in elongated positions is compromised.[1,2]

The precise anatomic location of injury within the hamstring muscle complex varies between injuries resulting from high-speed running and those resulting from slow excessive stretching.[13,14] During high-speed running, the terminal swing phase has been identified as the time of hamstring injury occurrence, most often involving the intramuscular tendon of the biceps femoris long head.[15,16] As the limb enters the terminal swing phase, the hamstrings are actively lengthening to decelerate the limb for initial contact with the ground.[16-19] The biceps femoris long head undergoes the greatest amount of musculotendon stretch and load, which may explain its high incidence of injury during these movements compared to the semitendinosus and semimembranosus.[17,18,20-22] In contrast, hamstring injuries during activities such as dance or kicking typically occur within the proximal tendon of the semimembranosus because of excessive musculotendon stretch.[13,21,23] Location of the injury within the hamstrings complex is associated with recovery time. Individuals with injuries to the intramuscular tendon of the biceps femoris long head (common during high-speed running) have a faster recovery time compared to those with injuries of the proximal free tendon of the semimembranosus.[13,14,23]

It is well documented in the literature that the greatest risk factor for an acute hamstring strain is a previous hamstring strain.[24-27] Within the first 3 weeks of returning to sport following a hamstring injury, athletes can be at 20 times greater risk for re-injury.[24] Another risk factor for hamstring injury is hamstring to quadriceps strength imbalance.[28,29] Croisier et al.[28] found that professional soccer players who demonstrated a strength imbalance during preseason testing were 4.7 times more likely to experience a hamstring injury during the regular season. Changes that occur following hamstring injury may contribute to the high rate of injury recurrence including poor musculotendon extensibility and alterations in movement patterns and biomechanics.[30] Although hamstring stretching is often a component of rehabilitation, the benefit of stretching and hamstring flexibility on the recovery or prevention of hamstring strains has been disputed.[31-33] Although older age may be considered a non-modifiable risk factor for hamstring strains, some skeletal muscle changes associated with aging may be reversible.[34,35] Changes in skeletal muscle with age include reduction in muscle cross-sectional area, decrease in muscle fiber size, and possible denervation of muscle fibers.[36] The exact timing of these changes is not known, but they may contribute to increased risk of hamstring strains in the older population. Gabbe et al.[25] found that Australian footballers older than 24 years with a history of a hamstring injury in the previous 12 months had 4 times greater risk of sustaining a second injury compared to younger peers. Additional risk factors for acute hamstring strains such as hamstring weakness, lumbopelvic weakness and incoordination, and quadriceps inflexibility should be addressed in the multifactorial treatment of athletes.[5,37,38]

Physical Therapy Patient/Client Management

An acute hamstring strain can be a challenging case for the physical therapist. A **detailed patient interview and thorough examination** allows the physical therapist to confirm an accurate physical therapy diagnosis, assess the severity of injury, and determine whether imaging is required. Imaging or physician referral may be warranted if there is concern for tendon avulsion or an apophyseal avulsion fracture. Relevant anatomy, an individualized and evidence-based rehabilitation plan, and prognosis should be discussed with the patient. The physical therapy goal is 2-fold: (1) return the patient to his prior level of sport performance without pain, and (2) prevent re-injury.

Examination, Evaluation, and Diagnosis

An athlete presenting with an acute hamstring strain frequently reports a sudden onset of posterior thigh pain secondary to a bout of high-speed movement, often sprinting, or extreme hip flexion and knee extension.[39] Other symptoms may include an audible pop,[23] antalgic gait with shortened stride length,[24,40] ecchymosis, posterior thigh swelling, and pain with sitting or direct pressure.[40] While the reported mechanism of injury may lead the athlete and physical therapist to assume the injury is an acute hamstring strain, a thorough subjective interview and examination assists in the differential diagnosis. Because signs and symptoms of hamstring strain may parallel conditions such as L5-S1 nerve root involvement, hamstring tendon avulsion, apophyseal avulsion fracture, proximal hamstring tendinopathy, adductor injury, and pelvic fracture, these pathologies need to be ruled out to allow for an individualized rehabilitation plan and quickest return to play for the athlete.[6,41] If there is concern for a tendon avulsion or apophyseal avulsion fracture following examination, imaging should be performed. Table 10-1 describes clinical and diagnostic findings to assist in differential diagnosis of posterior thigh pain.

Mechanism of injury, involved structures, location of tenderness, and time to return to pain-free walking are prognostic factors for injury recovery and should be determined during the examination.[3,14,24] Common physical examination findings of an acute hamstring strain include pain and weakness with resisted knee flexion and hip extension, pain with passive hip flexion and knee extension, pain with palpation, and an antalgic gait pattern.[5,24,54] These factors also assist in determining prognosis for injuries to the intramuscular tendon or aponeurosis seen during high-speed running.[4,14,24] Injuries to the proximal tendon require a much longer rehabilitation period. In fact, the location of the injury can provide important prognostic insight with recovery time increasing the closer the maximum pain is to the ischial tuberosity.[3,13,23]

A comprehensive physical examination of the hamstring complex and lumbopelvic region includes comparison to the uninvolved lower extremity. However, it is important to note that *bilateral* neuromuscular and strength deficits have been observed following a unilateral injury.[55] To account for the various

Table 10-1 DIFFERENTIAL DIAGNOSIS OF POSTERIOR THIGH PAIN

Condition	Common Findings	Clinical/Diagnostic Findings
Ischial apophyseal avulsions[42,43]	Age: 13-16 years MOI: sprinting or stretching, possible audible pop	Ischial pain and tenderness with sitting Increased motion with straight leg raise and active knee extension (compared to uninvolved side) Imaging recommended: AP pelvis radiograph
Hamstring tendon avulsion[6,44,45]	MOI: forceful hip flexion and knee extension (e.g., bull-riding, water skiing)	Distal bulge with knee flexion due to retraction Hematoma and ecchymosis Palpable defects Neurologic symptoms due to sciatic nerve compression Inability to bear weight on involved limb Imaging recommended: MRI
Referred posterior thigh pain[4,6,46-48]	MOI: gradual or sudden onset Minimal pain	Positive neurodynamic testing (e.g., slump test) Minimal symptoms with walking or running Abnormal sacroiliac and lumbar examination Symptoms proximal to ischial tuberosity and distal to knee (e.g., cramping, tingling, shooting pain) Positive lumbar quadrant test
Pelvic fracture[49]	More common in females MOI: traumatic event or insidious onset of asymmetric gluteal or low back pain	Tenderness over pubic symphysis and/or sacroiliac joint Painful hip ROM into flexion, abduction, and external rotation Possible radicular symptoms Imaging recommended: radiographs followed by MRI
Proximal hamstring tendinopathy[50-52]	Age: 29-37 years MOI: insidious onset Previous history of hamstring injuries Common in soccer players, middle and long distance runners, cross-country skiers	Normal hamstring strength Tenderness over ischial tuberosity Flexibility testing produces discomfort Positive modified bent knee stretch test (Sn: 89%; Sp: 91%; PPV: 0.91; NPV: 0.89) Imaging recommended for patients who do not respond to conservative treatment: MRI
Adductor strains[6,46,53]	MOI: acceleration or rapid change of direction; stretching into hip abduction and/or external rotation	Tenderness over pubic ramus Reproduction of pain with resisted hip adduction

Abbreviations: AP, anteroposterior; MOI, mechanism of injury; MRI, magnetic resonance imaging; NPV, negative predictive value; PPV, positive predictive value; ROM, range of motion; Sn, sensitivity; Sp, specificity.

musculotendinous lengths that occur with hip extension and knee flexion angles during sport, strength testing of the hamstrings should be performed in the prone position at varying hip and knee angles. With the hip stabilized at 0° of extension, bias toward the medial and lateral hamstring muscles is accomplished with internal and external tibial rotation, respectively, at 90° and 15° of knee flexion.[6] In addition to its role as a knee flexor, the hamstrings also contribute to hip extension. Hip extension strength should be assessed with the knee positioned at 90° and 0°, applying manual resistance to the distal posterior thigh and heel, respectively. Range of motion is measured with the passive straight leg raise test and the active knee extension test (Fig. 10-1).[6] Hamstring tightness is present if the hip joint angle is less than 80° during the passive straight leg raise[56] and if the knee flexion angle is greater than 20° during the active knee extension test.[57] The active knee extension test is a reliable measure of hamstring flexibility in patients with acute hamstring injury (<5 days).[58] There should be concern for an avulsion injury if there is significantly increased ROM on the involved side compared to the uninvolved.[46] Muscle atrophy may be noted in an athlete with a history of previous hamstring injuries. Palpation helps determine proximity of maximal pain to the ischial tuberosity, length of the painful region, muscles involved, and defects within the muscle.

Patient-related factors such as pain and apprehension may interfere with performing an accurate physical examination following an acute hamstring strain.

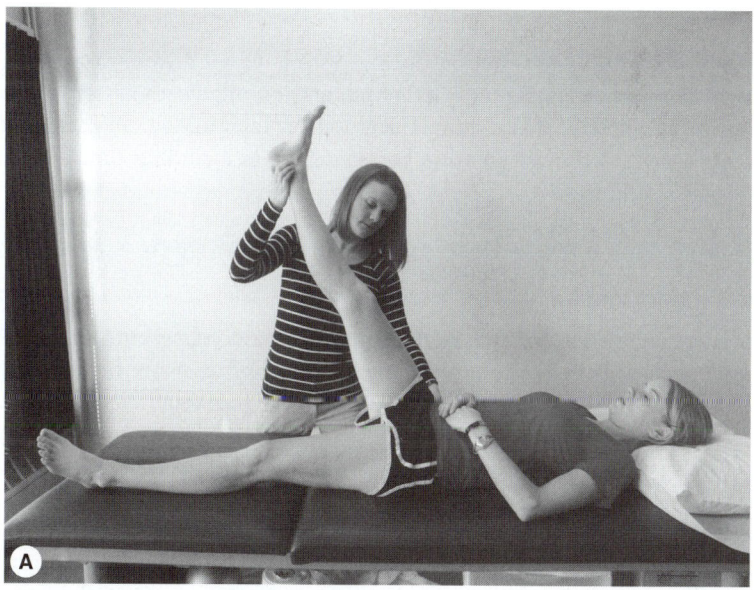

Figure 10-1. Straight leg raise test and active knee extension test. **A.** Straight leg raise test. The contralateral leg is maintained in extension on the table while the examiner passively flexes the involved hip with the knee in full extension and ankle in slight plantar flexion. The hip joint angle is measured at the end of the available range. Hamstring tightness is present if the hip joint angle is less than 80° despite pain and discomfort during testing.[56]

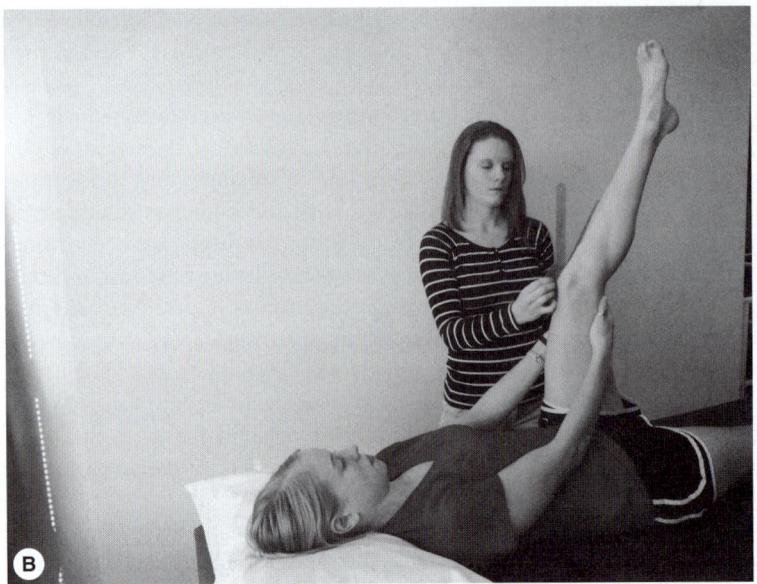

Figure 10-1. (*Continued*) Straight leg raise test and active knee extension test. **B.** Active knee extension test. The patient maintains the hip at 90° of flexion while actively extending the knee to maximal tolerance. Hamstring tightness is present if the knee flexion angle is greater than 20° despite pain and discomfort during testing.[57] The active knee extension test is a reliable measure of hamstring flexibility in patients with acute hamstring injury (<5 days).[58]

Pain may lead to muscle inhibition during testing. Clinical examination findings and magnetic resonance imaging (MRI) findings, if available, can assist in estimating the timeline of rehabilitation and return to sport. Table 10-2 highlights **prognostic factors for recovery following an acute hamstring strain** including clinical examination and MRI findings.

Plan of Care and Interventions

After performing a thorough physical examination and ruling out other potential sources of posterior thigh pain, initial management of an acute hamstring strain should focus on protection of the injured tissue. Protection should include avoidance of moderate to extreme passive or active hamstring lengthening because this may lead to pain, propagation of the injury, or increased scar tissue formation.[61] Modification of gait utilizing a shortened stride length or crutches should be encouraged to allow for protection and avoidance of increased tension across the damaged tissue.[6] Icing should occur multiple times per day to assist with pain control and inflammation. Early mobilization of the tissue while avoiding end-range stress to the hamstring complex may help to minimize muscle atrophy and neuromuscular control deficits, increase re-capillarization at the injury site, and minimize detrimental effects of scar tissue formation.[5,30,62,63] Goals during the early phase of rehabilitation (1-2 weeks after injury) should include normalization of gait, control of pain and swelling, and pain-free submaximal strengthening in a mid-length position of the hamstrings.

Table 10-2 PROGNOSTIC FACTORS FOR RECOVERY TIME FOLLOWING ACUTE HAMSTRING STRAINS

Examination Findings	Prognosis
Injury proximity to ischial tuberosity	The more proximal the injury is to the ischial tuberosity (determined via palpation), the more time required for return to sport.[3,14,23]
Mechanism of injury	Excessive stretching injuries seen in dancers require longer rehabilitation compared to injuries occurring during high-speed running.[3,13]
Location of injury within hamstring muscle complex	Injury to proximal free tendon is associated with longer recovery time compared to the musculotendon junction.[14]
Time to walk	Athletes taking >1 day to walk pain-free following injury are more likely to require >3 weeks of rehabilitation prior to 100% return to sport.[24]
Active knee extension test	This test is not associated with the time needed to return to sport or risk of hamstring re-injury.[24]
MRI Findings	
Craniocaudal length of injury	The greater the craniocaudal length, the more time required before returning to sport.[4,7,13]
Cross-sectional area	Increased cross-sectional area of injury on MRI is associated with a longer recovery period prior to returning to sport.[59,60]
Maximal T2 hypersensitivity	Greater edema on MRI assessed via T2 hypersensitivity is associated with longer recovery time.[59,60]
Distance from ischial tuberosity of maximal T2 hypersensitivity	Increased distance of maximal hypersensitivity on MRI is associated with longer recovery period.[13]

Because of the attachment sites of the hamstring muscles on the pelvis, neuromuscular control of the lumbopelvic region is needed to enable optimal function during normal sporting activities. This has led clinicians to increasingly utilize various trunk stabilization and progressive agility exercises for hamstring rehabilitation. For example, the **progressive agility and trunk stabilization (PATS) program initiated within the first week following acute hamstring strains** significantly decreased injury recurrence during the first 2 weeks and 1 year following return to sport compared to a program consisting of traditional hamstring stretching and strengthening.[5] The PATS program consisted primarily of neuromuscular control exercises, beginning with early active mobilization in the frontal and transverse planes, then progressing to movements in the sagittal plane. Although the exact neuromuscular changes that contributed to the re-injury reduction in the PATS group are unknown, the early neuromuscular control drills and motion in the frontal and transverse planes may improve lumbopelvic control. Improvement in lumbopelvic control may reduce re-injury risk by allowing the hamstrings to function at safe lengths during dynamic movements.[5,30] Examples of exercises in the PATS program include side-stepping (3 sets of 1 minute), cariocas (3 sets of 1 minute), boxer shuffle (3 sets of 1 minute), and rotating side planks (Fig. 10-2; 3 sets of 20 repetitions).

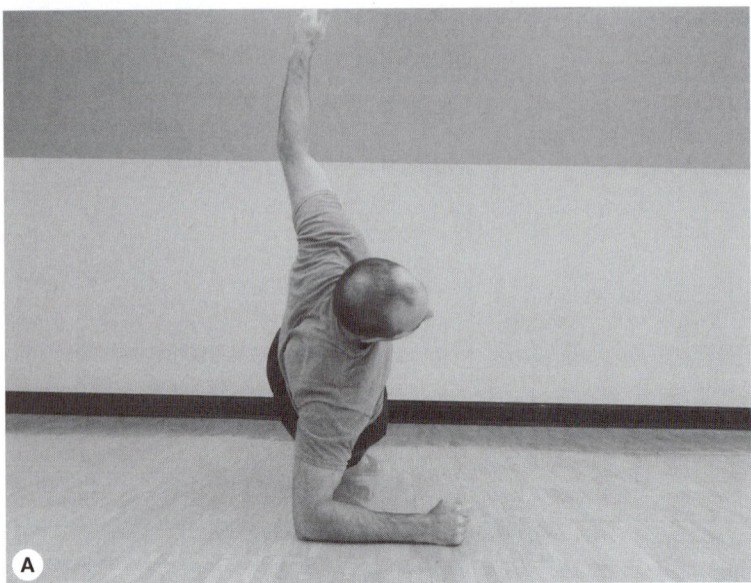

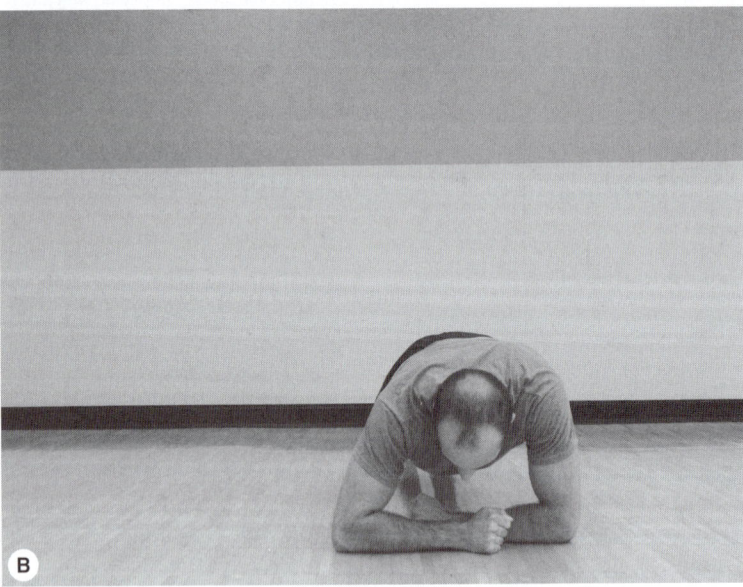

Figure 10-2. Rotating side plank exercise. **A.** The athlete starts in side plank position with the shoulders, hips, and ankles in a straight line on the right side, holding for 5 seconds. **B.** Maintaining hip position, the athlete rotates his body so chest is parallel to the floor.

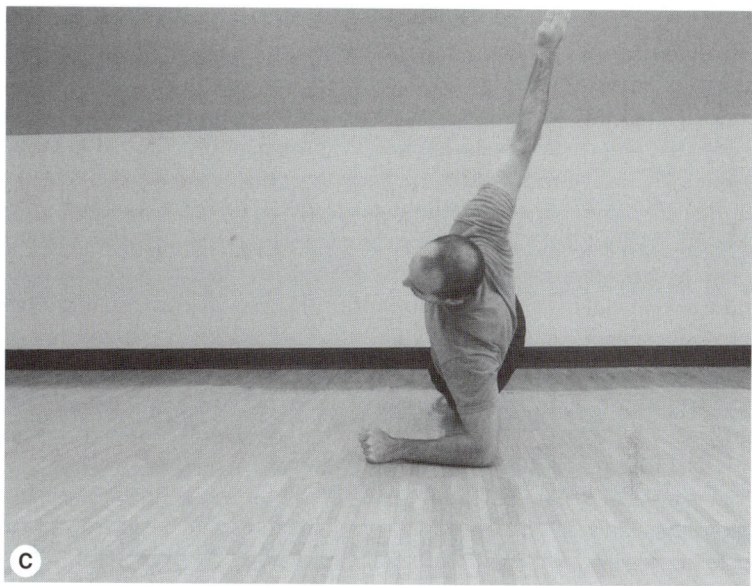

Figure 10-2. (*Continued*) Rotating side plank exercise. **C.** The athlete then rotates into a left side plank position holding again for 5 seconds. This exercise is repeated in reverse to the start position. This exercise can be progressed by adding dumbbells.

Patients in the PATS groups were asked to perform these exercises daily until they met the required criteria to return to sport, an average of 19 days.

Neuromuscular control deficits including altered muscle activation and decreased lower-limb proprioceptive awareness are present following a hamstring strain. In individuals with previous hamstring injuries, early activation of the biceps femoris and medial hamstrings on the involved and uninvolved sides was observed during a single-limb task.[55] The bilateral changes demonstrate the role of the central nervous system in neuromuscular control deficits.[55] In addition, poor proprioceptive awareness based on a leg swing movement discrimination test has been associated with hamstring injury in Australian League footballers.[64] To address the proprioceptive deficit, the HamSprint program was developed to incorporate neuromuscular re-education drills, single-limb balance, and progressive agility movements.[38] Examples of exercises from this program include ankle pops, forward running drills, skips, high knee marching, and quick starts.[38]

Eccentric strengthening has been shown to facilitate a shift in peak force development to longer musculotendon lengths. Allowing the muscle to generate more force at smaller angles of knee flexion potentially decreases the risk of injury during high-speed running when the eccentric loads are greatest near terminal extension.[21,22] Following an acute injury to the hamstrings, the optimal length for active tension becomes disrupted and shifts to a shortened position secondary to changes in neuromuscular control or scar tissue formation that begins as soon as 7 days post-injury.[12,55,63] Proske et al.[2] found the knee flexion angle of peak torque in the hamstrings to be 12° greater in previously injured versus uninjured athletes without any significant strength differences found between groups. In addition to scar tissue formation, a shorter optimal length for active tension following injury may be a training effect secondary to repetitive concentric strengthening exercises as part of injury rehabilitation or normal training.[6] Eccentric strengthening of the hamstrings can produce a shift toward a longer musculotendon length and restore the hamstring muscles optimal length for active tension to a longer position.[22] Eccentric flexor torque at lengthened positions (*i.e.*, approximately 25°-5° of knee flexion) was significantly less in individuals with a history of hamstring injury within the past 12 months compared to uninjured controls.[65] The combination of a shorter musculotendon length in the hamstring complex following injury,[2] decreased flexor torque in lengthened positions,[65] and the high inertial loads placed on the hamstrings during terminal swing phase of sprinting,[17] highlights the importance of eccentric strengthening at 25° to 5° of knee flexion.

The use of eccentric strengthening in successful hamstring injury prevention programs is supported by various studies.[21,31,66,67] Mjølsnes et al.[68] highlighted the benefit of an eccentric over a concentric strengthening program in developing maximal eccentric strength. The patient is ready to progress toward eccentric strengthening when he can perform a pain-free submaximal isometric hamstring contraction. Eccentric strengthening should focus on submaximal contractions at mid-range of motion. When the athlete demonstrates 5/5 strength at 90° of knee flexion, the therapist can progress him to end-range strengthening with increased loads.[5,21,65] Examples of end-range eccentric strengthening exercises include the single-limb windmill (Fig. 10-3), single-limb chair-bridge (Fig. 10-4), single-leg deadlift (Fig. 10-5), and supine bent knee walk out (Fig. 10-6).

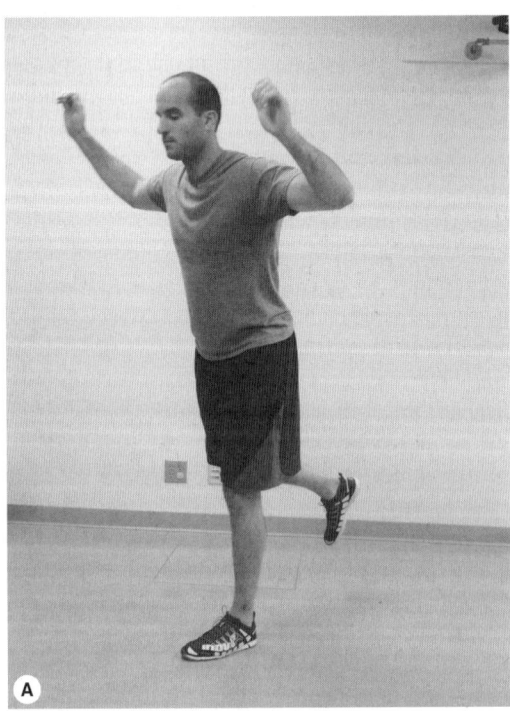

Figure 10-3. Single-leg windmills with opposite reaches. **A.** The athlete starts in single-limb stance on involved limb with shoulders abducted to 90° (handheld dumbbells can be added).

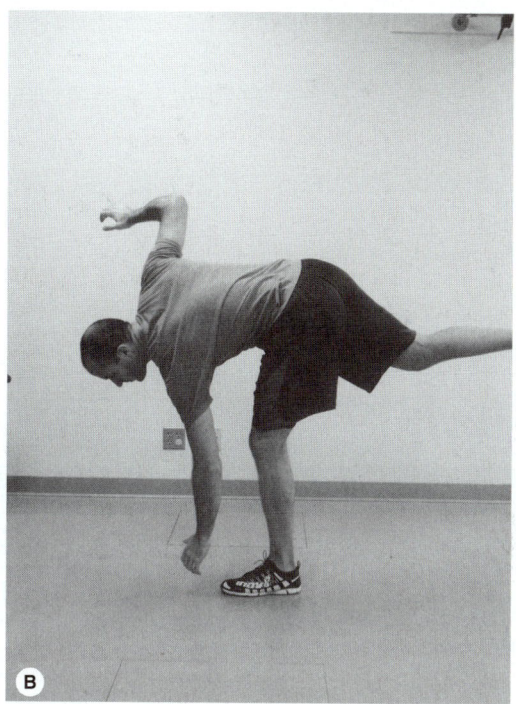

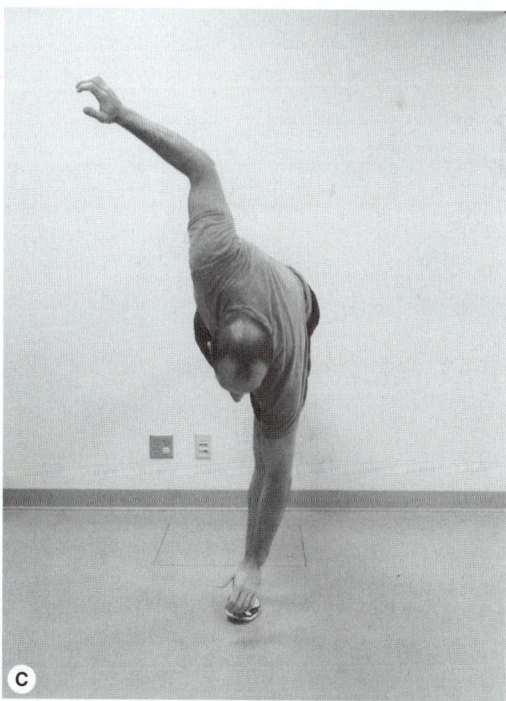

Figure 10-3. (*Continued*) Single-leg windmills with opposite reaches. **B. and C.** The athlete performs a windmill motion dropping his chest forward while rotating his arm to the floor. He should maintain slight hip and knee flexion with the goal of getting the trunk parallel to the floor. The athlete returns to the starting position and repeats the same movement with the opposite arm.

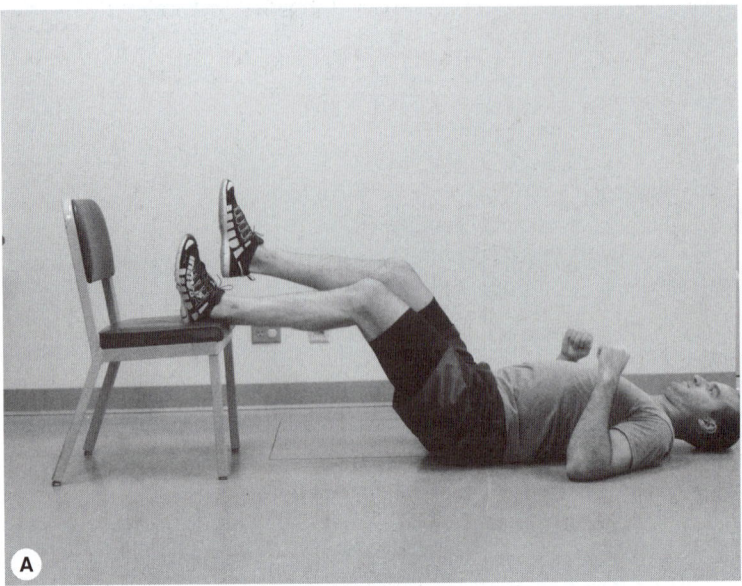

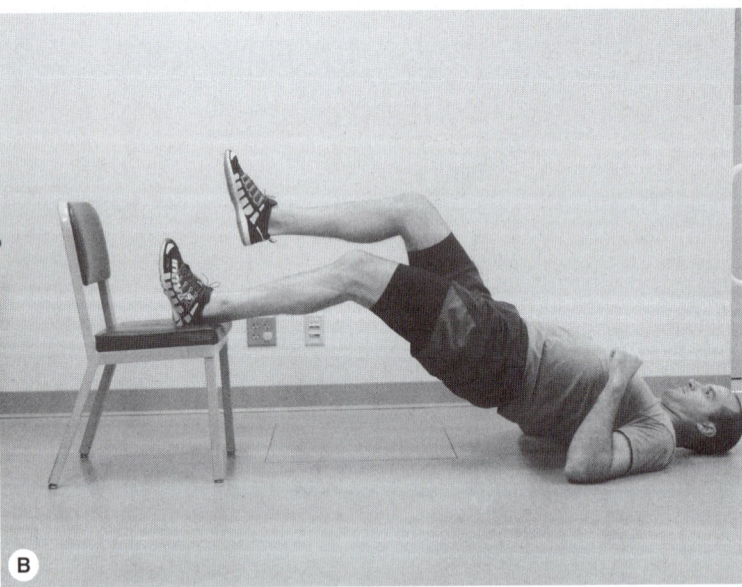

Figure 10-4. Single-limb chair-bridge. **A.** The athlete starts with involved leg on the chair. **B.** The athlete lifts his hips and pelvis off the ground, while maintaining a neutral spine and neutral hip position. He holds this position for 5 seconds and slowly lowers hips and pelvis to starting position. This movement can be performed at progressively faster speeds and at various knee flexion angles to alter hamstring length, using both legs if necessary.

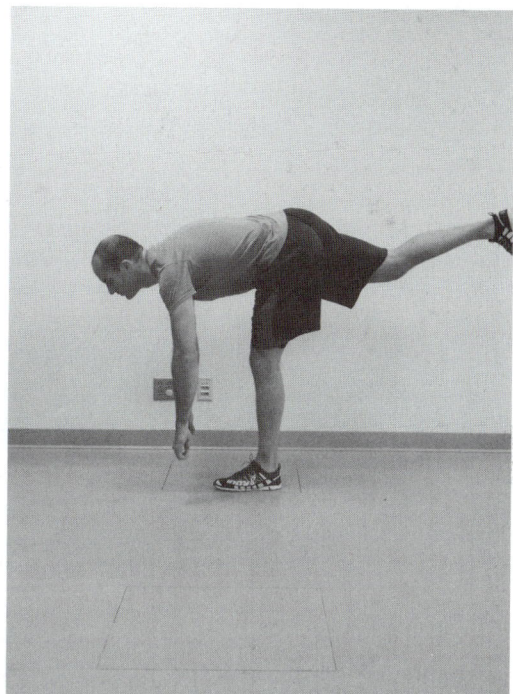

Figure 10-5. Single-limb dead lift. The athlete starts in single-limb stance position on involved extremity. While maintaining the same knee position, he flexes his trunk forward at the hips while the opposite hip extends in line with the trunk. Once tension is felt in the hamstrings, the athlete returns to the starting position.

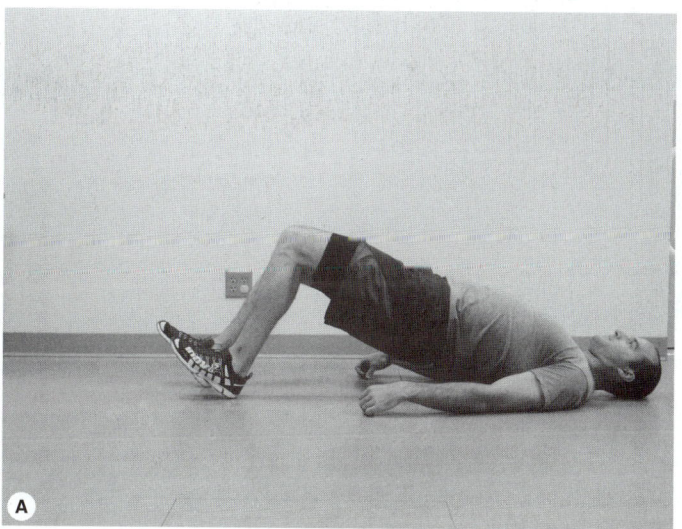

Figure 10-6. Supine bent knee walk out. **A.** The athlete starts in standard bridge position.

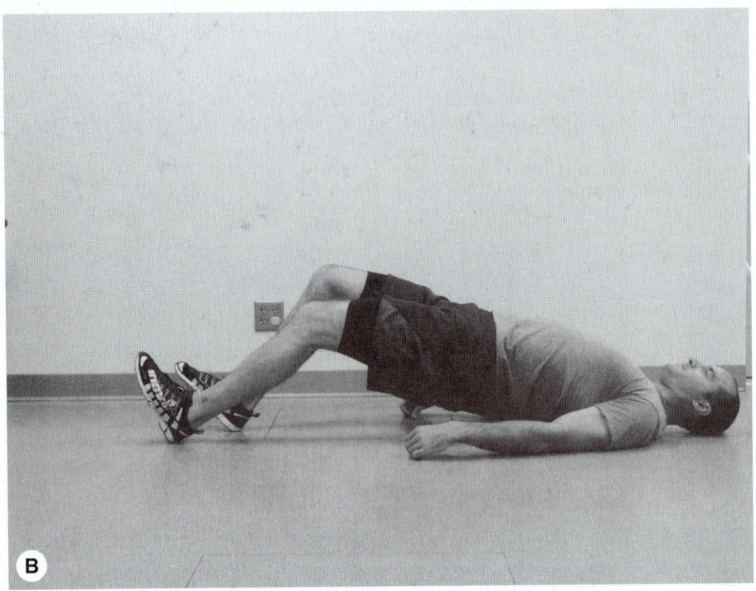

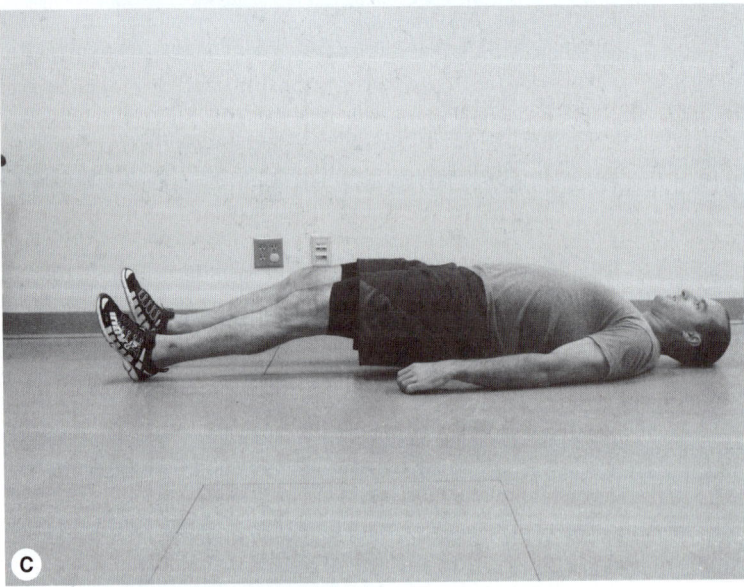

Figure 10-6. (*Continued*) Supine bent knee walk out. **B.** Athlete walks his feet away from his body, while **C.** maintaining his hips high.

The final steps in the rehabilitation process include sport-specific drills related to the athlete's sport and return-to-sport testing. Because of the high risk of re-injury when returning to sports following a hamstring strain, athletes should meet all specified criteria prior to returning to full participation.[5,7,8,26,69-71] These return-to-sport criteria include: (1) maximal, isometric strength of at least 4 repetitions at various degrees of knee flexion (*e.g.*, 90° and 15°) with medial and lateral tibial rotation bias; (2) full, pain-free hip and knee ROM; (3) isokinetic testing (if available) demonstrating less than 5% deficit of eccentric hamstring to concentric quadriceps ratio; (4) no palpable tenderness along the posterior thigh; (5) functional and sport-specific tasks without pain or apprehension; and (6) no pain or apprehension with active hamstring test. The active hamstring test is a ballistic hamstring flexibility test in which the patient is instructed to perform an active straight leg raise as fast as possible and to the greatest hip flexion angle possible without risking injury.[69] By rapidly stressing the musculotendinous structures near their end range, this test is useful in identifying an athlete's insecurities in performing the movement. For those individuals who passed a passive flexibility and standard clinical examination prior to returning to sport following a hamstring strain injury, 95% reported insecurity with the active hamstring test. Following repeated testing in 2-week increments, those who reported no insecurity with the active hamstring test remained injury-free 4 weeks after returning to sport.[69] The hop for height, hop for distance, and crossover hop have not been found to be effective return-to-sport criteria following hamstring injuries.[5] Despite the return-to-sport criteria presented in the literature, future research needs to be performed to determine the effectiveness of these criteria in preventing re-injury in addition to possible development of an evidence-based algorithm for return to sport following hamstring injuries.

The importance of return-to-sport criteria is reinforced in various imaging studies. Silder et al.[7] observed that 26% of the hamstring muscle complex's cross-sectional area based on MRI showed evidence of continued muscle injury at the time of returning to sport despite the individuals meeting the current standard criteria. Sanfilippo et al.[8] found not only residual edema on MRI at return to sport following hamstring strain injury, but also a reduction in isokinetic knee flexor torque. Both deficits resolved at 6 months following injury. The treating physical therapist must be aware that **continued morphologic and strength deficits in the muscle are likely present despite meeting or surpassing return-to-sport criteria.** Continuing with an independent progressive eccentric and lumbopelvic strengthening program following return to sport may assist the athlete in returning to prior level of performance while decreasing re-injury risk.

Evidence-Based Clinical Recommendations

SORT: Strength of Recommendation Taxonomy

A: Consistent, good-quality patient-oriented evidence
B: Inconsistent or limited-quality patient-oriented evidence
C: Consensus, disease-oriented evidence, usual practice, expert opinion, or case series

1. A thorough subjective interview and physical examination including strength testing, palpation, range of motion, and gait observation assists the physical therapist in developing a differential diagnosis, prognosis, and individualized rehabilitation plan following an acute hamstring strain. **Grade C**

2. Factors used to determine prognosis and time to return to sport following an acute hamstring strain include time to walk, distance of maximal tenderness to the ischial tuberosity, injury cross-sectional area, craniocaudal length of injury, and mechanism of injury. **Grade B**
3. Rehabilitation programs for athletes with acute hamstring injury should include exercises to improve lumbopelvic stabilization, lower extremity neuromuscular control, and eccentric hamstring strength. **Grade B**
4. Despite clearance for return to sport, athletes should continue an independent exercise program because of the persistence of morphologic changes present in the injured tissue. **Grade B**

COMPREHENSION QUESTIONS

10.1 Which of the following is the *most* appropriate treatment for an athlete following an acute hamstring strain?
   A. Eccentric hamstring strengthening from 25° to 5° of knee flexion and neuromuscular control exercises
   B. Maximal concentric hamstring strengthening
   C. Stretching exercises
   D. Passive hamstring stretching and isometric hip strengthening exercises

10.2 Based on factors demonstrated to be prognostic in estimating time needed to return to sport, which of the following athletes would you expect to return to sport the quickest?
   A. A 25-year-old male soccer player reporting a pop in the posterior thigh while kicking
   B. An 18-year-old male football player with 2 previous hamstring strain injuries reporting a sudden onset of posterior thigh pain while sprinting
   C. A 16-year-old female sprinter suffering her first hamstring strain in a 100-m race and walking off the track with a non-antalgic gait pattern
   D. A 21-year-old female ballet dancer reports a sudden onset of posterior thigh pain while moving into an extreme position of hip flexion and knee extension

10.3 A 14-year-old male presents to physical therapy with moderate right posterior thigh pain following a sprinting injury during soccer 5 days ago. He reports feeling a small pop at the time of injury, significant pain, and he was unable to continue playing. He demonstrates an antalgic gait pattern secondary to pain and reports increased pain with sitting. The active knee extension test was 35° on the uninvolved side and 20° on the involved side and straight leg raise was 80° on the uninvolved and 95° on the involved. The patient reports significant pain to palpation over the ischial tuberosity and shows no ecchymosis. Prone knee flexion strength testing at 90° and 15° was 4/5. Considering his examination findings, what would be the next step?

A. Place the patient on crutches for normalization of gait and protection of injury site, as well as refer the patient to another healthcare practitioner to obtain anteroposterior pelvic radiograph to rule out an ischial apophyseal avulsion.

B. Place the patient on crutches for normalization of gait and protection of injury site, as well as refer the patient to another healthcare practitioner to obtain anteroposterior pelvic MRI to rule out an ischial apophyseal avulsion.

C. Refer the patient to another healthcare practitioner to obtain an MRI to rule out a hamstring tendon avulsion.

D. Initiate gentle hamstring stretching and ROM exercises, and progress to concentric hamstring curl exercises as appropriate.

ANSWERS

10.1 **A.** Eccentric strengthening is needed to correct 2 commonly observed changes following hamstring strain injury: the shift in peak force development to shorter musculotendon lengths and the strength loss from 25° to 5° of knee flexion.[1,2,22] Neuromuscular control deficits including changes in muscle activation and limb proprioception occur following hamstring injury and should be addressed during physical therapy.[5,55,64] Concentric strengthening may encourage a shift toward a shorter optimal length for active tension possibly increasing injury recurrence (option B). Finally, the influence of hamstring stretching regarding injury recovery is unclear (option D).

10.2 **C.** The patient described in option C does not fit with any of the prognostic predictors for longer length of recovery and return to sport (see Table 10-2). First, she sustained the injury during sprinting, which has a shorter recovery time than excessive stretch-type injuries (options A and D). Second, this is the athlete's first hamstring injury. Recurrent hamstring injuries generally are more severe and take a longer period of time for recovery and return to sport (option B).[72,73] Finally, she immediately demonstrated a non-antalgic gait pattern; greater recovery time is expected when more than 1 day is needed for normal pain-free gait.[24]

10.3 **A.** The patient demonstrates an antalgic gait pattern due to pain so protection of the damaged tissue and normalization of gait through use of crutches is the first step when this patient is seen in clinic. Several factors present in the case are associated with the inclusion of ischial apophyseal avulsion in the differential diagnosis (see Table 10-1). First, ischial apophysis fusion occurs between the ages of 16 and 25 years, with the most likely time of injury to occur between the ages of 13 and 16 years.[5,42] Second, the patient reports tenderness and pain over the ischial tuberosity with sitting and has increased tenderness to palpation over this area.[46] Finally, he has increased motion with straight leg raising and active knee extension, which raises concern for displacement of the apophysis.

REFERENCES

1. Brockett CL, Morgan DL, Proske U. Predicting hamstring strain injury in elite athletes. *Med Sci Sports Exerc*. 2004;36:379-387.
2. Proske U, Morgan DL, Brockett CL, Percival P. Identifying athletes at risk of hamstring strains and how to protect them. *Clin Exp Pharmacol Physiol*. 2004;31:546-550.
3. Askling C, Saartok T, Thorstensson A. Type of acute hamstring strain affects flexibility, strength, and time to return to pre-injury level. *Br J Sports Med*. 2006;40:40-44.
4. Schneider-Kolsky ME, Hoving JL, Warren P, Connell DA. A comparison between clinical assessment and magnetic resonance imaging of acute hamstring injuries. *Am J Sports Med*. 2006;34:1008-1015.
5. Sherry MA, Best TM. A comparison of 2 rehabilitation programs in the treatment of acute hamstring strains. *J Orthop Sports Phys Ther*. 2004;34:116-125.
6. Heiderscheit BC, Sherry MA, Silder A, Chumanov ES, Thelen DG. Hamstring strain injuries: recommendations for diagnosis, rehabilitation, and injury prevention. *J Orthop Sports Phys Ther*. 2010;40:67-81.
7. Silder A, Sherry MA, Sanfilippo J, Tuite MJ, Hetzel SJ, Heiderscheit BC. Clinical and morphological changes following 2 rehabilitation programs for acute hamstring strain injuries: a randomized clinical trial. *J Orthop Sports Phys Ther*. 2013;43:284-299.
8. Sanfilippo JL, Silder A, Sherry MA, Tuite MJ, Heiderscheit BC. Hamstring strength and morphology progression after return to sport from injury. *Med Sci Sports Exerc*. 2013;45:448-454.
9. Feeley BT, Kennelly S, Barnes RP, et al. Epidemiology of National Football League training camp injuries from 1998 to 2007. *Am J Sports Med*. 2008;36:1597-1603.
10. Orchard J, Seward H. Epidemiology of injuries in the Australian Football League, seasons 1997-2000. *Br J Sports Med*. 2002;36:39-44.
11. Ekstrand J, Hagglund M, Walden M. Epidemiology of muscle injuries in professional football (soccer). *Am J Sports Med*. 2011;39:1226-1232.
12. Koulouris G, Connell D. Hamstring muscle complex: an imaging review. *Radiographics*. 2005;25:571-586.
13. Askling CM, Tengvar M, Saartok T, Thorstensson A. Acute first-time hamstring strains during slow-speed stretching: clinical, magnetic resonance imaging, and recovery characteristics. *Am J Sports Med*. 2007;35:1716-1724.
14. Askling CM, Tengvar M, Saartok T, Thorstensson A. Acute first-time hamstring strains during high-speed running: a longitudinal study including clinical and magnetic resonance imaging findings. *Am J Sports Med*. 2007;35:197-206.
15. Heiderscheit BC, Hoerth DM, Chumanov ES, Swanson SC, Thelen BJ, Thelen DG. Identifying the time of occurrence of a hamstring strain injury during treadmill running: a case study. *Clin Biomech (Bristol, Avon)*. 2005;20:1072-1078.
16. Schache AG, Wrigley TV, Baker R, Pandy MG. Biomechanical response to hamstring muscle strain injury. *Gait Posture*. 2009;29:332-338.
17. Chumanov ES, Heiderscheit BC, Thelen DG. The effect of speed and influence of individual muscles on hamstring mechanics during the swing phase of sprinting. *J Biomech*. 2007;40:3555-3562.
18. Chumanov ES, Heiderscheit BC, Thelen DG. Hamstring musculotendon dynamics during stance and swing phases of high-speed running. *Med Sci Sports Exerc*. 2011;43:525-532.
19. Thelen DG, Chumanov ES, Sherry MA, Heiderscheit BC. Neuromusculoskeletal models provide insights into the mechanisms and rehabilitation of hamstring strains. *Exerc Sport Sci Rev*. 2006;34:135-141.
20. Thelen DG, Chumanov ES, Best TM, Swanson SC, Heiderscheit BC. Simulation of biceps femoris musculotendon mechanics during the swing phase of sprinting. *Med Sci Sports Exerc*. 2005;37:1931-1938.

21. Askling CM, Tengvar M, Thorstensson A. Acute hamstring injuries in Swedish elite football: a prospective randomised controlled clinical trial comparing two rehabilitation protocols. *Br J Sports Med.* 2014;48:532-539.
22. Brockett CL, Morgan DL, Proske U. Human hamstring muscles adapt to eccentric exercise by changing optimum length. *Med Sci Sports Exerc.* 2001;33:783-790.
23. Askling CM, Tengvar M, Saartok T, Thorstensson A. Proximal hamstring strains of stretching type in different sports: injury situations, clinical and magnetic resonance imaging characteristics, and return to sport. *Am J Sports Med.* 2008;36:1799-1804.
24. Warren P, Gabbe BJ, Schneider-Kolsky M, Bennell KL. Clinical predictors of time to return to competition and of recurrence following hamstring strain in elite Australian footballers. *Br J Sports Med.* 2010;44:415-419.
25. Gabbe BJ, Bennell KL, Finch CF, Wajswelner H, Orchard JW. Predictors of hamstring injury at the elite level of Australian football. *Scand J Med Sci Sports.* 2006;16:7-13.
26. Verrall GM, Slavotinek JP, Barnes PG, Fon GT, Spriggins AJ. Clinical risk factors for hamstring muscle strain injury: a prospective study with correlation of injury by magnetic resonance imaging. *Br J Sports Med.* 2001;35:435-440.
27. Engebretsen AH, Myklebust G, Holme I, Engebretsen L, Bahr R. Intrinsic risk factors for hamstring injuries among male soccer players: a prospective cohort study. *Am J Sports Med.* 2010;38:1147-1153.
28. Croisier JL, Ganteaume S, Binet J, Genty M, Ferret JM. Strength imbalances and prevention of hamstring injury in professional soccer players: a prospective study. *Am J Sports Med.* 2008;36:1469-1475.
29. Yeung SS, Suen AM, Yeung EW. A prospective cohort study of hamstring injuries in competitive sprinters: preseason muscle imbalance as a possible risk factor. *Br J Sports Med.* 2009;43:589-594.
30. Orchard JW, Best TM. The managment of muscle strain injuries:an early return versus the risk of recurrence. *Clin J Sport Med.* 2002;12:3-5.
31. Arnason A, Andersen TE, Holme I, Engebretsen L, Bahr R. Prevention of hamstring strains in elite soccer: an intervention study. *Scand J Med Sci Sports.* 2008;18:40-48.
32. Bennell K, Tully E, Harvey N. Does the toe-touch test predict hamstring injury in Australian Rules footballers? *Aust J Physiother.* 1999;45:103-109.
33. Malliaropoulos N, Papalexandris S, Papalada A, Papacostas E. The role of stretching in rehabilitation of hamstring injuries: 80 athletes follow-up. *Med Sci Sports Exerc.* 2004;36:756-759.
34. Gabbe BJ, Bennell KL, Finch CF. Why are older Australian football players at greater risk of hamstring injury? *J Sci Med Sport.* 2006;9:327-333.
35. Orchard JW. Intrinsic and extrinsic risk factors for muscle strains in Australian football. *Am J Sports Med.* 2001;29:300-303.
36. Doherty TJ. The influence of aging and sex on skeletal muscle mass and strength. *Curr Opin Clin Nutr Metab Care.* 2001;4:503-508.
37. Gabbe BJ, Finch CF, Wajswelner H, Bennell KL. Predictors of lower extremity injuries at the community level of Australian football. *Clin J Sport Med.* 2004;14:56-63.
38. Cameron ML, Adams RD, Maher CG, Misson D. Effect of the HamSprint Drills training programme on lower limb neuromuscular control in Australian football players. *J Sci Med Sport.* 2007;12:24-30.
39. Clanton TO, Coupe KJ. Hamstring strains in athletes: diagnosis and treatment. *J Am Acad Orthop Surg.* 1998;6:237-248.
40. Cohen S, Bradley J. Acute proximal hamstring rupture. *J Am Acad Orthop Surg.* 2007;15:350-355.
41. Orchard JW, Farhart P, Leopold C. Lumbar spine region pathology and hamstring and calf injuries in athletes: is there a connection? *Br J Sports Med.* 2004;38:502-504.

42. Servant CT, Jones CB. Displaced avulsion of the ischial apophysis: a hamstring injury requiring internal fixation. *Br J Sports Med*. 1998;32:255-257.
43. Gidwani S, Bircher MD. Avulsion injuries of the hamstring origin - a series of 12 patients and management algorithm. *Ann R Coll Surg Engl*. 2007;89:394-399.
44. Konan S, Haddad F. Successful return to high level sports following early surgical repair of complete tears of the proximal hamstring tendons. *Int Orthop*. 2010;34:119-123.
45. Sarimo J, Lempainen L, Mattila K, Orava S. Complete proximal hamstring avulsions: a series of 41 patients with operative treatment. *Am J Sports Med*. 2008;36:1110-1115.
46. Sherry M. Examination and treatment of hamstring related injuries. *Sports Health*. 2012;4:107-114.
47. Turl SE, George KP. Adverse neural tension: a factor in repetitive hamstring strain? *J Orthop Sports Phys Ther*. 1998;27:16-21.
48. Kornberg C, Lew P. The effect of stretching neural structures on grade one hamstring injuries. *J Orthop Sports Phys Ther*. 1989;10:481-487.
49. Hosey RG, Fernandez MM, Johnson DL. Evaluation and management of stress fractures of the pelvis and sacrum. *Orthopedics*. 2008;31:383-385.
50. Cacchio A, Borra F, Severini G, et al. Reliability and validity of three pain provocation tests used for the diagnosis of chronic proximal hamstring tendinopathy. *Br J Sports Med*. 2012;46:883-887.
51. Cacchio A, Rompe JD, Furia JP, Susi P, Santilli V, De Paulis F. Shockwave therapy for the treatment of chronic proximal hamstring tendinopathy in professional athletes. *Am J Sports Med*. 2011;39:146-153.
52. Lempainen L, Sarimo J, Mattila K, Vaittinen S, Orava S. Proximal hamstring tendinopathy: results of surgical management and histopathologic findings. *Am J Sports Med*. 2009;37:727-734.
53. Maffey L, Emery C. What are the risk factors for groin strain injury in sport? A systematic review of the literature. *Sports Med*. 2007;37:881-894.
54. Malliaropoulos N, Isinkaye T, Tsitas K, Maffulli N. Reinjury after acute posterior thigh muscle injuries in elite track and field athletes. *Am J Sports Med*. 2011;39:304-310.
55. Sole G, Milosavljevic S, Nicholson H, Sullivan SJ. Altered muscle activation following hamstring injuries. *Br J Sports Med*. 2011;46:118-123.
56. Davis DS, Quinn RO, Whiteman CT, Williams JD, Young CR. Concurrent validity of four clinical tests used to measure hamstring flexibility. *J Strength Cond Res*. 2008;22:583-588.
57. Magee DJ. *Orthopedic Physical Assessment*. 5th ed. Philadelphia, PA: WB Saunders Company; 2008.
58. Reurink G, Goudswaard GJ, Oomen HG, et al. Reliability of the active and passive knee extension test in acute hamstring injuries. *Am J Sports Med*. 2013;41:1757-1761.
59. Connell DA, Schneider-Kolsky ME, Hoving JL, et al. Longitudinal study comparing sonographic and MRI assessments of acute and healing hamstring injuries. *AJR Am J Roentgenol*. 2004;183:975-984.
60. Slavotinek JP, Verrall GM, Fon GT. Hamstring injury in athletes: using MR imaging measurements to compare extent of muscle injury with amount of time lost from competition. *AJR Am J Roentgenol*. 2002;179:1621-1628.
61. Järvinen MJ, Lehto MU. The effects of early mobilisation and immobilisation on the healing process following muscle injuries. *Sports Med*. 1993;15:78-89.
62. Järvinen TA, Järvinen TL, Kääriäinen M, et al. Muscle injuries: optimising recovery. *Best Pract Res Clin Rheumatol*. 2007;21:317-331.
63. Kääriäinen M, Järvinen T, Järvinen M, Rantanen J, Kalimo H. Relation between myofibers and connective tissue during muscle injury repair. *Scand J Med Sci Sports*. 2000;10:332-337.
64. Cameron M, Adams R, Maher C. Motor control and strength as predictors of hamstring injury in elite players of Australian football. *Phys Ther Sport*. 2003;4:159-166.
65. Sole G, Milosavljevic S, Nicholson HD, Sullivan SJ. Selective strength loss and decreased muscle activity in hamstring injury. *J Orthop Sports Phys Ther*. 2011;41:354-363.

66. Askling C, Karlsson J, Thorstensson A. Hamstring injury occurrence in elite soccer players after preseason strength training with eccentric overload. *Scand J Med Sci Sports.* 2003;13:244-250.
67. Gabbe BJ, Branson R, Bennell KL. A pilot randomised controlled trial of eccentric exercise to prevent hamstring injuries in community-level Australian Football. *J Sci Med Sport.* 2006;9:103-109.
68. Mjølsnes R, Arnason A, Osthagen T, Raastad T, Bahr R. A 10-week randomized trial comparing eccentric vs. concentric hamstring strength training in well-trained soccer players. *Scand J Med Sci Sports.* 2004;14:311-317.
69. Askling CM, Nilsson J, Thorstensson A. A new hamstring test to complement the common clinical examination before return to sport after injury. *Knee Surg Sports Traumatol Arthrosc.* 2010;18:1798-1803.
70. Croisier JL, Forthomme B, Namurois MH, Vanderthommen M, Crielaard JM. Hamstring muscle strain recurrence and strength performance disorders. *Am J Sports Med.* 2002;30:199-203.
71. Orchard J, Best TM, Verrall GM. Return to play following muscle strains. *Clin J Sport Med.* 2005;15:436-441.
72. Koulouris G, Connell DA, Brukner P, Schneider-Kolsky M. Magnetic resonance imaging parameters for assessing risk of recurrent hamstring injuries in elite athletes. *Am J Sports Med.* 2007;35:1500-1506.
73. Brooks JH, Fuller CW, Kemp SP, Reddin DB. Incidence, risk, and prevention of hamstring muscle injuries in professional rugby union. *Am J Sports Med.* 2006;34:1297-1306.

Hamstring Tendinopathy: Postoperative Management

Daniel Cooper
Jonathan Eng
Jason James
Timothy Mansour

CASE 11

On New Year's Day, an active 35-year-old female suffered a proximal hamstring avulsion at the osteotendinous junction while cross-country skiing. The injury occurred when her ski suddenly crossed over a section of ice. She fell with her left lower extremity in extreme hip flexion and knee extension. She immediately experienced pain in her left posterior thigh and buttock and was unable to walk without assistance from another individual. A magnetic resonance imaging (MRI) scan performed 2 days after the injury revealed a complete avulsion of the left hamstring from the ischial tuberosity with retraction of 5 cm. Sixteen days after the injury, she underwent a left proximal hamstring repair. Two bioabsorbable anchors were placed into the ischial tuberosity, and 4 sutures were passed through the common proximal hamstring tendon to secure the hamstrings. The surgical team also performed a neurolysis of the sciatic nerve to remove scar tissue and free adhesions. She followed a proximal hamstring repair protocol outlined by her surgeon. Nine months after surgery, the patient presented for a physical therapy evaluation to address persistent focal pain at the left ischial tuberosity that she experiences with sitting and with exertion during running and cycling. At rest, she rates her pain as 0/10 on the numeric pain rating scale. However, during prolonged sitting or sport, the pain reaches 5/10 at its worst. She reports a sitting tolerance of less than 10 minutes. Her pain is relieved with cessation of provocative activity and with prolonged stretching of the affected hamstring. She currently participates in 4 group exercise boot-camp style classes per week. Prior to the injury, she was a competitive marathon runner and cyclocross racer. Her goals are to return to running and cycling without pain, with a focus on returning to cyclocross racing.

- Based on the patient's diagnosis, surgical intervention, and rehabilitation timeline, what do you anticipate may be the contributing factors to her condition?
- What examination signs may be associated with this diagnosis?
- What are the most appropriate physical therapy interventions at this stage of recovery?
- What complications may limit the effectiveness of physical therapy?

KEY DEFINITIONS

CYCLOCROSS RACING: Form of bicycle racing that blends road riding and mountain biking. Races typically last 45 minutes on a track that includes both paved and dirt sections, short steep climbs, and obstacles that can only be navigated by dismounting and carrying the bike. This is an aerobic event, but involves many bouts of anaerobic activity with sections that require significant lower extremity muscle power.

OSTEOTENDINOUS AVULSION: Tearing of the muscle tendon fibers from the bony insertion

TENDINOPATHY: Clinical term that encompasses all overuse conditions that affect tendons and is characterized by chronic pain and weakness; affected tendon presents with specific histological changes.

Objectives

1. Identify risk factors for a hamstring strain and an avulsion injury.
2. Identify appropriate medical referral and diagnostic imaging that should be performed to assess for a potential avulsion injury.
3. Describe evidence-based or best practice interventions for an individual with a hamstring avulsion repair and subsequent tendinopathy.
4. Describe appropriate criteria for advancement through return-to-sport testing protocol.

Physical Therapy Considerations

PT considerations for management of the individual with a surgically repaired hamstring after an avulsion injury:

- **General physical therapy plan of care/goals:** Decrease pain; restore pain-free range of motion (ROM) and muscular flexibility; increase hip muscular strength and endurance; maintain aerobic capacity
- **Physical therapy interventions:** Patient education related to anatomy, surgical procedure, and rehabilitation protocol; manual therapy to restore ROM and joint mobility; muscular flexibility exercises; resistance training to increase hip strength to improve dynamic stability; core and lower extremity strength and endurance training to improve stability and power
- **Precautions during physical therapy:** Consideration of postsurgical timeline regarding tissue healing properties and appropriate selection and dosage of therapeutic exercise
- **Complications interfering with physical therapy:** Patient noncompliance with initial precautions and subsequent plan of care; premature phase progression; poor tissue healing; psychosocial challenges (*e.g.*, influence from other athletes, fear

of re-injury, unrealistic view of current abilities, prior experience/knowledge of physical therapy)

Understanding the Health Condition

The hamstring muscle group consists of 3 muscles: semitendinosus, semimembranosus, and biceps femoris. These muscles originate proximally at the ischial tuberosity and insert distally at the medial tibia and lateral fibula. Table 11-1 lists the specific attachments of the individual muscles. In general, concentric hamstring activation flexes the knee or contributes to hip extension. If the lower extremities are fixed (*i.e.*, in contact with the ground), the hamstring muscle group can assist in posteriorly tilting the pelvis and extending the hips. When the knee is flexed, the hamstrings can either internally rotate (via contraction of the semitendinosus and semimembranosus) or externally rotate (via contraction of the biceps femoris) the lower leg. The long head of the biceps femoris can also assist in hip adduction.[1]

The primary mechanism for a hamstring injury is a sudden eccentric overload when the muscles are lengthened to their end range.[2-5] At maximum hip flexion and knee extension, significant tension is placed on the hamstrings as the knee decelerates. Hamstring tendon avulsions are observed in about 8% of all hamstring injuries.[6] The most common sports resulting in a hamstring avulsion include cross-country skiing, downhill skiing, and water skiing.[2,5] Hamstring avulsions have also been reported in American football and in sprinting.[2] In adolescents, it is more common to have an apophyseal avulsion fracture in which the ischial apophysis is displaced. Once the apophysis has fused (around the age of 25 years), it becomes more common for the tendon to avulse from the bone.[4,5]

When an ischial avulsion occurs, surgical reattachment is recommended if the avulsed mass is more than 2 cm retracted.[7-9] Individuals with complete tendon avulsions who have undergone surgical repair experience improvements in muscular

Table 11-1 ORIGINS AND INSERTIONS OF THE HAMSTRINGS

Muscle	Origin	Insertion	Concentric Muscle Action
Biceps femoris	Long head: ischial tuberosity Short head: linea aspera and lateral supracondylar line	Fibular head	Knee flexion Lateral rotation of the tibia on the femur Hip extension (long head)
Semimembranosus	Ischial tuberosity	Medial tibial condyle	Knee flexion Hip extension Medial rotation of tibia on the femur
Semitendinosus	Ischial tuberosity	Superior medial tibia	Knee flexion Hip extension Medial rotation of tibia on the femur

strength and endurance, report high patient satisfaction scores, and have a good chance to return to sport.[10-12] Surgical repair also decreases the incidence of chronic pain and disability resulting from this injury.[10-13] In a systematic review including 286 proximal hamstring avulsions managed surgically and 14 managed nonoperatively, 82% of those who had surgical intervention were able to return to sport at their pre-injury level compared to only 14% of those who were managed conservatively.[14]

Hamstring avulsions may initially be misdiagnosed as strains. If the therapist is concerned that a patient may have an avulsion, it is critical to refer the patient to an orthopaedist for requisite follow-up and imaging because early surgical repair (within the first month after avulsion) lessens the chance that the sciatic nerve will be damaged.[5,13] With chronic hamstring avulsions, sciatic nerve damage can occur due to the formation of scar tissue that can adhere the nerve to the tendon.[5,10,13] Whenever possible, the physical therapist should obtain an operative report to review the specific procedures performed and to gain an awareness of the state of the tissues involved. For example, it is common practice for the orthopaedic surgeon to identify the sciatic nerve during the surgery and to perform a neurolysis to remove scar tissue from the sciatic nerve.[4,13]

Physical Therapy Patient/Client Management

Rehabilitation considerations following a hamstring avulsion repair include the current state and health of the involved tissues and the patient's functional limitations, environmental factors, and sport-specific considerations. To determine the health of the healing tissue and facilitate prognosis, the physical therapist considers the patient's age and comorbidities, time since surgery, surgical report (noting the presence of adhesions or scar tissue), subsequent imaging, and subjective patient reports. In a retrospective cohort study of 11 adults with complete hamstring avulsions, 7 of 9 athletically active subjects returned to sport an average of 6 months following surgical repair and postoperative physical therapy.[10] More recently, Cohen et al.[12] reported on a case series of 52 adults who underwent proximal hamstring repair, with 40 having acute repairs and 12 having chronic repairs. All subjects participated in a 6- to 8-week rehabilitation protocol that included the use of a hip brace, progressive weightbearing, ROM exercises, and progressive isotonic exercises.[12] The average time for return to sport was 6.6 months after surgery. Return to sport should be based on functional outcome measures including hamstring strength, hamstring length, and sport-specific activities rather than a specific timeframe. By basing return to sport on the functional capacity of the individual's hamstrings, the risk of re-injury may be reduced.[15]

Examination, Evaluation, and Diagnosis

Acute hamstring injuries are painful and typically result in extensive bruising on the posterior thigh and the buttock. In complete rupture, patients often report that they felt the tendon rupture or heard a "pop" or "snap" immediately accompanied by pain and weakness. The physical therapist may be able to palpate a defect distal to the ischial tuberosity when the tendon has completely avulsed; however, this may be difficult to detect if there is significant edema. If an avulsion is suspected, the therapist should quickly refer the patient to an orthopaedic surgeon[5,10-13] to determine the integrity of the tendon and facilitate swift surgical repair, if indicated. The **gold standard to diagnose hamstring tissue injury** in adults is MRI.[16]

The initial physical therapy evaluation typically occurs 7 to 10 days after proximal hamstring tendon repair. At this time, the patient would still be following the surgeon's postoperative protocol and should be arriving to the physical therapy clinic with a brace and ambulating with an assistive device. The patient in this case failed to comply with the orthopaedic surgeon's referral to physical therapy and chose to self-manage her rehabilitation. Thus, she initially presented to physical therapy for an evaluation 9 months after surgery to address persistent pain and weakness. Because of the atypical timeframe of the evaluation, she had no post-surgical precautions and a standard orthopaedic evaluation was completed. The evaluation includes a detailed subjective examination, objective measures of impairments (strength, ROM, hamstring length, muscle girth), functional limitations, and functional assessments (single-leg balance and single-leg hop tests). Because of the close proximity and frequent involvement of the sciatic nerve in hamstring avulsions, a neurologic screen, including strength, sensation, and reflexes of the lower extremities, should be performed.

During the subjective portion of the examination, the therapist should inquire about pain frequency, intensity, duration, and location as well as sitting tolerance, current level of activity, general activity tolerance, sport-specific activity tolerance, and patient-specific goals. Strength assessment includes manual muscle testing (MMT) of hip and knee musculature as well as observation of functional movements. For example, observing a Trendelenburg sign during stance phase in gait, lack of lower extremity and lumbopelvic control with forward step-downs, and/or medial knee deviation with single-leg squats may indicate functional lower extremity, hip, and core weakness. ROM, strength, palpation, and functional stability should be compared to the unaffected side. Muscle length of the hamstrings can be assessed with a 90/90 hamstring test (Fig. 11-1). The 90/90 test is performed with the patient in the supine position. The therapist moves the lower extremity into 90° of hip flexion with a fully flexed knee and then extends the knee until a soft end feel is appreciated. The knee flexion angle is measured and represents hamstring length. Girth measurements of the thigh and palpation of the hamstrings from the popliteal fossa to the ischial tuberosity should be performed bilaterally. Table 11-2 presents subjective and objective findings for the patient in this case.

Sport-specific activities should be assessed. In this case, a running and cycling assessment would be appropriate because the patient's primary goal was to return to pain-free running and cyclocross racing. Initially, the single-leg squat and single-leg hop test were used to evaluate the dynamic control of her lower extremity and pelvis. A single-leg hop test was used to assess the highest level of dynamic lumbopelvic stability and lower extremity motor control under load of body weight impact. A single-leg squat was used to assess deliberate fine motor control and balance strategies of the pelvis and lower extremity more similar to the demands cycling. A bike fit and cycling assessment were performed during the next therapy session (see Case 13).

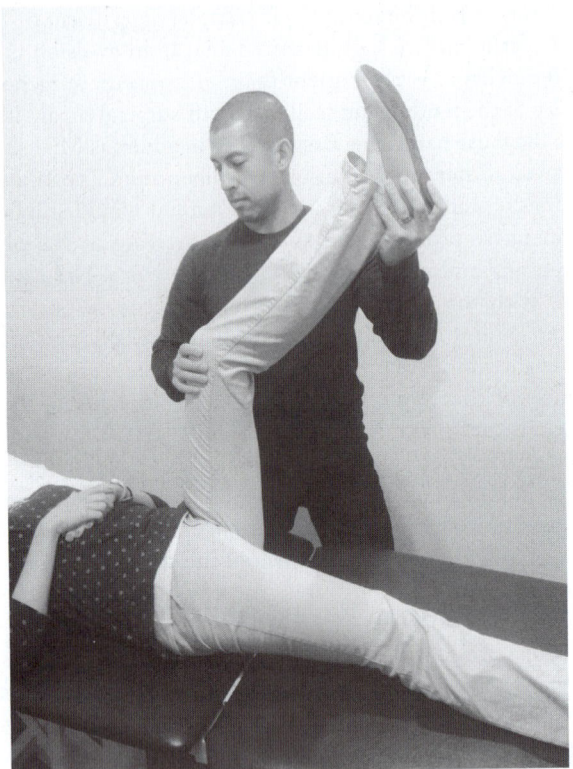

Figure 11-1. A 90-90 muscle length test for the hamstrings.

Table 11-2	FINDINGS FROM THE PHYSICAL THERAPY EXAMINATION
Subjective complaints	Decreased sitting tolerance (<10 minutes) Pain with exercise
Range of motion (ROM)	Decreased left hip extension, internal and external rotation Decreased left hamstring length
Flexibility	Decreased flexibility of left tensor fascia latae
Strength	Left hip abductors 4/5; left knee flexors 3/5
Functional movement	Increased lateral trunk lean and medial collapse of left lower extremity during single-leg squat
Palpation	Tender to palpation on left ischial tuberosity

Plan of Care and Interventions

The primary goal following surgical reattachment of the proximal hamstring is to promote successful healing and prevent re-injury. **Postoperative rehabilitation** programs are variable, primarily determined by surgeon preference. Most orthopaedic surgeons support immediate postoperative immobilization for 4 weeks (using a

Table 11-3 POSTOPERATIVE REHABILITATION PROTOCOL

Time After Surgery	Precautions/Progression
Days 1-10	NWB
Days 10-14	TTWB, initiation of PROM
Week 3	25% WB, initiation of AROM
Week 4	50% WB Discontinue use of spica brace Limited CKC resistance exercise and core pelvic strength training
Week 5	Full WB
Week 10	Initiation of jogging and sport-specific training program

Abbreviations: AROM, active range of motion; CKC, closed kinetic chain; NWB, non-weightbearing; PROM, passive range of motion; TTWB, toe-touch weightbearing; WB, weightbearing.

hip spica brace that prevents hip flexion) and non-weightbearing on the surgical limb with progression to weightbearing as tolerated (WBAT) at 4 to 6 weeks after surgery. Initiation of resistance training can usually commence 6 weeks after surgery. Table 11-3 outlines a general timelined postoperative rehabilitation protocol after surgical reattachment of the proximal hamstring.

The patient in this case progressed from non-weightbearing to full weightbearing after 5 weeks, began progressive closed kinetic chain (CKC) hamstring and core strengthening at 6 weeks, and at 10 weeks initiated sport-specific training. She progressed herself through exercises independently. At approximately 9 months after surgery, the patient's primary complaints were weakness, pain, and sitting intolerance. During the examination, the therapist noted palpable tenderness of the left ischial tuberosity, painful weakness of left knee flexion, weakness of left hip abduction, decreased left dorsiflexion and bilateral hip internal and external ROM, decreased left hamstring flexibility, and poor trunk stability during the single-leg squat (see Table 11-2). Thus, physical therapy interventions were designed to decrease tenderness, improve strength and ROM, and improve sitting tolerance to allow the patient to return to full participation in running and cyclocross.

On average, individuals can expect to return to sport 6 months after surgical repair of the proximal hamstring.[10,12] It is critical for the therapist to educate the patient that surgically repaired tendon will never regain its original tensile strength, but will reach its *optimal* strength 1 year after surgery.[17] One prospective study of 11 subjects reported an average of 91% return of hamstring muscle strength when compared to the healthy hamstring,[10] whereas another retrospective study of 15 subjects reported injured hamstring strength recovered only up to 78% of the contralateral side 3 years post-surgery.[11] To reduce the risk of re-injury, **return to sport** should be based on functional criteria, including hamstring strength, hamstring length, and sport-specific activities as opposed to a certain timeframe.[15] Thirty-seven sports medicine physicians from the French and Belgian male professional soccer clubs have ordinally ranked the following return-to-play criteria after hamstring injury: complete pain relief, muscle strength performance, subjective feeling reported by player, muscle flexibility, and sport-specific test performance.[18] Although this patient is not a soccer player, the previously discussed 5 criteria helped guide the therapist to make an informed decision in the best interest of the patient and her specific goals.

It is important to understand that individuals with surgical hamstring repairs are rehabilitating from significant tissue injury that can be associated with chronic complications such as tendinopathy. Tendinopathy is a common clinical condition characterized by pain during activity, localized tenderness upon palpation, swelling of the tendon, and impaired performance.[19] MRI studies have demonstrated **tendinopathy** in 25% of patients at an average of 3 years after proximal hamstring repair.[11,19] At the cellular level, tendinopathy is currently understood as tendon with matrix disturbances due to "failed healing" leading to focal hypervascularity, neoneuralization, and increased cytokine concentration.[20] Functionally, an individual with hamstring tendinopathy may present with pain, weakness, sitting intolerance, activity intolerance, and fatigue of the involved hamstring. Mild reports of pain in a sciatic nerve distribution, specifically the posterior buttock, and discomfort at the ischial tuberosity are common.[10-12]

In this case, the patient's symptoms are consistent with tendinopathy of the repaired tendon. **Eccentric loading** of the muscle and tendon during rehabilitation can increase collagen synthesis and upregulate collagen expression.[19] Optimal synthesis of collagen occurs between 2 and 4 days after exercise.[19] In soccer players, the Nordic hamstring curl exercise reduced hamstring injury risk and prevented hamstring re-injury by 70% compared to general training with no specific hamstring intervention.[21] To perform this exercise, the patient begins in tall kneeling with ankles plantar flexed and the feet held securely on the floor either by placing the feet under a fixed support or with someone kneeling over the feet to prevent them from lifting off the floor during the exercise. Maintaining erect posture from head to knees, the patient leans forward in a slow and controlled manner (Fig. 11-2A). The patient lowers the upper body toward the floor, keeping the trunk as straight as possible (Fig. 11-2B) and breaking impact with the floor by using outstretched hands to push up and return to the start position. This movement pattern is repeated for the desired number of repetitions.

While eccentric loading of the hamstring has the strongest level of evidence for treating tendinopathy[19] and reducing the risk of re-injury,[21] other interventions for the rehabilitation of hamstring injuries have been investigated. In a study of 24 athletes with acute hamstring strain, athletes were assigned to a protocol of static stretching, isolated progressive hamstring resistance exercise, and icing (STST group) or a protocol of progressive agility and trunk stabilization exercises and icing (PATS group). At both 2 weeks and 1 year after returning to sport, the STST group demonstrated a significantly greater re-injury rate compared to the PATS group,[22] indicating that incorporation of agility and trunk stabilization exercises was important in injury risk reduction. Progressive plyometric training has also been found to be effective in promoting return to sports and preventing recurrent injuries.[23] Thus, interventions should include eccentric loading on the affected limb, lumbopelvic control/proprioception exercises, and progressive agility/plyometric training.[22-24] Last, the physical therapist should consider incorporating sport-specific movements and demands required for a return to participation in sports.[15] For the patient in this case, eccentric loading using the Nordic hamstring exercise, rapid ankle-weighted kicks in standing with slight hip flexion

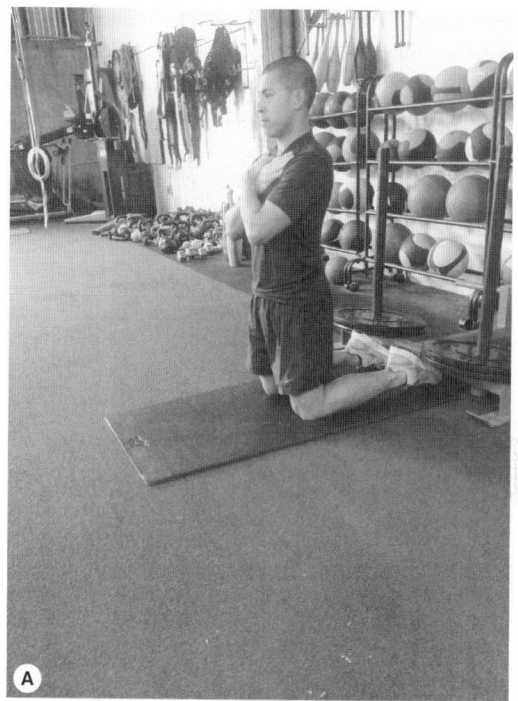
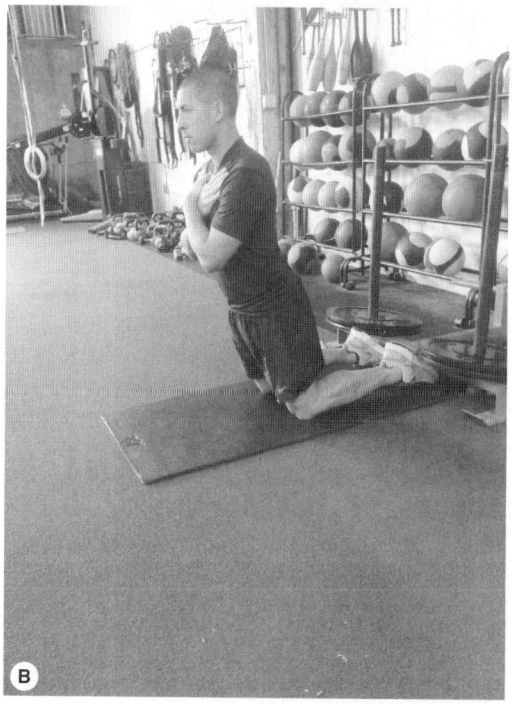

Figure 11-2. Nordic hamstring curl exercise. **A.** Starting position. **B.** Lowering body toward the floor.

(Fig. 11-3), and supine straight leg cable eccentrics (Fig. 11-4) were implemented. Single-leg stance exercises were prescribed to improve balance and lumbopelvic control. High hurdle lateral step-overs (Fig. 11-5) and a high-speed running overload program were prescribed near the end of the rehabilitation program to prepare the athlete to return to sport.[23]

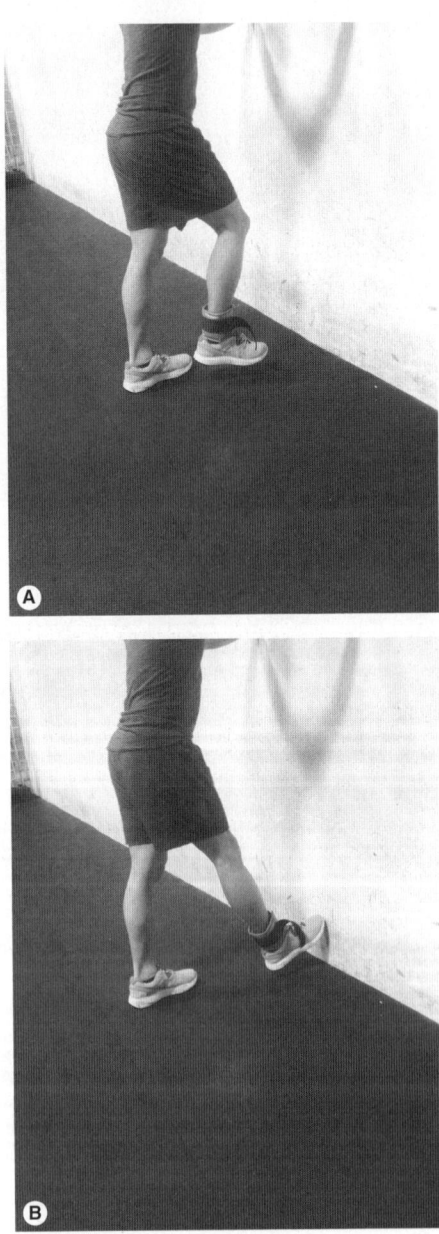

Figure 11-3. Rapid ankle-weighted kicks in standing. **A.** Starting position. **B.** Ending position.

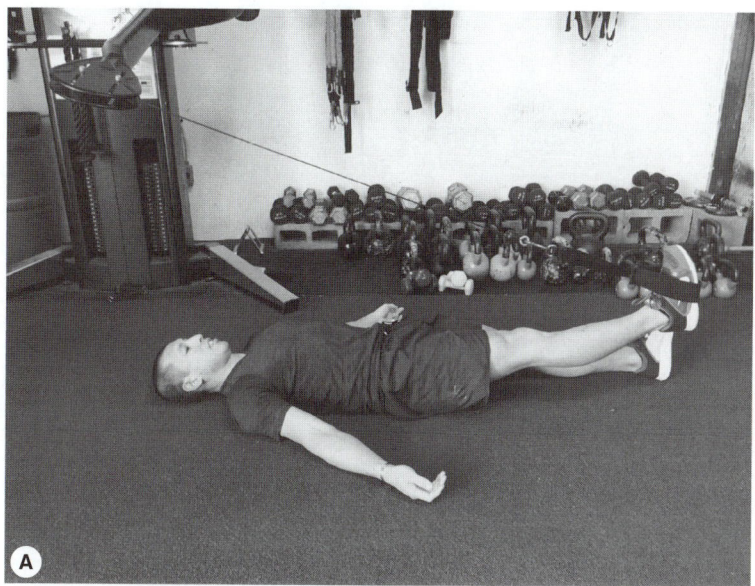
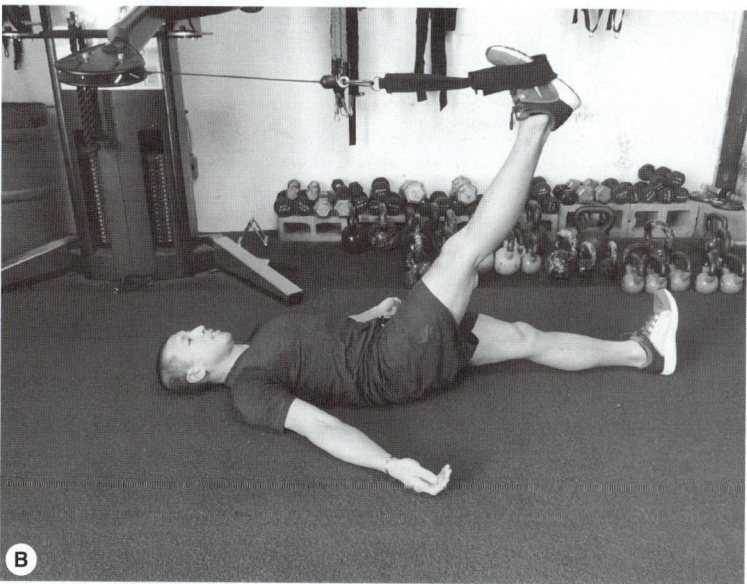

Figure 11-4. Supine straight leg cable eccentric exercise. **A.** Starting position. **B.** Ending position.

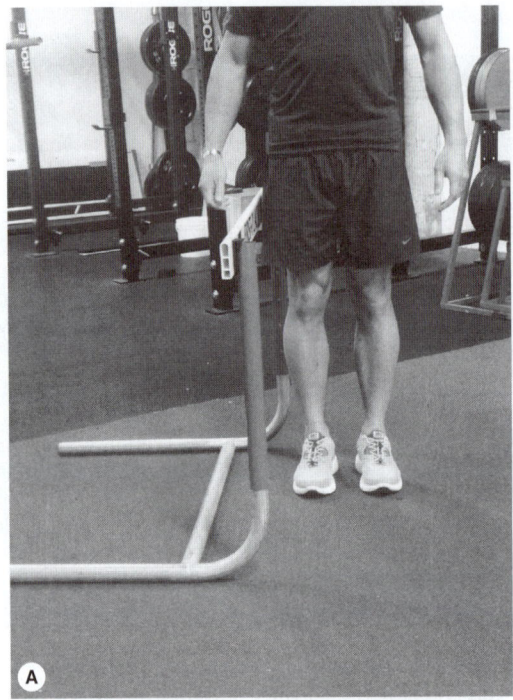

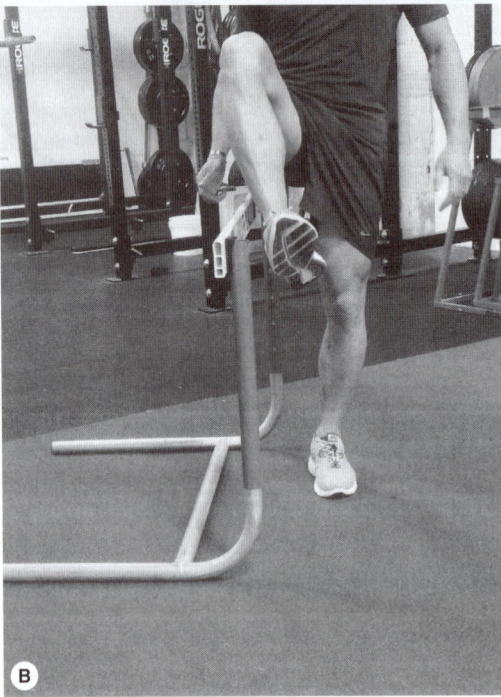

Figure 11-5. High hurdle lateral step-overs. **A.** Starting position. **B.** Step-over. The step-over is performed in a slow and controlled manner initially with focus on lumbopelvic control (a complete step-over is performed with each repetition). As the patient demonstrates adequate lumbopelvic control, the speed of the movement is progressed to simulate quick execution as if getting on/off a bike.

Evidence-Based Clinical Recommendations

SORT: Strength of Recommendation Taxonomy
A: Consistent, good-quality patient oriented evidence
B: Inconsistent or limited-quality patient-oriented evidence
C: Consensus, disease-oriented evidence, usual practice, expert opinion, or case series

1. The gold standard for diagnosis of a hamstring tissue injury is magnetic resonance imaging. **Grade A**
2. Physical therapists should consider tendinopathy as a complication after surgical repair of the proximal hamstring. **Grade B**
3. Eccentric exercises improve collagen synthesis and reduce the risk of subsequent injury. **Grade B**
4. Treatment for hamstring tendinopathy should include eccentric loading of the hamstrings. **Grade A**

COMPREHENSION QUESTIONS

11.1 Which treatment has been shown to be the *most* effective for treating tendinopathy?
   A. Cryotherapy
   B. Eccentric loading
   C. Ultrasound
   D. Manual soft tissue mobilization

11.2 Which of the following is *not* a common sequela of hamstring avulsion?
   A. Sciatic nerve damage
   B. Hamstring tendinopathy
   C. Sitting intolerance
   D. Quadriceps weakness

ANSWERS

11.1 **B.** Eccentric loading has been shown to effectively treat tendinopathy of the hamstrings. When properly dosed, it can provide a net positive effect on the musculotendinous unit.

11.2 **D.** Involvement of the sciatic nerve is common, particularly when surgical repair is not performed within 1 month of injury. Tendinopathy has been shown in 25% of patients 3 years after surgical repair. Sitting intolerance was a major complaint of this patient and has been commonly documented following hamstring avulsion.

REFERENCES

1. Moore K, Dalley A, Agur A. *Clinically Oriented Anatomy*. 6th ed. Baltimore, MD: Lippincott Williams & Wilkins; 2010.
2. Abebe ES, Moorman CT, Garrett WE. Proximal hamstring avulsion injuries: Injury mechanism, diagnosis and disease course. *Oper Techniq Sports Med*. 2009;17:205-209.
3. Porr J, Lucaciu C, Birkett S. Avulsion fractures of the pelvis - a qualitative systematic review of the literature. *J Can Chiropr Assoc*. 2011;55:247-255.
4. Gidwani S, Bircher MD. Avulsion injuries of the hamstring origin - a series of 12 patients and management algorithm. *Ann R Coll Surg Engl*. 2007;89:394-399.
5. Sarimo J, Lempainen L, Mattila K, Orava S. Complete proximal hamstring avulsions: a series of 41 patients with operative treatment. *Am J Sports Med*. 2008;36:1110-1115.
6. Koulouris G, Connell D. Evaluation of the hamstring muscle complex following acute injury. *Skeletal Radiol*. 2003;32:582-589.
7. Copland ST, Tipton JS, Fields KB. Evidence-based treatment of hamstring tears. *Curr Sports Med Rep*. 2009;8:308-314.
8. Wootton JR, Cross MJ, Holt KW. Avulsion of the ischial apophysis. The case for open reduction and internal fixation. *J Bone Joint Surg Br*. 1990;72:625-627.
9. Servant CT, Jones CB. Displaced avulsion of the ischial apophysis: a hamstring injury requiring internal fixation. *Br J Sports Med*. 1998;32:255-257.
10. Klingele KE, Sallay PI. Surgical repair of complete proximal hamstring tendon rupture. *Am J Sports Med*. 2002;30:742-747.
11. Chahal J, Bush-Joseph CA, Chow A, et al. Clinical and magnetic resonance imaging outcomes after surgical repair of complete proximal hamstring ruptures: does the tendon heal? *Am J Sports Med*. 2012;40:2325-2330.
12. Cohen SB, Rangavajjula A, Vyas D, Bradley JP. Functional results and outcomes after repair of proximal hamstring avulsions. *Am J Sports Med*. 2012;40:2092-2098.
13. Carmichael J, Packham I, Trikha SP, Wood DG. Avulsion of the proximal hamstring origin. Surgical technique. *J Bone Joint Surg Am*. 2009;91:249-256.
14. Harris JD, Griesser MJ, Best TM, Ellis TJ. Treatment of proximal hamstring ruptures - a systematic review. *Int J Sports Med*. 2011;32:490-495.
15. Thorborg K. Why hamstring eccentrics are hamstring essentials. *Br J Sports Med*. 2012;46:463-465.
16. Linklater JM, Hamilton B, Carmichael J, Orchard J, Wood DG. Hamstring injuries: anatomy, imaging, and intervention. *Semin Musculoskelet Radiol*. 2010;14:131-161.
17. Goodman C, Kuller K. *Pathology Implications for the Physical Therapist*. 3rd ed. St. Louis, MO: Saunders; 2009.
18. Delvaux F, Rochcongar P, Bruyère O, et al. Return-to-play criteria after hamstring injury: actual medicine practice in professional soccer teams. *J Sports Sci Med*. 2014;13:721-723.
19. Magnusson P, Langberg H, Kjaer M. The pathogenesis of tendinopathy: balancing the response to loading. *Nat Rev Rheumatol*. 2010;6:262-268.
20. Fu SC, Rolf C, Cheuk YC, Lui PP, Chan KM. Deciphering the pathogenesis of tendinopathy: a three-stages process. *Sports Med Arthrosc Rehabil Ther Technol*. 2010;2:30.
21. Petersen J, Thorborg K, Nielsen MB, Budtz-Jorgensen E, Holmich P. Preventive effect of eccentric training on acute hamstring injuries in men's soccer: a cluster-randomized controlled trial. *Am J Sports Med*. 2011;39:2296-2303.
22. Sherry MA, Best TM. A comparison of 2 rehabilitation programs in the treatment of acute hamstring strains. *J Orthop Sports Phys Ther*. 2004;34:116-125.

23. Kirkland A, Garrison JC, Singleton SB, Rodrigo J, Boettner F, Stuckey S. Surgical and therapeutic management of a complete proximal hamstring avulsion after failed conservative approach. *J Orthop Sports Phys Ther*. 2008;38:754-760.
24. Brukner P, Nealon A, Morgan C, Burgess D, Dunn A. Recurrent hamstring muscle injury: applying the limited evidence in the professional football setting with a seven-point programme. *Br J Sports Med*. 2014;48:929-938.

Patellofemoral Pain in a Cross-Country Runner

B.J. Lehecka
Robert C. Manske

CASE 12

A 17-year-old female high school cross-country runner with anterior right knee pain presents to physical therapy for evaluation and treatment. She noticed an insidious onset of the pain with concomitant swelling in her right knee joint after resuming regular running 2 months ago during preparation for the cross-country season. Two months ago, she was exercising on an elliptical trainer a few times per week for about 6 weeks, but she was not running. She has no previous history of lower extremity injury. Her symptoms occur after running approximately a quarter mile and intensify with increasing mileage. On the numeric pain rating scale, she rates her pain at baseline (rest) as 1/10 and at worst as 5/10 (associated with runs of 2 or more miles). With a few days of rest, the pain and swelling are largely absent. This is her first formal physical therapy session; however, she has been taking over-the-counter anti-inflammatory medication and stretching to help reduce her symptoms. Although her cross-country team began conditioning practices 2 weeks ago, she has been unable to participate due to pain. Her goal is to return to running symptom-free as soon as possible. Her physician referred her to physical therapy and recommended that she stop running.

▶ Based on her health condition, what do you anticipate may be the contributors to activity limitations?
▶ What are the examination priorities?
▶ What are the most appropriate physical therapy interventions?

KEY DEFINITIONS

PATELLOFEMORAL PAIN: One of the most common forms of chronic pain about the anterior knee (also known as anterior knee pain); usually has insidious onset

PES PLANUS: A lower than normal medial longitudinal arch of the foot, also called flatfoot

Q-ANGLE: Angle between the line of the rectus femoris coursing from the anterior inferior iliac spine to the patella and the line of the patellar tendon distal to the patella; represents the angle of quadriceps muscle force

REGIONAL INTERDEPENDENCE: Theory that dysfunction occurring either proximal or distal (or both) to the tibiofemoral joint may contribute to pathology at the knee

Objectives

1. Describe patellofemoral pain.
2. Identify methods to assess for regional interdependence.
3. Describe common muscle weaknesses that may contribute to producing patellofemoral pain.
4. Select appropriate treatment interventions for the individual with patellofemoral pain.
5. Implement a therapeutic exercise program that targets dysfunction in the lower extremities to treat patellofemoral pain.

Physical Therapy Considerations

PT considerations during management of the athlete with patellofemoral pain:

- **General physical therapy plan of care/goals:** Decrease pain; increase muscular flexibility; increase lower-quadrant strength; prevent or minimize loss of aerobic fitness capacity; return to cross-country running with team
- **Physical therapy interventions:** Patient education regarding functional anatomy and injury pathomechanics; modalities and manual therapy to decrease pain; muscular flexibility exercises; resistance exercises to increase muscular endurance capacity of the core and to increase strength of lower extremity muscles around the hip; aerobic exercise program; home exercise program with emphasis on strengthening symptomatic lower extremity in positions that do not allow compensatory patterns
- **Precautions during physical therapy:** Monitor vital signs; address precautions or contraindications for exercise, based on patient's preexisting condition(s)
- **Complications interfering with physical therapy:** Unremitting pain or swelling; excessive soft tissue damage

Understanding the Health Condition

Patellofemoral pain (PFP) is one of the most common chronic knee conditions in active adolescents and adults.[1] PFP is also one of the more common pathologies among runners, particularly females, accounting for up to 17% of running injuries.[2] PFP is characterized by diffuse anterior knee pain that is aggravated with activities that increase compressive forces across the knee. Several factors have been correlated with PFP, including patellar malalignment, increased Q-angle, lower extremity weakness, decreased lower extremity flexibility, lower extremity overuse, and muscle imbalances within the lower extremity.[2]

The patella is a large sesamoid bone within the quadriceps tendon. Its shape is that of an inverted triangle with its apex oriented inferiorly and its base located superiorly. Both superior and inferior aspects are roughened for the attachments of the quadriceps and the patellar ligament, respectively. The anterior patellar surface is convex in each direction, whereas the posterior surface has 2 slightly concave areas called facets (see Fig. 16-1A). The posterior surface is covered with articular cartilage that is roughly 6-mm thick in the mid-patellar region, but narrows to less than 1-mm thick along its periphery.[3-6]

In addition to acting as a bony shield for the anterior knee, the patella's primary functions are to guide the quadriceps tendon and increase the moment arm for the quadriceps muscle. Because of the patella, the moment arm of the quadriceps muscle is located at a further distance from the axis of knee motion. This longer moment arm facilitates knee extension by increasing the distance of the extensor mechanism from the center of knee joint. This extensor moment arm provides the greatest quadriceps torque between 20° and 60° of knee flexion.[7,8] This range coincides with the greatest amount of patellofemoral compressive force. When knee flexion increases during weightbearing, compressive forces increase as the angle between femur and tibia decreases. Contact forces on the posterior patella are 0.5 to 1.5 times one's body weight with walking, 3 times one's body weight with stair ascension, and up to 8 times one's body weight with squatting.[9]

Multiple studies have demonstrated a relationship between hip dysfunction and patellofemoral pathology. Dierks et al.[10] examined the relationship between hip strength and hip kinematics in runners with PFP during a prolonged run averaging 40 minutes in duration at each runner's self-selected pace. The authors concluded that runners with patellofemoral pain syndrome (PFPS) displayed weaker hip abductor muscles than uninjured runners before and after the prolonged run. More recently, Ferber et al.[11] investigated the relationship between hip abductor strength and frontal plane knee mechanics in runners with PFPS. Runners with PFPS demonstrated significantly less hip abduction strength than controls; moreover, **hip abductor strengthening in this population** decreased knee pain, increased strength, and normalized stride variability. In a study measuring isometric hip muscle torque production with a multimodal dynamometer, females with PFP demonstrated 14% less hip abductor strength and 17% less hip extensor strength than pain-free controls.[12] It is clear from these studies and others that **hip muscle strength, specifically that of the abductors and extensors, is intimately related with PFP.**[2,13]

Physical Therapy Patient/Client Management

A conservative approach is advocated for individuals with PFP. A physical therapy treatment program should include lower extremity strengthening and stretching exercises and manual therapy. Therapeutic exercises to address proximal muscular weakness effectively reduce PFP.[14] Strength training (quadriceps and hip abductors) and stretching exercises (quadriceps) are strongly supported as effective interventions for runners with PFPS.[1] Adjunct treatments such as taping and orthotic inserts have been shown to provide small additive benefits, but they do not show significant benefit when they are used alone.[1]

Examination, Evaluation, and Diagnosis

Highlights of the clinical examination include a review of the patient's history and symptoms followed by examination of the knee and its functional movements (including gait analysis), knee range of motion (ROM) and girth measurements, lower extremity strength measurements, a neurologic screen, and special tests. The clinical examination typically begins with a gait analysis to guide examination procedures (although some clinicians prefer to perform this toward the end of the examination), followed by observation of the knee and ROM measurements, lower extremity muscle strength testing, and a neurologic screen. During the gait analysis in this case, the therapist noted that the patient demonstrated mild pes planus bilaterally, but no other deviations. To determine whether the patient has edema in the affected knee joint, the therapist can perform girth measurements and the ballottement test. Girth should be measured circumferentially with a tape measure at the joint line. With the patient in long sitting (or supine with the knee extended) and the quadriceps muscles relaxed, the therapist can perform the patellar ballottement test (or, floating patella test). The therapist places one hand proximal to the knee and the other distal to it, moving both hands toward the knee. The therapist then pushes the patella downward into the trochlea and quickly releases it. A positive patellar ballottement test is indicated by palpation or observation of the patella flowing back to its original position, indicating the presence of knee joint effusion.[15] The ballottement test was found to have a sensitivity of 83% and specificity of 49% in patients with acute knee pain compared to effusion noted on magnetic resonance imaging (MRI).[15] These researchers also found sensitivity and specificity values of 80% and 45%, respectively, for knee joint swelling when the patient reported that he or she had noticed knee swelling upon questioning. **Patient report of swelling in addition to the ballottement test** produced a combined sensitivity of 67% and specificity of 82% for detecting knee joint swelling compared to MRI assessment.[15] For the current patient, the therapist noted that her right knee girth at the joint line equaled that of her left knee, and the ballottement test was negative, confirming the lack of joint effusion.

Next, the therapist measured the athlete's knee ROM in supine and prone because knee flexion ROM can vary due to tightness of the rectus femoris. In supine, the athlete's passive knee ROM was similar bilaterally with the unaffected left knee measuring 7°-0°-150° (7° of hyperextension and 150° of flexion) and the affected right knee measuring 7°-0°-147°. When measuring knee flexion in prone, the therapist must ensure that the patient's ipsilateral hip does not spontaneously flex, which indicates a tight rectus femoris (positive Ely's test). The current patient still demonstrated 150° of flexion on the left, but only 140° of flexion on the right. This signified a tighter rectus femoris on the right (limiting knee flexion by ~10°) and indicated a need for rectus femoris stretching in the plan of care.

The therapist next assesses patellar mobility with the patient in the long sitting position. Patellar mobility was equal bilaterally, with each patella gliding equally in all directions including medially, laterally, superiorly, and inferiorly. A lack of medial tilt was noted bilaterally, although greater hypomobility was noted on the right. For example, while the therapist was able to mobilize the lateral edge of her left patella into greater than 5° of medial tilt, the right patella could not be mobilized passed horizontal. This inability of the lateral edge of the patella to move beyond horizontal is indicative of tight fibers of the deep lateral retinaculum attaching to the patella.[16]

The therapist then assessed the athlete's lower extremity strength, first testing the uninvolved left side. The therapist graded most hip and knee muscles on the left side at 5/5 except her hip abductors, which were graded at 4+/5. On the patient's right side, the quadriceps, hamstrings, hip flexors, hip internal rotators, and hip adductors were graded at 5/5; however, her hip extensors, hip external rotators, and hip abductors were graded at 4/5. In addition to strength deficits noted with manual muscle testing, the patient demonstrated poor motor control during functional testing. Observation of the patient's single-leg vertical jump revealed significant valgus collapse upon landing, which has been suggested as a risk factor for PFP (Fig. 12-1).[17] During the Star Excursion Balance Test (SEBT; see Case 23),

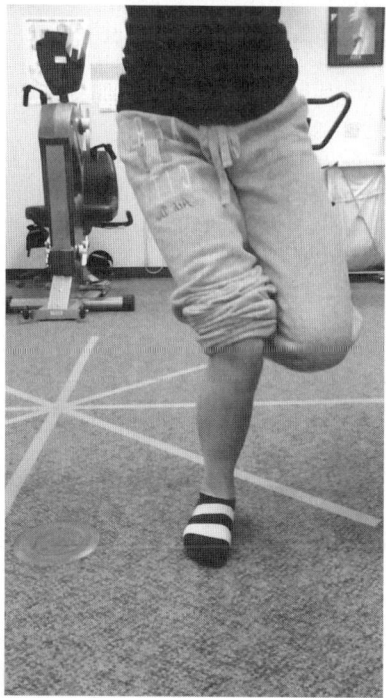

Figure 12-1. Knee valgus collapse upon landing from a single-leg vertical jump.

the athlete had a 6-cm deficit on the right side compared to the left, which has been shown to be a risk factor for injury.[18] Moreover, she demonstrated significant valgus collapse of the right knee during the SEBT with a compensatory trunk lean to the right. This collapse and compensation indicated right gluteal weakness due to the inability to control hip adduction and internal rotation during landing.

Last, a neurologic screen of the lower extremities was performed, including sensation and reflex testing. The patient had normal sensation bilaterally to light touch (tested with a cotton ball) and deep touch (tested with finger palpation) along lower extremity dermatomes. Patellar and Achilles deep tendon reflexes were normal and symmetrical at 2/3 bilaterally. Deep tendon reflexes were graded as follows: 0 = no reflex or absent; 1/3 = hypotonic reflex; 2/3 = normal reflex; 3/3 = hypertonic reflex.

Plan of Care and Interventions

There are several evidence-based interventions for the young, female runner with PFP. Interventions should target dysfunctions found during the clinical examination. For example, the current patient demonstrated weakness in right hip muscles (extensors, external rotators, abductors), right patellofemoral joint hypomobility (lack of patellar medial tilt), motor control deficits (right knee valgus collapse upon landing), and right rectus femoris tightness (10° of tightness measured via Ely's test). Therefore, intervention should target these deficits with a graded, increasingly demanding program, and consistent awareness of the patient's tolerance for the prescribed activities. The therapist should guide the patient in pain-free exercise and advise her to avoid activities that produce swelling at the knee. The therapist should routinely ask if the prescribed activities reproduce symptoms and monitor knee girth for swelling, which may indicate that exercise progression was too aggressive.

During the initial phase of rehabilitation, isometric strengthening and stretching are most appropriate given the patient's inability to perform single-limb exercises without valgus collapse of the affected limb. Isometric exercises for hip extension, hip external rotation, and hip abduction were prescribed in the form of static supine bridges, seated heel squeezes for hip external rotation, and supine hip abduction against a wall, with each repetition performed for 3 seconds. The therapist prescribed these exercises to be performed to fatigue twice per day to promote strengthening and endurance. The patient was also instructed in prone quadriceps stretching (30-second holds, 3 repetitions, 3 times per day) and medial patellar tilts to address the noted deficits in patellar mobility. The patient performed medial patellar tilts in long sitting with her right knee extended. With her thumbs stabilizing the medial border of the patella, she used her fingers to apply an anterior force under the lateral patellar border for a sustained duration of 30 seconds. She was instructed to perform this mobilization 3 times per session, 3 times per day.

The second phase of rehabilitation advanced the hip strengthening and continued the quadriceps stretching and patellar mobilization. Supine bridges with isometric holds at the top of the motion were advanced to isotonic bridging, including emphasis on both concentric and eccentric gluteus maximus contractions. These were done first bilaterally, then unilaterally (bridging with one knee extended) when 2 sets of 15 repetitions were achievable with good form and no pain. Isometric hip external rotation was advanced to hip external rotation in standing. For this exercise, the patient stood on her left leg with her right knee bent so that the leg was on a rolling stool. She was instructed to externally rotate her right hip by moving her right lower leg and foot medially. Resistance was applied by looping elastic tubing from a wall mount to the right of the patient at knee height to her right ankle. This exercise was performed in 2 sets of 15 repetitions each, using progressively stronger elastic tubing as tolerated. Strengthening exercises for hip abduction were progressed to the sidelying hip abduction position (with repetitions performed to fatigue) and hip hikes in standing. For hip hikes, the therapist instructed the patient to stand on the weaker right lower extremity and "hike up" the left hip. The latter 2 exercises not only elicit high hip muscle activity, but also minimize stress at the patellofemoral joint because they are performed with the knee fully extended.[19,20]

When the patient was able to perform higher-level exercises without exacerbation of symptoms or demonstration of compensatory patterns, the therapist replaced the previous exercises with multiple single-limb stance exercises. Single-limb squatting, single-limb deadlift, and lateral band walks with elastic resistance around the foot were used because they recruit high levels of activity in the gluteus medius and gluteus maximus.[19,21] These exercises should only be performed once the patient is able to perform them correctly without symptom exacerbation to prevent joint inflammation.[22]

After the patient's right hip strength increased to 5/5 in manual muscle testing and her rectus femoris and patellar mobility were restored to match the unaffected side, the therapist progressed her to sport-specific activities. Vertical, sagittal plane, and frontal plane hopping were performed for several weeks, progressing from bilateral to unilateral hops, to increase the patient's tolerance to increased loads (see Case 15). To help retrain her landing pattern and minimize patellofemoral stress, the therapist provided cues to avoid knee valgus and to land on the toes.

After approximately 8 therapy sessions (1-2 times per week for 6 weeks) and pain-free performance of exercises, the patient was instructed on a slow jogging progression and underwent multiple sessions of retraining on the treadmill. It has been shown that increasing step rate (*i.e.*, cadence) to 110% of the preferred step rate reduces patellofemoral joint force by 14% primarily by placing the knee in a more extended posture during midstance.[23,24] The patient's initial preferred step rate was 150 steps per minute, potentially inducing significant heel striking anterior to the frontal plane of the body. Therefore, the patient was instructed to increase her cadence to 165 steps per minute (with the aid of a metronome) and she was cued to heel strike nearer to the frontal plane of her body beneath her hip instead of using her initial anterior landing pattern (Fig. 12-2). The therapist provided cues such as "keep your kneecaps pointed forward" and "squeeze your gluteals" because these have also been shown to be helpful in improving running mechanics and reducing pain in subjects with PFPS.[25] The therapist incorporated mirror gait retraining into 2 sessions because this can reduce pain and improve mechanics in female runners with PFPS.[26]

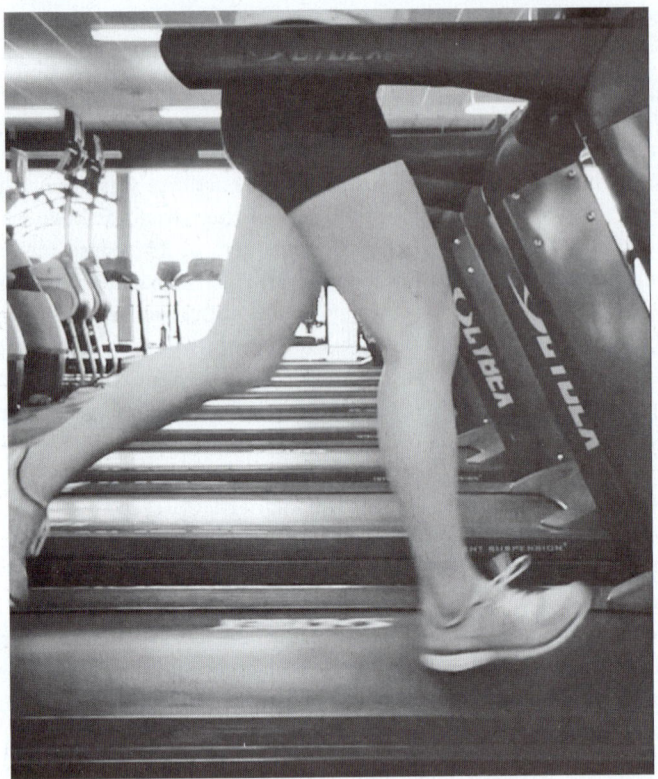

Figure 12-2. Patient with right anterior knee pain running on a treadmill. Note the right heel striking significantly anterior to the hip, which increases patellofemoral joint forces by increasing knee flexion at midstance.

Evidence-Based Clinical Recommendations

SORT: Strength of Recommendation Taxonomy
A: Consistent, good-quality patient-oriented evidence
B: Inconsistent or limited-quality patient-oriented evidence
C: Consensus, disease-oriented evidence, usual practice, expert opinion, or case series

1. Incorporation of hip strengthening exercises in the rehabilitation program for individuals with patellofemoral pain decreases knee pain and increases strength. **Grade B**
2. Individuals with patellofemoral pain syndrome (PFPS) demonstrate muscular weakness in the ipsilateral hip. **Grade B**
3. Patient report of knee joint swelling combined with the patella ballottement test allows therapists to detect the presence of knee joint swelling with moderate specificity. **Grade B**

COMPREHENSION QUESTIONS

12.1 During examination of a patient's single-leg squat and vertical jump, the therapist observed significant femoral internal rotation and valgus collapse at the knee. Which exercises would be *most* appropriate to address the associated weak muscle groups?

   A. Straight leg raises and marching
   B. Hip internal rotation and hip adduction with elastic resistance
   C. Sidelying hip abduction and lateral band walks
   D. Leg press and hamstring curls

12.2 When assessing the running pattern of the patient with patellofemoral pain, the therapist records her cadence as 145 steps per minute with significant heel strike anterior to the frontal plane. Which is the *most* appropriate cue for retraining?

   A. Increase running cadence to 160 steps per minute.
   B. Maintain running cadence of 145 steps per minute.
   C. Decrease running cadence to 140 steps per minute.
   D. Increase running cadence to 185 steps per minute.

ANSWERS

12.1 **C.** Femoral internal rotation and valgus collapse upon landing are especially indicative of weak hip abductors. Manual muscle testing of hip extensors and external rotators would also likely detect deficits. Sidelying hip abduction has been shown to produce relatively high activation of the gluteus medius in a group of runners. Lateral band walks also challenge the gluteus medius to a high degree; if elastic resistance is used around the foot, this exercise can significantly activate the gluteus maximus. Straight leg raises and marching primarily utilize quadriceps and hip flexors (option A). Leg press and hamstring curls primarily activate quadriceps and hamstrings (option D).

12.2 **A.** Subtle increases (5%-10%) in running cadence have been shown to substantially reduce loading at the knee and hip joints during running and, therefore, can be effective at helping reduce common running-related injuries such as PFP. Increasing running cadence by more than 10% (option D) may place too much demand on the metabolic system and prove to be too drastic of a change from a patient's preferred rhythm.

REFERENCES

1. Rixe JA, Glick JE, Brady J, Olympia RP. A review of the management of patellofemoral pain syndrome. *Phys Sportsmed*. Sep 2013;41:19-28.
2. Prins MR, van der Wurff P. Females with patellofemoral pain syndrome have weak hip muscles: a systematic review. *Aust J Physiother*. 2009;55:9-15.

3. Fulkerson JP. *Disorders of the Patellofemoral Joint*. 3rd ed. Baltimore, MD: Williams & Wilkins; 1997.
4. Fulkerson JP. Diagnosis and treatment of patients with patellofemoral pain. *Am J Sports Med*. 2002;30:447-456.
5. Grelsamer RP, Weinstein CH. Applied biomechanics of the patella. *Clin Orthop Rel Res*. 2001;389:9-14.
6. Heegaard J, Leyvraz PF, Curnier A, Rakotomanana L, Huiskes R. The biomechanics of the human patella during passive knee flexion. *J Biomech*. 1995;28:1265-1279.
7. Huberti HH, Hayes WC. Patellofemoral contact pressures. The incidence of q-angle and tendofemoral contact. *J Bone Joint Surg*. 1984;66:715-724.
8. Huberti HH, Hayes WC, Stone JL, Shybut GT. Force ratios in the quadriceps tendon and ligamentum patella. *J Orthop Res*. 1984;21:49-54.
9. Reilly DT, Martens M. Experimental analysis of the quadriceps muscle force and patellofemoral joint reaction force for various activities. *Acta Orthop Scan*. 1972;43:126-137.
10. Dierks TA, Manal KT, Hamill J, Davis IS. Proximal and distal influences on hip and knee kinematics in runners with patellofemoral pain during a prolonged run. *J Orthop Sports Phys Ther*. 2008;38:448-456.
11. Ferber R, Kendall KD, Farr L. Changes in knee biomechanics after a hip-abductor strengthening protocol for runners with patellofemoral pain syndrome. *J Athl Train*. 2011;46:142-149.
12. Souza RB, Powers CM. Differences in hip kinematics, muscle strength, and muscle activation between subjects with and without patellofemoral pain. *J Orthop Sports Phys Ther*. 2009;39:12-19.
13. Meira EP, Brumitt J. Influence of the hip on patients with patellofemoral pain syndrome: a systematic review. *Sports Health*. 2011;3:455-465.
14. Peters JS, Tyson NL. Proximal exercises are effective in treating patellofemoral pain syndrome: a systematic review. *Int J Sports Phys Ther*. 2013;8:689-700.
15. Kastelein M1, Luijsterburg PA, Wagemakers HP, et al. Diagnostic value of history taking and physical examination to assess effusion of the knee in traumatic knee patients in general practice. *Arch Phys Med Rehabil*. 2009;90:82-86.
16. Manske RC, Davies GJ. A nonsurgical approach to examination and treatment of the patellofemoral joint, part I: examination of the patellofemoral joint. *Crit Rev Phys Rehabil Med*. 2003;15:141-166.
17. Boling MC, Padua DA, Marshall SW, Guskiewicz K, Pyne S, Beutler A. A prospective investigation of biomechanical risk factors for patellofemoral pain syndrome: the Joint Undertaking to Monitor and Prevent ACL Injury (JUMP-ACL) cohort. *Am J Sports Med*. 2009;37:2108-2116.
18. Plisky PJ, Rauh MJ, Kaminski TW, Underwood FB. Star Excursion Balance Test as a predictor of lower extremity injury in high school basketball players. *J Orthop Sports Phys Ther*. 2006;36:911-919.
19. Boren K, Conrey C, Le Coguic J, Paprocki L, Voight M, Robinson TK. Electromyographic analysis of gluteus medius and gluteus maximus during rehabilitation exercises. *Int J Sports Phys Ther*. 2011;6:206-223.
20. McBeth JM, Earl-Boehm JE, Cobb SC, Huddleston WE. Hip muscle activity during 3 side-lying hip-strengthening exercises in distance runners. *J Athl Train*. 2012;47:15-23.
21. Cambridge ED, Sidorkewicz N, Ikeda DM, McGill SM. Progressive hip rehabilitation: the effects of resistance band placement on gluteal activation during two common exercises. *Clin Biomech (Bristol, Avon)*. 2012;27:719-724.
22. Distefano LJ, Blackburn JT, Marshall SW, Padua DA. Gluteal muscle activation during common therapeutic exercises. *J Orthop Sports Phys Ther*. 2009;39:532-540.
23. Heiderscheit BC, Chumanov ES, Michalski MP, Wille CM, Ryan MB. Effects of step rate manipulation on joint mechanics during running. *Med Sci Sports Exerc*. 2011;43:296-302.

24. Lenhart RL, Thelen DG, Wille CM, Chumanov ES, Heiderscheit BC. Increasing running step rate reduces patellofemoral joint forces. *Med Sci Sports Exerc*. 2014;46:557-564.
25. Noehren B, Scholz J, Davis I. The effect of real-time gait retraining on hip kinematics, pain and function in subjects with patellofemoral pain syndrome. *Br J Sports Med*. 2011;45:691-696.
26. Willy RW, Scholz JP, Davis IS. Mirror gait retraining for the treatment of patellofemoral pain in female runners. *Clin Biomech (Bristol, Avon)*. 2012;27:1045-1051.

Patellofemoral Pain in the Cyclist

Christine Panagos
Emily Ohlin

CASE 13

A 32-year-old male cyclist consulted with an orthopaedic physician for right knee pain that had been progressively worsening over the previous 3 months of the spring cycling season. X-rays of the knee performed in the physician's office were negative for bony abnormalities. The patient was referred to physical therapy. In your clinic, the patient states that he rides his bike an average of 150 miles per week in the winter and more than 250 miles per week in the spring and fall. He is a Cat 3 level road racer. He reports a history of right knee pain that occurred when he played high school varsity basketball. Past medical history includes left clavicle fracture 2 years ago and right distal tibia and fibula fractures with open reduction internal fixation (ORIF) 13 months ago. The patient reports that his current knee symptoms worsen after cycling approximately 35 miles and improve when he rises out of the saddle to pedal. He also reports knee pain when descending stairs, but only when preceded by cycling activity the same day or the previous day. Adjusting his bike saddle height has not improved his symptoms.

▶ Based on the patient's history and current condition, what abnormal movement patterns could be contributing to his patellofemoral symptoms?
▶ What are the most appropriate examination tests?
▶ What impairments would you expect to find?
▶ What are possible complications that may limit the effectiveness of physical therapy?
▶ What are the most appropriate physical therapy interventions?

KEY DEFINITIONS

ANATOMY OF A BIKE: Fig. 13-1.

CADENCE: Number of pedal revolutions per minute

CAT 3 ROAD RACER: CAT (abbreviation for category) is a level assigned to amateur and professional cyclists to rate level of competitive success; CAT 5 is considered beginner level and CAT 1 is considered elite level. A cyclist must successfully compete and place in the top tier of their category in a minimum of 10 races prior to being allowed to progress to the next higher category.

CLIPLESS PEDALS: Shoe and pedal system in which a cleat on the sole of the cycling shoe clips onto the top of the pedal; different systems allow for varying degrees of "float," which is the amount of internal and external rotation available at the cleat-pedal interface.

DYNAMIC STABILIZERS: Joint stability that is created by *active* muscular contraction

HANDLEBAR REACH: Distance from the front end of the saddle to the center of the handlebars (Fig. 13-1)

INSEAM OF THE CYCLIST: Measurement from the floor to the crotch while the cyclist is standing barefoot

MAXIMUM VOLUNTARY CONTRACTION (MVC): Greatest amount of tension a muscle can generate and sustain (however briefly) during testing

PEDAL STROKE: Full revolution of the pedal 360 degrees through the sagittal plane

REGIONAL INTERDEPENDENCE: The concept that regions proximal or distal to a body segment can contribute to pain localized in or around that specific structure

SADDLE: Bike seat

SEAT HEIGHT: Distance from the center of the crank to the top of the saddle (Fig. 13-1)

STATIC STABILIZERS: Passive structures in and around a joint that provide stability (*e.g.*, ligaments, joint capsule, menisci, bony congruity)

STEM RISE: Angle between top of the head tube and top of the handlebar grip area (Fig. 13-1)

TRAINER: Device that holds the bicycle in place and allows the cyclist to pedal the bike while remaining stationary

Objectives

1. Describe patellofemoral pain syndrome.
2. Describe how to perform a lower extremity screen specific to the cyclist.
3. Identify contributing factors to lower-quarter injuries in the cyclist.

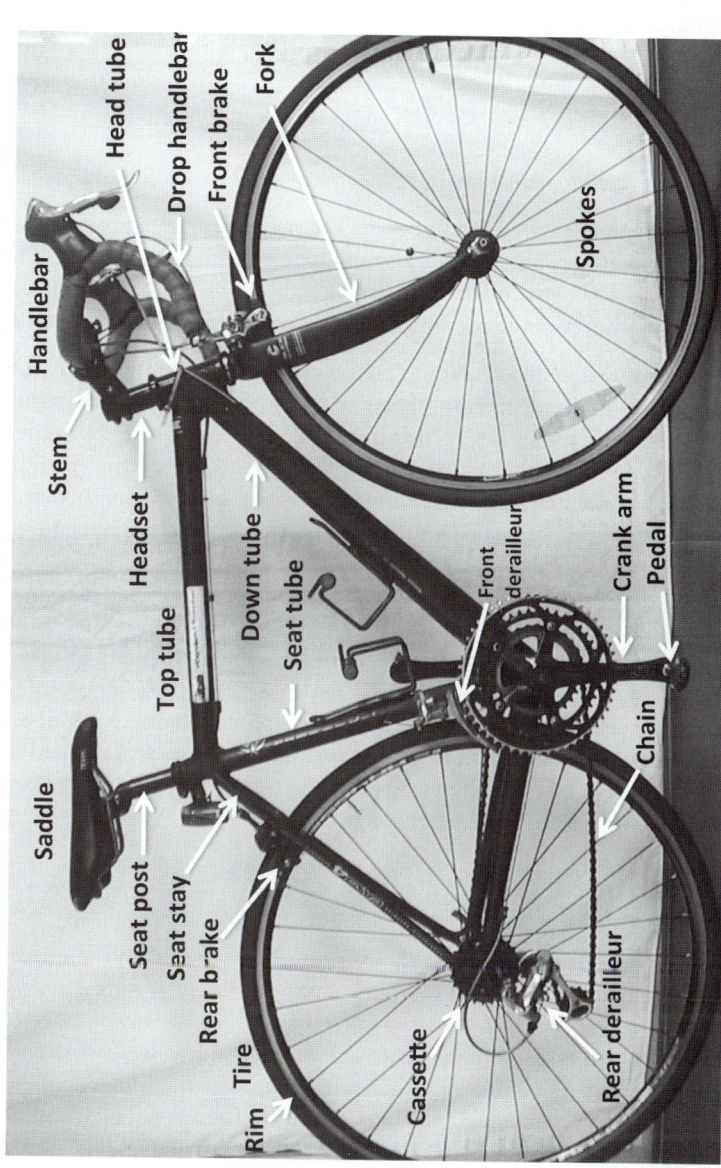

Figure 13-1. Anatomy of a bike.

4. Identify how saddle, cleat position, and improper pedaling mechanics can contribute to patellofemoral pain syndrome in the cyclist.
5. Identify key markers for bike fit and pedal stroke analysis.
6. Prescribe appropriate treatment interventions to decrease knee pain by addressing potential contributing sources proximal and/or distal to the knee.

Physical Therapy Considerations

PT considerations during management of the cyclist with patellofemoral knee pain:

- **General physical therapy plan of care/goals:** Decrease pain; improve pedal stroke to allow for bilateral lower extremity symmetry; restore normal ankle and hip range of motion (ROM); increase proximal stability at the hip in frontal and transverse planes; prevent or minimize loss of cardiovascular conditioning
- **Physical therapy interventions:** Patient education regarding lumbopelvic and hip stabilization and pathomechanics of injury; manual therapy and stretching to normalize ankle, knee, and hip ROM; resistance exercises to improve strength, balance, and endurance; neuromuscular re-education to promote joint and muscular control; patient education regarding the importance of off-the-bike training to address cycling-specific health issues; bike fit and pedal stroke analysis
- **Precautions during physical therapy:** Close monitoring of current movement patterns to avoid reinforcing improper cycling technique; monitor vital signs; address precautions or contraindications for exercise based on patient's pre-existing condition(s)
- **Complications interfering with physical therapy:** Lack of adherence to recommended cycling restrictions until severity of symptoms decreases; potentially permanent impairments due to prior injuries; inability to make suggested modifications to the bike or replace worn equipment in a timely manner

Understanding the Health Condition

The patella is a triangular-shaped sesamoid bone that rests within the quadriceps tendon. The primary biomechanical function of the patella is to create a mechanical advantage for the quadriceps by increasing the length of the quadriceps tendon from the joint axis of rotation of the knee. This allows the quadriceps to create greater force through the knee. The patella also serves to protect the quadriceps tendon from excessive friction during flexion and extension of the knee. The undersurface of the patella is covered with a 4- to 7-mm thick layer of articular cartilage that is thicker laterally to help maintain the patella's position within the trochlear groove.[1] The underlying patellar surface is divided into medial and lateral facets that accommodate the concave surface of the trochlear groove of the femur (see Fig. 16-1). The stability of this gliding synovial joint depends on proper balance between the static and dynamic stabilizers of the knee as well as the dynamic stability provided at the hip, foot, and ankle. The static resting position of the patella depends on the depth of the femoral sulcus, height of the lateral femoral condyle wall, shape of the patella, and the tautness of the lateral retinaculum. Dynamically, the quadriceps muscle group influences patellar position. Normally, the patella sits midway between the medial and lateral femoral condyles when the knee is flexed 20°.[2]

Patellofemoral pain (PFP) is a type of anterior knee pain that occurs when the static and dynamic stabilizers fail to maintain proper patellar alignment within the trochlear groove.[2-6] Often, PFP occurs during activities that increase compressive forces such as ascending and descending stairs, jumping, and prolonged sitting.[7] The quadriceps are able to produce the greatest amount of force between 20° and 60° of knee flexion.[4] It is through this ROM that the greatest amount of patellofemoral compressive forces occurs.[3]

Cycling-related knee pain is the most frequently reported injury that results in training time lost by professional road cyclists.[8] The pedal stroke occurs primarily in the sagittal plane and is generally considered a non-weightbearing activity. The professional cyclist averages 90 to 100 revolutions per minute (RPM) on long, flat terrain, performing up to 6000 revolutions per hour.[9] Even the competitive amateur cyclist can spend between 2 and 6 hours per day training on the bike. Although dynamic in nature, cycling requires limited ROM at the hip, knee, and ankle. At the knee, approximately 25° to 112° is required to make a full revolution.[10] This ROM corresponds with the range in which the quadriceps produces the greatest amount of force. Because of the repetitive nature of the sport and the hours athletes spend training or competing, overuse cycling injuries are increasingly prevalent in amateur and recreational populations.[8]

Physical Therapy Patient/Client Management

"Bike fit specialists" at cycle shops offer varying levels of expertise and utilize general guidelines to improve rider comfort and minimize risk of injury. However, sports physical therapists with training in bicycle fitting have the expertise to address both the bike and the cyclist. When evaluating the cyclist with PFP, it is important for the physical therapist to assess the patient both on and off the bike. On the bike, there are ROM standards for the road cyclist to be able to properly fit into the riding position. Average hip flexion angle in the forward flexed position is approximately 133°.[11] Maximal knee flexion is 112° and maximal ankle dorsiflexion has been shown to be 13°.[10] The knee is also influenced proximally and distally by the hip, foot, and ankle.[5,6,12-14] This concept of regional interdependence implies that symptoms localized to one region of the body can be influenced by the motion, strength, and neuromuscular control deficits proximally and/or distally from the affected area of the body. Therefore, the physical therapist must also evaluate ROM and strength at the hip, ankle, and foot, patellar tracking patterns, and any excessive lower extremity movement patterns outside the sagittal plane in the cyclist with PFP. PFP can be caused by a combination of inadequate preparation for long hours of cycling, faulty equipment, poor technique, inappropriate training techniques, and overuse. Prevention of chronic anterior knee pain should be a focus of therapeutic interventions with particular attention to bicycle fit, the cyclist's body alignment on the bike, appropriate equipment, pedaling mechanics, and appropriate training. The most effective management of PFP includes patient education, correction of lower extremity alignment, activity modification, rest, and therapeutic exercise progression.[15] In contrast, ultrasound, cross-friction massage, iontophoresis, glucocorticoid injections, and oral nonsteroidal anti-inflammatories have not been shown to be effective.[15-17]

Examination, Evaluation, and Diagnosis

The main goal of the therapist's examination of the patient who is a regular cyclist is to identify impairments—both off and on the bike—that may be contributing to his knee pain. The primary goal for the patient is to return to pain-free cycling.

The examination begins off the bike. First, the physical therapist performs a lower-body movement screen to assess for dysfunction in both stability and mobility. The off-the-bike assessment begins with observation of a double-leg squat. The cyclist in this case demonstrated a proper hip hinge with a double-leg squat (*i.e.*, initiation of the squat with a posterior movement at the hips), but a lateral pelvic shift to the left was observed (Fig. 13-2). Next, the single-leg squat is performed

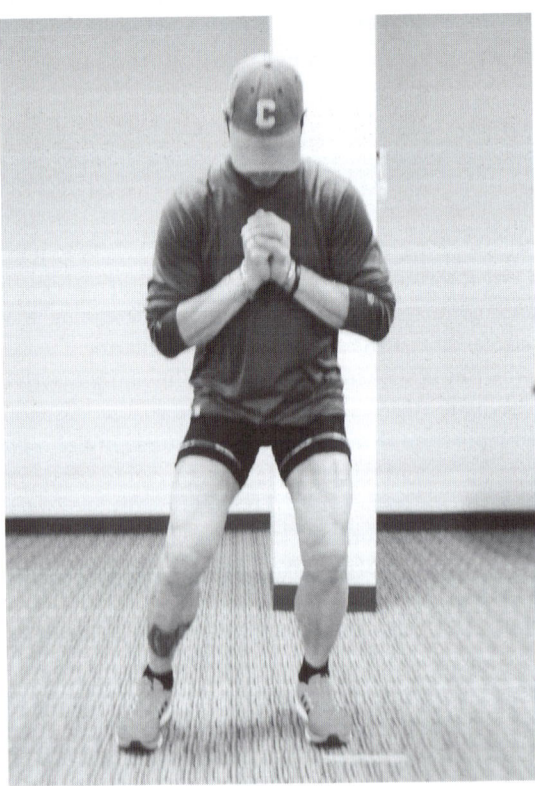

Figure 13-2. Double-leg squat. Note the left lateral pelvic shift and right knee valgus.

to observe each lower extremity in isolation. The patient demonstrated good alignment in the frontal and transverse planes, a proper hip hinge, forward motion of the tibia over the foot, and no loss of balance when performing the single-leg squat on the left. However, during the single-leg squat on the right lower extremity, the patient demonstrated a right lateral shift of the pelvis, valgus collapse at the knee (Fig. 13-3A), limited hip hinge, no forward movement of the tibia over the foot, and loss of balance (Fig. 13-3B). On a second attempt using his upper extremity for balance, the quality of the right single-leg squat did not change. Next, static single-leg standing balance is assessed. The patient was able to maintain controlled single-leg balance for 30 seconds on the left and 8 seconds on the right. Observation of single-leg stance on the right side also revealed excessive pronation of the foot, valgus collapse of the knee, lateral pelvic shift in the frontal plane, and increased trunk sway. Next, closed-chain dorsiflexion should be measured (Fig. 13-4) because limited closed chain dorsiflexion ROM will result in compensations further up the kinetic chain at the knee and hip. To measure closed-chain dorsiflexion, the patient was asked to face the wall, placing his toes 8 cm from the wall. He was then instructed to dorsiflex the left ankle by moving the knee toward the wall until contact was made between the knee and the wall. He was cued to maintain heel contact with the floor and avoid any lower body movement outside the sagittal plane. The same maneuver was repeated on the right side. The patient was able to properly perform the task with the toes only 3 cm from the wall, indicating a loss

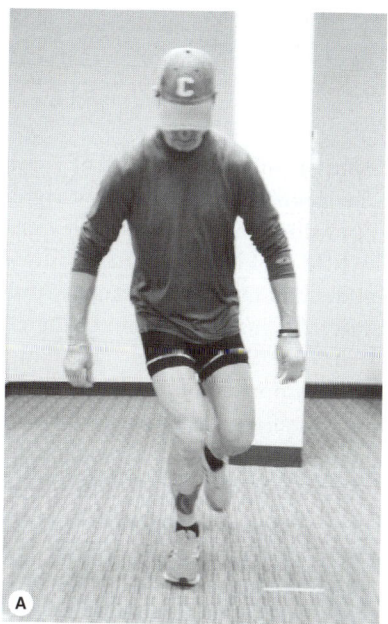
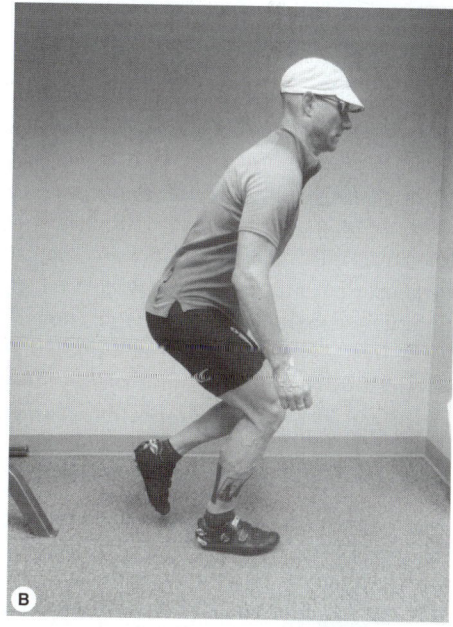

Figure 13-3. Single-leg squat. **A.** Front view: Note the lateral pelvic shift to the right and valgus collapse at the knee. **B.** Side view: Note the lack of hip hinge and decreased anterior translation of the tibia over the foot.

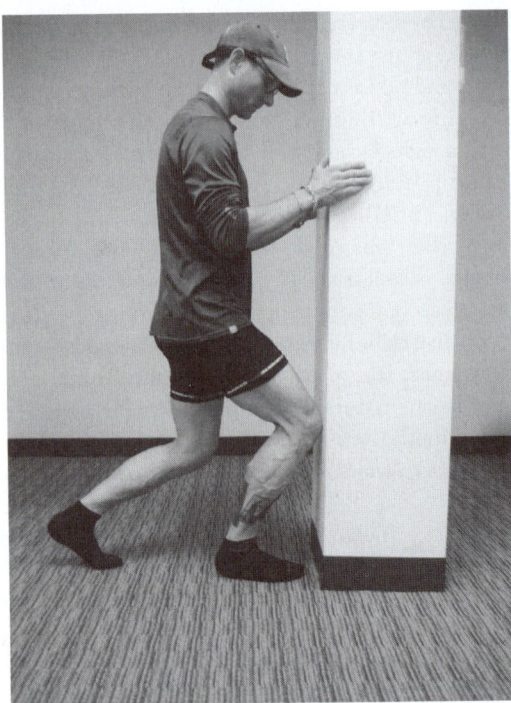

Figure 13-4. Closed-chain dorsiflexion assessment. With the toes placed just over 3 cm from the wall, note the inability of the patient's knee to touch the wall without elevating the heel off the floor. This demonstrates a loss of closed-chain dorsiflexion.

of closed-chain dorsiflexion in the right ankle. The patient's impairment level measurements are listed in Table 13-1.

The impairments noted on the objective examination included loss of right passive ankle dorsiflexion (open- and closed-chain positions), decreased right ankle strength (manual muscle testing [MMT] of dorsiflexors, plantar flexors, inverters, and everters), and right hip strength (MMT of hip extensors, abductors, internal and external rotators), functional deficits in single-leg squat, and diminished balance on the right lower extremity (22 seconds less in single-leg stance). Knee ROM was equal bilaterally and quadriceps and hamstring strength were normal, highlighting the absence of abnormal objective findings in the patient's right symptomatic knee. These cumulative objective findings support the concept of regional interdependence and the work of Powers[3] and Powers et al.,[5] affirming that deficits in structures both proximal and distal to the knee can contribute to PFP syndrome. **A strong correlation has been found between restricted dorsiflexion and anterior knee pain.**[18-20] Further up the kinetic chain, it has also been shown that the inability to correctly perform a single-leg squat by isolating motion to the frontal plane indicates functional hip abductor muscle weakness.[21]

The off-the-bike evaluation gives the therapist insight into the biomechanics of the pedal stroke when assessing the patient on his bike. Thorough inspection of

Table 13-1 RANGE OF MOTION AND MANUAL MUSCLE TEST RESULTS FOR CASE PATIENT

	PROM/AROM		Strength	
	L	R	L	R
Hip flexion	130°/125°	130°/125°	5/5	5/5
Hip extension	30°/20°	30°/20°	5/5	4⁻/5
Hip abduction	45°/40°	45°/40°	5/5	4⁻/5
Hip external rotation	45°/35°	40°/30°	5/5	4⁻/5
Hip internal rotation	25°/20°	30°/25°	5/5	4⁻/5
Knee PROM	0°-140°	3°-0°-142°	–	–
Knee extension	–	–	5/5	5/5
Knee flexion	–	–	5/5	5/5
Ankle dorsiflexion	14°/10°	6°/4°	5/5	3⁻/5
Ankle plantar flexion	60°/60°	48°/48°	5/5	3⁻/5
Ankle inversion	30°/30°	16°/16°	5/5	2⁺/5
Ankle eversion	14°/14°	8°/8°	5/5	3⁻/5
Straight leg raise	75°/75°	80°/80°	–	–

Abbreviations: AROM, active range of motion; PROM, passive range of motion.

the patient's bike can provide valuable information about the rider's pedal stroke. First, the therapist must ensure that the bike is mounted level on the trainer. The saddle should be level. If one side of the saddle is more worn than the other, this could indicate pelvic shifting during the pedal stroke. The saddle should support the rider's ischial tuberosities and pubic bone, but avoid pressure on the perineal soft tissue and pudendal nerve. Various saddle designs and materials are designed to improve rider comfort and decrease saddle paresthesia (*e.g.*, cut-out saddles). All saddles have a width measurement listed that should coincide with ischial tuberosity width. Selection of design and materials is based on the distance between the ischial tuberosities and on rider comfort or preference. The rider should be encouraged to visit his local bike shop to be measured for the proper saddle width and to test-ride multiple saddles. Once the cyclist has chosen the best saddle for his specific anatomy and comfort, the therapist can make the appropriate height and fore/aft adjustments. The chain stays and cycling shoes should also be inspected for signs of wear. If there is an asymmetry in the cyclist's pedal stroke, wearing will be noted on the medial side of the shoe where the cyclist has rubbed his heel on the chain stay. The therapist should measure the length of the crank arm (Fig. 13-1) and determine whether it is consistent with recommendations for the cyclist's inseam (Table 13-2). Although the crank arm length is important for optimal positioning on the bike,[10,22,23] changes in crank arm length do not correlate to changes in peak power output.[23] Last, the therapist should inspect the front end of the bike.

Table 13-2 SUGGESTED CRANK ARM LENGTH ASSOCIATED WITH CYCLISTS' INSEAM LENGTH[10]

Crank Length	Inseam
170 mm	74-80 cm
172.5 mm	81-86 cm
175 mm	87-93 cm

The tips of the brake levers should be in line with the bottom of the drops to allow the rider to properly engage the brakes[10] (Fig. 13-5).

After the therapist performs a thorough investigation of the rider and the bike, the on-the-bike analysis can commence. With the patient wearing the shorts and shoes that he typically wears while riding, he mounts the bike and begins pedaling for approximately 10 minutes. This allows the patient to perform an aerobic warm-up and settle into his preferred riding position. During this time, the therapist observes the mechanics of the cyclist's riding posture and pedaling mechanics in all 3 planes of movement. We recommended beginning the observation at the pelvis. A stable pelvis produces optimal efficiency and power with each pedal stroke and reduces the risk of injury due to poor body alignment and altered biomechanics. Ideally, the rider should maintain the pelvis in a neutral position rather than excessively rotating posteriorly or anteriorly. The therapist should assess whether lateral shifting of the pelvis occurs during the pedal stroke; this "rocking" on the saddle may indicate a saddle height that is too high or a limitation in hip or ankle ROM

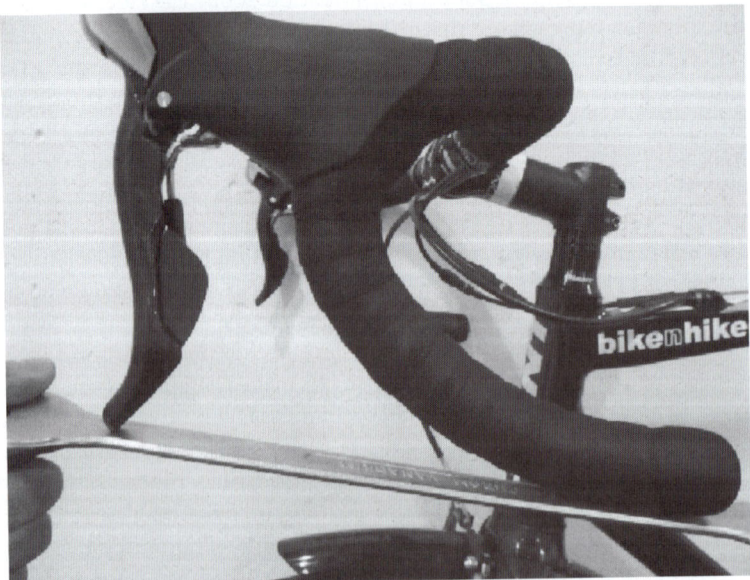

Figure 13-5. Proper placement of brake levers on handlebars. Note the tips of the brake levers are parallel to the bottom of the handlebar drops.

and/or strength. From the side view, the therapist measures the shoulder position, trunk angle, knee angle, and elbow position with the wrist in neutral (Fig. 13-6). To start these measurements, the saddle should be positioned fore and aft to align the inferior patellar pole over the pedal spindle. Trunk angle is measured relative to a horizontal femur with hands on the hoods. Elbow flexion angle is measured with

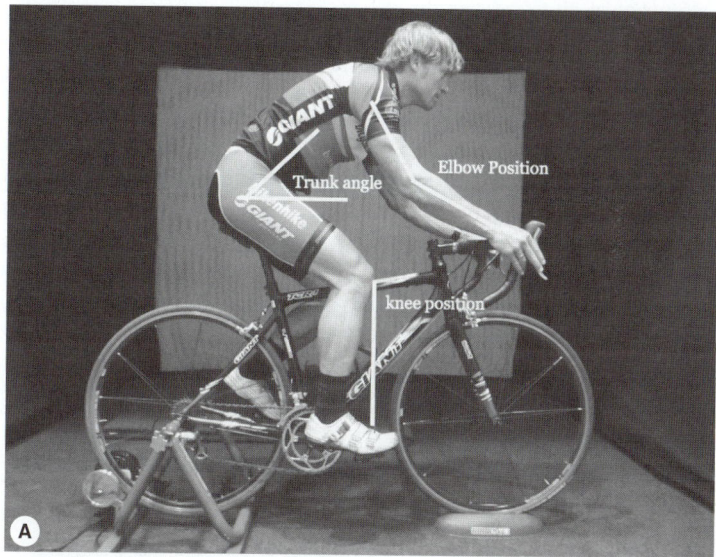

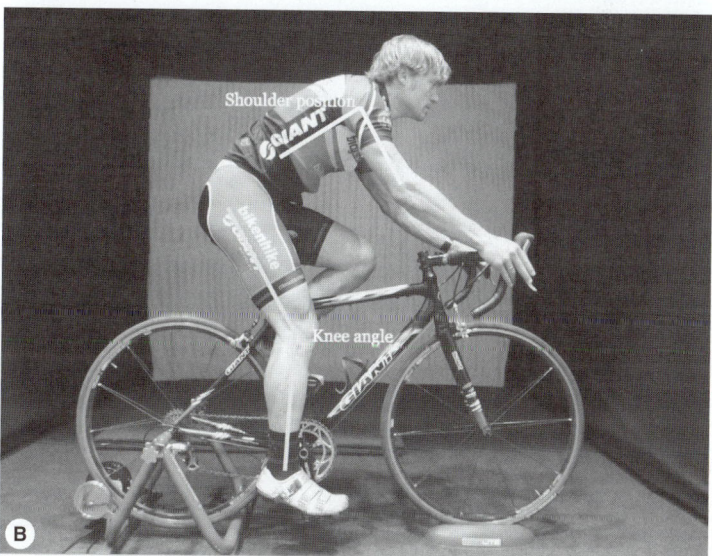

Figure 13-6. **A.** Side view of rider on a trainer in which trunk and knee angles, shoulder and elbow position, and knee position over pedal spindle can be assessed. **B.** With the crank arm in the 6-o'clock position, the knee should be in 25° to 30° flexion with the ankle slightly plantar flexed. Shoulders should be in approximately 90° flexion.

the wrist in neutral. The amount of plantar flexion and dorsiflexion through each revolution is easily observed from the side view. Observing the rider from the front, the knee should track directly over the foot throughout the pedal stroke. The therapist should ensure that the rider does not display knee varus and/or valgus at the 12-o'clock and 3- to 6-o'clock positions of the pedal stroke. Excessive femoral internal or external rotation and abnormal ankle and foot motion should not occur. Although the clipless pedal system allows for some tibial rotation, the foot should remain in subtalar joint neutral, with toes forward and heel not in contact with the chain stay.

The patient in this case demonstrated right knee valgus and decreased right ankle dorsiflexion from the 9-o'clock through the 3-o'clock crank position during the revolution (Fig. 13-7). During the same phase of the pedal stroke, he also demonstrated increased right hip internal rotation and increased right foot pronation. The patient's limited ankle dorsiflexion resulted in a valgus alignment at the knee, which was apparent as he came up and over the top of the pedal stroke. This is the ROM at which the quadriceps begin to generate the greatest amount of downward force through the pedal.[24,25]

Plan of Care and Interventions

Physical therapy management should include interventions both off and on the bike. Off the bike interventions include manual therapy, therapeutic exercise prescription, and balance retraining. On the bike interventions include ergonomic assessment and bike fitting.

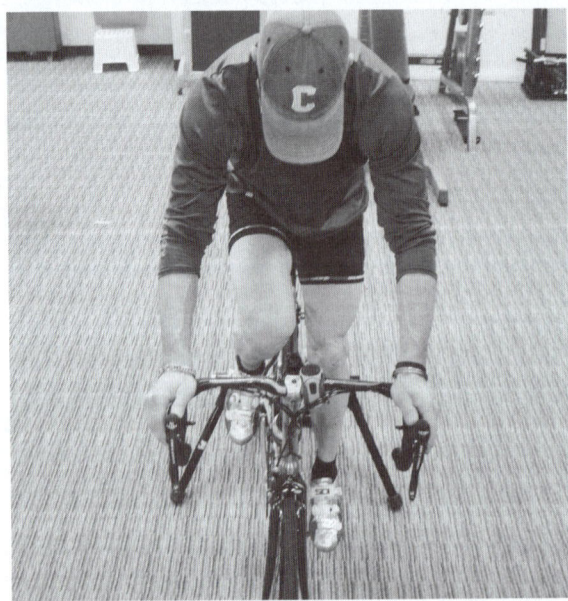

Figure 13-7. Improper pedal stroke. Note the valgus collapse at the right knee.

For the patient in this case, off-the bike treatments should be focused on addressing identified joint and soft tissue restrictions (in the right ankle) as well as right hip weakness and neuromuscular control deficits. It should be noted that attention to ROM and strength alone have been shown to be insufficient in returning an athlete to sport safely.[26] For this cyclist, the therapist placed heavy emphasis on educating the patient on his current deficits and their implications because he was attempting to increase his training time on the bike.

Foot and ankle deficits need to be addressed through manual therapy techniques, therapeutic exercise, and proprioceptive retraining. To promote gains in right dorsiflexion, Mulligan mobilization with movement (MWM) was applied to the ankle joint with a combined posterior talar glide mobilization and active dorsiflexion movement (Fig. 13-8).[27-29] It is believed that closed kinetic chain application of this technique results in greater gains in motion due to the arthrokinematic principle that the talus glides posteriorly during dorsiflexion.[29-31] This movement has been shown to improve dorsiflexion by 26% of the pre-application deficit between affected and unaffected sides in individuals with recurrent ankle sprains.[30]

The cyclist was then instructed on standing gastrocnemius and soleus stretching as well as dorsiflexion self-mobilization. Stretching was prescribed to improve soft tissue and muscular mobility within the gastrocnemius-soleus complex, and joint mobilizations were performed to facilitate posterior talar glide. Both interventions

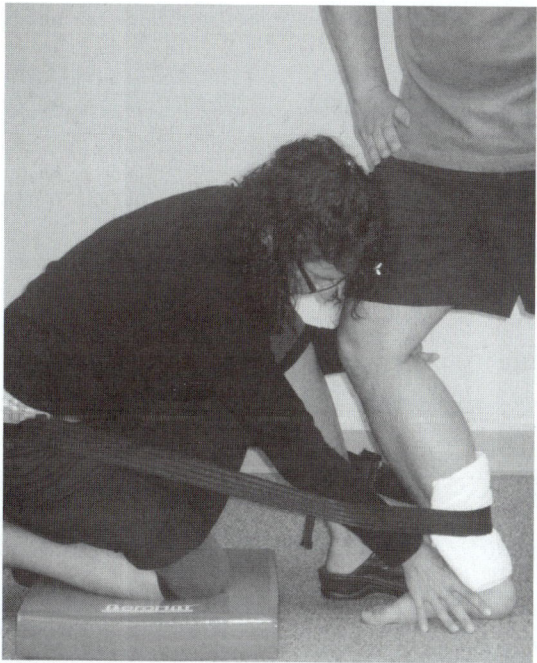

Figure 13-8. Mulligan mobilization to increase ankle dorsiflexion. A strap is placed around the posterior tibia of the patient and then around the therapist's pelvis. The therapist applies a posterior force on the talus and leans back on the strap to provide an anterior force on the tibia while the patient lunges forward. This maneuver is repeated for 3 sets of 10 repetitions in a pain-free range of motion.

were aimed at increasing dorsiflexion to allow sufficient ROM through the top of the pedal stroke where the greatest amount of dorsiflexion is required. Restrictions in dorsiflexion at the top of the pedal stroke will create compensation further up the kinetic chain at the knee, hip, and pelvis. The dorsiflexion self-mobilization was performed in a half-kneeling stance facing the wall (Fig. 13-9). To perform this activity, the patient is instructed to kneel on the unaffected limb and place the ankle to be mobilized with the foot flat on the floor. He is asked to shift his weight forward until his knee contacts the wall, which dorsiflexes the ankle. If his knee is able to contact the wall without compensation further up the kinetic chain (e.g., pelvic rotation), he is asked to move the foot further from the wall to allow for a larger mobilization. The therapist compares the distance between the toes and the wall on the affected side versus the distance between his toes and the wall on his unaffected side. This comparison allows the patient to monitor his progress and compare the motion between the two sides.

Strengthening of the foot and ankle off the bike is imperative to provide the cyclist with the strength necessary to maintain the foot and ankle in a subtalar joint neutral alignment through the pedal stroke. Because the patient demonstrated right ankle weakness in all directions and decreased single-limb balance, he was instructed on 4-way ankle strengthening exercises with Theraband, "short-foot" exercises for intrinsic strengthening, and a single-foot stance progression for intrinsic strengthening and balance retraining. For short-foot intrinsic strengthening, the patient can sit or stand. The therapist cues the patient to elevate the arch of the foot while maintaining the ends of the toes and heel in contact with the floor

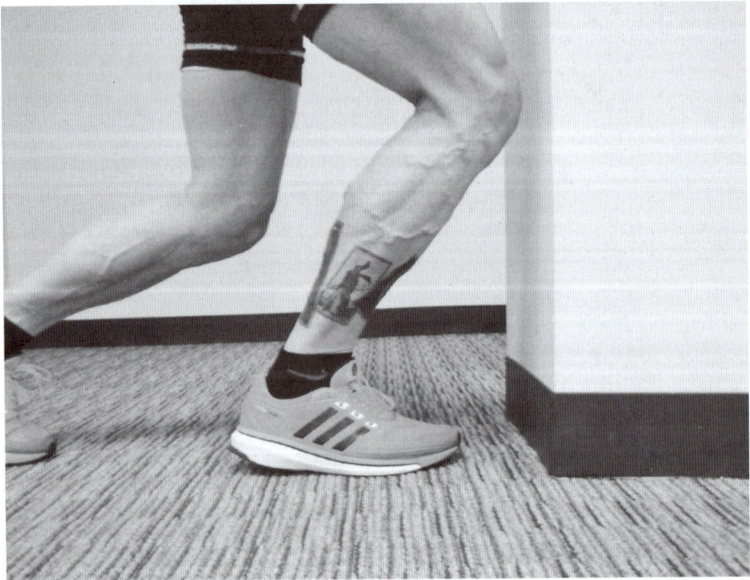

Figure 13-9. Self-mobilization to increase ankle dorsiflexion. To facilitate posterior talar glide in the right ankle, the patient is in a half-kneeling position with the right knee facing the wall. The patient moves the knee toward the wall while maintaining heel contact with the floor, thus dorsiflexing the ankle. This mobilization is performed for 3 sets of 10 repetitions at least twice daily.

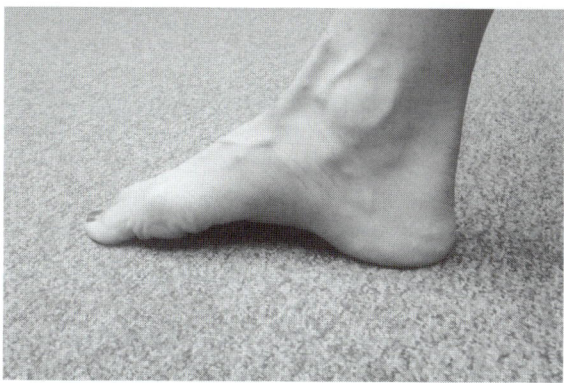

Figure 13-10. Short foot intrinsic strengthening. The patient is asked to elevate the arch of the foot while maintaining the ends of the toes and heel in contact with the floor. This exercise should be performed for 3 sets of 10 repetitions, three times daily.

(Fig. 13-10). The single-foot stance progression involves single-leg static standing on a stable surface first with eyes open, then eyes closed, then eyes open with head turns and head nods. As the patient improves in his ability to perform these activities, he is progressed to an unstable surface with the same progression of activity with added internal and external perturbations.

The patient's hip weakness and lack of neuromuscular control were treated with a variety of strengthening, stabilization, and proprioceptive/balance exercises. Hip abductor weakness causes small alterations in frontal plane knee mechanics. An 8-week program of **isolated hip abductor and external rotator muscle strengthening** has been shown to improve pain and health status in females with PFP.[12,32] This patient was prescribed the following exercises targeted at strengthening the gluteus maximus, gluteus medius, and trunk muscles: clamshell, sidelying hip abduction, side plank, quadruped arm and leg lift, single-leg bridging, and Pallof press or half-kneeling isometric oblique exercise (Figs. 13-11 through 13-14). Clamshell exercises,

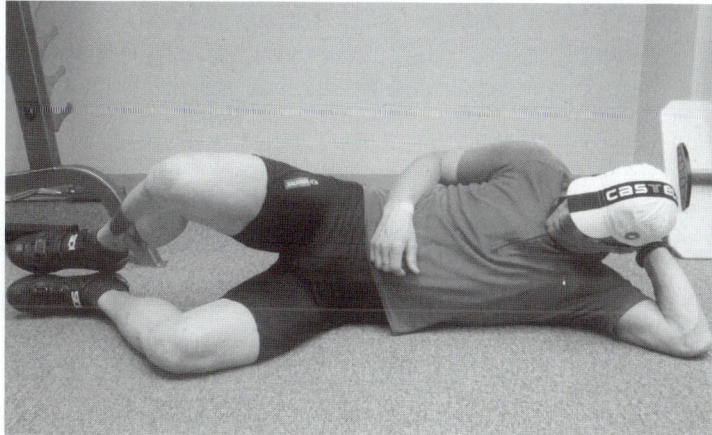

Figure 13-11. Sidelying clamshell exercise.

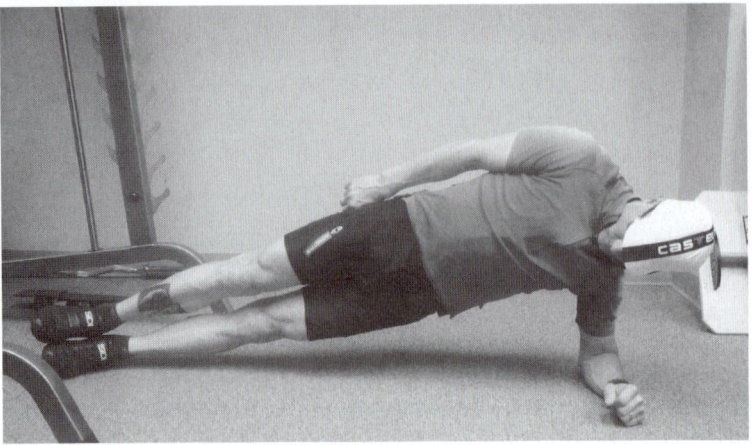

Figure 13-12. Side plank exercise.

sidelying hip abduction, and side plank (with involved side down) have been shown to produce high levels of gluteus medius muscle activation.[33,34] To address strength impairments in the gluteus maximus, several positions can be used. The quadruped position provides weightbearing input to the hip, whereas the half-kneeling position (with the involved knee down) improves proprioception and activates gluteus maximus and the obliques.[35] In the half-kneeling position, performance in front of a mirror provides visual feedback to ensure that the patient keeps his knee, hip, and shoulder in a straight line in the frontal and sagittal planes. Because the patient was able to maintain this position well with perturbation at the shoulders and pelvis in all directions, he was progressed to half-kneeling lifts and chops (Fig. 13-15). The chop and lift exercises require instant muscle activity and promote balance retraining.[36] When the patient is able to stabilize his position in the half-kneeling position,

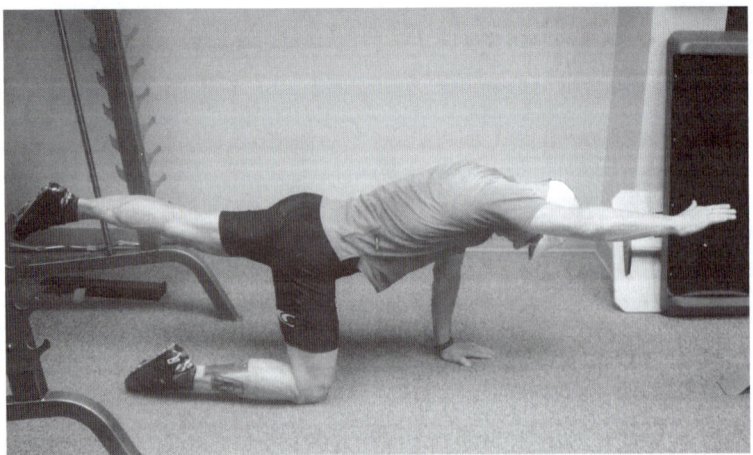

Figure 13-13. Quadruped alternating arm and leg lift exercise.

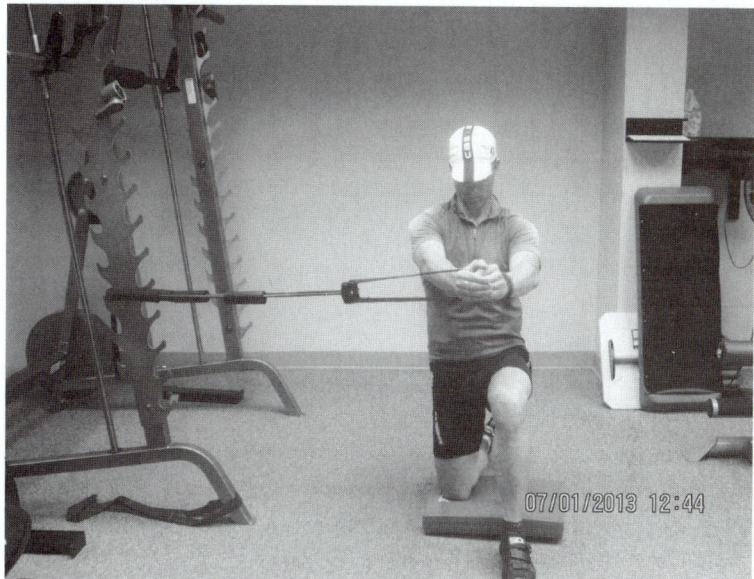

Figure 13-14. Pallof press. Position the patient with the affected limb down in a half-kneeling position, with the weighted pulley in line with the shoulder axis. With the arms extended, there should be a direct lateral line of pull from the weighted pulley. The exercise is initiated by asking the patient to hold the weight in midline against his chest and then fully extend his elbows while maintaining gluteal activation and upright posture. This exercise targets the gluteal muscles as well as hip and trunk rotational stabilizers. The patient should hold the end position for 10 seconds and perform 5 to 10 repetitions.

he is progressed to performing these exercises in the standing position. Right single-foot stance with upper extremity proprioceptive neuromuscular facilitation (PNF) patterns can be incorporated to integrate ankle proprioception, hip, trunk, and lumbopelvic stabilization for training the whole kinetic chain.

Because the patient was eager to resume high-level cycling activities, the therapist treated the joint and tissue mobility dysfunctions and hip impairments concurrently. He gained strength and stability through greater ranges of motion as his ankle joint mobility improved. The physical therapist advised the patient to limit riding to 30 miles per day or less to prevent provocation of knee pain and until the majority of his impairments were fully resolved.

To fully address the cyclist's goal of pain-free long distance cycling, the physical therapist's expertise in treating his off-the-bike impairments must be accompanied by on-the-bike interventions. **On-the-bike corrections of body alignment and pedaling mechanics** are part of the comprehensive management of the cyclist with PFP. Because body position affects force profiles and joint movement patterns throughout the kinetic chain, a proper bike fit is critical.[23] The guidelines for fitting the cyclist to the bike presented here are based on experts in the field of bike fitting[10] and the authors' clinical experience. The bicycle is a static machine, but many components are adjustable. The human body is a dynamic machine, but adaptable. Therefore, it is imperative to address the ergonomics of the cyclist on the bike to

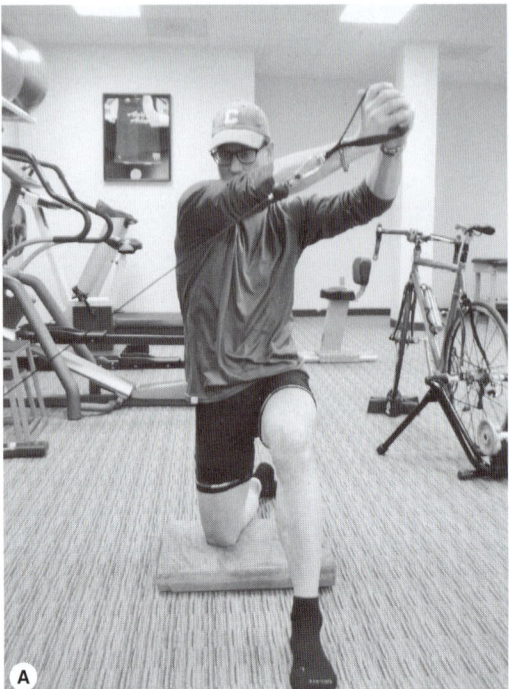

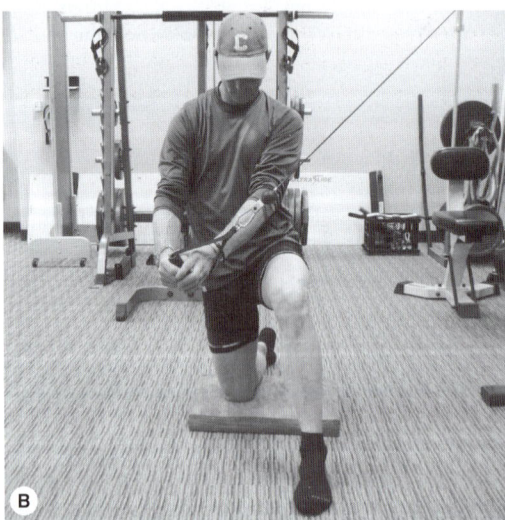

Figure 13-15. **A.** Half-kneeling lifts. Position the pulley at the floor with the patient in half kneeling with the affected knee down. Ensure that the patient has his knee, hip, and shoulder in straight alignment in both the sagittal and frontal planes. The patient grasps the pulley handle with both hands at the affected hip. While maintaining upright posture in all planes, he pulls up and diagonally above the opposite shoulder. This exercise strengthens the gluteals and anterior and rotational stabilizers of the trunk. **B.** Half-kneeling chops. Position the patient on the opposite side of the pulley weight. The patient grasps the pulley with the fulcrum above his head height and pulls the handle down and across the body to the opposite hip while maintaining upright posture in all planes. This exercise targets the gluteals and rotational trunk stabilizers.

Table 13-3 GUIDELINES FOR BIKE FITTING (WITH HANDS PLACED ON BRAKE LEVER HOODS)

Knee flexion	25°-30° when the crank arm is in the 6-o'clock position
Patellar position	Left inferior pole directly over pedal spindle when the left crank arm is in the 9-o'clock position
Trunk angle	25°-35°
Shoulder flexion	90°
Saddle to bar position	≤5 cm
Elbow flexion	25°
Wrist position	Neutral

prevent abnormal, repetitive stresses to the body. By adjusting the bike to position the cyclist in optimal muscle length-tension relationships, the physical therapist can optimize positional tolerance, improve power output, and promote injury prevention. For a perfect union, both the bike and the cyclist need to be addressed. It is important to recognize the limitations of the cyclist (*e.g.*, short hamstring length) and adjust the bike accordingly. Table 13-3 lists guidelines for positioning the rider on the bike that do not take into account individual athlete's limitations.

Before starting the bike fit, the therapist must make sure that the bike is level on the trainer and that the saddle is also level. Wearing the appropriate cycling gear, the cyclist mounts and pedals for approximately 10 minutes, settling into his riding position. It is during this time that the therapist observes the cyclist's body mechanics while he is pedaling, as previously described. Any changes to the bike should begin at the cleat/pedal interface and proceed up the kinetic chain. The cleat/pedal interface is the point of contact for the closed-chain transfer of energy between the cyclist and the bike. Poor positioning at the cleat/pedal interface will result in misalignment at the foot, ankle, and knee. The cleat should be positioned at the first metatarsal head, in line with the pedal spindle, avoiding tibial rotation (Fig. 13-16). Next, the saddle height is adjusted to create 25° to 30° of knee flexion angle when the crank arm is in the 6-o'clock position (Fig. 13-6B). The saddle should also be adjusted fore and aft to align the inferior pole of the patella over the pedal spindle when the crank arm is in the 9-o'clock position. All upper-body positional measurements are performed with the cyclist's hands on the break lever hoods. Trunk-to-thigh angle should be between 25° and 35° when the thigh is parallel to the floor. Shoulder flexion angle should be 90° and elbow flexion angle should be 25°. Wrists should rest in neutral position—avoiding flexion, extension, ulnar, and radial deviations. The authors recommend documenting saddle height and reach before and after the bike fitting adjustments have been made to identify baseline values and record all changes made to the bike.

A correct bike fit and education on posture and pedal stroke should be performed using visual feedback by placing a mirror in front of the patient. During gait, real-time visual feedback improves neuromuscular control.[37] Although similar studies on the bike have yet to be published, visual feedback enhances the cyclist's and therapist's understanding of impairments and the ability to correct them. Video analysis

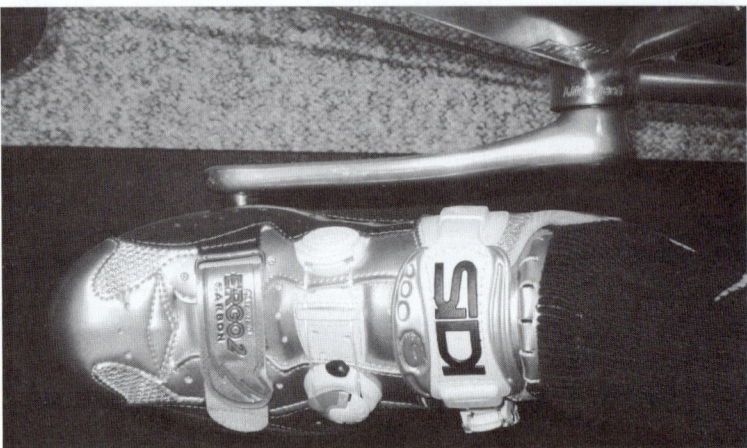

Figure 13-16. Optimal cleat position. Note the cleat is positioned with the first metatarsal head in line with the pedal spindle.

of the rider prior to and following the fitting is helpful and can be used to modify the pedal stroke and posture of the rider after the fitting is complete. Modifying the bike without addressing weakness, joint restrictions, and neuromuscular control will not address the current injury or prevent future injury. These objective deficits should be addressed with a home program off the bike and from visual feedback the rider can gain riding the trainer in front of a mirror to improve neuromuscular control.

Evidence-Based Clinical Recommendations

SORT: Strength of Recommendation Taxonomy
A: Consistent, good-quality patient-oriented evidence
B: Inconsistent or limited-quality patient-oriented evidence
C: Consensus, disease-oriented evidence, usual practice, expert opinion, or case series

1. Patellofemoral pain is often associated with a loss of ankle dorsiflexion. **Grade B**
2. Strengthening the gluteus maximus and medius decreases patellofemoral pain. **Grade B**
3. Correction of body alignment and pedaling mechanics and proper training techniques reduce the incidence of patellofemoral pain in the competitive cyclist. **Grade C**

COMPREHENSION QUESTIONS

13.1 Which of the following strength deficits would *most* likely be identified in the examination of a cyclist with knee pain?
    A. Hip flexion, hip abduction
    B. Hip abduction, hip external rotation
    C. Hip extension, hip abduction
    D. Hip internal rotation, hip abduction

13.2 A female cyclist comes into the physical therapy clinic with complaints of low back pain while riding. Which of these possibilities would *most* likely be contributing to her symptoms?
   A. Saddle height too low
   B. Decreased hip flexion
   C. Decreased abdominal strength
   D. Decreased quadriceps length

ANSWERS

13.1 **B.** Cycling involves movement of the lower extremity through the sagittal plane. Deviation from the sagittal plane can lead to injury at the foot/ankle, knee, hip, and low back, due to its repetitive nature. It is important to be able to maintain neutral alignment in the lower extremity through 360° of the pedal stroke. The hip abductors and external rotators assist in keeping the pelvis and lower leg in neutral alignment as the cyclist motions through the pedal stroke. Cyclists are prone to weakness in the hip abductors and external rotators because they are seldom strengthened outside the sagittal plane.

13.2 **B.** Decreased hip flexion will cause a pelvic shift as the cyclist comes over the top of the pedal stroke, contributing to low back pain. Low saddle position (option A) will have greater impact on knee symptoms. In cyclists, abdominal musculature has been shown to function mainly as an accessory breathing muscle[38] rather than a pelvic stabilizer (option C). The quadriceps remain in a shorted position throughout the pedal stroke (option D).

REFERENCES

1. Standring S. *Gray's Anatomy. The Anatomical Basis of Clinical Practice*. 40th ed. London: Churchill Livingstone; 2009.
2. Fulderson JP. Diagnosis and treatment of patients with patellofemoral pain. *Am J Sports Med*. 2002;30:447-456.
3. Powers CM. Rehabilitation of patellofemoral joint disorders: a critical review. *J Orthop Sports Phys Ther*. 1998;28:345-354.
4. Huberti HH, Hayes WC, Stone JL, Shybut GT. Force ratios in the quadriceps tendon and ligamentum patella. *J Orthop Res*. 1984;21:49-54.
5. Powers CM, Bolgia LA, Callaghan MJ, Collins N, Sheehan FT. Patellofemoral pain: proximal, distal, and local factors, 2nd International Research Retreat. *J Orthop Spors Phys Ther*. 2012;42:A1-A54.
6. Piva SF, Goodnite EA, Childs JD. Strength around the hip and flexibility of soft tissue in individuals with and without patellofemoral pain syndrome. *J Orthop Sports Phys Ther*. 2005;35:793-801.
7. Yamaguchi GT, Zajac FE. A planar model of the knee joint to characterize the knee extensor mechanism. *J Biomech*. 1989;22:1-10.
8. Clarsen B, Krosshaug T, Bahr R. Overuse injuries in professional road cyclists. *Am J Sports Med*. 2010;38:2492-2501.
9. Abbiss CR, Peiffer JJ, Laursen PB. Optimal cadence selection during cycling. *Int J Sports Med*. 2009;10:1-15.

10. Burke ER. *The Science of Cycling*. Champaign, IL: Human Kinetics; 1988.
11. Lajam C, Bharam S, Hall G, Hadley S. Evaluation of hip flexion angle in cyclists and hip impingement. Poster presentation at *International Society for Hip Arthroscopy*. NYU Langone Medical Center; 2012.
12. Khayambashi K, Mohammadkhani Z, Ghaznayi K, Lyle MA, Powers CM. The effects of isolated hip abductor and external rotator muscle strengthening on pain, health status, and hip strength in females with patellofemoral pain: a randomized controlled trial. *J Orthop Sports Phys Ther*. 2012;41:22-29.
13. Cook G. *Movement*. 1st ed. Santa Cruz, CA: On Target Publications; 2010.
14. Wainner RS, Whitman JM, Cleland JA, Flynn TW. Regional interdependence: a musculoskeletal examination model whose time has come. *J Orthop Sports Phys Ther*. 2007;37:658-660.
15. JOSPT perspectives for patients. Anterior knee pain: a holistic approach to treatment. *J Orthop Sports Phys Ther*. 2012;42:573.
16. Stasinopoulos D, Stasinopoulos I. Comparison of effects of exercise program, pulsed ultrasound and transverse friction in the treatment of chronic patellar tendinopathy. *Clin Rehabil*. 2004;18:347-352.
17. Speed CA. Fortnightly review: Corticosteroid injections in tendon lesions. *BMJ*. 2001;323:382-386.
18. Witvrouw E, Lysens R, Bellemans J, Cambier D, Vanderstraaeten G. Intrinsic risk factors for the development of anterior knee pain in an athletic population. A two-year prospective study. *Am J Sports Med*. 2000;28:480-489.
19. Backman LJ, Danielson P. Low range of ankle dorsiflexion predisposes patellar tendinopathy in junior elite basketball players: a 1-year prospective study. *Am J Sports Med*. 2011;39:2626-2633.
20. Burton CJ, Bananno D, Levinger R, Menz HB. Foot and ankle characteristics in patellofemoral pain syndrome: a case control and reliability study. *J Ortho Sports Phys Ther*. 2010;40:286-296.
21. Crossley KM, Zhang WJ, Schache AG, Bryant A, Cowan SM. Performance on the single-leg-squat task indicates hip abductor muscle function. *Am J Sports Med*. 2011;39:866-873.
22. Smith D, Searle B, Thomas S. *The Racing Bike Book*. 3rd ed. London: Haynes Publications; 2008.
23. Barratt PR, Korff T, Elmar SJ, Martin JC. Effect of crank length on joint-specific power during maximal cycling. *Med Sci Sports Exerc*. 2011;43:1689-1697.
24. Cavanaugh PR, Sanderson DJ. *The Biomechanics of Cycling: Studies of the Pedaling Mechanics of Elite Pursuit Riders*. Champaign, IL. Human Kinematics; 1986:105.
25. Gregor RJ, Broker JP, Ryan MM. The biomechanics of cycling. *Exerc Sports Sci Rev*. 1991;19:127-169.
26. Baer G, Heidersheit B. ACL Reconstruction: Third Time's the Charm for Wisconsin Athlete When Professionals Collaborate. *JBJS-JOSPT*. Special Report. 2013:1-6.
27. Mulligan B. *Manual Therapy: "NAGS," "SNAGS," "MWM," etc*. 4th ed. Wellington, NZ: Plane View Services Ltd; 1999.
28. Vincenzino B, Branjerdporn M, Teys P, Jordan K. Initial changes in posterior talar glide and dorsiflexion of the ankle after mobilization with movement in individuals with recurrent ankle sprain. *J Ortho Sports Phys Ther*. 2006;36:464-471.
29. Vincenzino B, O'Brien T. A study of the effects of Mulligan's mobilization with movement. *Manual Therapy*. 1998;3:78-84.
30. Trevino SG, Davis P, Hecht PJ. Management of acute and chronic lateral ankle injuries of the ankle. *Orthop Clin North Am*. 1994;25:1-16.
31. Youdas JW, Krause DA, Egan KS, Theeau TM, Laskowski ER. The effect of static stretching of the calf muscle-tendon unit on active ankle dorsiflexion range of motion. *J Orthop Sports Phys Ther*. 2003;33:408-417.
32. Geiser CF, O'Connor KM, Earl JE. Effects of isolated hip abductor fatigue on frontal plane knee mechanics. *Med Sci Sports Exerc*. 2010;42:535-545.

33. McBeth JW, Earl-Boehm JE, Cobb SC, Huddleston WE. Hip muscle activity during 3 sidelying hip strengthening exercises in distance runners. *J Athl Train*. 2012;47:15-23.
34. Boren K, Conrey C, LeCoguic J, Paprocki L, Voight M, Robinson TK. Electromyographic analysis of gluteus medius and maximus during rehab exercises. *Int J Sports Phys Ther*. 2011;6:206-223.
35. Ekstrom RA, Donatelli RA, Carp KC. Electromyographic analysis of core trunk, hip, and thigh muscle during 9 rehabilitation exercises. *J Orthp Sports Phys Ther*. 2007;37:754-762.
36. Voight ML, Hoogenboom BJ, Cook G. The chop and lift reconsidered: integrating neuromuscular principles into orthopedic and sports rehabilitation. *N Am J Sports Phys Ther*. 2008;3:151-159.
37. Teran-Yengle P, Birkhofer R, Weber MA, Patton K, Thatcher E, Yack HJ. Efficacy of gait training in real-time biofeedback in correcting knee hyperextension patterns in young women. *J Orthop Sports Phys Ther*. 2011;12:948-952.
38. Usabiaga J, Crespo R, Iza I, Aramendi J, Terrados N, Poza JJ. Adaptations of the lumbar spine to different positions of bicycle racing. *Spine*. 1997;22:1965-1969.

Patellar Tendinosis in Volleyball Player With Female Athlete Triad

Jill Thein-Nissenbaum

CASE 14

A 15-year-old competitive female volleyball player with progressively worsening left knee pain over the past 6 months is referred to physical therapy by her pediatrician. She is an outside hitter and her left leg is her take-off leg. Her pain is "right below her kneecap." During volleyball practice, hitting, jumping, running and squatting make her knee pain worse. Her pain is minimally alleviated by ice. She has rested completely and avoided any pain-provoking activity for 3 weeks only to have the pain return immediately upon resumption of activity. The patient reports she grew 4 inches last year; she is now 5 feet 10 inches and weighs 121 lb (body mass index 17.4 kg/m^2). Because of her height, she was moved from junior varsity to the varsity volleyball team. She reports the coach "depends" on her to win, which she finds very stressful. In addition, varsity practices are much longer and she has had a difficult time fitting homework into her schedule. She reports doing "extra" training on an elliptical trainer 60 to 75 minutes every evening. Since starting high school last year, her periods have become more irregular. In the past 12 months, she has had only 4 periods and her last cycle was 4 months ago. She reports the lack of menstruation as "very convenient." In the past 2 years, she has experienced several overuse injuries, including Achilles tendinosis, a metatarsal stress fracture, and a chronic hamstring strain. She reports that each of these conditions took a very long time to heal, even with rest. When the patient walked into the clinic, the physical therapist noted a normal gait pattern, with visible left quadriceps atrophy. Based on the patient's sport, medical history, description of symptoms, and brief observation, the physical therapist suspects the patient presents with chronic patellar tendinosis due to a poor healing environment related to female athlete triad components.

▶ What examination signs are associated with the diagnosis of patellar tendinosis?
▶ Identify referrals to other medical team members.

KEY DEFINITIONS

FEMALE ATHLETE TRIAD: Condition originally identified in 1992[1] as an association between disordered eating, amenorrhea, and osteoporosis; because of strict diagnostic criteria, many females with triad-related conditions were not identified or properly treated.[2] In 2007, the terms were changed to energy availability, menstrual function, and bone mineral density.[2]

SECONDARY AMENORRHEA: Cessation of menstruation for 3 consecutive months in the post-menarche female[2]

TENDINOPATHY: Broad term encompassing any painful condition occurring in and around tendons in response to overuse; tendinitis and tendinosis are both forms of tendinopathy.[3]

TENDINOSIS: Chronic cellular degeneration of a tendon *without* inflammation; classical characteristics include degenerative changes in collagen matrix, hypercellularity, hypervascularity, and a lack of inflammatory cells; thought to be caused by microtears in connective tissue in and around the tendon, leading to reduced tensile strength and increased risk of tendon rupture[3]

Objectives

1. Identify the components of the female athlete triad and describe their interrelatedness.
2. Utilize appropriate screening tools for an individual with suspected female athlete triad.
3. Describe appropriate management of patellar tendinosis.
4. Explain how the female athlete triad is associated with musculoskeletal overuse disorders and how the presence of this condition influences or changes patient/client management.

Physical Therapy Considerations

PT considerations during management of the female athlete with patellar tendinosis and a suspected diagnosis of female athlete triad:

- ▶ **General physical therapy plan of care/goals:** For patellar tendinosis: decrease knee pain; increase lower extremity flexibility; increase lower extremity strength; return to sport and functional activities with minimal pain. For triad-related symptoms: screen for all 3 components of the triad; refer to pediatrician or primary care physician (PCP) for follow-up testing and interprofessional team management.

- ▶ **Physical therapy interventions:** For patellar tendinosis: patient education regarding functional anatomy and injury pathomechanics; modalities and manual therapy to decrease pain; mobilization and passive stretching to improve joint mobility and lower extremity flexibility; eccentric exercise to increase muscular strength and endurance of the quadriceps and remodel the patellar tendon; home exercise instruction. For triad-related symptoms: education regarding adequate rest and recovery for normal tissue healing; education regarding importance of cross-training and anaerobic sport-specific exercise.

▶ **Precautions during physical therapy:** For patellar tendinosis: monitor for signs and symptoms of overuse and overtraining; educate patient about delayed-onset muscle soreness and how to appropriately manage the condition. For triad-related symptoms: monitor signs of delayed or unusually slow healing, fatigue, and resumption of menses.

▶ **Complications interfering with physical therapy:** Patient noncompliance with activity modification, specifically with decrease in exercise regimen and volleyball practice; inability of family to provide emotional support such as transportation to therapy sessions; lifestyle habits (e.g., diet, sleep hygiene) that interfere with optimal tissue healing

Understanding the Health Condition

Patellar tendinosis (jumper's knee) is an overuse condition characterized by pain with jumping and landing. The condition is frequently identified in volleyball players and can affect 38% to 50% of players[4] and can significantly decrease sports performance.[5] Although rest from sport may reduce symptoms, a return to training and competition is often accompanied by worsening symptoms.[6] One-third of volleyball players with patellar tendinosis required at least 6 months of rest prior to resumption of activity.[5] The treatment of patellar tendinosis requires a structured, well-supervised rehabilitation program due to the fact that it is a chronic condition with potentially poor outcomes. Clinical diagnosis is frequently based on individuals' subjective reports of pain during activity. The most common location of the pain is the proximal patellar attachment, just under the apex of the patella.[5] Tenderness during palpation of the tendon confirms the clinical diagnosis, which can be further verified by ultrasound imaging or magnetic resonance imaging (MRI).[3,5] Many risk factors influence the initiation of degenerative changes in the patellar tendon. Intrinsic factors include decreased muscle flexibility in the hamstrings, quadriceps, and gastrocnemius-soleus complex as well as decreased joint mobility at the talocrural joint, limiting dorsiflexion.[5] Extrinsic factors include inadequate footwear and inappropriate training—especially a rapid increase in frequency and intensity of activity.[5]

For more than a decade, **eccentric exercise has been a cornerstone of rehabilitation for tendinosis** and a substantial body of evidence supports its effectiveness.[4-9] In particular, painful eccentric decline squats have been shown to be a superior therapeutic exercise intervention compared to standard eccentric squats.[9] However, outcomes after rehabilitation are still less than ideal. In a study comparing surgical versus conservative management in 35 athletes with patellar tendinosis, athletes in the conservative management group performed decline eccentric training twice per day, 3 × 15 repetitions each session for 12 weeks.[4] The athletes slowly resumed activity after the 12-week intervention and continued the eccentric training program twice weekly. While the authors concluded that eccentric strength training for 12 weeks was prudent because surgical treatment offered no advantage over eccentric strength training, only 55% of the athletes achieved either excellent or good outcomes at the 12-month follow-up.[4] Strength training such as heavy, slow resistance training (double-leg exercises) has also proven to be as effective as eccentric training.[8] In a study by Kongsgaard et al.,[8] subjects were divided into 3 groups: a decline squat group, a heavy, slow resistance training group, and a glucocorticoid injection group. The decline squat was performed twice per day, every day for 12 weeks at home. The resistance training group trained 3 times per week for 12 weeks at a gymnasium. At 6-month follow-up, subjects in both exercise groups achieved outcomes superior to those of the steroid injection group; however, the outcomes between the 2 exercise groups were not statistically different.[8] Extracorporeal shock wave therapy (ESWT) is a noninvasive treatment using strong sound waves directed at connective tissues for a variety of musculoskeletal conditions. In Europe, ESWT has been evaluated for its effectiveness in treating patellar tendinopathy. In a randomized controlled trial of 62 symptomatic jumping athletes, ESWT treatment delivered during the competitive season was no more effective than placebo treatment for patellar tendinopathy.[10] Other treatments such as massage, injections of platelet-rich plasma or glucocorticoids, dry needling, and arthroscopic debridement are not as effective as eccentric squats.[7]

The female athlete triad (Triad) is a syndrome describing the interrelatedness of 3 conditions: energy availability, menstrual function, and bone mineral density. Its prevalence and traits have been extensively examined in adolescent females.[11-16] Although previously thought to occur primarily in athletes whose sports require leanness such as gymnastics, diving, and cheer, the triad components have been identified in females participating in nearly all sports, including volleyball, basketball, and swimming. Energy availability is defined as energy intake minus energy expenditure. The resulting post-exercise energy must be utilized for the regulation of body homeostasis, including tissue healing, cardiovascular functioning, and menstruation.[2,17] Low energy availability may occur intentionally (through excessive exercise, dramatic decrease in caloric intake, or a combination of both) or unintentionally (athletes are unaware of their caloric needs and neglect to eat enough calories to off-set the calories burned through physical activity).[2] In a sample of 311 female high school athletes, those with disordered eating behaviors were twice as likely to be injured during the sports season compared to those reporting normal eating behaviors.[16] **Energy availability may also affect healing rates of overuse injuries.** If the amount of post-exercise energy is decreased, there may not be sufficient energy available to promote a positive healing environment. Menstrual function occurs along a spectrum, ranging from eumenorrhea (normal menses) to amenorrhea. Menstrual dysfunction includes primary amenorrhea, secondary amenorrhea, and oligomenorrhea. Primary amenorrhea is the lack of onset of menses by the age of 15 years.[2,11] Secondary amenorrhea is a cessation of menstruation for 3 consecutive months in the post-menarche female. Oligomenorrhea is menstrual cycles occurring more than 35 days apart.[2] The prevalence of menstrual dysfunction in female high school athletes ranges from 27% to 54%.[13,16] The third Triad component is bone mineral density (BMD). BMD ranges from optimal bone health to osteoporosis. Although osteopenia and osteoporosis are well-defined terms in post-menopausal women, there are numerous challenges in determining the ideal BMD in the adolescent female athlete.[18] An athlete's BMD reflects numerous variables, including energy availability, menstrual status, genetic composition, and environmental factors, (e.g., amount of sunlight exposure, vitamin D absorption).[19] A one-time "snapshot" of the adolescent female athlete's BMD may not provide as much information as changes in BMD over time.[2,20] Although studies related to BMD in young females are limited, the prevalence of low BMD has been reported to be approximately 22% in high school female athletes.[13,14]

Physical Therapy Patient/Client Management

The athlete presenting with an overuse injury benefits from education regarding the nature of the pathology, including variables that are amenable to change through physical therapy interventions. In this case, the athlete with patellar tendinosis may benefit from changes in her training regimen, increasing lower extremity flexibility, and increasing eccentric quadriceps strength. She presents with a history of menstrual irregularity, an abrupt increase in training, a rapid change in body composition (requiring additional energy to support tissue growth and new homeostasis), and external stressors, including performance pressure from her coach and time management for academics. Menstrual irregularity is a concern; the athlete may be falling into a negative energy balance (unintentionally) due to the rapid increase in activity that may not be offset by an increase in caloric consumption. In addition, the recent growth spurt warrants additional energy to support the growth of tissue and new homeostasis. The physical therapist can treat the athlete for the patellar tendinosis, but referral to the patient's pediatrician or PCP for further examination of secondary amenorrhea is warranted. The athlete's report of slow or delayed healing of previous overuse injuries may be directly related to the negative energy balance; her body may simply not have enough "left-over" energy available to support tissue healing and menstruation. Further testing of her menstrual dysfunction, as well as further screening for other Triad-related components, is indicated.

Examination, Evaluation, and Diagnosis

The examination of this particular athlete is 2-fold: the left lower extremity and issues related to the Triad. Physical examination of the lower extremity should begin in standing with observation for quadriceps atrophy and circumferential girth measurements to document differences between limbs. Patellar alignment, foot position (pronation or supination), and any transverse plane alterations in the tibia and femur should be noted. In non-weightbearing positions, active and passive range of motion of the hip, knee, and ankle should be assessed. In addition, lower extremity flexibility should be examined. **Decreased flexibility in the quadriceps and hamstrings** has been identified as a contributing factor to patellar tendinosis.[21,22] In this patient, lower extremity flexibility testing revealed bilateral hamstring tightness with the left hamstring tighter than the right. Ely's test, Ober test, and the

Thomas test were all positive on the left. In long sitting, patellar tracking with isometric quadriceps setting ("quad sets") can be assessed. If the patella is tracking laterally, the increased lateral pull on the patellar tendon may contribute to the athlete's pain. Tightness in the lateral structures, including the iliotibial (IT) band and lateral patellar retinaculum, may be contributing factors to the lateral tracking of the patella. With quad sets, this athlete demonstrated a laterally tracking patella, which was painful. Isolated strength assessment of the quadriceps, hamstrings, gluteus maximus, and gluteus medius should be performed. Some evidence has suggested that **decreased quadriceps strength** is associated with patellar tendinosis.[21] Gluteal weakness may also contribute to femoral internal rotation, which may cause irritation of the patellar tendon in closed-chain activities such as squatting and jumping.[23] This athlete's left lower extremity strength was decreased in hip abduction, external rotation, and knee extension. Palpation of the patellar tendon should be performed with the athlete in long sitting with the knees flexed to approximately 20° to allow for better access of the inferior pole of the patella. In patellar tendinosis, **point tenderness is noted along the length of the patellar tendon, especially proximally, at the insertion into the patella**.[21] In this athlete, the therapist noted mild thickening of the left patellar tendon with point tenderness at its inferior pole.

Last, function should be assessed. The physical therapist can first ask the athlete to perform double-limb squats, noting any frontal plane weight shifting, increased femoral rotation, knee valgus, and/or foot pronation. Next, the athlete should perform single-limb squats, starting with the uninvolved side to provide the examiner what "normal" movement is for the athlete. On the involved limb, the examiner should note where in the range of motion the athlete experiences pain. In addition, the therapist should note if the pain is primarily with a concentric or eccentric contraction. During performance of the double-leg squat, the patient demonstrated reliance (*i.e.*, increased weightbearing) on her right lower extremity. When performing the single-leg squat on her left leg, she reported pain at 25° of knee flexion that worsened with continued knee flexion (eccentric phase of the squat). She also demonstrated increased knee valgus and hip internal rotation during the single-limb squat on the left as compared to the right.

Because of the athlete's history of secondary amenorrhea, recent stress fracture, and delayed healing of overuse injuries, increased physical activity, physical and emotional stress, and recent rapid growth, screening for the female athlete triad is indicated. Although management of Triad-related symptoms is beyond the scope of the physical therapist, appropriate screening and referral to the proper healthcare professional is paramount. Numerous screening tools exist, many of which focus primarily on disordered eating behaviors.[24-28] One relatively brief screening tool that addresses all Triad components is the Female Athlete Triad Coalition Screening Questionnaire.[29] The questionnaire consists of 12 questions, most of which can be answered "yes" or "no". The questionnaire addresses issues such as body image, eating behaviors, age at menarche, and stress fracture history. The questionnaire takes less than 5 minutes for the athlete to complete (Fig. 14-1).[29] There is no set number of questions that must be answered "yes" or "no" to warrant a referral; rather, the questionnaire should be reviewed by the clinician and used to start a discussion with the athlete related to the female athlete triad. Because of her irregular menstruation, increased activity and

FEMALE ATHLETE TRIAD SCREENING QUESTIONNAIRE

This tool can be given to female athletes during the pre-season evaluation, known as the pre-participation examination. Positive responses to these questions should trigger concern for the evaluating physician, thus identifying the female athlete at risk for the Female Athlete Triad. Upon identification of an "at-risk" athlete, the physician can investigate further by completing a second level, more in-depth, questionnaire, physical examination and laboratory evaluation found following this screening questionnaire.

1) Do you worry about your weight or body composition?
   Yes   No

2) Do you limit or carefully control the foods that you eat?
   Yes   No

3) Do you try to lose weight to meet weight or image/appearance requirements in your sport?
   Yes   No

4) Does your weight affect the way you feel about yourself?
   Yes   No

5) Do you worry that you have lost control over how much you eat?
   Yes   No

6) Do you make yourself vomit, use diuretics or laxatives after you eat?
   Yes   No

7) Do you currently or have you ever suffered from an eating disorder?
   Yes   No

8) Do you ever eat in secret?
   Yes   No

9) What age was your first menstrual period?
   _____

10) Do you have monthly menstrual cycles?
    Yes   No

11) How many menstrual cycles have you had in the last year?
    _____

12) Have you ever had a stress fracture?
    Yes   No

Figure 14-1. Female athlete triad screening questionnaire. (Reproduced with permission from the Female Athlete Triad Coalition including Drs. Margo Mountjoy, Mark Hutchinson, Laura Cruz, and Connie Lebrun.)

stress, history of a stress fracture and overuse injuries, this athlete should be referred to an appropriate healthcare provider for further assessment. The Female Athlete Triad Coalition has developed guidelines to assist physicians and primary care providers when performing an in-depth examination for a patient at risk for female athlete triad (Fig. 14-2).[29] The physical therapist, in cooperation with the athlete, her

FEMALE ATHLETE TRIAD SCREENING QUESTIONNAIRE
Physician Follow-up

This document outlines the guidelines for the physician that should be undertaken once a female athlete has been identified at risk for the female athlete triad in the initial screening process. A detailed nutritional analysis of energy availability can be completed in cooperation with a registered sports nutritionist.

DETAILED HISTORY

Please circle the response that best matches your situation.

Never = 1
Rarely = 2
Occasionally = 3
More often than not = 4
Regularly = 5
Always = 6

1. Do you want to weigh more or less than you do?
   1 2 3 4 5 6

2. Do you lose weight regularly to meet weight requirements for your sport?
   1 2 3 4 5 6
   How do you do it?_____

3. Is weight/body composition an issue for you?
   1 2 3 4 5 6

4. Are you satisfied with your eating habits?
   1 2 3 4 5 6

5. Do you think your performance is directly affected by your weight?
   1 2 3 4 5 6
   If so how?_____

6. Do you have forbidden foods?
   1 2 3 4 5 6

7. Are you a vegetarian?
   1 2 3 4 5 6
   Since what age?_____

Figure 14-2. In-depth Triad questionnaire, completed if the screening questionnaire (Fig. 14-1) raises concern. (Reproduced with permission from the Female Athlete Triad Coalition including Drs. Margo Mountjoy, Mark Hutchinson, Laura Cruz, and Connie Lebrun.)

8. Do you miss meals?
   1 2 3 4 5 6
   If so, how often? For what reason?_____

9. Do you have rapid increases of decreases in your body weight?
   1 2 3 4 5 6

10. What do you consider your ideal competitive weight? _____

11. Has anyone ever suggested you lose weight or change your eating habits?
    1 2 3 4 5 6

12. Has a coach, judge, or family member ever called you fat?
    1 2 3 4 5 6

13. What do you do to control your weight?_____
    _____

14. Do you worry if you have missed a workout?
    1 2 3 4 5 6

15. Do you exercise or are you physically active as well as training for your sport?
    1 2 3 4 5 6

16. Do you have stress in your life outside sport?
    1 2 3 4 5 6
    What are these stresses?_____

17. Are you able to cope with stress?
    1 2 3 4 5 6
    How?_____

18. What is your family structure?_____

19. Do you use or have you use(d) these ways to lose weight?
    a. Laxatives   1 2 3 4 5 6
    b. Diuretics   1 2 3 4 5 6
    c. Vomiting   1 2 3 4 5 6
    d. Diet pills   1 2 3 4 5 6
    e. Saunas   1 2 3 4 5 6
    f. Plastic bags or wrap during training   1 2 3 4 5 6
    g. Other methods (please state)_____ 1 2 3 4 5 6

Figure 14-2. (*Continued*)

Review of systems: (headaches/visual problems, galactorrhea/acne/male pattern hair distribution)

Complete history of injuries.

Nutritional analysis assessing energy balance and nutrient balance.

PHYSICAL EXAMINATION

Height: _____

Weight: _____

Blood Pressure: _____

Pulse: _____

Physical signs of Eating Disorder: (lanugo, parotid gland enlargement, carotonemia): _____
_____

Skin: Acne/Male Pattern Hirsutism: _____

Tanner Staging: _____

Percent Body Fat (fat callipers): _____

Musculoskeletal Injury Assessment: _____

Figure 14-2. (*Continued*)

parents, the pediatrician, sports nutritionist or dietician, sports psychologist, and her coaches can establish a well-defined interprofessional team that can assist the athlete to achieve the goals of decreased knee pain, improved sports performance, resumption of menses, and decreased stress.

Plan of Care and Interventions

In this case, the athlete will need to be treated and referred. Because her medical history raises some concerns, the athlete should be referred back to her pediatrician for follow-up of signs and symptoms related to the female athlete triad. However, she can concurrently be treated for her patellar tendinosis.

Successful management of patellar tendinosis includes many published strategies. Several authors have suggested that comprehensive patellar tendinosis rehabilitation include eccentric exercises, exercises performed in closed kinetic chain, maintenance of aerobic capacity, and incorporation of functional (multiplanar) stretching of shortened muscles.[3,30] Patients should be informed that moderate pain during eccentric exercise is acceptable. Specifically, using the numeric pain rating scale in which 0 represents no pain and 10 is maximal pain, a level of 3 to 4 is acceptable.[3]

The athlete in this case presented with decreased lower extremity flexibility, particularly in the quadriceps and hamstrings. Stretching of these muscles as well as other lower extremity muscles, such as the IT band and gastrocnemius-soleus complex, should be performed frequently throughout the day. Hamstring stretching can be performed using a doorjamb (Fig. 14-3) or with a towel so that the quadriceps remain passive. Hold-relax stretching, using the rationale of autogenic inhibition, may be useful. Quadriceps stretching can be performed in prone with a posterior pelvic tilt using a towel draped around the foot or in standing with

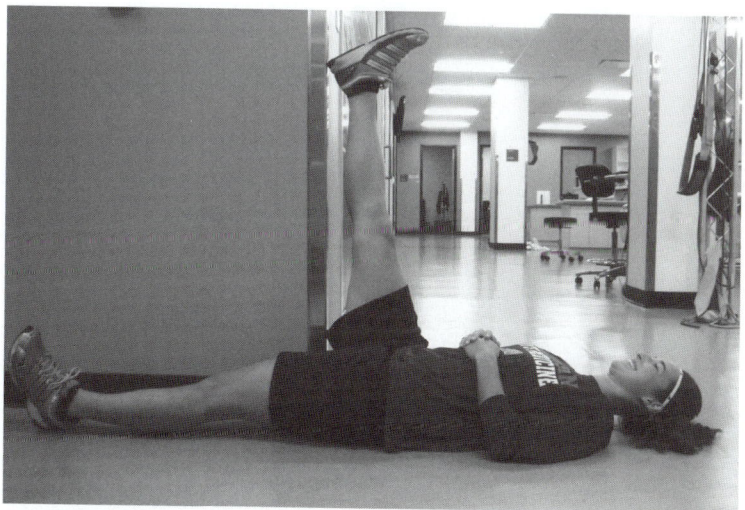

Figure 14-3. Hamstring stretching in a doorjamb. Prolonged stretching in this position allows the muscle fibers to remodel into a lengthened position.

the use of a chair (Fig. 14-4). Stretching of the gastrocnemius-soleus complex can be performed in standing. Stretching of the IT band can be performed in sidelying with the use of a foam roller. A substitute for a foam roller can be a 2-L beverage bottle, filled with water, then frozen. The ice provides both a firm and cold surface. In this author's experience, stretching, regardless of the mode, should be performed frequently throughout the day, at least 5 to 7 times per day, with each stretch held for approximately 30 seconds. In addition to the static stretching described previously, the athlete should perform dynamic warm-up stretching that includes multiplanar movements such as forward and backward leg swings that incorporate some rotation, as well as high knees (Fig. 14-5) and donkey kicks. These dynamic stretching activities can be performed after the athlete is aerobically warmed up, but before the start of practice or competition. Static stretching is intended to increase muscle length by taking the muscle to its end range and maintaining this position for a specified duration. Unfortunately, some studies have demonstrated that acute static stretching immediately prior to performance may negatively affect performance outcomes.[31] In contrast, most research studies have shown that dynamic stretching has a positive effect on performance.[31] Thus, static stretching can be safely performed at home with the intent to increase muscle

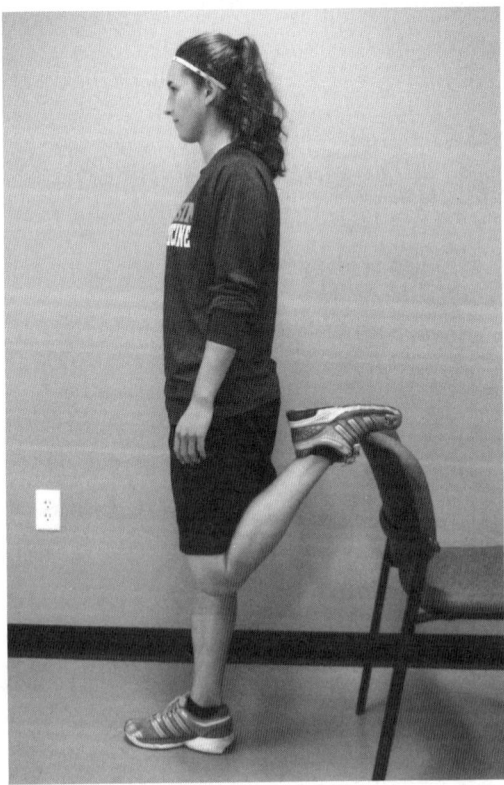

Figure 14-4. Standing quadriceps stretching with a chair to support the ankle. The athlete is performing a concurrent posterior pelvic tilt to incorporate the rectus femoris into the stretch.

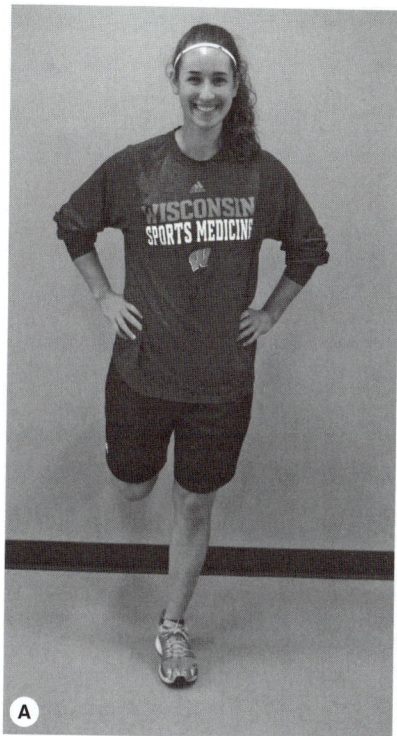 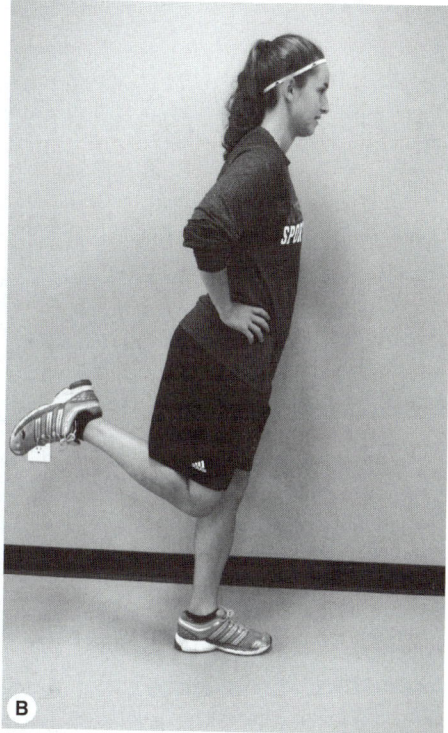

Figure 14-5. Donkey kicks from the front (**A.**) and side (**B.**). This dynamic warm-up requires concentric contraction of the hamstrings, thereby creating reciprocal inhibition of the quadriceps muscle, resulting in a dynamic quadriceps stretch.

length, whereas dynamic stretching performed prior to sports participation can positively affect performance.[31]

Strengthening of the quadriceps, particularly eccentric strength training, is critical. Eccentric exercise on a decline board of an angle of 25° should be utilized.[5] This position limits the use of plantar flexors and allows the athlete with decreased dorsiflexion mobility to perform the squat throughout a greater range of motion without altering body mechanics. The eccentric phase is performed with the athlete lowering to 60° of knee flexion while standing only on the involved lower extremity (Fig. 14-6). The concentric phase of the squat should be done using both lower extremities, making sure the trunk is maintained in a vertical position. Biernat et al.[5] investigated the effectiveness of eccentric squat strength training during volleyball season in male volleyball players with patellar tendinosis. The athletes performed the eccentric squats for 3 sets of 15 repetitions once per day. On match days, or days when the training session was very intense, the volleyball players did not perform the exercises. Each athlete only performed the exercises if his pain level did not exceed 4 points on the visual analog scale (0-10 points). At week 4 of the 12-week training program, the authors had the players perform the eccentric decline squat exercises on an unstable surface. The results showed that athletes with patellar tendinosis had a decrease in pain when performing the eccentric

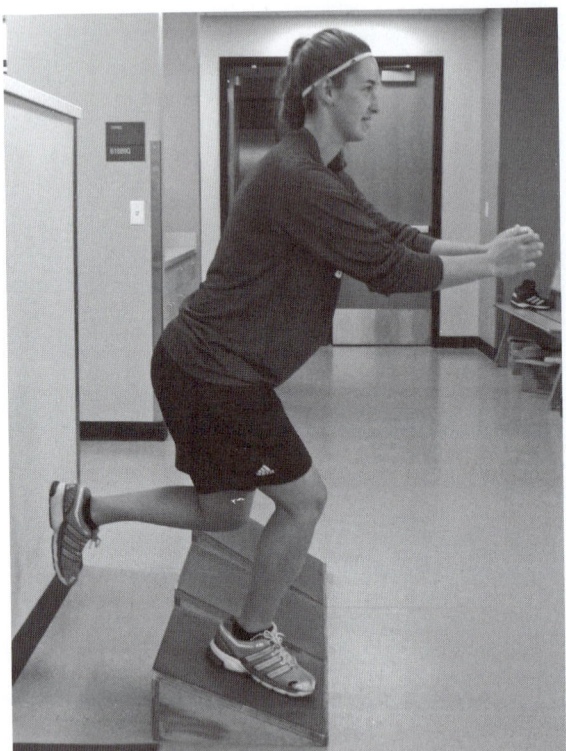

Figure 14-6. The eccentric phase of a single-limb squat on a 25° decline board. The athlete lowers to 60° of knee flexion on the affected leg, then uses both legs to come out of the squat (the concentric phase).

training program during the volleyball season.[5] Based on these findings, the athlete in this case could start with the guideline of 3 sets of 15 repetitions performed daily if her pain level is less than 5 points and it is not a match or heavy practice day. Progression could occur through the addition of an unstable surface, or through increasing the load by having the patient hold weights or dumbbells (Fig. 14-7).

General lower extremity strengthening of the hamstrings, hip abductors, and hip extensors should be performed, starting with isolated open-chain strengthening and progressing to functional closed-chain strengthening. The patient can be instructed to perform these exercises at home with weights or resistive tubing. Sidelying hip abduction with the leg against the wall (Fig. 14-8) is an open-chain hip abduction exercise that has been proven particularly effective at recruiting the gluteus medius.[32] Other exercises that bias the gluteus medius include side plank abduction with dominant leg on top or bottom and single-limb squat.[33] Hamstring strengthening can be achieved through seated hamstring curls against resistance or roll-ups with the affected limb on a physioball (Fig. 14-9). Exercises that bias the gluteus maximus include single-limb squat, single-limb deadlift, front plank with hip extension, gluteal squeeze, side plank abduction with dominant leg on top or bottom, and single-limb squat (Fig. 14-10).[32,33] The frequency of these activities depends on the resistance and the intent of the exercise. If the exercise is designed

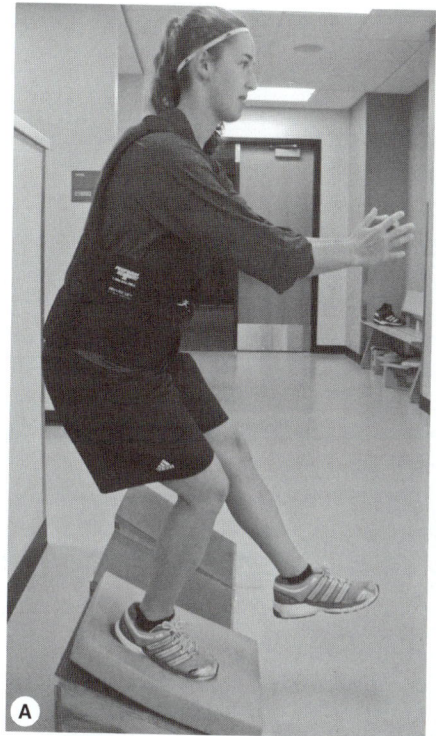 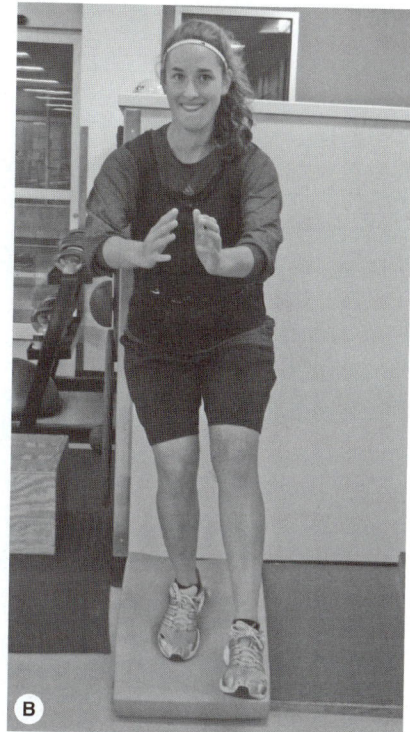

Figure 14-7. Single-limb squat progression with the patient wearing a weight vest and standing on an unstable surface. **A.** Side view. **B.** Front view.

primarily for neuromuscular retraining, or teaching the athlete how to recruit specific muscles, the resistance should be low, but can be performed daily. On the other hand, if the intent is to increase force production, the activity should be performed against higher resistance, but less often, such as 3 times per week.

Deep friction massage (DFM) to the patellar tendon can also be performed. The theory behind the utilization of DFM is to increase the mechanical load to the tendinopathic tissue, as well as to reduce molecular cross-linking. With tendinosis, scar tissue is laid down in a disorganized fashion. DFM, followed by stretching and eccentric strength training, can help scar tissue remodel along the lines of load.[34] The clinician can perform DFM and also teach the athlete to perform this skill at home for 5 to 7 minutes prior to her exercise sessions. Although the evidence supporting the use of DFM in tendinosis is limited, there is anecdotal evidence and a rationale for its use that fits the current understanding of tendinosis.[34]

Last, aerobic capacity needs to be maintained.[3,30] This patient is currently performing additional cardiovascular activity outside the scheduled volleyball practice. Because volleyball is primarily an anaerobic sport, additional aerobic conditioning beyond that completed in regular practice sessions is not necessary and may be aggravating her patellar tendinosis. The activity she is performing in practice is most likely enough activity to maintain a healthy aerobic capacity. At the initial

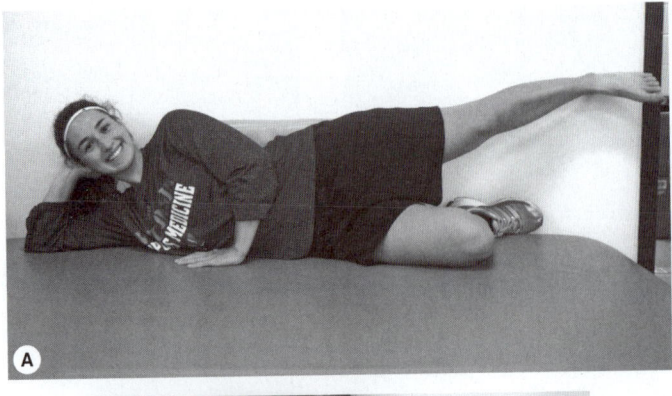
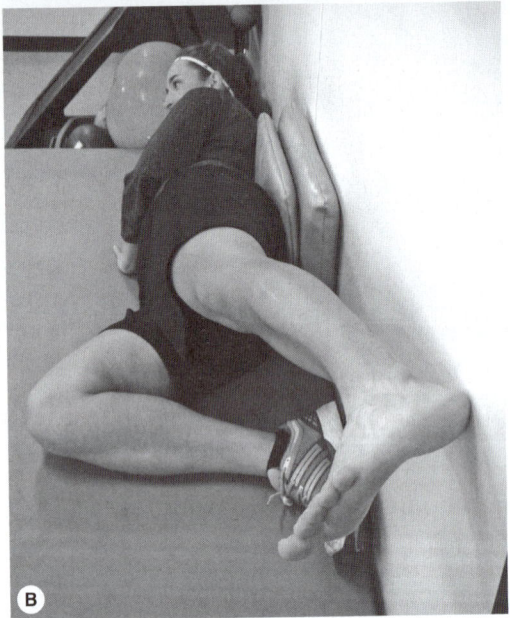

Figure 14-8. Sidelying hip abduction using a wall as a tactile cue. The athlete puts a pillow behind her back, places her heel on the wall (biasing her into hip extension), and pushes her top hand into the mat or floor, increasing core activation. The heel of the top leg is maintained against the wall while the athlete performs hip abduction. **A.** Front view. **B.** Side view. Note how the use of pillows behind the back biases the hip into extension.

evaluation, the physical therapist recommended that the "extra" conditioning she is performing on the elliptical trainer every day should be discontinued. An interval program consisting of short bursts (30-45 seconds) of high-intensity activity followed by a 30-second recovery may be more beneficial and can slowly be reintroduced as the athlete's symptoms subside.

In addition to implementation of the program for patellar tendinosis, this athlete requires **referral back to her PCP** for follow-up examination testing of the conditions related to the female athlete triad. The physical therapist will need to work

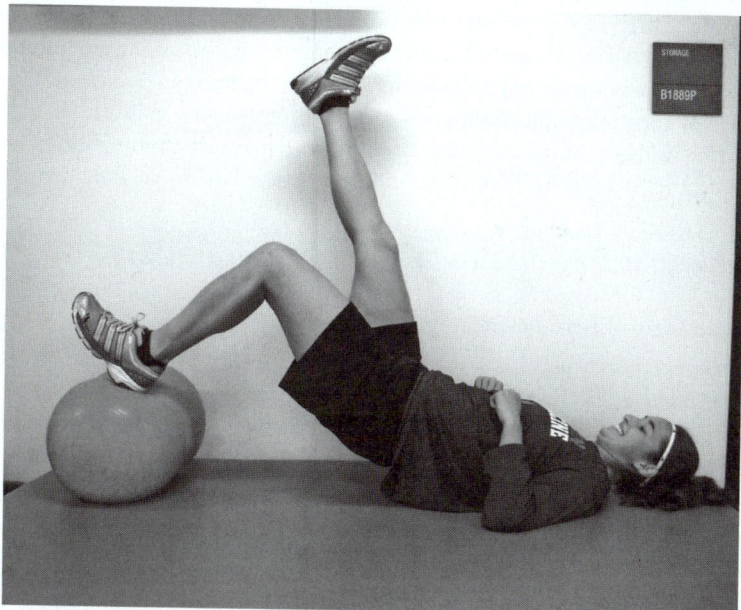

Figure 14-9. Single-leg hamstring strengthening using a ball.

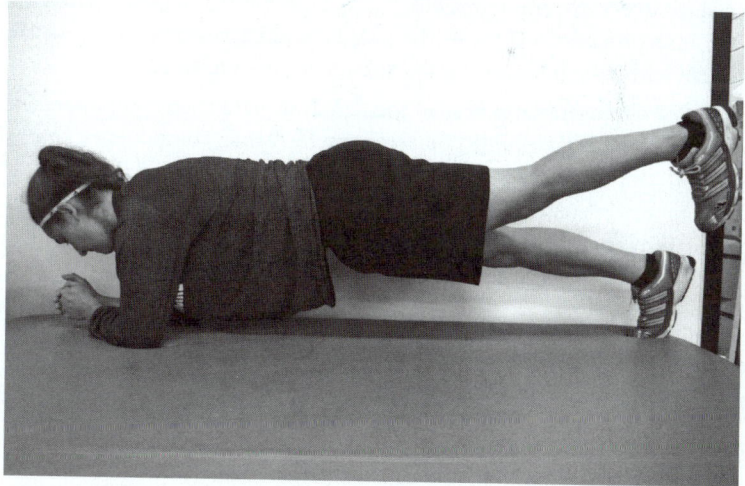

Figure 14-10. Front plank with leg lift with hip extension. The athlete can alternate the leg lift.

closely with the PCP, reporting signs and symptoms observed during the therapy visit. Once the PCP has examined and developed a plan of care for this athlete, the role of the physical therapist is to monitor physical activity and tendinosis symptoms. The physical therapist will need to observe the athlete for signs of fatigue, delayed healing, and additional or subsequent injuries, all of which are signs that the athlete is not improving and may have continued issues related to the Triad. Education of the athlete as well as her parents is critical; they must understand the importance of adequate caloric intake as well as rest to promote a good healing environment for overuse injuries. As with any overuse injury, patients must be educated about the high rate of recurrence and symptoms to watch for. Because this athlete has a history of amenorrhea and chronic overuse injuries, she must thoroughly understand the importance of cross-training, rest, and recovery for her overall long-term health.

Evidence-Based Clinical Recommendations

SORT: Strength of Recommendation Taxonomy
A: Consistent, good-quality patient-oriented evidence
B: Inconsistent or limited-quality patient-oriented evidence
C: Consensus, disease-oriented evidence, usual practice, expert opinion, or case series

1. Successful management of the athlete with patellar tendinosis includes activity modification, eccentric strengthening of the quadriceps using a decline board, maintaining aerobic capacity, and incorporating functional (multiplanar) stretching of inflexible muscles. **Grade B**
2. Females with decreased caloric intake and negative energy balance may experience slow or delayed healing. **Grade C**
3. Physical examination of individuals with patellar tendinosis typically reveals decreased lower extremity flexibility, pain with palpation of the patellar tendon at the insertion on the apex of the patella, and decreased eccentric quadriceps strength with no current signs of acute inflammation. **Grade B**
4. Because of the interrelatedness of the female athlete triad components, females with one component should be screened for other components and referred back to their primary care provider for further testing. **Grade B**

COMPREHENSION QUESTIONS

14.1 Evidence supports that patients with patellar tendinosis will benefit most from what type of muscle contraction of the quadriceps?
   A. Concentric
   B. Eccentric
   C. Isometric
   D. Isokinetic

14.2 When menstrual dysfunction occurs in the female adolescent athlete, she must be screened for the other Triad components, which include:
   A. Disordered eating and bone mineral density
   B. Disordered eating and osteoporosis
   C. Energy availability and bone mineral density
   D. Energy availability and osteoporosis

ANSWERS

14.1 B. Eccentric exercise has been a cornerstone of tendinopathy rehabilitation for more than a decade, and a substantial body of evidence supports its effectiveness.[7] It is acceptable to experience mild pain during this activity; because this may be counterintuitive, the physical therapist should educate the athlete regarding this training.

14.2 C. The female athlete triad is the interrelatedness of energy availability, menstrual function, and bone mineral density.[11-16] Terms such as disordered eating and osteoporosis are too exclusive (options A, B, and D); they do not "capture" all individuals who suffer from Triad components. An athlete may have decreased energy availability because she is unaware of her caloric needs and is simply not consuming enough calories for the energy she is expending. This individual does not have disordered eating, but does have decreased energy availability. She would not be identified as having a Triad component if disordered eating were the defining term.

REFERENCES

1. Otis CL, Drinkwater B, Johnson M, Loucks A, Wilmore J. American College of Sports Medicine position stand. The Female Athlete Triad. *Med Sci Sports Exerc*. 1997;29:i-ix.
2. Nattiv A, Loucks AB, Manore MM, Sanborn CF, Sundgot-Borgen J, Warren MP. American College of Sports Medicine position stand. The female athlete triad. *Med Sci Sports Exerc*. 2007;39:1867-1882.
3. Peers KH, Lysens RJ. Patellar tendinopathy in athletes: current diagnostic and therapeutic recommendations. *Sports Med*. 2005;35:71-87.
4. Bahr R, Fossan B, Loken S, Engebretsen L. Surgical treatment compared with eccentric training for patellar tendinopathy (Jumper's Knee). A randomized, controlled trial. *J Bone Joint Surg Am*. 2006;88:1689-1698.
5. Biernat R, Trzaskoma Z, Trzaskoma L, Czaprowski D. Rehabilitation protocol for patellar tendinopathy applied amongst 16-19 year old volleyball players. *J Strength Cond Res*. 2014;28:43-52.
6. Kountouris A, Cook J. Rehabilitation of Achilles and patellar tendinopathies. *Best Pract Res Clin Rheumatol*. 2007;21:295-316.
7. Gaida JE, Cook J. Treatment options for patellar tendinopathy: critical review. *Curr Sports Med Rep*. 2011;10:255-270.
8. Kongsgaard M, Kovanen V, Aagaard P, et al. Corticosteroid injections, eccentric decline squat training and heavy slow resistance training in patellar tendinopathy. *Scand J Med Sci Sports*. 2009;19:790-802.
9. Purdam CR, Jonsson P, Alfredson H, Lorentzon R, Cook JL, Khan KM. A pilot study of the eccentric decline squat in the management of painful chronic patellar tendinopathy. *Br J Sports Med*. 2004;38:395-397.
10. Zwerver J, Hartgens F, Verhagen E, van der Worp H, van den Akker-Scheek I, Diercks RL. No effect of extracorporeal shockwave therapy on patellar tendinopathy in jumping athletes during the competitive season: a randomized clinical trial. *Am J Sports Med*. 2011;39:1191-1199.
11. Barrack MT, Rauh MJ, Nichols JF. Prevalence of and traits associated with low BMD among female adolescent runners. *Med Sci Sports Exerc*. 2008;40:2015-2021.
12. Barrack MT, Rauh MJ, Nichols JF. Cross-sectional evidence of suppressed bone mineral accrual among female adolescent runners. *J Bone Miner Res*. 2010;25:1850-1857.

13. Hoch AZ, Pajewski NM, Moraski L, et al. Prevalence of the female athlete triad in high school athletes and sedentary students. *Clin J Sport Med.* 2009;19:421-428.
14. Nichols JF, Rauh MJ, Lawson MJ, Ji M, Barkai HS. Prevalence of the female athlete triad syndrome among high school athletes. *Arch Pediatr Adolesc Med.* 2006;160:137-142.
15. Rauh MJ, Nichols JF, Barrack MT. Relationships among injury and disordered eating, menstrual dysfunction, and low bone mineral density in high school athletes: a prospective study. *J Athl Train.* 2010;45:243-252.
16. Thein-Nissenbaum JM, Rauh MJ, Carr KE, Loud KJ, McGuine TA. Associations between disordered eating, menstrual dysfunction, and musculoskeletal injury among high school athletes. *J Orthop Sports Phys Ther.* 2011;4:60-69.
17. Rumball JS, Lebrun CM. Preparticipation physical examination: selected issues for the female athlete. *Clin J Sport Med.* 2004;14:153-160.
18. World Health Organization. Assessment of fracture risk and its application to screening for postmenopausal women. *World Health Organ Tech Rep Ser.* 1994;843:1-129.
19. Pekkinen M, Viljakainen H, Saarnio E, Lamberg-Allardt C, Makitie O. Vitamin D is a major determinant of bone mineral density at school age. *PLoS One.* 2012;7:e40090.
20. Khan KM, Liu-Ambrose T, Sran MM, Ashe MC, Donaldson MG, Wark JD. New criteria for female athlete triad syndrome? As osteoporosis is rare, should osteopenia be among the criteria for defining the female athlete triad syndrome? *Br J Sports Med.* 2002;36:10-13.
21. van der Worp H, van Ark M, Roerink S, Pepping GJ, van den Akker-Scheek I, Zwerver J. Risk factors for patellar tendinopathy: a systematic review of the literature. *Br J Sports Med.* 2011;45:446-452.
22. Witvrouw E, Bellemans J, Lysens R, Danneels L, Cambier D. Intrinsic risk factors for the development of patellar tendinitis in an athletic population. A two-year prospective study. *Am J Sports Med.* 2001;29:190-195.
23. Willson JD, Kernozek TW, Arndt RL, Reznichek DA, Scott Straker J. Gluteal muscle activation during running in females with and without patellofemoral pain syndrome. *Clin Biomech (Bristol, Avon).* 2011;26:735-740.
24. Binford RB, Le Grange D, Jellar CC. Eating disorders examination versus eating disorders examination-questionnaire in adolescents with full and partial-syndrome bulimia nervosa and anorexia nervosa. *Int J Eat Disorders.* 2005;37:44-49.
25. Carter JC, Stewart DA, Fairburn CG. Eating disorder examination questionnaire: norms for young adolescent girls. *Behav Res Ther.* 2001;39:625-632.
26. Celio AA, Wilfley DE, Crow SJ, Mitchell J, Walsh BT. A comparison of the binge eating scale, questionnaire for eating and weight patterns-revised, and eating disorder examination questionnaire with instructions with the eating disorder examination in the assessment of binge eating disorder and its symptoms. *Int J Eat Disorders.* 2004;36:434-444.
27. Goldfein JA, Devlin MJ, Kamenetz C. Eating Disorder Examination-Questionnaire with and without instruction to assess binge eating in patients with binge eating disorder. *Int J Eat Disorders.* 2005;37:107-111.
28. Passi VA, Bryson SW, Lock J. Assessment of eating disorders in adolescents with anorexia nervosa: self-report questionnaire versus interview. *Int J Eat Disorders.* 2003;33:45-54.
29. Mountjoy M, Hutchinson M, Cruz L, Lebrun C. Screening the female athlete algorithm. http://www.sunnjenteidrett.no/media/6680/ppe_for_website.pdf. Accessed August 14, 2015.
30. Cook JL, Khan KM. What is the most appropriate treatment for patellar tendinopathy? *Br J Sports Med.* 2001;35:291-294.
31. Amiri-Khorasani M, Abu Osman NA, Yusof A. Acute effect of static and dynamic stretching on hip dynamic range of motion during instep kicking in professional soccer players. *J Strength Cond Res.* 2011;25:1647-1652.
32. Distefano LJ, Blackburn JT, Marshall SW, Padua DA. Gluteal muscle activation during common therapeutic exercises. *J Orthop Sports Phys Ther.* 2009;39:532-540.

33. Boren K, Conrey C, Le Coguic J, Paprocki L, Voight M, Robinson TK. Electromyographic analysis of gluteus medius and gluteus maximus during rehabilitation exercises. *Int J Sports Phys Ther*. 2011;6:206-223.

34. Joseph MF, Taft K, Moskwa M, Denegar CR. Deep friction massage to treat tendinopathy: a systematic review of a classic treatment in the face of a new paradigm of understanding. *J Sport Rehabil*. 2012;21:343-353.

Knee Anterior Cruciate Ligament: Injury Prevention

Kevin R. Ford
Jeffrey B. Taylor

CASE 15

The coach of a competitive girls soccer team has heard about the high prevalence of anterior cruciate ligament (ACL) ruptures in female athletes. He was referred to a sports physical therapist for assistance in designing an injury prevention program for his team that he can implement during the upcoming season. The physical therapist agreed to assist, pending the results of a preseason screening session formulated to identify risk factors for ACL injury. During the screening session, the therapist noticed a 13-year-old left-footed dominant kicker that displayed a "high" risk of ACL rupture. The coach commented that she is one of the better players on the team, with aspirations of playing college soccer. Her health history form indicates that she has recently gone through a major growth spurt and she has a sister who ruptured her ACL when she was 15 years old. Static testing revealed that the athlete stands with 10° of bilateral genu recurvatum and abnormally low foot arches. Dynamically, she exhibits a visually obvious valgus collapse of both lower extremities (right > left) during landing and cutting maneuvers. In addition, when performing single-leg landings, she displays increased levels of lateral trunk lean toward the right leg.

- What parts of an athlete's history are important to help identify high risk for ACL injuries?
- What tests should be included in the screening battery to identify risk factors?
- What are the major risk factors for ACL injury that should be addressed during ACL prevention program design?
- What are the most effective physical therapy interventions for the prevention of ACL injuries?

KEY DEFINITIONS

MODIFIABLE RISK FACTORS: Characteristics that can be changed or controlled because of an intervention

NON-MODIFIABLE RISK FACTORS: Variables that cannot be changed

Objectives

1. Describe an objective screening battery of tests to determine whether an individual has an increased risk of non-contact ACL injury.
2. Describe appropriate exercise prescription, including neuromuscular interventions, which may address the modifiable risk factors for ACL injury.
3. Identify key therapeutic progressions that address poor lower extremity neuromuscular control, deficits in core and hip strength, and side-to-side asymmetries during jump landing tasks.
4. Describe the expected effectiveness of ACL injury prevention programs and the prognosis for participating athletes.

Physical Therapy Considerations

PT considerations during the design and implementation of an ACL injury prevention program:

- **General physical therapy plan of care/goals:** Educate coach and athletes about proper technique and ACL injury risk; improve strength of hamstrings and posterolateral hip musculature; improve landing and cutting techniques by reducing dynamic lower extremity valgus collapse; reduce the incidence of ACL injury
- **Physical therapy tests and measures:** Drop vertical jump, tuck jump, single-leg hop, triple hop, lower extremity strength testing
- **Physical therapy interventions:** Neuromuscular interventions including strength and plyometric training; feedback on technique; dynamic warm-up
- **Precautions during physical therapy:** Feedback must be given during exercise training to increase the likelihood that optimal technique is followed.

Understanding the Health Condition

Females who participate in sports such as basketball and soccer experience a higher rate of ACL injuries than their male counterparts.[1] Increased injury risk, combined with dramatic increases in sports participation, has led to a significant number of ACL injuries in females. These injuries result in short- and long-term consequences that may include surgery, rehabilitation, and a high likelihood of debilitating knee osteoarthritis. As a result, ACL injury prevention strategies have been thoroughly investigated over the last decade. A theoretical model toward preventing ACL injuries is the "Sequence of Prevention" model.[2,3] This model targets commonly recognized modifiable risk factors that are biomechanical and neuromuscular in nature.[2,3] Using this framework, an intervention program that emphasizes detailed movement technique feedback during a combination of plyometric and resistance training may provide the best success for reducing ACL injury risk in young female athletes.[4]

ACL injury prevention programs reduce knee and/or ACL injury incidence in female athletes.[4-12] A review of 5 neuromuscular training programs designed to prevent non-contact ACL injuries in female athletes concluded that the pooled relative risk reduction was 70% (95% confidence interval, 54%-80%), with a pooled numbers needed to treat of 89 (95% confidence interval, 66-136).[13] Several prevention approaches have been utilized that include neuromuscular training implemented with a combination of a comprehensive preseason component and/or a focused in-season warm-up component. Regardless of how individual programs are implemented, it appears that athlete compliance with the exercise program is a major factor in their ultimate success. In a recent meta-analysis of neuromuscular training programs, Sugimoto et al.[5] suggest that compliance rates should be greater than 66% in order for these programs to exhibit prophylactic effects.

Physical Therapy Patient/Client Management

Physical therapists play an integral role in ACL injury prevention. Prior to designing an ACL injury prevention program, screening for potential risk factors needs to be performed in the form of history taking, physical performance tests, and movement analysis. Interventions most frequently consist of neuromuscular training and the education of athletes, coaches, and parents. Education of coaches is especially important, because these programs may not be consistently performed under the direct supervision of the sports physical therapist. Because managing preventative programs in athletes can be an interprofessional endeavor, communication among the sports medicine team (*e.g.*, physician, physical therapist, athletic trainer, strength and conditioning coaches) is essential for ideal athlete care.

Examination, Evaluation, and Diagnosis

Screening and examination should incorporate both subjective and objective components to help identify intrinsic risk factors for ACL injury (Table 15-1). Information that is gained throughout the screening process should then be addressed as part of the prevention program. Specific questioning regarding the athlete's medical history (especially previous ACL or lower extremity injuries) can help identify athletes who may be more susceptible to ACL rupture. Prior injuries to the lower extremity often lead to altered neuromuscular movement strategies resulting from incomplete rehabilitation or compensational patterns. For example, Paterno et al.[14] identified that limb asymmetries in landing ground reaction force are still present

Table 15-1 KEY RISK FACTORS TO ASSESS IN AN ACL INJURY PREVENTION SCREENING EXAMINATION

Subjective evaluation
- Past injuries to back or lower extremity
- Family history of ACL tear
- Recent growth spurt

Anatomical characteristics
- Generalized joint laxity
- Genu recurvatum
- Anterior knee laxity
- Excessive navicular drop

Neuromuscular characteristics
- Decreased quadriceps and/or hamstrings strength
- Decreased core and/or posterolateral hip strength

Movement strategies during a drop vertical jump (bilateral and unilateral), lateral hop, or tuck jump
- Dynamic lower extremity valgus
- Asymmetrical landing

2 years following ACL reconstruction and rehabilitation. In addition, individuals with patellofemoral pain syndrome may demonstrate similar risk factors to those that predict ACL injury.[15] It may also be important to ask about a family history of ACL tear, because ACL injury risk has been linked to familial predisposition and genetics.[16,17]

In addition to a thorough subjective history, **pre-competition screening tests** that identify abnormal postural characteristics and neuromuscular movement strategies may help clinicians target athletes that are at higher risk for ACL injury. Postural screening is performed to identify alignment abnormalities that may place athletes at higher risk of injury. Researchers have hypothesized that abnormal knee anatomical characteristics may lead to higher ACL injury rates by promoting larger levels of dynamic valgus during sport activities.[18] Currently, no definitive relationships between static measures and faulty biomechanics to ACL injury risk have been identified. However, measures of foot structure may be helpful because of the role of the feet in dynamic function of the lower extremity. Navicular drop is the difference in height of the navicular tubercle between relaxed stance and stance in subtalar neutral, and excessive navicular drop has been linked to higher ACL injury rates.[19] This may be because higher levels of navicular drop are associated with subtalar joint overpronation, producing anterior tibial translation and ACL strain.[20]

Increases in knee laxity are predictive of non-contact ACL injury.[21,22] The therapist can determine whether an individual has generalized joint laxity (GJL) by assessing the presence of: bilateral hyperextension of the fifth MCP joint, bilateral elbow and knee hyperextension, the ability to touch the thumb to the volar aspect of the forearm bilaterally, and the ability to bend forward and place the palms flat on the ground while keeping the knees straight. This test is graded on a 0 to 9 scale, with higher scores indicating greater GJL.[22] Of particular interest are levels of knee hyperextension (genu recurvatum). Whether measured passively or actively, higher levels of genu recurvatum alter movement strategies, placing athletes at higher risk of ACL injury.[23,24] In particular, larger anterior knee laxity (AKL) values are typically found in females and may be predictive of ACL injury.[21,25] A knee arthrometer (*e.g.*, KT-2000) can be used to quantify levels of passive AKL.

While the use of external supports such as knee braces or foot orthoses may limit knee laxity or foot pronation, these anatomical characteristics are typically thought of as non-modifiable risk factors for ACL injury. While anatomical characteristics help the clinician with early identification of at-risk athletes, prevention programs must be designed to target modifiable neuromuscular characteristics (*e.g.*, poor movement strategies, weakness) for optimal injury risk reduction. High-risk biomechanics during jumping and landing activities, including high levels of dynamic lower extremity valgus, have been reported as strong predictors of ACL injury.[26] Dynamic lower extremity valgus is operationally defined as a combination of motions and rotations at all 3 lower extremity joints, potentially including hip adduction and internal rotation, knee abduction, tibial external rotation and anterior translation, and ankle eversion.[27] During athletic movements, dynamic lower extremity valgus often presents as a knocked-knee posture (Fig. 15-1).

Identification of dynamic lower extremity valgus is especially important during injury risk screening, and can be assessed in real time, or through the use of 2-dimensional video using a video camera, tablet computer, or equivalent. This movement pattern can be observed during a variety of athletic tasks.[27-30] Most

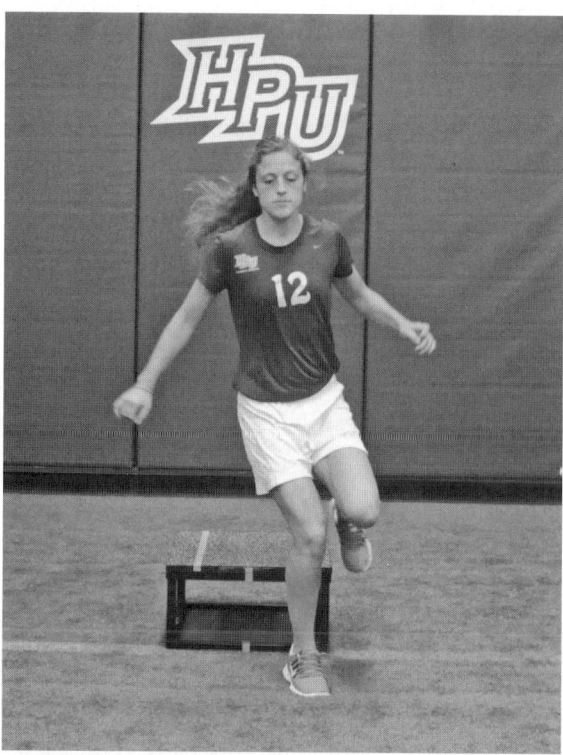

Figure 15-1. Athlete exhibiting dynamic right lower extremity valgus during a single-leg landing.

commonly, a drop vertical jump (DVJ) is performed. In the DVJ, the athlete drops straight down onto both feet from a box 30 cm in height and immediately performs a maximal vertical jump. The first landing of this activity is typically analyzed for the presence of dynamic valgus or asymmetry (in motion or timing) during landing. Other bilateral landing tasks, such as the tuck jump, can also be used in combination or in place of the DVJ.[31] The tuck jump assessment requires the athlete to perform 10 seconds of repetitive tuck jumps. The challenging nature of the tuck jump may force the athlete to focus more specifically on the performance of the activity as opposed to the landing mechanics, allowing the examiner to more clearly identify abnormal mechanics, asymmetries, or performance decrements.

Depending on the demands of the athlete's sport, other assessments may be warranted. In sports such as basketball or volleyball where single-leg landings are prevalent, the therapist can modify the DVJ by instructing the athlete to drop off the box and land on only one leg. However, because of the difficulty of the task, an athlete may not be able to perform a subsequent maximal vertical jump on one leg, as seen in a double-leg DVJ. Thus, characterization of the athlete's movement pattern during the landing may be sufficient. In addition, any form of the triple hop test may be useful to identify performance discrepancies and limb asymmetries. These tests are often used in conjunction with ACL reconstruction rehabilitation protocols in the criteria for return to play.[31] Sport-specific demands may also warrant the inclusion of landing tasks that are performed out of the sagittal plane. In the frontal plane, the therapist can analyze the athlete's landing mechanics during a single-leg lateral hop. In this test, the therapist asks the athlete to stand on one leg and hop laterally over a small barrier and land on the same leg (*e.g.*, the athlete would stand on her left leg and hop to the left direction). In the transverse plane, a similar assessment can be performed by having the athlete perform various types of cutting maneuvers.[32]

While analysis of biomechanics during sport activities is the crux of the screening battery, more standard clinical measures can also be incorporated. The ratio of strength between the quadriceps and hamstring muscle groups can have implications for ACL injury risk.[27] The quadriceps can act as an ACL antagonist by producing anterior tibial shear and ACL strain during isolated forceful contractions. The hamstrings can act to oppose the force of the quadriceps by limiting the amount of anterior shear during co-contraction. Therefore, while an optimal quadriceps to hamstrings strength ratio has not been defined, addressing any noticeable weakness in the hamstrings may be appropriate. In addition, deficits in posterolateral hip strength can lead to poor lower extremity control and increased valgus collapse during closed-chain activities. Quantifying the strength of hip abductors, extensors, and external rotators through manual muscle testing, a handheld dynamometer, or isokinetic dynamometer may provide beneficial information for the individualized design of an ACL injury prevention program.

Plan of Care and Interventions

Many injury prevention programs have been successful at reducing the incidence of knee and/or ACL injury.[4-12,33] Multiple aspects of these published programs may be useful to integrate into a new injury prevention program for young female athletes.[4,5] Interventions for injury prevention must address relevant results from the screening and examination of an individual athlete or team of athletes. Targeting deficits at the most appropriate time may be a key component to reducing risk of non-contact ACL injury.[30] To appropriately progress an uninjured athlete through a series of exercises, it is important that the physical therapist understand the underlying theory behind the selection of each component.[34-37]

Several common deficits or asymmetries have been identified in screening batteries of athletes: lack of neuromuscular control, asymmetries in landing forces, and decreased strength (in the "core," hip musculature, and hamstrings). Examples of exercise progressions that target the underlying mechanisms potentially responsible for dynamic lower extremity valgus are detailed in this section.[38-40]

To address the lack of neuromuscular control identified in the DVJ as excessive frontal plane knee motion, a simple progression of exercises starting with a wall jump (Fig. 15-2) is useful. The wall jump is a relatively low-intensity bilateral exercise in which the athlete is asked to repeatedly jump vertically with minimal knee flexion and focus on ankle plantar flexion/dorsiflexion. As the athlete lands during repeated wall jumps, real-time consistent feedback of technique should be given. **Feedback was found to be crucial component** in successful ACL injury prevention programs.[4] To help identify neuromuscular activation patterns during the *take-off* phase of the jump that results in dynamic lower extremity valgus, a broad jump and hold exercise is useful (Fig. 15-3).[40] This moderate-intensity exercise can also be used to reinforce proper landing posture. Progression to a broad jump and vertical or broad-broad jump may be utilized to challenge the athlete throughout a preseason ACL injury prevention protocol. Additional progressions from sagittal

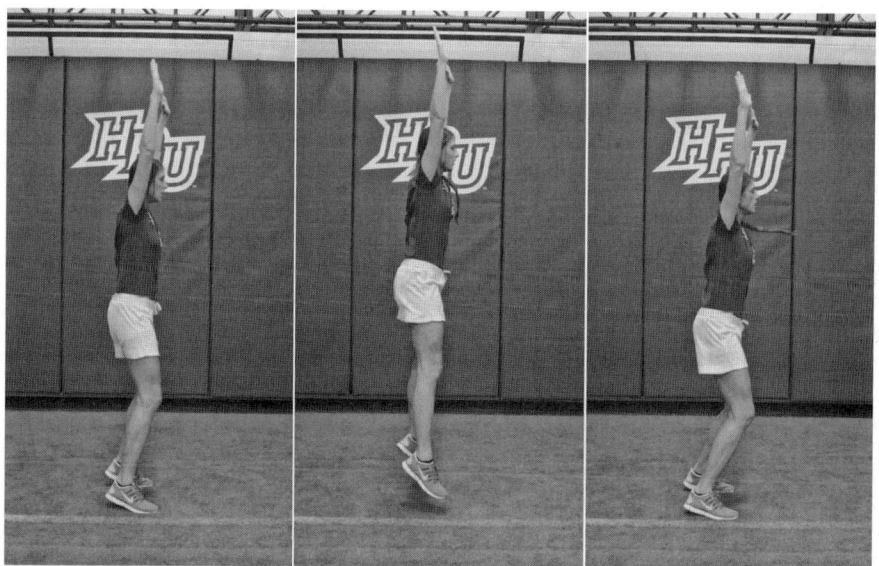

Figure 15-2. Wall jump exercise. The therapist should view the exercise from the front and side and provide constant feedback regarding performance.

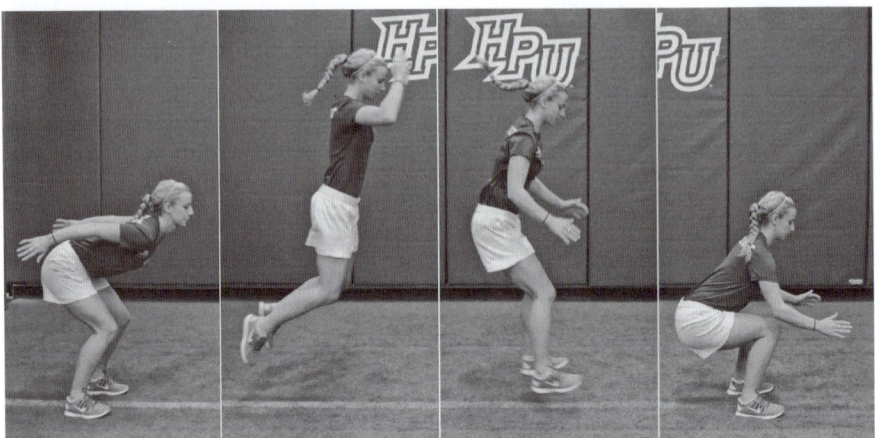

Figure 15-3. Broad jump and hold exercise. The athlete is instructed to jump forward as far as possible with both legs while striving for a "soft" landing and minimizing frontal plane knee motion during both the take-off and landing. Once the athlete lands, she is instructed to hold this position for 2 seconds.

plane movements to frontal plane movements (*i.e.*, barrier jumps) and transverse plane movements (*i.e.*, 180° jump) are typically incorporated throughout a program to challenge multidirectional neuromuscular control.

While a DVJ is frequently used to identify side-to-side asymmetries, single-leg activities are typically used for screening asymmetries in landing forces. For example, the difference in total distanced traveled between the left and right sides during a single-leg triple hop will be apparent if the athlete has a functional side-to-side imbalance. Transitioning from double-leg to single-leg exercises is an important component in comprehensive ACL injury prevention programs to correct these imbalances.[40] A tuck jump (Fig. 15-4) with a soft landing is useful to identify a potentially "weaker" leg because the athlete will often position this leg slightly posterior to the "stronger" leg during landing. Proper landing is an important baseline

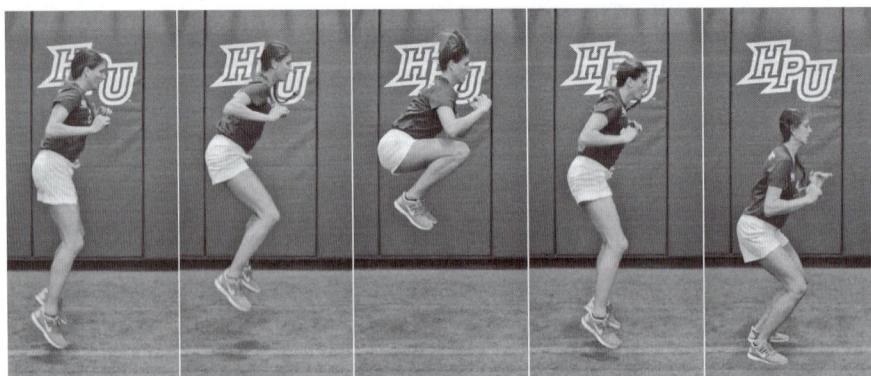

Figure 15-4. Repeated tuck jump exercise. The therapist should view the exercise from the front and side during this challenging exercise. The athlete is instructed to pull her knees up toward her chest during the jump and perform another jump immediately upon ground contact.

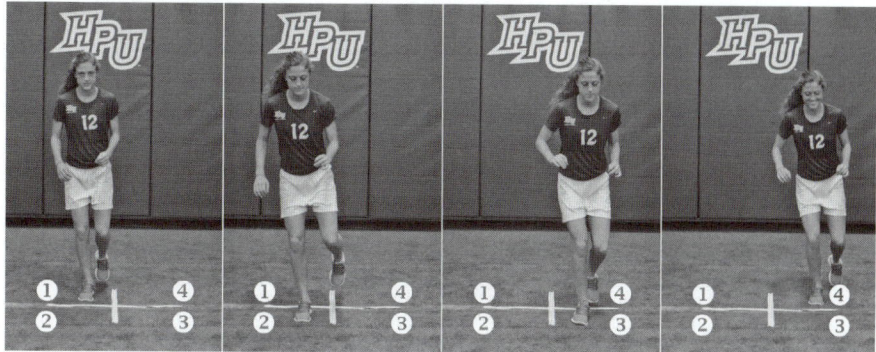

Figure 15-5. Single-leg X-hop. This balancing exercise requires the athlete to hop and land on one leg from positions 1 through 4.

skill because the task will be progressed to higher-intensity plyometric repeated tuck jumps with focus on balanced landing.[40] The tuck jump can be used to train and measure improvements in neuromuscular imbalances.[41] To help transition from bilateral to unilateral tasks, single-leg X-hops (Fig. 15-5) and balancing activities are helpful. During the single-leg X-hop, the athlete moves in the medial/lateral and anterior/posterior directions by hopping, landing, and immediately holding each position while controlling the knee in the frontal plane. Progression to bounding exercises (Fig. 15-6) focuses on single-leg landing and take-off movements in a controlled manner. The therapist can provide feedback on jump height and power during these movements, which is important because these aspects may directly translate to a variety of sports.[40]

The last common deficit identified in pre-participation injury screens is decreased strength. Isokinetic testing may be used to identify not only hamstrings/quadriceps imbalances but also decreased hip abduction strength.[36,42] A single-leg squat while standing on a box can be a valuable component to a screening battery that may identify a lack of core, hip, and/or hamstrings strength in maturing females. As female athletes reach the end of their pubertal growth spurt, the changes that occur in height and mass may result in difficulties controlling the lower extremities and trunk if a concomitant increase in core/hip/hamstrings strength is not present. For example, deficits in hip strength may be noted with increased dynamic lower extremity valgus and trunk motion when the athlete steps down from the

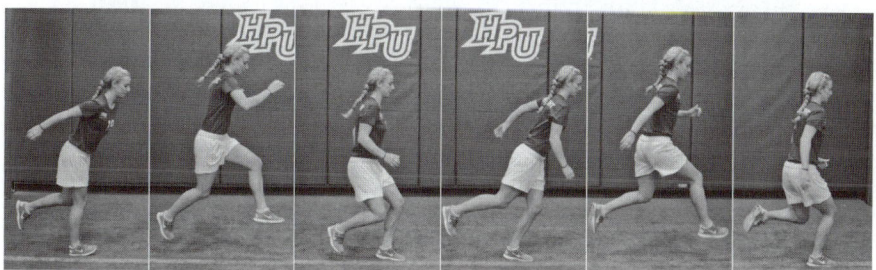

Figure 15-6. Bounding exercise. The athlete is asked to run in a bounding manner and may be instructed to focus on height and/or distance during the bounding.

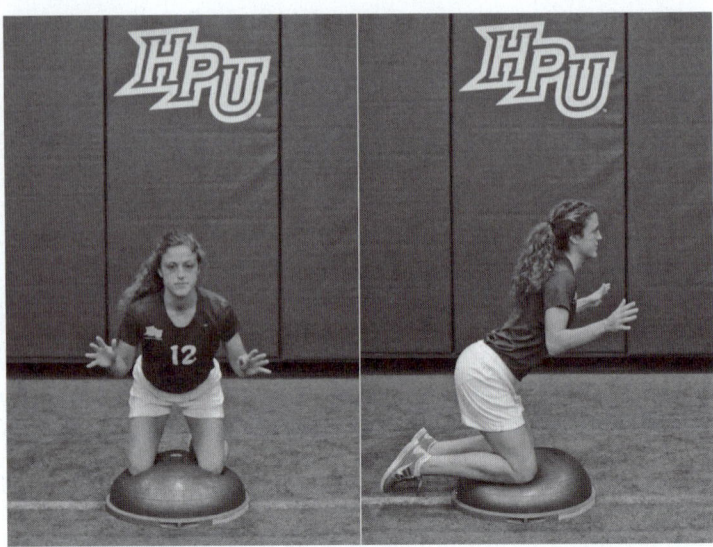

Figure 15-7. Double-kneeling hold exercise. The athlete is positioned on a BOSU trainer in an athletic posture with hip flexion and chest up. The athlete is instructed to hold this position for 10 seconds with an emphasis on control of thigh and trunk motion.

box with one limb. Improving the strength of the core, hip, and hamstrings muscles can be accomplished with a variety of exercise progressions that have been shown to improve hip strength in female athletes.[36] In a pilot study to assess the effect of trunk and hip focused training exercises on hip and knee strength, Myer et al.[36] presented numerous progressions. An example involves kneeling exercises on unstable devices. The athlete may begin in a double-kneeling hold position (Fig. 15-7) on the round surface of a BOSU trainer and transition to a single-kneeling hold position (Fig. 15-8). Attention to an athletic posture with hip flexion should be encouraged

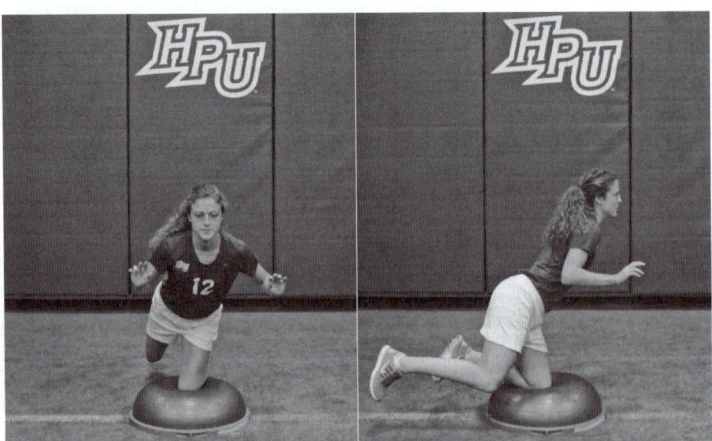

Figure 15-8. Single-kneeling hold exercise. The athlete is positioned on a BOSU trainer on a single knee in an athletic posture with hip flexion and chest up. The athlete is instructed to hold this position for 10 seconds with an emphasis on control of thigh and trunk motion.

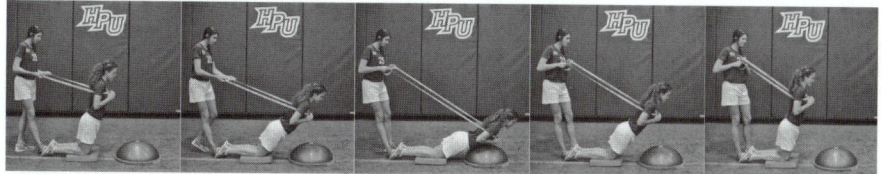

Figure 15-9. Russian hamstrings curl exercise with resistance band. In a double-kneeling position, the athlete leans forward (eccentric hamstring contraction) until the chest touches the BOSU trainer. At the end of this move, the athlete moves back to the starting position (concentric hamstring contraction). Assistance during both phases is provided with a resistance band around the athlete's chest.

throughout these exercises. Perturbations and ball tosses may also be included to challenge the athlete throughout the program. Russian hamstring curls (Fig. 15-9) provide a focused hamstrings strengthening exercise in which the athlete works eccentrically and concentrically with an elastic band to provide assistance.[39]

ACL injury prevention programs may consist of a comprehensive preseason and/or an in-season protocol. Table 15-2 provides an example of an in-season progression of plyometric and strengthening components that was developed from published literature.[11,35,36,40] Consistent feedback on technique during each of the exercises is emphasized. The program includes a dynamic warm-up lasting approximately 5 to 8 minutes with sport-related movement patterns. For example, the authors typically include a jog with internal/external hip rotations for soccer players, and for basketball players, we typically include bounding with a reach. Usually,

Table 15-2 EXAMPLE IN-SEASON WARM-UP PROGRAM

Phase 1	Phase 2	Phase 3	Phase 4
Diagonal cut hold	Jog jog diagonal cut hold	Jog jog diagonal cut	Sprint cut
Broad jump hold	Squat jump	Broad jump, squat jump (2 times) hold	Broad jump (2 times), squat jump (2 times) hold
Jump single-leg hold	Hop hold	180 hop hold	Hop hop hold
Single tuck jump hold with soft landing	Double tuck hold	Repeated tucks	Side to side tucks
Walking lunge	Walking lunge with jump	Lunge jumps	Scissor jumps
Side lunge	Side walking lunge	Side walking lunge ball hold	Side hop hold
Double crunch ball hold	Swivel double crunch ball hold	Ball half V (while holding a ball, flex upper body to a "half V" position)	Ball full V (while holding a ball, flex upper body and lower body to a "full V" position)
Forearm alternate leg hold	Prone alternate hand and leg extension	Prone double leg	Prone "Supermans"
Russian hamstring curls	Russian hamstring curls	Russian hamstring curls	Russian hamstring curls

the authors focus on only 4 to 5 key exercises during each practice by alternating the first and last halves of the exercises within each phase (Table 15-2). Each phase is implemented for 2 or 3 weeks and is progressive in nature.

Evidence-Based Clinical Recommendations

SORT: Strength of Recommendation Taxonomy
A: Consistent, good-quality patient-oriented evidence
B: Inconsistent or limited-quality patient-oriented evidence
C: Consensus, disease-oriented evidence, usual practice, expert opinion, or case series

1. ACL prevention programs that incorporate a combination of plyometric and strength training are effective in reducing the risk of ACL injury in female athletes. **Grade A**
2. Pre-competition screening tests that identify abnormal postural characteristics and neuromuscular movement strategies can help clinicians target athletes who are at higher risk for ACL injury. **Grade B**
3. Detailed feedback on movement technique and performance reduces high-risk biomechanics during sport-related movement tasks. **Grade B**

COMPREHENSION QUESTIONS

15.1 Which of the following has the *least* amount of evidence to be included in a screening battery to identify potential risk factors related to non-contact ACL injury in female athletes?
   A. Drop vertical jump test
   B. Tuck jump test
   C. 40-m linear speed run
   D. Hip strength assessment

15.2 Which of the following components has the *least* amount of evidence for inclusion in a comprehensive preseason ACL injury prevention program?
   A. Detailed technique feedback
   B. Strengthening of hamstrings and musculature of the core and hip
   C. Plyometric exercises
   D. Flexibility exercises

ANSWERS

15.1 **C.** An athlete who exhibits greater linear speed may be considered a higher-performing athlete; however, this test does not clearly identify known risk factors for non-contact ACL injury in females.

15.2 **D.** Neuromuscular training programs that have reduced ACL injury incidence in females support the inclusion of detailed technique feedback, plyometric training, and strengthening of the core/hip/hamstrings.

REFERENCES

1. Agel J, Arendt EA, Bershadsky B. Anterior cruciate ligament injury in national collegiate athletic association basketball and soccer: a 13-year review. *Am J Sports Med.* 2005;33:524-530.
2. van Mechelen W, Hlobil H, Kemper HC. Incidence, severity, aetiology and prevention of sports injuries. A review of concepts. *Sports Med.* 1992;14:82-99.
3. Hewett TE, Myer GD, Ford KR, Paterno MV, Quatman CE. The 2012 ABJS Nicolas Andry Award: the sequence of prevention: a systematic approach to prevent anterior cruciate ligament injury. *Clin Orthop Relat Res.* 2012;470:2930-2940.
4. Hewett TE, Ford KR, Myer GD. Anterior cruciate ligament injuries in female athletes: part 2, a meta-analysis of neuromuscular interventions aimed at injury prevention. *Am J Sports Med.* 2006;34:490-498.
5. Sugimoto D, Myer GD, Bush HM, Klugman MF, Medina McKeon JM, Hewett TE. Compliance with neuromuscular training and anterior cruciate ligament injury risk reduction in female athletes: a meta-analysis. *J Athl Train.* 2012;47:714-723.
6. Hewett TE, Lindenfeld TN, Riccobene JV, Noyes FR. The effect of neuromuscular training on the incidence of knee injury in female athletes. A prospective study. *Am J Sports Med.* 1999;27:699-706.
7. Petersen W, Braun C, Bock W, et al. A controlled prospective case control study of a prevention training program in female team handball players: the German experience. *Arch Orthop Trauma Surg.* 2005;125:614-621.
8. Heidt RS Jr, Sweeterman LM, Carlonas RL, Traub JA, Tekulve FX. Avoidance of soccer injuries with preseason conditioning. *Am J Sports Med.* 2000;28:659-662.
9. Myklebust G, Engebretsen L, Braekken IH, Skjolberg A, Olsen OE, Bahr R. Prevention of anterior cruciate ligament injuries in female team handball players: a prospective intervention study over three seasons. *Clin J Sport Med.* 2003;13:71-78.
10. Mandelbaum BR, Silvers HJ, Watanabe DS, et al. Effectiveness of a neuromuscular and proprioceptive training program in preventing anterior cruciate ligament injuries in female athletes: 2-year follow-up. *Am J Sports Med.* 2005;33:1003-1010.
11. Walden M, Atroshi I, Magnusson H, Wagner P, Hagglund M. Prevention of acute knee injuries in adolescent female football players: cluster randomised controlled trial. *BMJ.* 2012;344:e3042.
12. LaBella CR, Huxford MR, Grissom J, Kim KY, Peng J, Christoffel KK. Effect of neuromuscular warm-up on injuries in female soccer and basketball athletes in urban public high schools: cluster randomized controlled trial. *Arch Pediatr Adolesc Med.* 2011;165:1033-1040.
13. Grindstaff TL, Hammill RR, Tuzson AE, Hertel J. Neuromuscular control training programs and noncontact anterior cruciate ligament injury rates in female athletes: a numbers-needed-to-treat analysis. *J Athl Train.* 2006;41:450-456.
14. Paterno MV, Ford KR, Myer GD, Heyl R, Hewett TE. Limb asymmetries in landing and jumping 2 years following anterior cruciate ligament reconstruction. *Clin J Sport Med.* 2007;17:258-262.
15. Boling MC, Padua DA, Marshall SW, Guskiewicz K, Pyne S, Beutler A. A prospective investigation of biomechanical risk factors for patellofemoral pain syndrome: the Joint Undertaking to Monitor and Prevent ACL Injury (JUMP-ACL) cohort. *Am J Sports Med.* 2009;37:2108-2116.
16. Hewett TE, Lynch TR, Myer GD, Ford KR, Gwin RC, Heidt RS Jr. Multiple risk factors related to familial predisposition to anterior cruciate ligament injury: fraternal twin sisters with anterior cruciate ligament ruptures. *Br J Sports Med.* 2010;44:848-855.
17. Posthumus M, September AV, O'Cuinneagain D, van der Merwe W, Schwellnus MP, Collins M. The COL5A1 gene is associated with increased risk of anterior cruciate ligament ruptures in female participants. *Am J Sports Med.* 2009;37:2234-2240.

18. Sutton KM, Bullock JM. Anterior cruciate ligament rupture: differences between males and females. *J Am Acad Orthop Surg*. 2013;21:41-50.
19. Loudon JK, Jenkins W, Loudon KL. The relationship between static posture and ACL injury in female athletes. *J Orthop Sports Phys Ther*. 1996;24:91-97.
20. Trimble MH, Bishop MD, Buckley BD, Fields LC, Rozea GD. The relationship between clinical measurements of lower extremity posture and tibial translation. *Clin Biomech*. 2002;17:286-290.
21. Uhorchak JM, Scoville CR, Williams GN, Arciero RA, St Pierre P, Taylor DC. Risk factors associated with noncontact injury of the anterior cruciate ligament: a prospective four-year evaluation of 859 West Point cadets. *Am J Sports Med*. 2003;31:831-842.
22. Myer GD, Ford KR, Paterno MV, Nick TG, Hewett TE. The effects of generalized joint laxity on risk of anterior cruciate ligament injury in young female athletes. *Am J Sports Med*. 2008;36:1073-1080.
23. Kawahara K, Sekimoto T, Watanabe S, et al. Effect of genu recurvatum on the anterior cruciate ligament-deficient knee during gait. *Knee Surg Sports Traumatol Arthrosc*. 2012;20:1479-1487.
24. Ramesh R, Von Arx O, Azzopardi T, Schranz PJ. The risk of anterior cruciate ligament rupture with generalised joint laxity. *J Bone Joint Surg Br*. 2005;87:800-803.
25. Pollard CD, Braun B, Hamill J. Influence of gender, estrogen and exercise on anterior knee laxity. *Clin Biomech*. 2006;21:1060-1066.
26. Hewett TE, Myer GD, Ford KR, et al. Biomechanical measures of neuromuscular control and valgus loading of the knee predict anterior cruciate ligament injury risk in female athletes: a prospective study. *Am J Sports Med*. 2005;33:492-501.
27. Hewett TE, Myer GD, Ford KR. Anterior cruciate ligament injuries in female athletes: part 1, mechanisms and risk factors. *Am J Sports Med*. 2006;34:299-311.
28. Ford KR, Myer GD, Hewett TE. Valgus knee motion during landing in high school female and male basketball players. *Med Sci Sports Exerc*. 2003;35:1745-1750.
29. Ford KR, Myer GD, Toms HE, Hewett TE. Gender differences in the kinematics of unanticipated cutting in young athletes. *Med Sci Sports Exerc*. 2005;37:124-129.
30. Ford KR, Shapiro R, Myer GD, van den Bogert AJ, Hewett TE. Longitudinal sex differences during landing in knee abduction in young athletes. *Med Sci Sports Exerc*. 2010;42:1923-1931.
31. Myer GD, Ford KR, Hewett TE. Tuck jump assessment for reducing anterior cruciate ligament injury risk. *Athl Ther Today*. 2008;13:39-44.
32. McLean SG, Walker KB, van den Bogert AJ. Effect of gender on lower extremity kinematics during rapid direction changes: an integrated analysis of three sports movements. *J Sci Med Sport*. 2005;8:411-422.
33. Taylor JB, Waxman JP, Richter SJ, Shultz SJ. Evaluation of the effectiveness of anterior cruciate ligament injury prevention programme training components: a systematic review and meta-analysis. *Br J Sports Med*. 2015;49:79-87.
34. Chmielewski TL, Myer GD, Kauffman D, Tillman SM. Plyometric exercise in the rehabilitation of athletes: physiological responses and clinical application. *J Orthop Sports Phys Ther*. 2006;36:308-319.
35. Myer GD, Ford KR, Brent JL, Hewett TE. The effects of plyometric versus dynamic balance training on power, balance and landing force in female athletes. *J Strength Cond Res*. 2006;20:345-353.
36. Myer GD, Brent JL, Ford KR, Hewett TE. A pilot study to determine the effect of trunk and hip focused neuromuscular training on hip and knee isokinetic strength. *Br J Sports Med*. 2008;42:614-619.
37. Myer GD, Chu DA, Brent JL, Hewett TE. Trunk and hip control neuromuscular training for the prevention of knee joint injury. *Clin Sports Med*. 2008;27:425-448.
38. Myer GD, Ford KR, Brent JL, Hewett TE. An integrated approach to change the outcome Part II: targeted neuromuscular training techniques to reduce identified ACL injury risk factors. *J Strength Cond Res*. 2012;26:2272-2292.

39. Myer GD, Ford KR, Brent JL, Hewett TE. An integrated approach to change the outcome Part I: neuromuscular screening methods to identify high ACL injury risk athletes. *J Strength Cond Res.* 2012;26:2265-2271.
40. Myer GD, Ford KR, Hewett TE. Rationale and clinical techniques for anterior cruciate ligament injury prevention among female athletes. *J Athl Train.* 2004;39:352-364.
41. Myer GD, Ford KR, Hewett TE. Tuck jump assessment for reducing anterior cruciate ligament injury risk. *Athl Ther Today.* 2008;13:39-44.
42. Brent J, Myer GD, Ford KR, Paterno M, Hewett T. The effect of sex and age on isokinetic hip abduction torques. *J Sport Rehabil.* 2013;22:41-46.

Knee Anterior Cruciate Ligament: Reconstruction

Angela H. Smith
David Logerstedt

CASE 16

A 17-year-old female is referred to physical therapy 2 weeks after right anterior cruciate ligament (ACL) reconstruction with hamstring autograft. Six weeks ago, the patient was injured during a soccer game when she planted her right foot and changed direction to go around a defender. She heard a "pop" and had immediate pain in her right knee. She attempted to walk off the field but experienced a "giving way" episode and had to be carried off the field. On the sidelines, she noticed significant knee swelling. The patient consulted an orthopaedic surgeon the following day. The surgeon's examination revealed limited and painful knee flexion range of motion (ROM) and 2+ joint effusion. The patient's pivot shift test was equivocal because of muscle guarding; however, the Lachman test was positive as noted by an absent end feel. Subsequent magnetic resonance imaging (MRI) scan demonstrated a full-thickness tear of the ACL with associated contusions of the lateral femoral condyle and posterolateral (PL) tibia. The medial and lateral menisci were intact. To address the current impairments and improve postoperative outcomes, the patient had 5 physical therapy visits before she underwent right ACL reconstruction. Postoperative instructions for the first week after surgery included active ROM for knee flexion and extension, quad sets, cryotherapy for effusion management, and weightbearing as tolerated. One week after surgery, the patient was referred to physical therapy with an order to "evaluate and treat." The patient entered the clinic in a knee immobilizer, ambulating with bilateral axillary crutches. She rates her pain on the numeric pain rating scale as 2/10 at rest and 7/10 while performing ROM exercises. The patient's medical history is otherwise unremarkable. Her goals are to return to playing soccer for her high school soccer team the following season.

- Based on the patient's diagnosis and history, what do you anticipate may be the contributors to her activity limitations?
- What are the most appropriate examination tests?
- What are the most appropriate physical therapy interventions?
- What is her rehabilitation prognosis?

KEY DEFINITIONS

ACL RECONSTRUCTION: Arthroscopic surgical technique whereby the ACL is replaced using a tendon graft, either from the patient's own body or from a cadaveric donor

AUTOGRAFT: Tissue transferred from one part of a patient's body to another; common autografts used in ACL reconstruction include part of the hamstring or patellar tendon (PT).

EFFUSION: Presence of increased fluid in the synovial cavity of a joint

GIVING WAY EPISODE: Event commonly associated with knee instability in the ACL-deficient knee in which the patient experiences tibiofemoral shifting with associated pain and swelling

LACHMAN TEST: Considered the gold standard for clinical assessment of ACL deficiency; test is performed by placing the patient's knee in 30° flexion and applying an anterior translatory force to the tibia while stabilizing the femur; the examiner assesses for the amount of excursion and type of end feel; a positive test is indicated by increased excursion and/or an absent or "mushy" end feel.

Objectives

1. Identify postoperative clinical milestones for early, intermediate, and late functional progression and return-to-sport (RTS) phases of rehabilitation.
2. Identify evidence-based physical therapy interventions that can safely be applied in each postoperative phase based on healing timeframes.
3. Understand the effusion grading scale and soreness rules and describe how they relate to rehabilitation progression.

Physical Therapy Considerations

PT considerations during management of the athlete with an ACL reconstruction using soft tissue autograft or allograft:

- **General physical therapy plan of care/goals:** Decrease pain; increase active and passive knee ROM; normalize patella mobility; improve quadriceps strength and activation; normalize gait without assistive device; eliminate joint effusion
- **Physical therapy interventions:** Patient education regarding general precautions to avoid stressing graft; modalities to decrease pain; manual therapy and patient education to decrease joint effusion; active and passive ROM and patellar mobilizations to increase knee ROM; progressive strengthening exercises to improve quadriceps and lower extremity strength; gait training to normalize gait pattern; home exercise instruction
- **Precautions during physical therapy:** Choose appropriate open- and closed-chain strengthening exercises to minimize graft stress in early and intermediate

postoperative phases; address precautions based on graft selection and/or secondary surgeries performed (*e.g.*, meniscal repair or microfracture)

▶ **Complications interfering with physical therapy:** Arthrofibrosis, cyclops lesion, anterior knee pain, persistent knee joint effusion

Understanding the Health Condition

The ACL is one of the 4 major ligaments of the knee and plays a vital role in dynamic stability of the knee. The primary function of the ACL is to prevent anterior translation of the tibia on the femur; however, it also serves as a secondary restraint to tibial internal rotation, particularly when the knee is near full extension.[1] The ACL is a thick band of connective tissue that can be divided into 2 sections: the anteromedial (AM) bundle and the PL bundle,[2] named for where they insert on the tibia (Fig. 16-1). The ligament originates proximally on the femur and courses anteriorly, medially, and inferiorly to attach on the tibia.[3] More specifically, the ACL originates on the posterior medial surface of the lateral femoral condyle and inserts on the anterior portion of the tibial plateau, with the smaller AM bundle attaching more anteromedially and the PL bundle attaching more posterolaterally.[4] Each bundle plays a different role in knee stability dependent on the angle of knee flexion. The AM bundle lengthens and becomes tauter with greater angles of knee flexion, whereas the PL bundle becomes tauter with greater angles of knee extension.[4,5]

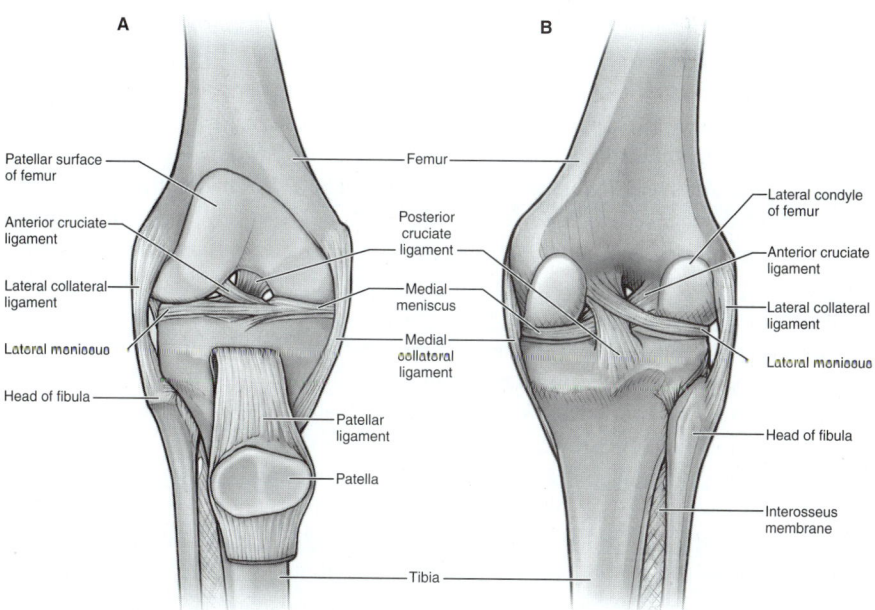

Figure 16-1. Primary ligaments of the knee. **A.** Anterior view. **B.** Posterior view. (Reproduced with permission from Morton DA, Foreman KB, Albertine KH. *The Big Picture: Gross Anatomy.* New York: McGraw-Hill Education; 2011. Figure 36-5.)

Because of its significant role in providing dynamic knee stability, ACL injuries are quite common across a variety of cutting and pivoting sports. ACL injuries constitute 20% of all athletic knee injuries and 45% of internal knee lesions occurring in sports.[6] Injuries can occur in both contact and non-contact situations, with incidence estimates ranging between 80,000 and 250,000 injuries occurring each year in the United States.[7] Non-contact ACL injuries are more common, occurring 70% of the time, whereas contact injuries account for the remaining 30%.[8] Non-contact injuries occur most frequently during cutting and pivoting activities that require rapid deceleration,[9] change of direction,[10] or when landing from a jump on one leg.[10] There are many proposed risk factors and various mechanisms of injury commonly associated with non-contact ACL injuries. The 2005 Hunt Valley II Meeting Consensus statement classified risk factors for non-contact injuries into 4 categories: environmental, anatomical, hormonal, and biomechanical.[7] Furthermore, this group identified that combined loading patterns in the frontal, sagittal, and transverse planes lead to dynamic loading of the ACL, putting the athlete at risk for injury, particularly when the knee is near full extension.[7] Female athletes are at higher risk for non-contact ACL injuries, with 6 to 8 times higher incidence than males partaking in the same activity.[10] There is still much debate regarding why ACL injuries occur more frequently in females; however, common risk factors associated with female athletes include hormonal changes related to menstrual cycle, decreased intercondylar notch width, and increased knee valgus moments upon landing.[11]

Although some ACL tears can be managed nonoperatively, ACL reconstruction is recommended for the majority of injuries occurring in young, active individuals in order to restore knee function and dynamic stability. More than 127,000 ACL reconstructions are performed annually in the United States.[12] For athletes undergoing this procedure, the goal is to return them to their preoperative level of sports activity. The ruptured ACL does not heal spontaneously, and it is not amenable to surgical repair; instead, a soft tissue autograft or cadaveric allograft is used to *reconstruct* the ACL during arthroscopic surgery. The PT remains the most commonly utilized graft selection to replace the ACL.[13] However, hamstring tendon (HT) autografts, which generally consist of a combined semitendinosus-gracilis bundle, are quickly growing in popularity.[14] There is much debate about the superiority of the PT versus the HT autograft. PT grafts have long been associated with increased graft stability due to bone-to-bone fixation.[15] However, recent research has shown that this correlation may not exist.[16] PT grafts are also linked to anterior knee pain (particularly with kneeling),[17,18] as well as clinical, radiographic, and histologic abnormalities at the donor site.[13] On the other hand, HT autografts are associated with potential complications including tunnel widening and problematic fixation, and poor postoperative functioning of the partially harvested hamstring tendon.[14] Regardless of the many speculated advantages and disadvantages associated with either PT or HT autografts, mid- and long-term outcomes regarding strength, ROM, knee stability, subjective reports, and patient performance are similar across both graft types.[14,18-20] With the advances in surgical techniques and rehabilitation protocols, it appears that graft selection does not have an impact on long-term postoperative success.[17]

Physical Therapy Patient/Client Management

Postoperative rehabilitation of athletes who have undergone ACL reconstruction is important to restore normal knee function and prepare the individual for eventual RTS. Both strength and neuromuscular training exercises should be included in postoperative care in order to maximize function.[21] Literature supports that muscle strengthening programs after ACL reconstruction should include both open and closed kinetic chain (CKC) exercises.[22-24] The physical therapist should be familiar with healing timeframes and graft stresses to prescribe proper exercises at appropriate intervals. Clinical milestones, effusion grading, and soreness rules are used to aid clinical decision making regarding exercise progression. Functional testing and outcome measures are performed to assess the athlete's readiness to begin a RTS progression.

Examination, Evaluation, and Diagnosis

Physical therapy evaluation following ACL reconstruction should occur in the first 1 to 2 weeks following surgery. Examination includes observation and palpation of the knee joint and assessment of incision integrity, knee ROM, patella mobility, joint effusion, quadriceps function, lower extremity strength, and gait. Palpation of the knee joint and surrounding structures can provide insight into sources of postoperative pain. Elevated temperature, combined with increased redness of the skin or drainage from the incision, can indicate an infection. Once sutures have been removed and incision sites have closed, mobility of the scar should be assessed because adhesions can contribute to postoperative pain. The therapist should identify areas of pain or adherent tissue adjacent to and/or under the scar and note any discoloration or puckering of the scar. The therapist measures both active and passive knee ROM, as well as patella mobility in all directions because patellofemoral joint restrictions can contribute to ROM loss in knee flexion and extension. Knee joint effusion should be graded using a quantifiable outcome measure. The modified stroke test (Table 16-1), which has demonstrated good inter-rater reliability, quantifies joint effusion on a 5-point grading scale.[25]

Table 16-1 EFFUSION GRADING SCALE OF THE KNEE JOINT BASED ON THE MODIFIED STROKE TEST[25]	
Grade	Test Result
Absent	No wave produced on downstroke
Trace	Small wave on medial side with downstroke
1+	Larger bulge on medial side with downstroke
2+	Effusion spontaneously returns to medial side after upstroke (no downstroke necessary)
3+	So much fluid that it not possible to move the effusion out of the medial aspect of the knee

Reproduced with permission from Sturgill L, Snyder-Mackler L, Manal TJ, Axe MJ. Interrater reliability of a clinical scale to assess knee joint effusion. *J Orthop Sports Phys Ther.* 2009;39:845-849.

To perform the modified stroke test, the therapist applies several upward strokes from the medial joint line toward the suprapatellar pouch in an attempt to move any interstitial fluid away from the knee (Fig. 16-2A). If no immediate return of fluid is seen, the therapist applies a downward stroke to the lateral side of the knee from the suprapatellar pouch toward the lateral joint line (Fig. 16-2B). The effusion is graded as "absent" if no wave of fluid is seen with the downstroke, "trace" if a small wave of fluid is seen on the medial side with the downstroke, "1+" if a large wave of fluid is seen on the medial side with the downstroke, "2+" if there is spontaneous return of the fluid on the medial side without a downstroke, and "3+" if there

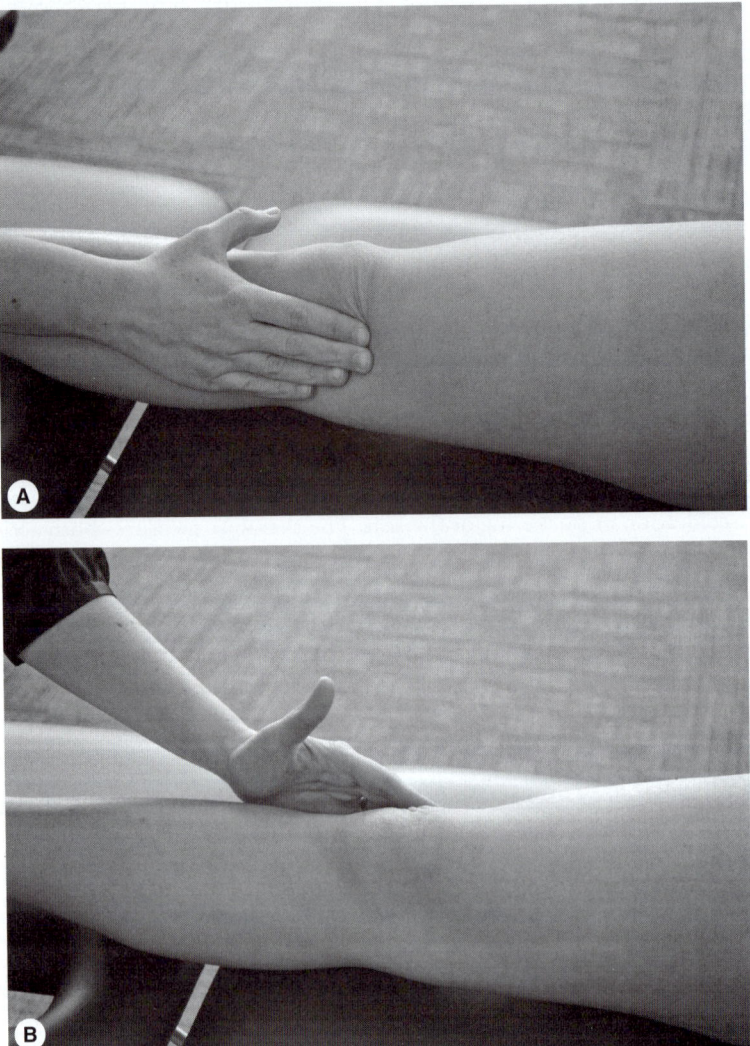

Figure 16-2. Modified stroke test. **A.** The therapist applies several upward strokes from medial joint line toward suprapatellar pouch. **B.** If no immediate return of fluid is seen, the therapist applies downward stroke to lateral side of the knee from suprapatellar pouch toward lateral joint line.

is too much fluid to move out of the knee. Early after surgery, most patients present with a 2+ or 3+ joint effusion related to the trauma associated with surgery.

Quadriceps function can be established by assessing the quality of a "quad set" (isometric contraction of the quadriceps muscles) with the patient's knee in full extension. The therapist should be able to observe the patella glide superiorly; the quad set can be clinically described as poor, fair, or good based on the quality of contraction observed. Asking the patient to perform a straight leg raise (SLR) can identify if the patient demonstrates a "quad lag" (an inability to maintain full knee extension), which indicates poor quadriceps strength/activation. Quadriceps strength can be quantified using an electromechanical dynamometer during a patient's maximum voluntary isometric contraction. Gait should be assessed using an appropriate assistive device and following the surgeon's prescribed weightbearing precautions. In the case of an isolated ACL reconstruction without concomitant injuries, the patient is typically allowed to weightbear as tolerated. It is now commonly accepted that immediate weightbearing following surgery is appropriate, and in fact can reduce the incidence of anterior knee pain and help overcome postoperative reflex inhibition of the quadriceps.[26] Common postoperative gait issues include absence of heel strike at initial contact, lack of terminal knee extension in stance phase, and decreased knee flexion excursion in swing phase. Further lower extremity strength should be assessed as necessary via manual muscle testing; hip abduction and ankle plantar flexion are of particular importance because deficits in these muscle groups can contribute to postoperative gait deviations. However, resisted muscle testing of the hamstring complex should be avoided if the patient had a hamstring autograft. As the patient transitions toward the RTS phase of rehabilitation, further evaluation will be necessary. Performance-based testing is important to assess a patient's readiness to return to higher level, sport-specific activities.

Plan of Care and Interventions

Postoperative ACL rehabilitation can be divided into 5 phases: early, intermediate, late, functional progression, and RTS. The athlete's readiness to progress to the next phase can be assessed by utilizing established clinical milestones such as those in the surgeon's postoperative protocol or the University of Delaware's Rehabilitation Practice Guidelines for ACL Reconstruction (Table 16-2).[27]

The early phase occurs in postoperative weeks 1 to 2 and the focus is on increasing knee ROM and improving quadriceps activation in order to facilitate ambulation without an immobilizer or assistive device. ROM milestones are important to achieve early on; the patient should attain full active knee extension and at least 90° of knee flexion by the end of week 1 and greater than 110° of flexion by the end of week 2.[27,28] Restoring full knee extension equal to the contralateral side is of vital importance because ROM deficits can lead to long-term functional impairments including pain and gait deviations,[29-31] as well as increased risk of developing osteoarthritis.[30,32] Mauro et al.[33] found that 25% of patients experienced loss of knee extension ROM at 4 weeks after ACL reconstruction, and 48% of those with deficits had to go on to have arthroscopic debridement of the knee to improve

Table 16-2 UNIVERSITY OF DELAWARE REHABILITATION PRACTICE GUIDELINES FOR ACL RECONSTRUCTION[27]

Postsurgery Timeframe	Interventions	Milestones
Week 1 (Early phase)	Wall slides, patellar mobilizations, gait training, NMES, bike for ROM	Knee A/PROM 0°-90° Active quadriceps contraction with superior patellar glide
Week 2 (Early phase)	Step-ups in pain-free range; incision mobilization as needed, if skin is healed (Fig. 16-3); wall sits/squats to 45°; prone hangs if lacking extension; inferior patellar mobilizations in flexion, if flexion is limited; transition to functional brace as swelling allows	Knee flexion ROM >110° Ambulation without crutches and using full knee extension Straight leg raise without a lag
Weeks 3-5 (Intermediate phase)	Tibiofemoral rotation mobilizations, if joint mobility is restricted; begin balance and proprioceptive activities; CV activities including bike or stepper for at least 10 min; knee extension from 90°-45°; leg press from 0°-45°; lateral step-downs	Knee flexion to within 10° of uninvolved side Quadriceps index > 60%
Weeks 6-8 (Late phase)	Progress therapeutic exercise in intensity and duration; progress CKC exercise toward 0°-90°; progress OKC exercise toward 90°-30°; forward step-downs; begin running progression at 8 weeks and transition to gym program as milestones are met	Full knee ROM Normal gait pattern Quadriceps index > 80% Knee effusion trace or less
Weeks 9-12 (Functional progression phase)	Sport-specific activities, agility drills, functional testing	Maintaining or gaining quadriceps strength Hop tests > 85% of uninvolved side at 12 weeks
Follow-up functional testing (4 months, 5 months, 6 months, and 1 year postsurgery)	Treatment modified based on current deficits; may include continued unilateral strengthening and explosive activities such as cutting, jumping, plyometrics, or landing training	Meeting all RTS criteria: Quadriceps index > 90% Hop tests > 90% KOS-ADL score > 90% Global rating of knee function score > 90%

Abbreviations: A/PROM, active/passive range of motion; CKC, closed kinetic chain; CV, cardiovascular; KOS-ADL, Knee Outcome Survey-Activities of Daily Living; NMES, neuromuscular electrical stimulation; OKC, open kinetic chain; ROM, range of motion RTS, return-to-sport.
Reproduced with permission from University of Delaware Physical Therapy Clinic. Rehab practice guidelines for: ACL reconstruction. http://www.udptclinic.com/downloads/knee/ACL_Protocol_2015.pdf. Accessed September 3, 2015.

ROM. **Rehabilitation programs** that include early weightbearing and emphasize achieving full active knee ROM lead to less pain and help prevent scar tissue formation and capsular contractures that can limit knee joint motion.[28,34-37] Bynum et al.[34] also found that accelerated rehabilitation programs reduced the incidence of postoperative flexion or extension loss and patellofemoral pain without any adverse effects. The beginning phase of rehabilitation should include initiation of strengthening exercises such as quad sets and straight leg raises.[38] **Neuromuscular electrical**

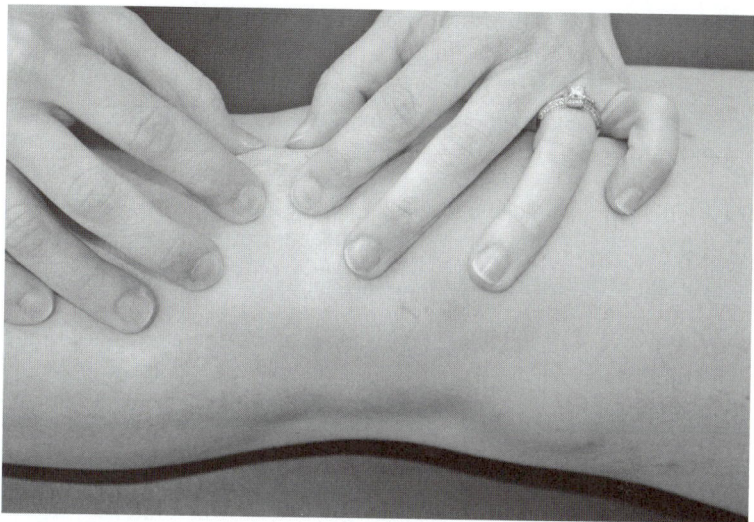

Figure 16-3. Incision mobilization.

stimulation (**NMES**) should be started in the early phase to facilitate quadriceps activation and supplement active strengthening exercises. When combined with exercise, the use of high-intensity NMES leads to greater quadriceps strength gains than exercise alone.[39,40] Gait training to address gait deviations must be incorporated into this phase. This is a critical intervention because individuals who have undergone ACL reconstruction are at higher risk for developing knee osteoarthritis and there is growing evidence that this risk may be associated with changes in gait mechanics and joint loading following surgery.[41,42]

The intermediate phase constitutes weeks 3 to 5 of postoperative rehabilitation. At the end of this phase, it is expected that the athlete should achieve active knee flexion to within 10° of the uninvolved side and a quadriceps index (QI) of at least 60%.[28] At this stage, quadriceps strength can be assessed with an electromechanical dynamometer when the athlete performs a maximum voluntary isometric contraction (MVIC). The athlete's QI is calculated by dividing the MVIC of the involved side by the MVIC of the uninvolved side and multiplying by 100. The ideal angle to test quadriceps strength is 60° to 70° of knee flexion.[43] If the therapist does not have access to an electromechanical dynamometer, strength indices can be calculated using a handheld dynamometer at a fixed angle or with one repetition maximum (1RM) testing on a leg press machine. It is important to establish strength milestones during ACL rehabilitation because quadriceps weakness can persist for 2 years after surgery.[44] Restoring muscle strength is especially critical for the athlete because increased strength is associated with positive long-term functional outcomes of the ACL reconstructed knee.[45] Recovery of quadriceps strength should be accomplished with both **open kinetic chain (OKC) and CKC exercises**.[21,24] In a 2004 systematic review, Risberg et al.[46] determined that quadriceps strengthening CKC exercises at knee joint angles less than 60° and OKC exercises at knee flexion angles greater than 40° can be performed without increasing strain on the ACL and without increased stresses on the patellofemoral joint. Throughout the course of ACL rehabilitation, the therapist should prescribe exercises considering the graft strength and fixation based on the stages of graft incorporation and maturation (as the graft starts to vascularize and mature, its strength increases).[47] Because one of the primary goals of ACL rehabilitation is to restore dynamic knee joint stability, balance and proprioception activities should also begin in this phase. Altered movement patterns persist after ACL reconstruction,[48] suggesting that neuromuscular training activities should be included in postoperative rehabilitation programs because these activities may lead to improvements in limb symmetry and movement patterns.[49]

The late phase of ACL rehabilitation occurs in postoperative weeks 6 to 8. This phase functions as a transitional period to prepare the athlete to begin an independent gym program. The milestones in this phase include achievement of full knee ROM, QI greater than 80%, knee effusion of trace or less, and normal gait pattern. Both CKC[47] and OKC[50] strengthening activities can be used to progress toward performance through the full ROM. At 8 weeks after surgery, the athlete's quadriceps activation and strength may be tested via a burst superimposition method. This method of testing is performed using an electromechanical dynamometer and a square pulse stimulator. The therapist asks the patient to perform an MVIC of the quadriceps while a burst of electrical stimulation is superimposed during the contraction (Fig. 16-4). This provides a valuation of quadriceps muscle activation by calculating a ratio of the force produced during the MVIC to the force produced with the electrical stimulation.[51,52] An activation ratio of 95% indicates that the athlete's active quadriceps force output is 95% of the total muscle capability as measured by the superimposed electrical stimulation. An activation ratio of 95% indicates normal muscle functioning.[52,53] The testing is performed on both legs, after which a QI can be calculated as described previously. Although

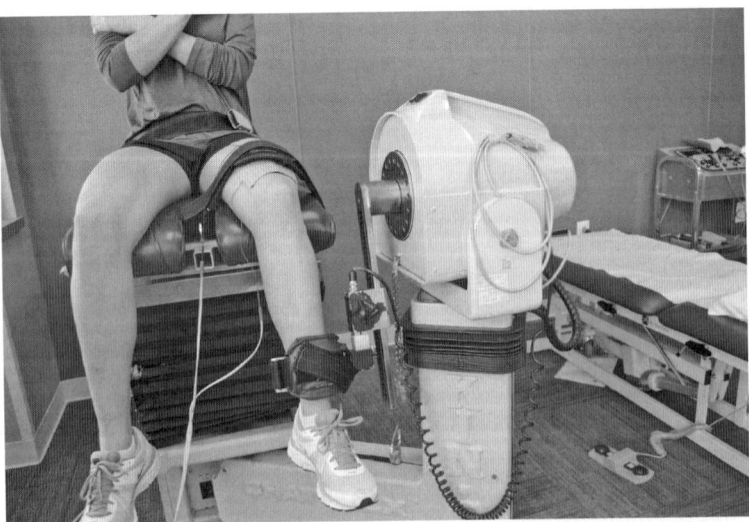

Figure 16-4. Testing quadriceps strength with burst superimposition method.

handheld dynamometry can also be used to quantify quadriceps strength, the burst superimposition method is superior because it assesses muscle activation[52] and does not rely on the ability of the examiner to provide sufficient resistive force during testing. If the athlete has yet to achieve the 80% QI milestone, supervised physical therapy and NMES should continue. Lewek et al.[54] found that individuals with ACL-reconstructed knees and a QI less than 80% demonstrated walking and jogging patterns similar to patients with ACL-deficient knees, which may be detrimental to joint health. If the athlete has a QI greater than 80% and other milestones for this phase have been met, it is recommended that unilateral strengthening and neuromuscular control activities be continued until strength is at least 90% of the contralateral leg.[28] The patient may also begin a running progression in the late phase[27] (Table 16-3). The running progression should be completed on a treadmill or a track in order to maintain a level surface and to provide some shock absorption. The University of Delaware's rehabilitation program consists of 8 levels, beginning with walk/jog intervals for a total of 2 miles and concluding with a 3-mile jog/run. The athlete is advised to progress to the next level when she is able to perform the activity for 2 miles without increased effusion or pain. The athlete should not perform the program more than 4 times in 1 week and no more frequently than every other day. In addition, the athlete should not progress more than 2 levels in a 7-day period. It is suggested that all athletes complete the running progression because the unilateral loading that occurs during running provides dynamic lower extremity strengthening.[28]

The functional progression phase occurs during postoperative weeks 9 to 12. The goals of this phase are to maintain or gain quadriceps strength and to attain hop test scores greater than 85% compared to the contralateral side when tested at 12 weeks.[27,28] During this phase, the athlete may either be participating in an

Table 16-3   RUNNING PROGRESSION

Level	Treadmill	Track
1	Alternate 0.1 mile walk/0.1 mile jog, repeat 10 times	Jog straights/walk curves (2 miles)
2	Alternate 0.1 mile walk/0.2 mile jog (2 miles total)	Jog straights, jog 1 curve every other lap (2 miles)
3	Alternate 0.1 mile walk/0.3 mile jog (2 miles total)	Jog straights, jog 1 curve every lap (2 miles)
4	Alternate 0.1 mile walk/0.4 mile jog (2 miles total)	Jog 1.75 laps/walk curve (2 miles)
5	Jog full 2 miles	Jog all laps (2 miles)
6	Increase to 2.5 miles	Increase workout to 2.5 miles
7	Increase to 3 miles	Increase workout to 3 miles
8	Alternate running/jogging every 0.25 mile	Increase speed on straights/jog curves

Reproduced with permission from University of Delaware Physical Therapy Clinic. Rehab practice guidelines for: ACL reconstruction. http://www.udptclinic.com/downloads/knee/ACL_Protocol_2015.pdf. Accessed September 3, 2015.

independent rehabilitation program or one supervised by another professional such as a certified athletic trainer or strength and conditioning coach. The running progression can be continued. If the athlete has not experienced any increase in knee pain or effusion with running, then she may start agility, plyometric, and sport-specific activities.[28] The physical therapist should instruct the patient in these activities and may add them to the home program. It is important for the athlete or the supervising healthcare professional to utilize guidelines for activity progression during this phase. Modified soreness rules (Table 16-4) provide a systematic approach to activity progression and may be applied to each phase of rehabilitation.[28,55] These rules should be combined with effusion monitoring to direct the athlete's participation in high-demand functional activities. If progression to loading activities leads to adverse responses such as joint pain, increased effusion, or muscle soreness, a change in the current program is necessary. Appropriate activity modification depends on when in the rehabilitation session the patient experiences such a response. For example, if the athlete reports increased knee pain or experiences knee effusion *during* a treatment session, the intensity of the next session should be decreased until the impairments are resolved. If the same signs and symptoms occurred the day *after* a treatment session, the program should not be advanced, but rather maintained at that same level. If the athlete can complete a workout with no soreness during or after the session, it is appropriate to advance to the next level of training. However, it is suggested that the athlete complete 2 to 3 sessions at the same intensity without any adverse responses before the intensity of the program is progressed.[56] As the athlete reaches the 12-week postoperative mark, she can move forward to the RTS phase of rehabilitation, and should undergo functional testing when appropriate milestones have been met.

The RTS phase of ACL rehabilitation tends to have the most variability because treatment is based on the athlete's current deficits and sport of choice. Functional

Table 16-4 MODIFIED SORENESS RULES

Timing of Soreness Encountered During Training	Presence of Soreness	Action Plan
Soreness encountered during warm-up	Soreness goes away	Patient continues at the same intensity level.
Soreness encountered during exercise	Soreness continues	Patient takes off 2 days and drops off the training intensity 1 level.
Soreness encountered 1 day after exercise (not muscle soreness)	Soreness continues	Patient takes 1 day off, continues at the same intensity level (does not advance to next volume or intensity level).
Soreness not encountered	No soreness	Patient either advances to the next volume or intensity level or follows training progression prescribed by healthcare provider.

Reproduced with permission from Zakariya Nawasreh.

Table 16-5 CRITERIA FOR HOP TESTING AFTER ACL RECONSTRUCTION[28]
Minimum of 12 weeks after ACL reconstruction:
≥80% quadriceps index
Trace or less effusion
Full knee ROM
No pain with single-legged hopping in place

testing usually occurs 3 to 6 months after surgery, based on the patient's desire to RTS and healing timeframes.[28] When the athlete is ready, it is important to utilize a battery of functional tests and outcome measures to assess the athlete's readiness to begin RTS activities.[57-59] A specific battery of tests that includes quadriceps strength testing, single-legged hop testing, and 2 patient-report questionnaires has been utilized to assess readiness to RTS following ACL injury and reconstruction.[43,60,61] Quadriceps strength testing should be completed as described previously. A minimum QI of 90% as compared to the uninvolved limb is required for RTS. If all appropriate criteria are met, the athlete may undergo hop testing no earlier than 12 weeks after ACL reconstruction (Table 16-5).

Hop testing is a reliable and valid performance-based outcome measure following ACL reconstruction.[62,63] In fact, postoperative single-legged hop tests performed at 6 months can predict the likelihood of a successful outcome after ACL reconstruction at 1 year.[63] Noyes et al.[58] described a series of single-limb hop testing commonly utilized for functional testing. This sequence of tests includes the single hop for distance, the crossover hop for distance, the triple hop for distance, and the 6-m timed hop (Fig. 16-5). Hop testing is performed on a line that is 6 m in length by 15 cm in width.[63] In order to be considered a valid trial, the athlete must achieve a stable landing on one foot when testing the single, crossover, and triple hops. The distance hopped is measured to the nearest centimeter (measured from the starting line to the athlete's heel upon landing). For the timed hop, time is recorded with a

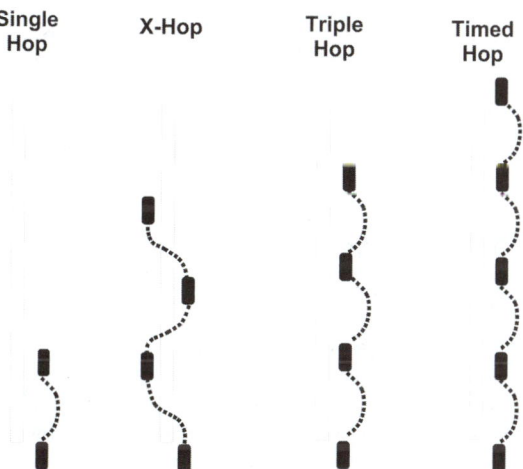

Figure 16-5. Schematic for hop tests.

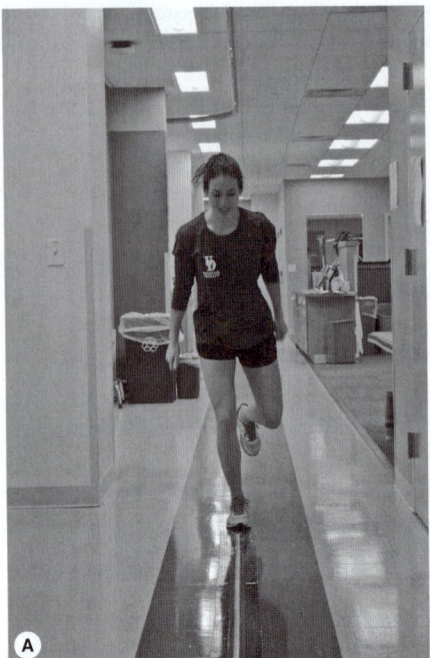 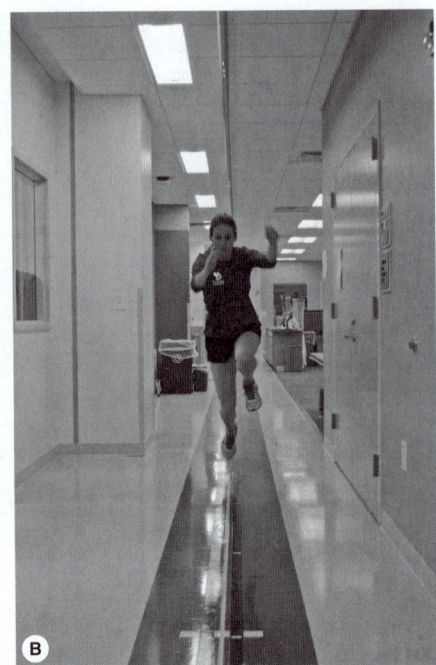

Figure 16-6. A 6-m timed hop. **A.** Starting position. **B.** Time is started when the athlete's heel leaves the floor at the starting line and stopped when the athlete crosses the finish line.

standard stopwatch, starting when the athlete's heel leaves the floor at the starting line and stopping when the athlete crosses the finish line (Fig. 16-6). Each hop is completed on the uninvolved limb first, with 1 practice trial followed by 2 measured trials; this sequence is then repeated on the involved limb in order to determine a limb symmetry index (LSI). The mean distance of the 2 measured trials is calculated for each leg for the single, crossover, and triple hops, and then the LSI is determined by the ratio of the mean distance on the involved limb to the mean distance on the uninvolved limb, multiplied by 100. For the timed hop, the LSI is calculated as a ratio of the uninvolved limb mean time over the involved limb mean time multiplied by 100. In addition to strength and hop testing, 2 self-report outcome measures are utilized in this test battery. The Knee Outcome Survey-Activities of Daily Living Scale (KOS-ADLS) is a valid, reliable, and responsive measurement tool used to assess functional limitations for a varied population with knee injuries and impairments.[64] The Global Rating Scale of Perceived Function (GRS) is a single question that asks the patient to rate the function of his/her knee on a scale of 0 to 100 with 100 being the function before injury.[65] In order to begin a RTS progression, the athlete must achieve 90% or more on each of the following criteria: QI, all 4 single-legged hop tests, KOS-ADLS, and the GRS.[29] However, meeting these criteria does not indicate that the athlete is ready for unrestricted return to activity; instead, she may begin a phased progression back toward her sport. The athlete should begin with full-speed agility training, progressing to unopposed practice of sport-specific skills, followed by one-on-one opposed practice of sport-specific skills and then full practice activity with the team.[66] Progression of these activities should be based on soreness rules, as well as the athlete's confidence.

Evidence-Based Clinical Recommendations

SORT: Strength of Recommendation Taxonomy
A: Consistent, good-quality patient-oriented evidence
B: Inconsistent or limited-quality patient-oriented evidence
C: Consensus, disease-oriented evidence, usual practice, expert opinion, or case series

1. Accelerated ACL reconstruction rehabilitation programs that emphasize early weightbearing and achievement of full active knee ROM lead to less pain, scar tissue formation, and contractures. **Grade A**
2. The combination of exercise and high-intensity neuromuscular electrical stimulation (NMES) after ACL reconstruction improves quadriceps strength gains. **Grade A**
3. In the ACL reconstructed knee, a combination of closed and open kinetic chain exercises at specific knee joint angles optimizes outcomes without increasing strain on the ACL graft. **Grade A**

COMPREHENSION QUESTIONS

16.1 The ACL is the passive restraint to _____ translation and _____ rotation of the tibia on the femur.
   A. Posterior, internal
   B. Posterior, external
   C. Anterior, internal
   D. Anterior, external

16.2 _____ athletes are more likely to suffer a _____ ACL injury.
   A. Female, non-contact
   B. Male, non-contact
   C. Male, contact
   D. Female, contact

16.3 The minimum quadriceps index (QI) needed to hop test an athlete following ACL reconstruction is:
   A. 60%
   B. 70%
   C. 80%
   D. 90%

16.4 After ACL reconstruction, closed kinetic chain strengthening exercises of the quadriceps muscles should:

A. Be discouraged
B. Be performed in combination with open kinetic chain strengthening exercises
C. Be initiated after the ACL graft has fully healed
D. Be performed after the individual has passed all return-to-sport criteria

ANSWERS

16.1 **C.** The primary function of the ACL is to prevent anterior translation of the tibia on the femur; however, it also serves as a secondary restraint to tibial internal rotation, particularly when the knee is near full extension.

16.2 **A.** Female athletes have 6 to 8 times greater risk of sustaining a non-contact ACL injury than male athletes.

16.3 **C.** Eighty percent QI ensures that the individual has adequate quadriceps strength that reduces the risk of giving way or injury during hop testing. The other criteria for hop testing include trace or less knee effusion, full knee ROM, and no pain with single-legged hopping in place (Table 16-5).

16.4 **B.** Recovery of quadriceps strength should be accomplished with both open kinetic chain (OKC) and closed kinetic chain (CKC) exercises.

REFERENCES

1. Duthon VB, Barea C, Abrassart S, Fasel JH, Fritschy D, Menetrey J. Anatomy of the anterior cruciate ligament. *Knee Surg Sports Traumatol Arthrosc.* 2006;14:204-213.
2. Girgis FG, Marshall JL, Monajem A. The cruciate ligaments of the knee joint. Anatomical, functional and experimental analysis. *Clin Orthop Relat Res.* 1975;106:216-231.
3. Bicer EK, Lustig S, Servien E, Selmi TA, Neyret P. Current knowledge in the anatomy of the human anterior cruciate ligament. *Knee Surg Sports Traumatol Arthrosc.* 2010;18:1075-1084.
4. Dodds JA, Arnoczky SP. Anatomy of the anterior cruciate ligament: a blueprint for repair and reconstruction. *Arthroscopy.* 1994;10:132-139.
5. Amis AA, Gupte CM, Bull AM, Edwards A. Anatomy of the posterior cruciate ligament and the meniscofemoral ligaments. *Knee Surg Sports Traumatol Arthrosc.* 2006;14:257-263.
6. Majewski M, Susanne H, Klaus S. Epidemiology of athletic knee injuries: a 10-year study. *Knee.* 2006;13:184-188.
7. Griffin LY, Albohm MJ, Arendt EA, et al. Understanding and preventing noncontact anterior cruciate ligament injuries: a review of the Hunt Valley II meeting, January 2005. *Am J Sports Med.* 2006;34:1512-1532.
8. Griffin LY, Agel J, Albohm MJ, et al. Noncontact anterior cruciate ligament injuries: risk factors and prevention strategies. *J Am Acad Orthop Surg.* 2000;8:141-150.
9. Shimokochi Y, Shultz SJ. Mechanisms of noncontact anterior cruciate ligament injury. *J Athl Train.* 2008;43:396-408.

10. Hughes G, Watkins J. A risk-factor model for anterior cruciate ligament injury. *Sports Med.* 2006;36:411-428.
11. Renstrom P, Ljungqvist A, Arendt E, et al. Non-contact ACL injuries in female athletes: an International Olympic Committee current concepts statement. *Br J Sports Med.* 2008;42:394-412.
12. Kim S, Bosque J, Meehan JP, Jamali A, Marder R. Increase in outpatient knee arthroscopy in the United States: a comparison of National Surveys of Ambulatory Surgery, 1996 and 2006. *J Bone Joint Surg Am.* 2011;93:994-1000.
13. Kartus J, Movin T, Karlsson J. Donor-site morbidity and anterior knee problems after anterior cruciate ligament reconstruction using autografts. *Arthroscopy.* 2001;17:971-980.
14. Herrington L, Wrapson C, Matthews M, Matthews H. Anterior cruciate ligament reconstruction, hamstring versus bone-patella tendon-bone grafts: a systematic literature review of outcome from surgery. *Knee.* 2005;12:41-50.
15. Brown CH Jr, Hecker AT, Hipp JA, Myers ER, Hayes WC. The biomechanics of interference screw fixation of patellar tendon anterior cruciate ligament grafts. *Am J Sports Med.* 1993;21:880-886.
16. Poolman RW, Abouali JA, Conter HJ, Bhandari M. Overlapping systematic reviews of anterior cruciate ligament reconstruction comparing hamstring autograft with bone-patellar tendon-bone autograft: why are they different? *J Bone Joint Surg Am.* 2007;89:1542-1552.
17. Spindler KP, Kuhn JE, Freedman KB, Matthews CE, Dittus RS, Harrell FE Jr. Anterior cruciate ligament reconstruction autograft choice: bone-tendon-bone versus hamstring: does it really matter? A systematic review. *Am J Sports Med.* 2004;32:1986-1995.
18. Hui C, Salmon LJ, Kok A, Maeno S, Linklater J, Pinczewski LA. Fifteen-year outcome of endoscopic anterior cruciate ligament reconstruction with patellar tendon autograft for "isolated" anterior cruciate ligament tear. *Am J Sports Med.* 2011;39:89-98.
19. Carter TR, Edinger S. Isokinetic evaluation of anterior cruciate ligament reconstruction: hamstring versus patellar tendon. *Arthroscopy.* 1999;15:169-172.
20. Keays SL, Bullock-Saxton JE, Keays AC, Newcombe PA, Bullock MI. A 6-year follow-up of the effect of graft site on strength, stability, range of motion, function, and joint degeneration after anterior cruciate ligament reconstruction: patellar tendon versus semitendinosus and gracilis tendon graft. *Am J Sports Med.* 2007;35:729-739.
21. Risberg MA, Holm I. The long-term effect of 2 postoperative rehabilitation programs after anterior cruciate ligament reconstruction: a randomized controlled clinical trial with 2 years of follow-up. *Am J Sports Med.* 2009;37:1958-1966.
22. Mikkelsen C, Werner S, Eriksson E. Closed kinetic chain alone compared to combined open and closed kinetic chain exercises for quadriceps strengthening after anterior cruciate ligament reconstruction with respect to return to sports: a prospective matched follow-up study. *Knee Surg Sports Traumatol Arthrosc.* 2000;8:337-342.
23. Glass R, Waddell J, Hoogenboom B. The effects of open versus closed kinetic chain exercises on patients with ACL deficient or reconstructed knees: a systematic review. *N Am J Sports Phys Ther.* 2010;5:74-84.
24. Fleming BC, Oksendahl H, Beynnon BD. Open- or closed-kinetic chain exercises after anterior cruciate ligament reconstruction? *Exerc Sport Sci Rev.* 2005;33:134-140.
25. Sturgill L, Snyder-Mackler L, Manal TJ, Axe MJ. Interrater reliability of a clinical scale to assess knee joint effusion. *J Orthop Sports Phys Ther.* 2009;39:845-849.
26. Tyler TF, McHugh MP, Gleim GW, Nicholas SJ. The effect of immediate weightbearing after anterior cruciate ligament reconstruction. *Clin Orthop Relat Res.* 1998;357:141-148.
27. University of Delaware Physical Therapy Clinic. Rehab practice guidelines for: ACL reconstruction. Updated 2014 ed. http://www.udptclinic.com/downloads/knee/ACL_Protocol_2015.pdf. Accessed August 11, 2015.
28. Adams D, Logerstedt DS, Hunter-Giordano A, Axe MJ, Snyder-Mackler L. Current concepts for anterior cruciate ligament reconstruction: a criterion-based rehabilitation progression. *J Orthop Sports Phys Ther.* 2012;42:601-614.

29. Shelbourne KD, Patel DV, Martini DJ. Classification and management of arthrofibrosis of the knee after anterior cruciate ligament reconstruction. *Am J Sports Med*. 1996;24:857-862.
30. Mayr HO, Weig TG, Plitz W. Arthrofibrosis following ACL reconstruction--reasons and outcome. *Arch Orthop Trauma Surg*. 2004;124:518-522.
31. Paulos LE, Rosenberg TD, Drawbert J, Manning J, Abbott P. Infrapatellar contracture syndrome. An unrecognized cause of knee stiffness with patella entrapment and patella infera. *Am J Sports Med*. 1987;15:331-341.
32. Shelbourne KD, Urch SE, Gray T, Freeman H. Loss of normal knee motion after anterior cruciate ligament reconstruction is associated with radiographic arthritic changes after surgery. *Am J Sports Med*. 2011;40:108-113.
33. Mauro CS, Irrgang JJ, Williams BA, Harner CD. Loss of extension following anterior cruciate ligament reconstruction: analysis of incidence and etiology using IKDC criteria. *Arthroscopy*. 2008;24:146-153.
34. Bynum EB, Barrack RL, Alexander AH. Open versus closed chain kinetic exercises after anterior cruciate ligament reconstruction. A prospective randomized study. *Am J Sports Med*. 1995;23:401-406.
35. Beynnon BD, Johnson RJ. Anterior cruciate ligament injury rehabilitation in athletes. Biomechanical considerations. *Sports Med*. 1996;22:54-64.
36. MacDonald PB, Hedden D, Pacin O, Huebert D. Effects of an accelerated rehabilitation program after anterior cruciate ligament reconstruction with combined semitendinosus-gracilis autograft and a ligament augmentation device. *Am J Sports Med*. 1995;23:588-592.
37. Beynnon BD, Johnson RJ, Abate JA, Fleming BC, Nichols CE. Treatment of anterior cruciate ligament injuries, part 2. *Am J Sports Med*. 2005;33:1751-1767.
38. Shaw T, Williams MT, Chipchase LS. Do early quadriceps exercises affect the outcome of ACL reconstruction? A randomised controlled trial. *Aust J Physiother*. 2005;51:9-17.
39. Snyder-Mackler L, Delitto A, Stralka SW, Bailey SL. Use of electrical stimulation to enhance recovery of quadriceps femoris muscle force production in patients following anterior cruciate ligament reconstruction. *Phys Ther*. 1994;74:901-907.
40. Kim KM, Croy T, Hertel J, Saliba S. Effects of neuromuscular electrical stimulation after anterior cruciate ligament reconstruction on quadriceps strength, function, and patient-oriented outcomes: a systematic review. *J Orthop Sports Phys Ther*. 2010;40:383-391.
41. Butler RJ, Minick KI, Ferber R, Underwood F. Gait mechanics after ACL reconstruction: implications for the early onset of knee osteoarthritis. *Br J Sports Med*. 2009;43:366-370.
42. Di Stasi SL, Logerstedt D, Gardinier E, Snyder-Mackler L. Differing gait patterns Between ACL-reconstructed athletes who do and do not pass return to sport criteria. *Am J Sports Med*. 2013;41:1310-1318.
43. Kong PW, van Haselen J. Revisiting the influence of hip and knee angles on quadriceps excitation measured by surface electromyography. *Int Sport Med J*. 2010;11:313-323.
44. Risberg MA, Holm I, Tjomsland O, Ljunggren E, Ekeland A. Prospective study of changes in impairments and disabilities after anterior cruciate ligament reconstruction. *J Orthop Sports Phys Ther*. 1999;29:400-412.
45. Moisala AS, Jarvela T, Kannus P, Jarvinen M. Muscle strength evaluations after ACL reconstruction. *Int J Sports Med*. 2007;28:868-872.
46. Risberg MA, Lewek M, Snyder-Mackler L. A systematic review of evidence for anterior cruciate ligament rehabilitation: how much and what type? *Phys Ther in Sport*. 2004;5:125-145.
47. Escamilla RF, Macleod TD, Wilk KE, Paulos L, Andrews JR. Anterior cruciate ligament strain and tensile forces for weight-bearing and non-weight-bearing exercises: a guide to exercise selection. *J Orthop Sports Phys Ther*. 2012;42:208-220.
48. Ingersoll CD, Grindstaff TL, Pietrosimone BG, Hart JM. Neuromuscular consequences of anterior cruciate ligament injury. *Clin Sports Med*. 2008;27:383-404.

49. Hartigan E, Axe MJ, Snyder-Mackler L. Perturbation training prior to ACL reconstruction improves gait asymmetries in non-copers. *J Orthop Res.* 2009;27:724-729.

50. Perry MC, Morrissey MC, King JB, Morrissey D, Earnshaw P. Effects of closed versus open kinetic chain knee extensor resistance training on knee laxity and leg function in patients during the 8- to 14-week post-operative period after anterior cruciate ligament reconstruction. *Knee Surg Sports Traumatol Arthrosc.* 2005;13:357-369.

51. Snyder-Mackler L, Delitto A, Bailey SL, Stralka SW. Strength of the quadriceps femoris muscle and functional recovery after reconstruction of the anterior cruciate ligament. A prospective, randomized clinical trial of electrical stimulation. *J Bone Joint Surg Am.* 1995;77:1166-1173.

52. Chmielewski TL, Stackhouse S, Axe MJ, Snyder-Mackler L. A prospective analysis of incidence and severity of quadriceps inhibition in a consecutive sample of 100 patients with complete acute anterior cruciate ligament rupture. *J Orthop Res.* 2004;22:925-930.

53. Lynch AD, Logerstedt DS, Axe MJ, Snyder-Mackler L. Quadriceps activation failure after anterior cruciate ligament rupture is not mediated by knee joint effusion. *J Orthop Sports Phys Ther.* 2012;42:502-510.

54. Lewek M, Rudolph K, Axe M, Snyder-Mackler L. The effect of insufficient quadriceps strength on gait after anterior cruciate ligament reconstruction. *Clin Biomech.* 2002;17:56-63.

55. University of Delaware Physical Therapy. Soreness rules. http://www.udptclinic.com/downloads/handouts/SorenessRule_2015.pdf. Accessed August 11, 2015.

56. Chmielewski TL, Myer GD, Kauffman D, Tillman SM. Plyometric exercise in the rehabilitation of athletes: physiological responses and clinical application. *J Orthop Sports Phys Ther.* 2006;36:308-319.

57. Myer GD, Paterno MV, Ford KR, Quatman CE, Hewett TE. Rehabilitation after anterior cruciate ligament reconstruction: criteria-based progression through the return-to-sport phase. *J Orthop Sports Phys Ther.* 2006;36:385-402.

58. Noyes FR, Barber SD, Mangine RE. Abnormal lower limb symmetry determined by function hop tests after anterior cruciate ligament rupture. *Am J Sports Med.* 1991;19:513-518.

59. Hartigan EH, Axe MJ, Snyder-Mackler L. Timeline for noncopers to pass return-to-sports criteria after anterior cruciate ligament reconstruction. *J Orthop Sports Phys Ther.* 2010;40:141-154.

60. Fitzgerald GK, Axe MJ, Snyder-Mackler L. A decision-making scheme for returning patients to high-level activity with nonoperative treatment after anterior cruciate ligament rupture. *Knee Surg Sports Traumatol Arthrosc.* 2000;8:76-82.

61. Reid A, Birmingham TB, Stratford PW, Alcock GK, Giffin JR. Hop testing provides a reliable and valid outcome measure during rehabilitation after anterior cruciate ligament reconstruction. *Phys Ther.* 2007;87:337-349.

62. Paterno MV, Greenberger HB. The test-retest reliability of a one legged hop for distance in young adults with and without ACL reconstruction. *Isokinetics Exer Sci.* 1996;6:1-6.

63. Logerstedt D, Grindem H, Lynch A, et al. Single-legged hop tests as predictors of self-reported knee function after anterior cruciate ligament reconstruction: the Delaware-Oslo ACL cohort study. *Am J Sports Med.* 2012;40:2348-2356.

64. Irrgang JJ, Snyder-Mackler L, Wainner RS, Fu FH, Harner CD. Development of a patient-reported measure of function of the knee. *J Bone Joint Surg Am.* 1998;80:1132-1145.

65. Irrgang JJ, Ho H, Harner CD, Fu FH. Use of the International Knee Documentation Committee guidelines to assess outcome following anterior cruciate ligament reconstruction. *Knee Surg Sports Traumatol Arthrosc.* 1998;6:107-114.

66. Fitzgerald GK, Axe MJ, Snyder-Mackler L. Proposed practice guidelines for nonoperative anterior cruciate ligament rehabilitation of physically active individuals. *J Orthop Sports Phys Ther.* 2000;30:194-203.

Functional Testing to Return Athlete Back to Sport After ACL Reconstruction

Phil Plisky

CASE 17

A 16-year-old female basketball player underwent bone-patellar tendon-bone anterior cruciate ligament (ACL) reconstruction 5 months ago. Her orthopaedic medical history includes grade II lateral ankle sprain 2 years ago and occasional low back pain. Immediately after her ACL reconstruction, the physical therapist initiated basic range of motion (ROM) and strengthening exercises and then progressed her through a myriad of exercises (from low to high level). Five months after surgery, the physical therapist initiated plyometric training in her rehabilitation sessions. The patient and her mother ask when she can return to sports including track, soccer, and basketball.

- What are the most appropriate tests to determine her readiness for return to sport?
- Are criteria for return to sport the same as criteria for discharge from physical therapy?
- What patient and clinician values may be in conflict with each other?

KEY DEFINITIONS

LIMB SYMMETRY INDEX (LSI): Method to determine the performance of one limb compared to the other; typically calculated as uninvolved side divided by involved side multiplied by 100 and expressed as a percentage. An LSI of 100% would mean that the involved and uninvolved limbs performed the same on a given test.

MODIFIABLE RISK FACTOR: Characteristic that can be changed through training or behavioral modification[1]

MOTOR CONTROL: Ability to regulate and direct mechanisms essential to movement.[2] Motor control encompasses how the central nervous system coordinates muscles and joints to produce movement. Abnormal motor control after injury has been shown in electromyographic (EMG) studies that demonstrate changes in timing and firing patterns and biomechanical studies that demonstrate kinematic changes during performance of functional tasks.

Objectives

1. Describe risk factors for future injury in sports and the motor control changes that occur after injury.
2. Describe the psychometric properties of commonly used return-to-sport tests.
3. Arrange evidence-based return-to-sport tests in a hierarchical fashion from least complicated movements to most complicated movement (e.g., ROM and strength testing prior to movement testing prior to hop testing).
4. Define passing criteria for discharge from physical therapy and return to sport.
5. Describe how the patient's values for sport participation may conflict with the physical therapist's values for the patient's long-term musculoskeletal health and potential strategies to reconcile this conflict.

Physical Therapy Considerations

PT considerations during treatment and return-to-sport testing of the individual with a diagnosis of postoperative bone-patella, tendon-bone ACL reconstruction:

- ▶ **General physical therapy plan of care/goals:** Ensure athlete can safely return to sport and confirm modifiable risk factors for injury have been removed.
- ▶ **Physical therapy interventions:** Patient education regarding return-to-sport and discharge requirements including minimizing the risks of re-injury; comprehensive, step-wise return-to-sport testing procedure that identifies modifiable motor control changes after injury, as well as deficits related to future injury risk
- ▶ **Precautions during physical therapy:** Ensure medical history and current injury status do not present contraindications to testing; progress patient through tests

in hierarchical fashion from least complicated to most complicated movements because more complicated movements place greater stress on the knee joint and therefore increase potential for injury; monitor for pain and instability episodes and discontinue testing if either is present.

▶ **Complications interfering with physical therapy:** Pressure for the athlete to return to sport as soon as possible (*e.g.*, to maintain a sports scholarship) requires the therapist to balance the athlete's desire to return to participation with the risk of returning to sport too soon and increasing the potential for future disability.

Understanding the Health Condition

To improve outcomes after ACL reconstruction, it is critical to understand the pathoanatomical and biomechanical considerations of ACL reconstruction (see Case 16), as well as current rehabilitation outcomes. In a systematic review of the outcomes of athletes with ACL reconstruction (48 studies evaluating 5770 participants with a mean follow-up of 3.4 years), only 63% returned to pre-injury level of participation and only 44% returned to competitive sport at final follow-up.[3] However, based on the traditional impairment measures such as strength, approximately 90% achieved normal knee function after completing their rehabilitation programs.[4] In addition, 10% to 20% of athletes who have had an ACL reconstruction will go on to tear the reconstructed or contralateral ACL.[5,6] Lack of systematic, rigorous return-to-sport and discharge criteria may contribute to these poor outcomes and high re-injury rates. Multiple systematic reviews and surveys have concluded that return-to-sport testing criteria are at best highly variable and frequently nonexistent.[7-10]

More than 25 prospective cohort studies have identified previous injury as the most commonly reported risk factor for future injury.[5,11-14] After ACL reconstruction, athletes are 4 to 15 times more likely to tear the same or contralateral ACL.[5,14] Increased injury risk applies not only to re-injury of the same site, but also to injury elsewhere in the body.[11,12] There is a plethora of literature describing the motor control changes that remain after injury.[15-19] For example, loading asymmetry remains even 2 years after ACL reconstruction[20] and predicts second ACL tear.[5] Thus, while it is tempting to consider a previous injury as a non-modifiable risk factor, training to improve motor control after injury may decrease the risk of future injuries.

The ankle and low back pain (LBP) literature provide substantial evidence documenting underlying motor control changes that occur after injury.[15-19] These studies provide insight for the necessity of proper motor control–oriented testing. For example, in individuals with chronic ankle instability, significant muscle activation latency differences occur in the hip, knee, and ankle muscles in response to a simple inversion perturbation or in transition from double- to single-limb stance.[15,18] These motor control changes can be identified through simple tests such as the Star Excursion Balance Test.[21-24] Individuals with chronic ankle instability do not reach as far and use different strategies at the hip and knee (*e.g.*, less hip and knee range of motion). Motor control changes also occur after LBP in athletes even when the pain has resolved. Cholewicki et al.[16,17] showed that athletes with a history of LBP demonstrated altered activation in outer core muscles (*e.g.*, external obliques, rectus abdominis, erector spinae) even when they were pain-free at the time they were tested and this altered control increased re-injury risk.[16,17] Further, in 277 collegiate athletes who were followed for more than 3 years, poor trunk proprioception, trunk displacements in response to sudden unloading, and a history of LBP predicted knee ligament injury with 91% sensitivity and 68% specificity.[17]

Given the potential for motor control changes after an injury and the increased risk of re-injury to the same or even anatomically remote region, physical therapists must identify residual motor control deficits and address these in physical therapy discharge criteria and return-to-sport criteria. It is imperative that physical therapists screen for all modifiable risk factors that may increase patients' risk of future injury prior to discharge from physical therapy, especially after ACL reconstruction.

Physical Therapy Patient/Client Management

The current patient's history of ankle sprain and LBP may have been risk factors for her grade III ACL tear. During the initial evaluation, the physical therapist should begin to delineate return-to-sport testing and therapy discharge criteria and communicate this plan of care to the patient. By thoroughly explaining the goals for return-to-sport and the specific discharge criteria at the beginning and throughout the rehabilitation process, both therapist and patient are "on the same page" which may minimize future potential conflict if the patient feels "ready to go" when testing reveals that modifiable risk factors remain.

Examination, Evaluation, and Diagnosis

Each test performed in the rehabilitation setting should be reliable, modifiable, have discriminant validity (*i.e.*, distinguish between those with and without the disorder), and be predictive of the outcome desired. For each patient, the chosen tests should be able to predict who returns to sport (based on normative data) and identify who is at increased risk of injury.

Three key concepts need to be considered for return-to-sport and discharge testing. First, each test should be clinically feasible. While there is some research supporting the results from complex, time-consuming biomechanical testing (*e.g.*, assessment of drop jump landing using a 3-dimensional motion capture system) relating to injury risk,[25] most clinicians do not have access to expensive equipment or the patient cannot afford the associated time or expense. However, it should be noted that there are times (*e.g.*, after a second ACL reconstruction or history of multiple injuries in an athlete returning to high-level sport) that a thorough biomechanical assessment is warranted and extremely useful.[26] Second, each test within the battery needs to be performed in a hierarchical fashion. Therapists may assume (often unconsciously) that if an athlete can hop, cut, and/or run well, then she possesses normal ROM, strength, fundamental movement patterns, and balance. If there are identifiable impairments in movement or balance at lower

Table 17-1 CHECKLIST OF DOMAINS TO INCLUDE IN RETURN-TO-SPORT TESTING
Movement
Pain
Strength and range of motion[a]
Coordination
Balance
Neuromuscular control
Power
Sport-specific movements
Self-report measures (*e.g.*, International Knee Documentation Committee, Lower Extremity Functional Scale, etc.)

[a]This domain was not included in Haines et al.,[27] but is important for risk of future dysfunction.

levels of function, there is little need to administer tests of higher levels of function. In addition, an athlete is placed at risk of injury during higher-level testing if lower-level tests are not performed that could identify that she is not ready for higher-level testing. A failure to systematically and hierarchically conduct testing can inadvertently return an athlete to sport with modifiable risk factors for future injury or re-injury. Because athletes who have been previously injured are more likely to be injured again and since motor control changes frequently remain after injury, it is necessary that athletes' test results are close to normal prior to discharge.[15-19] The minimum criterion for discharge from physical therapy should be the achievement of test scores comparable to an individual who does not possess risk factors for injury. For example, it is common for researchers (and those who interpret the research) to compare an athlete's return-to-sport LSI to normative criteria. While this allows comparison of the injured athlete to a general athletic population, it does not provide information regarding the particular athlete's risk of re-injury or whether her long-term participation in the sport may be compromised. Thus, physical therapists need to look at how healthy subjects (*e.g.*, uninjured athletes) perform on each test.

While it is clear that the test should be reliable, valid, and predict return to sport as well as re-injury, it should also measure the domain of function the therapist is interested in assessing. Using a Delphi study method, Haines et al.[27] created a checklist of domains that an expert panel felt were important to include in return-to-sport testing. Table 17-1 presents the domains that experts have suggested testing should include.

Plan of Care and Interventions

Within the first few therapy sessions, the physical therapist should provide a clear list of physical therapy discharge and return-to-sport requirements. This strategy can improve patient compliance with the rehabilitation program, provide goals for the patient and therapist, and allow the sports medicine team to work toward the same short- and long-term goals. Further, it can reduce debate that can occur in the "heat of the battle" when the return-to-sport decision is made.

Throughout the physical therapy episode of care, the physical therapist conducts traditional and functional tests to assess the patient's ability to progress from one stage to the next and to assess readiness to return to sport. While Case 16 presented a rehabilitation program for an athlete with a reconstructed ACL, the current case focuses on appropriate tests and measures as the athlete is preparing to return to sport and minimum test scores for the postoperative athlete with a bone-patellar tendon-bone ACL-reconstructed knee.

For some physical therapists, it has been common clinical practice to establish knee ROM goals of 0° or even 5° of hyperextension post-ACL reconstruction. However, researchers have found that the key component to patient satisfaction and to return to higher-level functional tasks is *symmetrical* hyperextension and full flexion ROM after ACL reconstruction.[28] In an average follow-up of 5 years after ACL reconstruction, researchers found an association between loss of knee ROM and osteoarthritic changes on radiographs.[28] Thus, full and symmetrical knee ROM would be prudent to include in the return-to-sport and discharge criteria.

Once ROM is examined, the physical therapist should test strength. In examining isokinetic strength, peak knee extensor torque: body weight ratio should be 90%.[29] These researchers concluded this is a characteristic of the athletes who return to sport, not necessarily those who have removed any modifiable risk factors for injury. Because strength ratio asymmetry is a risk factor for injury,[30] it would be prudent to expect 95% or greater LSI prior to discharge from rehabilitation.

Because motor control changes occur after injury, the physical therapist must attempt to identify those changes through clinical movement testing. However, clinical movement testing can be difficult to perform in a reliable manner. One option to help quantify movement testing is the Functional Movement Screen (discussed in detail in Case 23). The **Functional Movement Screen** has been found to be reliable,[31-34] modifiable,[35] and predictive of injury in professional football players,[36] marine officer candidates,[37] female collegiate athletes,[38] and firefighters.[39]

The next higher-level testing is dynamic balance testing, which can be accomplished with the Star Excursion/Y Balance Test. In a systematic review of the **Star Excursion Balance Test (SEBT) and Y Balance Test** (a testing protocol designed to improve the reliability and ease of administration of the SEBT), the authors concluded that it is a reliable and modifiable test of dynamic balance that can identify balance deficits after injury and predict injury risk.[40] While numerous studies have indicated that the SEBT/YBT can identify deficits after ankle injury, 2 studies have examined individuals' performance after ACL tear and at return to sport after ACL reconstruction.[22,23] Even at return to sport, performance on the SEBT was impaired and concurrent biomechanical analysis demonstrated kinematic abnormalities.[22,23] Thus, the SEBT/YBT is an excellent, clinically based tool that can be used to demonstrate functional symmetry after ACL reconstruction. Using the SEBT/YBT, Plisky et al.[41] and Lehr et al.[42] found that asymmetries of greater than 4 cm in the anterior reach direction and composite score less than the age, sex, and sport risk cut-off increased the risk of lower extremity injury in high school and collegiate athletes. In a randomized controlled trial, Steffen et al.[43] found that if the SEBT is improved in soccer players using the FIFA 11+ injury prevention program, injury risk is reduced.

While it is clinically important to use double-limb hopping as part of the progression in rehabilitation, it may be unnecessary for return-to-sport and discharge testing. In a study by Myer et al.,[44] double-limb activities did *not* identify the unilateral deficits found after ACL reconstruction. **Unilateral hop tests** can identify the deficits that remain after ACL reconstruction. The 4 commonly used unilateral hop tests include the single-leg hop for distance, 6-m timed hop, triple hop, and triple crossover hop; these unilateral hop tests are reliable, valid, clinically feasible, and modifiable.[44-46] For hop testing, the most common return-to-sport criterion is 85% to 90% LSI.[7,45,46] Two studies have found that healthy subjects had an average LSI for the 4 hop tests of 100%, whereas those athletes who returned to sport scored on average around 90% LSI.[45,46] Thus, while 90% LSI may identify those who have successfully returned to sport in the short term, it does not appear to indicate that motor control has been normalized in the involved limb or that these athletes will successfully remain in their sport in the long term. Another observation from the research is that at 6 months post-ACL reconstruction, the participants' average LSI was 88.5% and their average Lower Extremity Functional Scale (LEFS) score was 69.3.[45,46] To score 69.3 on the LEFS, the athlete would likely report "moderate difficulty" with one or more of the following activities: "Your usual hobbies, recreational or sporting activities"; "Running on even ground"; "Running on uneven ground"; "Making sharp turns while running fast"; and "Hopping." From a face validity perspective, the physical therapist should consider whether it seems appropriate for a patient to return to sport if she reported this much difficulty with these activities. While the initial return-to-sport criterion might be as low as an LSI of 90%, it is this author's opinion that 97% to 100% LSI should be the recommended discharge criterion to help minimize the risk of future injury and potential long-term disability.

The next level of testing is examination of landing mechanics with jumping. Landing in a valgus collapse position has been reported as a risk factor for ACL tear[23] as well as re-tear.[5] These studies were performed in a biomechanics laboratory with equipment that is not universally available in patient care. Two popular methods for clinically assessing the high-risk landing positions are the **tuck jump assessment** (see Case 15) **and the Landing Error Scoring System**. While the reliability, clinical feasibility, and predictive validity of these measures are uncertain,[46] it is apparent from the biomechanical literature that some form of clinical assessment of landing position is warranted once the patient has passed the lower-level tests (*e.g.*, ROM, strength, fundamental movement, balance, etc.). In some cases (*e.g.*, after second ACL tear, returning quickly to high-level athletics), full biomechanical assessment may be warranted.

Because injury risk is multifactorial, the current trend in injury prevention is to categorize athletes using multiple risk factors. As discussed in the preparticipation case study (see Case 23), multiple tests and injury history can be used to place an athlete in an injury risk category.[42] In Lehr et al.,[42] the athletes provided an injury history report and were tested on the Y Balance Test Lower Quarter (YBT-LQ) and Functional Movement Screen. Results of the tests and the subjects' injury history were placed into the injury risk algorithm and each athlete was categorized according to future injury risk. If athletes were in the moderate or substantial risk category, they were 3.4 times (95% confidence interval, 2.0-6.0) more likely to get injured over the course of their season compared to those who were in the lower-risk categories. In a subsequent analysis, there were 4 non-contact ACL injuries: 3 were in the high-risk group (moderate and substantial risk categories), and 1 was in the slightly increased risk group.[42] This algorithm of utilizing multiple risk factors to get a comprehensive risk profile should be applied to the athlete prior to return to sport.

Whatever the sport or activity, the athlete must be able to complete graded sport-specific progressions without pain or compensation. In this case, a basketball player needs to be able to jog, sprint, cut, jump, and maneuver on the court in order to compete effectively. Simulated drills should be performed in a progressive manner (straight ahead jogging prior to cutting) and at progressive speed (50%, 75%, 90%, to 100% of maximum) prior to return to practice. Also, the therapist should consider that the athlete might be able to participate in conditioning prior to full participation in practice and match play.

It is important to consider the patient's values regarding returning to sport. While it is ideal to have all the described criteria met prior to return to sport, the patient's specific circumstances and values need to be considered. For example, if the patient is a high school senior and needs to return to sport in order to be eligible for collegiate scholarship athletics, the criteria of 97% LSI might be lowered to 90%. However, the physical therapist must inform the patient and her parent or guardian of the risks of returning to sport prior to achieving the criteria and that rehabilitation should continue until the modifiable risk factors for injury have normalized.

Evidence-Based Clinical Recommendations

SORT: Strength of Recommendation Taxonomy
A: Consistent, good-quality patient-oriented evidence
B: Inconsistent or limited-quality patient-oriented evidence
C: Consensus, disease-oriented evidence, usual practice, expert opinion, or case series

1. The Functional Movement Screen is a reliable and clinically feasible assessment that should be performed prior to return to sport because it can predict injury in certain populations. **Grade B**
2. The Star Excursion Balance Test and Y Balance Test (SEBT/YBT) are reliable and clinically feasible tests that can identify dynamic balance deficits and determine functional symmetry after ACL reconstruction and may predict future injury risk. **Grade A**
3. Hop testing is reliable and clinically feasible and can differentiate between athletes who have had ACL reconstruction and those who have not. **Grade B**
4. Drop jump landing and tuck jumps assess high-risk landing positions such as knee valgus collapse that may be associated with initial ACL tear and can also be used to predict a second ACL tear. **Grade C**

COMPREHENSION QUESTIONS

17.1 For the athlete preparing to return to sport after unilateral ACL reconstruction, which of the following would be considered an appropriate order of testing considering level of demand and load on the knee?

A. Functional Movement Screen, single-leg hop testing, double-leg drop jump landing

B. Star Excursion Balance Test, ROM, strength

C. Functional Movement Screen, Star Excursion Balance Test, single-leg hop testing

D. ROM, strength, sport-specific testing, Functional Movement Screen

17.2 Which of the following is considered a passing criterion for return to sport?

A. 89% LSI in triple crossover hop

B. 5-cm anterior asymmetry in Star Excursion Balance Test

C. 85% LSI in strength testing

D. Composite Star Excursion Balance Test Score or Y Balance Test score greater than age, sex, and sport-specific risk cut point

ANSWERS

17.1 **C.** Return-to-sport testing should be performed in order of complexity/demand from lowest level to highest level. From a body weight impact perspective, ROM and strength are the lowest, followed by the Functional Movement Screen and SEBT, and finally hop and sport-specific testing.

17.2 **D.** Appropriate return-to-sport criteria are LSI for hop testing at least greater than 90% and preferably greater than 97%, strength LSI greater than 90%, no greater than a 4-cm left/right Star Excursion Balance Test or Y Balance Test asymmetry, and composite Star Excursion Balance Test Score or Y Balance Test score greater than age, sex, and sport-specific risk cut point.

REFERENCES

1. Bahr R, Holme I. Risk factors for sports injuries—a methodological approach. *Br J Sports Med.* 2003;37:384-392.

2. Shumway-Cook A, Woollacott M. *Motor Control: Translating Research into Clinical Practice.* Philadelphia, PA: Wolters Kluwer Health/Lippincott Williams & Wilkins; 2012.

3. Ardern CL, Webster KE, Taylor NF, Feller JA. Return to sport following anterior cruciate ligament reconstruction surgery: a systematic review and meta-analysis of the state of play. *Br J Sports Med.* 2011;45:596-606.

4. Ardern CL, Taylor NF, Feller JA, Webster KE. Return-to-sport outcomes at 2 to 7 years after anterior cruciate ligament reconstruction surgery. *Am J Sports Med.* 2012;40:41-48.

5. Paterno MV, Rauh MJ, Schmitt LC, Ford KR, Hewett TE. Incidence of contralateral and ipsilateral anterior cruciate ligament (ACL) injury after primary ACL reconstruction and return to sport. *Clin J Sport Med*. 2012;22:116-121.
6. Ververidis A, Verettas D, Kazakos K, Xarchas K, Drosos G, Psillakis I. Anterior cruciate ligament reconstruction: outcome using a patellar tendon bone (PTB) autograft (one bone block technique). *Arch Orthop Trauma Surg*. 2009;129:323-331.
7. Barber-Westin SD, Noyes FR. Factors used to determine return to unrestricted sports activities after anterior cruciate ligament reconstruction. *Arthroscopy*. 2011;27:1697-1705.
8. Narducci E, Waltz A, Gorski K, Leppla L, Donaldson M. The clinical utility of functional performance tests within one-year post-ACL reconstruction: a systematic review. *Int J Sports Phys Ther*. 2011;6:333-342.
9. Petersen W, Zantop T. Return to play following ACL reconstruction: survey among experienced arthroscopic surgeons (AGA instructors). *Arch Orthop Trauma Surg*. 2013;133:969-977.
10. Shultz R, Bido J, Shrier I, Meeuwisse WH, Garza D, Matheson GO. Team clinician variability in return-to-play decisions. *Clin J Sport Med*. 2013;23:456-461.
11. de Visser HM, Reijman M, Heijboer MP, Bos PK. Risk factors of recurrent hamstring injuries: a systematic review. *Br J Sports Med*. 2012;46:124-130.
12. Hagglund M, Walden M, Ekstrand J. Previous injury as a risk factor for injury in elite football: a prospective study over two consecutive seasons. *Br J Sports Med*. 2006;40:767-772.
13. Walden M, Hagglund M, Ekstrand J. High risk of new knee injury in elite footballers with previous anterior cruciate ligament injury. *Br J Sports Med*. 2006;40:158-162.
14. Wright RW, Magnussen RA, Dunn WR, Spindler KP. Ipsilateral graft and contralateral ACL rupture at five years or more following ACL reconstruction: a systematic review. *J Bone Joint Surg Am*. 2011;93:1159-1165.
15. Beckman SM, Buchanan TS. Ankle inversion injury and hypermobility: effect on hip and ankle muscle electromyography onset latency. *Arch Phys Med Rehabil*. 1995;76:1138-1143.
16. Cholewicki J, Greene HS, Polzhofer GK, Galloway MT, Shah RA, Radebold A. Neuromuscular function in athletes following recovery from a recent acute low back injury. *J Orthop Sports Phys Ther*. 2002;32:568-575.
17. Cholewicki J, Silfies SP, Shah RA, et al. Delayed trunk muscle reflex responses increase the risk of low back injuries. *Spine*. 2005;30:2614-2620.
18. Van Deun S, Staes FF, Stappaerts KH, Janssens L, Levin O, Peers KK. Relationship of chronic ankle instability to muscle activation patterns during the transition from double-leg to single-leg stance. *Am J Sports Med*. 2007;35:274-281.
19. Zazulak BT, Hewett TE, Reeves NP, Goldberg B, Cholewicki J. Deficits in neuromuscular control of the trunk predict knee injury risk: a prospective biomechanical-epidemiologic study. *Am J Sports Med*. 2007;35:1123-1130.
20. Paterno MV, Ford KR, Myer GD, Heyl R, Hewett TE. Limb asymmetries in landing and jumping 2 years following anterior cruciate ligament reconstruction. *Clin J Sport Med*. 2007;17:258-262.
21. Aminaka N, Gribble PA. Patellar taping, patellofemoral pain syndrome, lower extremity kinematics, and dynamic postural control. *J Athl Train*. 2008;43:21-28.
22. Delahunt E, Chawke M, Kelleher J, et al. Lower limb kinematics and dynamic postural stability in anterior cruciate ligament-reconstructed female athletes. *J Athl Train*. 2013;48:172-185.
23. Herrington L, Hatcher J, Hatcher A, McNicholas M. A comparison of Star Excursion Balance Test reach distances between ACL deficient patients and asymptomatic controls. *Knee*. 2009;16:149-152.
24. Hertel J, Braham RA, Hale SA, Olmsted-Kramer LC. Simplifying the star excursion balance test: analyses of subjects with and without chronic ankle instability. *J Orthop Sports Phys Ther*. 2006;36:131-137.
25. Hewett TE, Myer GD, Ford KR, et al. Biomechanical measures of neuromuscular control and valgus loading of the knee predict anterior cruciate ligament injury risk in female athletes: a prospective study. *Am J Sports Med*. 2005;33:492-501.

26. Paterno MV, Schmitt LC, Ford KR, et al. Biomechanical measures during landing and postural stability predict second anterior cruciate ligament injury after anterior cruciate ligament reconstruction and return to sport. *Am J Sports Med.* 2010;38:1968-1978.
27. Haines S, Baker T, Donaldson M. Development of a physical performance assessment checklist for athletes who sustained a lower extremity injury in preparation for return to sport: a delphi study. *Int J Sports Phys Ther.* 2013;8:44-53.
28. Shelbourne KD, Urch SE, Gray T, Freeman H. Loss of normal knee motion after anterior cruciate ligament reconstruction is associated with radiographic arthritic changes after surgery. *Am J Sports Med.* 2012;40:108-113.
29. Schmitt LC, Paterno MV, Hewett TE. The impact of quadriceps femoris strength asymmetry on functional performance at return to sport following anterior cruciate ligament reconstruction. *J Orthop Sports Phys Ther.* 2012;42:750-759.
30. Soderman K, Alfredson H, Pietila T, Werner S. Risk factors for leg injuries in female soccer players: a prospective investigation during one out-door season. *Knee Surg Sports Traumatol Arthrosc.* 2001;9:313-321.
31. Minick KI, Kiesel KB, Burton L, Taylor A, Plisky P, Butler RJ. Interrater reliability of the functional movement screen. *J Strength Cond Res.* 2010;24:479-486.
32. Schneiders AG, Davidsson A, Horman E, Sullivan SJ. Functional movement screen normative values in a young, active population. *Int J Sports Phys Ther.* 2011;6:75-82.
33. Teyhen DS, Shaffer SW, Lorenson CL, et al. The Functional Movement Screen: a reliability study. *J Orthop Sports Phys Ther.* 2012;42:530-540.
34. Frohm A, Heijne A, Kowalski J, Svensson P, Myklebust G. A nine-test screening battery for athletes: a reliability study. *Scand J Med Sci Sports.* 2012;22:306-315.
35. Kiesel K, Plisky P, Butler R. Functional movement test scores improve following a standardized off-season intervention program in professional football players. *Scand J Med Sci Sports.* 2011;21:287-292.
36. Kiesel K, Plisky PJ, Voight ML. Can serious injury in professional football be predicted by a preseason Functional Movement Screen? *N Am J Sports Phys Ther.* 2007;2:147-158.
37. O'Connor FG, Deuster PA, Davis J, Pappas CG, Knapik JJ. Functional movement screening: predicting injuries in officer candidates. *Med Sci Sports Exerc.* 2011;43:2224-2230.
38. Chorba RS, Chorba DJ, Bouillon LE, Overmyer CA, Landis JA. Use of a functional movement screening tool to determine injury risk in female collegiate athletes. *N Am J Sports Phys Ther.* 2010;5:47-54.
39. Butler RJ, Contreras M, Burton LC, Plisky PJ, Goode A, Kiesel K. Modifiable risk factors predict injuries in firefighters during training academies. *Work.* 2013;46:11-17.
40. Gribble PA, Hertel J, Plisky P. Using the Star Excursion Balance Test to assess dynamic postural-control deficits and outcomes in lower extremity injury: a literature and systematic review. *J Athl Train.* 2012;47:339-357.
41. Plisky PJ, Rauh MJ, Kaminski TW, Underwood FB. Star Excursion Balance Test as a predictor of lower extremity injury in high school basketball players. *J Orthop Sports Phys Ther.* 2006;36:911-919.
42. Lehr ME, Plisky PJ, Butler RJ, Fink ML, Kiesel KB, Underwood FB. Field-expedient screening and injury risk algorithm categories as predictors of noncontact lower extremity injury. *Scand J Med Sci Sports.* 2013;23(4):e225-e232.
43. Steffen K, Emery CA, Romiti M, et al. High adherence to a neuromuscular injury prevention programme (FIFA 11+) improves functional balance and reduces injury risk in Canadian youth female football players: a cluster randomised trial. *Br J Sports Med.* 2013;47:794-802.
44. Myer GD, Schmitt LC, Brent JL, et al. Utilization of modified NFL combine testing to identify functional deficits in athletes following ACL reconstruction. *J Orthop Sports Phys Ther.* 2011;41:377-387.
45. Munro AG, Herrington LC. Between-session reliability of four hop tests and the agility T-test. *J Strength Cond Res.* 2011;25:1470-1477.
46. Reid A, Birmingham TB, Stratford PW, Alcock GK, Giffin JR. Hop testing provides a reliable and valid outcome measure during rehabilitation after anterior cruciate ligament reconstruction. *Phys Ther.* 2007;87:337-349.

Return to Rugby Following Posterior Cruciate Ligament Reconstruction

Kaan Celebi
Airelle O. Hunter-Giordano

CASE 18

A 28-year-old rugby player was examined by the physical therapist following an injury to his right knee. He was playing Sevens Rugby when he was tackled and fell on another player with his knee bent underneath him. The athlete reported instant pain and heard a "pop" at the time of the injury with swelling that slowly developed in his knee that night. The athlete's previous health history is unremarkable. When evaluated by the physical therapist 3 days after the injury, he presented with an antalgic gait pattern with his knee in a slightly flexed position. He reported feeling unsteady when walking and anterior knee pain with stair descent. The knee examination revealed a 3+ joint effusion, knee extension range of motion (ROM) limited by pain, a positive sag sign, positive posterior drawer and quadriceps activation tests, and a negative Lachman test. The player did not have any imaging performed because he was evaluated by the physical therapist as a direct access client. Based on the history and physical examination findings, the physical therapist was concerned about the possibility of a posterior cruciate ligament (PCL) tear. The therapist referred the patient to an orthopaedic surgeon and a PCL tear was confirmed through diagnostic imaging. The athlete completed a 6-session prehabilitation program prior to surgery. The goals of this program were aimed at restoring full active and passive knee ROM, decreasing effusion, and improving quadriceps strength and activation. Interventions to resolve impairments included passive and active ROM activities, retrograde message, icing with elevation, neuromuscular electrical stimulation (NMES), straight leg raises, and knee extensions. The patient had PCL reconstruction 1 month after the initial injury and initiated physical therapy 5 days after surgery.

- What examination signs may be associated with the diagnosis of a PCL injury?
- What are the examination priorities?
- Describe a physical therapy plan of care after PCL reconstruction.
- What is his rehabilitation prognosis?
- What is his prognosis regarding returning to rugby?

KEY DEFINITIONS

PEEL-OFF INJURY: A tearing away of the posterior cruciate ligament (PCL) from the tibia; "peel-off" acknowledges that the ligament literally pulls clean away from the bone.

POSTERIOR CRUCIATE LIGAMENT (PCL): Knee ligament that serves as the primary restraint to posterior tibial translation and the secondary restraint to external rotation of the tibia on the femur; the PCL proximally attaches to the medial aspect of the femoral intercondylar notch and distally attaches onto the superior aspect of the posterior tibia.

POSTEROLATERAL CORNER: Includes the lateral head of the gastrocnemius, popliteus tendon, popliteofibular ligament, lateral collateral ligament, and the arcuate ligament; these structures serve as the primary restraint to both varus and external rotation forces of the tibia on the femur.

QUADRICEPS INDEX (QI): Volitional quadriceps strength comparison between limbs; measured with an isokinetic dynamometer during a series of isolated isometric contractions

SEVENS RUGBY: Also known as Rugby Sevens; variant of rugby union in which matches are longer and teams are made up of 7 players, instead of the usual 15

TIBIOFEMORAL JOINT: Synovial hinge joint between tibia and femur

Objectives

1. Describe the anatomy and biomechanics of the PCL and the common mechanisms of injury.
2. Identify appropriate diagnostic imaging that should be completed to rule in or rule out intracapsular injuries at the knee (*e.g.*, PCL lesion).
3. Describe the most appropriate physical therapy interventions for the athlete following PCL reconstruction.
4. Determine the prognosis for an athlete returning to sport following reconstructive surgery of the PCL.

Physical Therapy Considerations

PT considerations during postoperative management of the athlete with a surgically reconstructed PCL:

- ▶ **General physical therapy plan of care/goals:** Decrease pain; increase active and passive knee ROM; increase lower extremity strength; follow orthopaedic surgeon's postoperative rehabilitation guidelines; meet clinical milestones throughout the guidelines (*e.g.*, full active knee extension by second postoperative week)
- ▶ **Physical therapy interventions:** Patient education regarding functional anatomy, injury pathomechanics, and surgical intervention; modalities to decrease pain

and swelling; manual therapy to improve joint mobility; therapeutic exercises to restore ROM, improve cardiovascular fitness, and increase lower extremity strength

- **Precautions during physical therapy:** No posterior force to the tibia during early phases of stretching into knee flexion; physical therapist should establish rehabilitation guidelines with the surgeon and follow throughout the program
- **Complication interfering with physical therapy:** Operative complications including vascular or nerve injury, infection, compartment syndrome, tourniquet and wound complications, deep vein thrombosis, graft failure, knee flexion ROM loss[1]

Understanding the Health Condition

PCL injuries account for 3% to 37% of all ligamentous knee injuries.[2,3] The 2 most common causes of PCL injuries are motor vehicle accidents (dashboard injuries) and contact injuries during sport.[4] The most common mechanism of PCL injury in athletic events is a fall on a flexed knee with the ankle in plantar flexion. A PCL injury can also occur with a sudden, violent hyperextension of the knee joint.[5] Because the majority of PCL injuries result from contact injuries, predisposing risk factors have not been characterized. This contrasts with the well-recognized risk factors for the more commonly injured anterior cruciate ligament (see Case 15). Therefore, no known factors could be addressed with a PCL injury prevention program.

An isolated PCL injury can be classified into 3 types based on the intracapsular structures that are damaged (isolated vs. combined) and the degree of instability.[6] Tibiofemoral laxity is defined by the amount of translation between the tibial plateau and femoral condyle. In a grade I PCL injury, the ligament is stretched, laxity is less than 5 mm, and the tibial plateau is 5 to 10 mm anterior to the femoral condyle. With a grade II injury, the PCL is torn, but the meniscofemoral ligaments are intact. Ligament laxity is between 5 and 10 mm, and the tibial plateau is 0 to 5 mm anterior to the femoral condyle. Grade III PCL injuries involve tearing of the PCL and the meniscofemoral ligaments. Laxity exceeds 10 mm, and this injury results in the tibial plateau being even with the femoral condyle.

Physical Therapy Patient/Client Management

If there is a concern for a PCL tear based on patient history and physical examination findings, the physical therapist should educate the patient on functional anatomy and injury pathomechanics. The physical therapist should provide a knee immobilizer and axillary crutches, train the patient in a protected gait pattern on the affected lower extremity, and refer the patient to an orthopaedic surgeon for further evaluation. Therapists should be aware that a PCL reconstruction is a technically difficult procedure, and the majority of these surgeries are performed by a limited number of surgeons. Therefore, optimal referral should be to a surgeon who specializes in PCL reconstructions. If the diagnosis of PCL rupture is confirmed, then appropriate nonoperative and/or surgical options can be considered in a timely manner. The primary goal following surgery is to return to pain-free activity as quickly and safely as possible in a manner that follows postoperative guidelines.

Examination, Evaluation, and Diagnosis

Examination begins with a thorough subjective report, including history of trauma and a review of the specific mechanism of injury (MOI). The MOI provides key information that guides the examination. After an acute PCL injury, most patients complain of pain in the retropatellar area and medial compartment of the knee, effusion, and an inability to bear weight.[6-8] Associated functional complaints may include difficulty ambulating (due to an inability to extend the knee during stance) and an apprehension descending stairs secondary to unsteadiness or a feeling of sliding of the joint.[6-9] However, it is important to note that this feeling of unsteadiness differs from "giving way" or buckling episodes that are hallmark complaints of a patient with an injury to the anterior cruciate ligament. Giving way episodes are rarely seen with an isolated PCL rupture.[6] Thus, when instability is a major complaint, other injuries such as combined ligament instabilities may be present.

The physical examination should include observation of the knee joint, gait assessment, ROM testing, and special tests. The examiner should observe for any abrasions and/or ecchymosis over the anterior tibia and effusion within the joint. Compensatory gait patterns such as a flexed knee gait should be identified.[6,10] The special test with the **best overall diagnostic accuracy for determining PCL deficiency is the posterior drawer test** (Table 18-1).[6,10,11] Two other special tests that may be performed to identify PCL lesions are the quadriceps activation test and the reverse pivot shift.[6,12-14] In addition to PCL testing, a comprehensive physical examination for the knee should include special tests to determine the integrity of the other main ligamentous structures and corners of the knee. If the patient has an injury to the posterolateral corner (PLC), additional surgery may be necessary to stabilize this area. The hallmark test for the PLC (and the PCL) is the prone dial test.[6] In addition, the therapist should assess for meniscal and patellofemoral pathology.

Diagnostic imaging to rule out or confirm any ligamentous injury may be ordered by a physician or primary care provider. The Ottawa Knee Rules were developed and validated to assist clinicians in determining when to order radiographs for individuals with acute knee injury.[16,17] According to these criteria, a knee radiograph series is required for any patient with acute knee injury who presents with any of the following 5 criteria: patient is 55 years or older, inability to flex the knee to 90°, tenderness at the fibular head, isolated tenderness of the patella, and inability to bear weight both immediately after injury as well as in the emergency department for 4 steps, regardless of limping. Although traditional radiographs are important to rule out any bony lesions, magnetic resonance imaging (MRI) is the gold standard for imaging ligamentous injury.[16,17]

With respect to the diagnosis of cruciate, collateral, or anatomic quadrant lesions of the knee, it should be noted that examination by well-trained clinicians

Table 18-1 SPECIAL TESTS FOR POSTERIOR CRUCIATE LIGAMENT INJURIES

Special Test	Description	Diagnostic Accuracy[15]
Posterior drawer test (Fig. 18-1)	The patient is supine with involved knee flexed to 90° and hip flexed to 45°. The therapist is seated on the foot of the involved limb and applies the thenar eminences of both hands on the anterior aspect of the proximal tibia. The therapist applies a posteriorly directed force to displace the tibia. Increased posterior tibial translation with a soft end point compared to the uninvolved side constitutes a positive test, indicating disruption of PCL.	Sensitivity: 90% Specificity: 99%
Quadriceps activation test (or, active quadriceps test)	The patient is supine with involved knee flexed to 90° and foot flat on the table. The therapist holds patient's foot flat against the table and asks the patient to try to slide his foot along the table, while the therapist provides manual resistance against the anterior tibia (causing isometric contraction of quadriceps that produces anterior tibial translation). Test is positive if proximal tibia shifts anteriorly greater than 2 mm.	Sensitivity: 54%-98% Specificity: 97%-100%
Reverse pivot shift	The patient is supine on treatment table with hip flexed 20°-30°. While grasping the tibia laterally and the ankle medially, the therapist flexes the knee 70°-80° while externally rotating the lower leg, which may cause a posterior subluxation of the lateral tibial plateau. Next, the therapist extends the knee while imparting a valgus stress to the knee. Test is positive if the lateral tibial tubercle translates anteriorly, reducing the posterior subluxation.	Sensitivity: 26% Specificity: 59%
Prone dial test (Fig. 18-2)	The patient may be tested in supine or prone. The therapist tests the amount of tibial ER at 30° and 90° of knee flexion. Increased tibial ER at 30° and *not* at 90° indicates isolated posterolateral corner injury. Increased tibial ER at *both* 30° and 90° indicates PLC and PCL injuries.	Sensitivity: 79% Specificity: 100%

Abbreviations: ER, external rotation; PCL, posterior cruciate ligament; PLC, posterolateral corner.

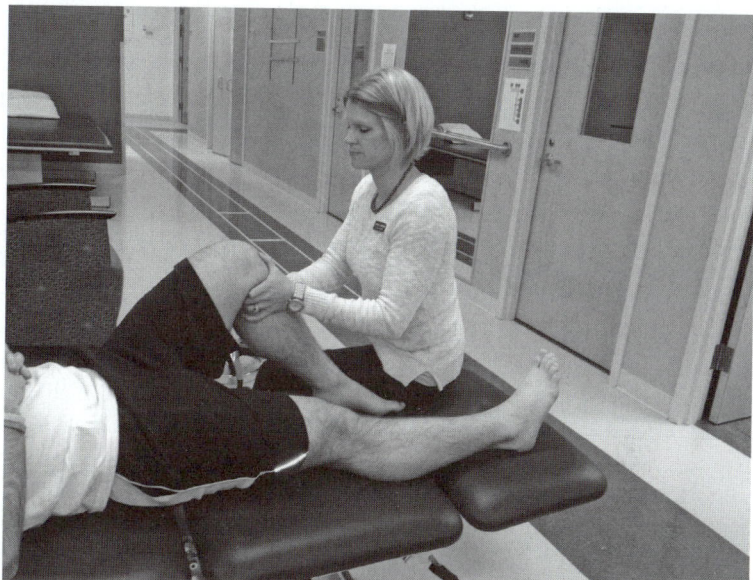

Figure 18-1. Posterior drawer test.

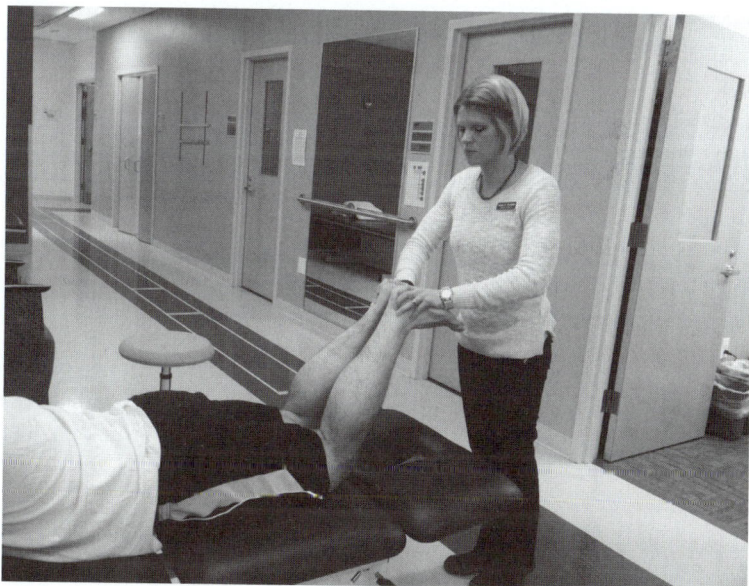

Figure 18-2. Prone dial test.

(*e.g.*, physicians, physical therapists) has been shown to be as accurate as MRI.[18-20] Thus, when considering the recommendation of pursuing further imaging, MRI may be reserved for combined injuries or more complicated cases and for assisting an orthopaedic surgeon in preoperative planning and predicting prognosis.[19,20]

Plan of Care and Interventions

Once a diagnosis is made, treatment is based on the site of the injury and the degree of instability. Immediate surgery is indicated if the PCL lesion is located at its attachment sites, causing either a bony avulsion of the tibial insertion or a "peel off" injury from the femoral origin.[6,21]

If the degree of PCL laxity is minimal (grade I or II intrasubstance tear), the best treatment choice is nonoperative conservative management.[6] If a grade III lesion is present, the best management option tends to be more controversial. If not repaired or reconstructed, there is a low to medium likelihood that these patients will continue to develop laxity that may increase forces across the knee, particularly on the medial and anterior articular surfaces, leading to earlier degenerative changes.[22,23] Early surgery may be the best preventative measure to inhibit the development of osteoarthritis after PCL tear; individuals with acutely reconstructed PCL injuries have demonstrated better results than those with chronic PCL injuries.[22] On the other hand, PCL reconstruction for an isolated injury has only been recommended for those with grade III lesions who have had a full course of physical therapy yet continue to remain symptomatic.[24]

Following an isolated PCL reconstruction, the patient's knee is locked at 0° of extension in a **protective brace or knee immobilizer and advised to maintain partial weightbearing during gait.** Full knee extension prevents the effects of gravity and posterior hamstring forces from adding excessive stresses to the newly reconstructed PCL. The athlete remains in the locked brace (Fig. 18-3) for up to 6 weeks and is slowly weaned out of the brace as he progressively tolerates more weight through the extremity.[6,25] During the first week, the patient may slowly increase the number of hours per day that he ambulates without the brace, gradually increasing the number of hours until he is brace-free. In order to discontinue the use of the knee immobilizer, the patient must demonstrate a straight leg raise (SLR) without a quad lag (*i.e.*, he must be able to maintain the knee extended during an isometric quadriceps contraction).[26] As the patient's strength improves and he returns to higher-level activities, the surgeon may recommend that he wear a different lower-profile functional brace. Once patients attain a **QI of 80%,**[27] **they can stop wearing the functional brace for activities of daily living (ADLs) and may only have to wear it during higher-level activities.** The QI is often measured with maximal volitional isometric contraction (MVIC) using an isometric dynamometer or isokinetic testing device (Fig. 18-4).

Throughout the postoperative phases of rehabilitation, there are specific exercises that are not included because of the potential shearing forces and injury to the graft. Two examples of exercises that are contraindicated early in therapy are the open kinetic chain hamstring curl (not allowed until the 12th week) and closed kinetic chain exercises (not allowed until the 6th week). These exercises are contraindicated early in the rehabilitation process because hamstring activation causes a posterior shearing force of the tibia on the femur. During the first postoperative week, the patient begins isometric quadriceps contractions and SLRs while wearing the protective immobilizer brace. The therapist should begin patella mobilizations to restore patella mobility and NMES to

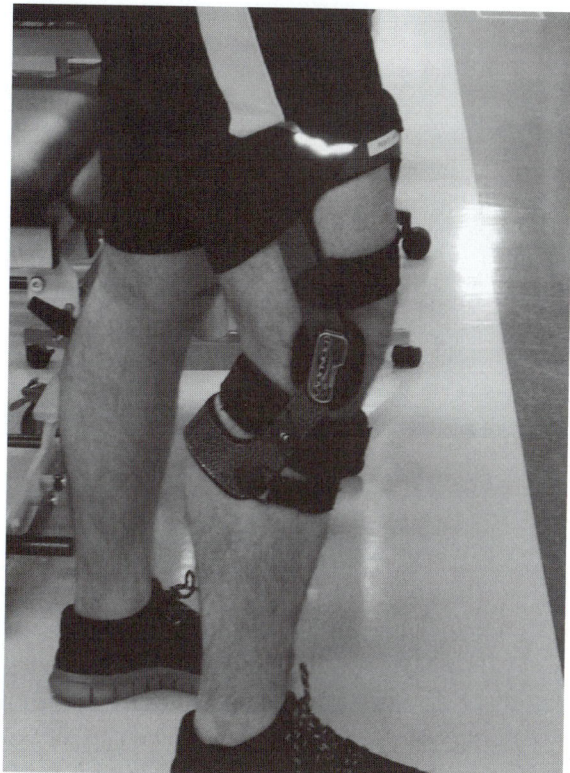

Figure 18-3. Posterior cruciate ligament (PCL) post-surgical brace.

the quadriceps muscle to decrease muscular inhibition and increase quadriceps muscular strength. Optimally, NMES should be performed in 30° of knee flexion, which places the hamstring muscles in a shortened (e.g., relaxed) position. Co-contraction of the hamstrings during NMES is avoided to prevent stressing of the graft.

By the end of the second postoperative week, full active and passive knee extension should be achieved. Open kinetic chain knee extension can be performed from 45° to full extension. When the athlete demonstrates proper quadriceps control, closed chain exercises such as leg presses and mini wall squats (0°-45°) may be slowly initiated. By the third week, active knee flexion should be progressed to achieve 90° to 100°. Passive ROM activities to increase flexion may be performed with the patient in a supine or seated position. The therapist uses one hand on the anterior tibia to help guide flexion, while the other hand remains on the posterior tibia (close to the tibiofemoral joint line) to limit the posterior tibial glide on the femur. Passive flexion motion may also be performed with the patient prone. In this position, gravity helps to limit unwanted posterior shearing of the tibia on the femur. Passive flexion may also begin in the supine or seated position with hand placement supporting the posterior tibia as close to the joint line as possible. The anterior support by the rehab specialist protects from unwanted posterior

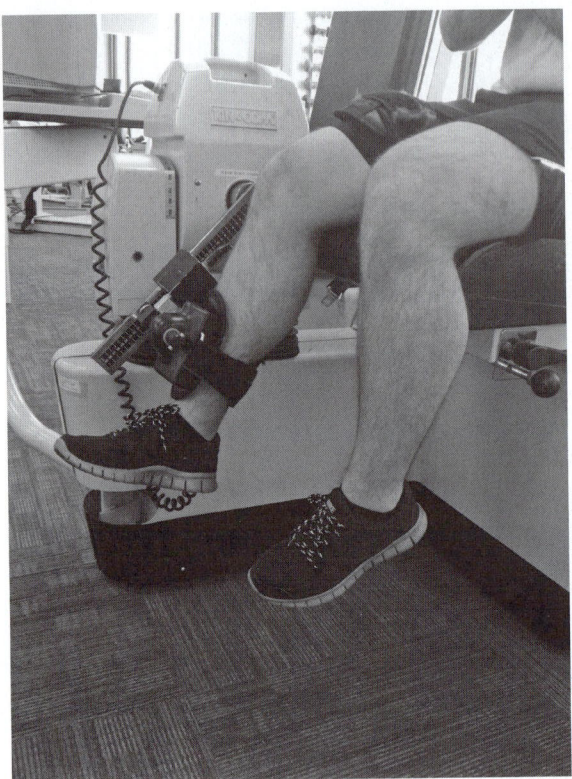

Figure 18-4. Isokinetic testing of the quadriceps to measure maximal volitional isometric contraction (MVIC).

translation to avoid stressing the graft. Passive motion may also be initiated in the prone position, in which gravity would provide the same support to the graft.

By the end of week 10, the goals are pain-free normal gait without crutches, quadriceps strength 80% of the nonsurgical knee, and flexion ROM within 10° of the nonsurgical knee. By the third month of postoperative rehabilitation, a walking program should be initiated. At this time, hamstring exercises against gravity in a 0° to 90° range may also begin.

At 4 months post-surgery, the athlete may begin a running program with a functional brace if he meets the following criteria: symmetrical knee ROM, QI is 90% or greater, and trace (or less) effusion within the joint.[27] By 5 months, a return-to-play progression may begin if the patient has maintained the previously mentioned criteria, has a QI of at least 95% with no other impairments, and has clearance from the surgeon. Table 18-2 outlines the postoperative rehabilitation protocol for PCL reconstruction (an isolated PCL injury with or without PLC injury).[27] The expected number of supervised physical therapy visits ranges from 30 to 44.

When returning the rugby player back to sport, the physical therapist must consider how his PCL injury and reconstruction will impact his position and what he

Table 18-2 POSTOPERATIVE REHABILITATION PROTOCOL FOR PCL RECONSTRUCTION (WITH OR WITHOUT PLC REPAIR/RECONSTRUCTION)

Weeks	Treatment	Milestones
Week 1 1 visit	NMES (see guidelines)[a] Quad sets SLRs Patellar mobilization Home program: patellar mobilizations 30-50 repetitions; quad sets and SLRs 3 sets × 10 repetitions each (3 times per day)	Good quadriceps contraction Superior patellar glide Ambulating PWB with crutches with postoperative orthosis locked
Week 2 2-3 visits (Total visits: 3-4)	Portal/incision mobilization as needed SAQ 30°-0°	Knee ROM: full extension, flexion to 60° SLR without lag (full quadriceps contraction)
Weeks 3-5 2-3 visits/week (Total visits: 9-13)	Therapist-assisted prone knee flexion or 0°-60° Therapist-assisted supine knee flexion (with hand placed behind posterior tibia to limit posterior tibial glide) OKC exercises 60°-0° Stationary bike for ROM (low or no resistance) Gait training: PWB with crutches and no orthosis	Knee flexion to 110° Quad strength >60% of uninvolved side Wean from orthosis Normalize gait with crutches
Weeks 6-10 2-3 visits/week (Total visits: 19-28)	Stationary bike (low or no resistance) Begin CKC exercises, if good quad control (wall sits, wall squats 0°-45°)	Normal gait without crutches Quad strength >80% of uninvolved side
Week 12 2 visits per week to reassess progress	Begin running progression with functional brace (Fig. 18-3) PRE hamstring curls 0°-90° Transfer to fitness facility (if all milestones are met)	Full ROM (compared to uninvolved side) Maintain quadriceps strength ≥95% of the uninvolved side

Week 20
Reassess progress
Total visits 25-44
	Return-to-sport transition
	Proprioceptive, static and dynamic balance, and functional activities:
	  Slow to fast speed
	  Low to high force
	  Controlled to uncontrolled
		Global report >70%
		KOS-ADLS >90%

(Continued)

Table 18-2 POSTOPERATIVE REHABILITATION PROTOCOL FOR PCL RECONSTRUCTION (WITH OR WITHOUT PLC REPAIR/RECONSTRUCTION) (*CONTINUED*)

Weeks	Treatment	Milestones
Precautions: 1. Partial meniscectomy: no modifications required, progress per patient tolerance and protocol 2. Meniscal repair: no modification required, progress per patient tolerance and protocol. Weightbearing in full extension appropriate. 3. Chondroplasty: restricted weightbearing for 4 weeks, no weightbearing exercise for 4 weeks. Consider tibiofemoral-unloading brace to help facilitate earlier participation in functional rehabilitation activities, if limited by pain. 4. MCL injury: restrict motion to sagittal plane until weeks 4-6 to allow healing of MCL 5. ACL injury: follow PCL guidelines	MVIC: Patient is asked to volitionally extend involved leg as hard as possible while knee is maintained isometrically at 30° knee flexion (Fig. 18-4) Side-to-side comparison: involved/uninvolved × 100 = % MVIC	Running progression: 1. Treadmill walking 2. Treadmill walk/run intervals 3. Treadmill running 4. Track: run straights, walk turns 5. Track: run straights and turns 6. Run on road Progress to next level when patient is able to perform activity for 2 miles without increased effusion or pain. Perform no more than 4 times in 1 week and no more frequently than every other day. Do not progress more than 2 levels in a 7-day period.

Abbreviations: ACL, anterior cruciate ligament; CKC, closed kinetic chain; KOS-ADLS, Knee Outcome Survey-Activities of Daily Living Scale; MCL, medial collateral ligament; MVIC, maximal volitional isometric contraction; NMES, neuromuscular electrical stimulation; OKC, open kinetic chain; PCL, posterior cruciate ligament; PRE, progressive resistance exercise; PWB, partial weightbearing; ROM, range of motion; SAQ, short arc quad; SLR, straight leg raise.
[a]Electrodes placed over proximal lateral quadriceps and distal medial quadriceps. (Modify distal electrode placement by not covering superior medial arthroscopy portal or incision until stitches have been removed.) Stimulation parameters: 2500 Hz, 75 bursts, 2 sec ramp, 12 sec on, 50 sec rest, intensity to max tolerable (at least 50% MVIC), 10 contractions per session. Three sessions per week until quadriceps strength MVIC is 80% of uninvolved side. Stimulation performed isometrically at 30° of knee flexion.

needs to do in order to perform at a high level. When athletes return from major reconstructive surgery, earlier restrictions on uncontrolled/forced movements need to be progressed back into their rehabilitation program in a pain-free and effusion-free manner in order to prevent further injury and pathology. Not only do movements need to be pain-free, but the athlete also needs to feel stable and confident when performing each exercise or he may not return to his same level of play and may be at increased risk of further injury or re-injury.

In this case, the patient was a Rugby Sevens player, which entails extreme amounts of running, changes of direction, and cutting/pivoting maneuvers. Each of these places a high demand of stress on the knee complex and supporting structures. At this stage of the athlete's rehabilitation, a running progression is underway and it is assumed that his cardiovascular conditioning has been mostly maintained. The player is typically allowed to participate in rugby practice with his knee braced, but often is not permitted to wear a "hard" functional brace (plastic or metal with hinges) during matches. The physician and player need to discuss this concern prior to returning to play.

Light agility training is introduced with forward/backward running, side shuffles, and cariocas at low speed with changes of direction at the player's discretion. Once this training is comfortable and pain-free, the intensity can be increased and changes of direction can be performed on verbal or auditory command, generating challenges in response time. As movements become easier, more intense activities can be introduced such as high speeds of running, 45° and 90° cutting drills, and introduction of pivoting on the involved lower extremity.

Activity progression should be based on symptoms and joint effusion levels. Knee effusion levels should be monitored before and after each training session to ensure appropriate demand is being put on the knee joint. It is ideal to keep joint effusion to a trace or less. If there are any changes from baseline effusion, time off should be incorporated until the effusion returns to baseline. If activities are pain-free and swelling is minimal, the player may be introduced to light non-contact practice with the team, eventually incorporating the athlete into light contact and progressing to full contact in order to prepare for game readiness. Modified soreness rules are a simple-to-follow protocol that may be used for progression or reduction of exercise if knee soreness or effusion occurs.[26]

Evidence-Based Clinical Recommendations

SORT: Strength of Recommendation Taxonomy
A: Consistent, good-quality patient-oriented evidence
B: Inconsistent or limited-quality patient-oriented evidence
C: Consensus, disease-oriented evidence, usually practice, expert opinion, or case series

1. A diagnosis of a grade II or grade III injury of the PCL can be made with a reasonable level of certainty when the patient presents with a mechanism of injury including: (1) a posteriorly directed force on the proximal tibia, a fall on the flexed knee with the foot in plantar flexion or a sudden violent hyperextension of the knee joint; (2) abrasions or ecchymosis on anterior aspect of proximal tibia; and (3) positive posterior drawer test at 90° with a non-discrete end feel or increased posterior tibial translation. **Grade A**
2. A protective knee brace locked in full extension minimizes the effects of gravity and the forces applied by the hamstrings to the newly reconstructed PCL. **Grade C**
3. To transition to a functional brace for use with higher-level activities, the athlete should be at least 6 weeks after PCL reconstruction, have decreased knee effusion, full knee extension, and a quadriceps index of at least 80% compared to the other lower extremity. **Grade C**

COMPREHENSION QUESTIONS

18.1 A physical therapist is evaluating a 16-year-old soccer player who just sustained a knee injury 1 hour ago. The player reports being slide tackled, with the opposing player's cleat driving his knee into a hyperextended position. Physical examination reveals knee joint effusion, limited extension ROM, a positive posterior drawer test, and localized tenderness on the fibular head. Which one of these knee findings would indicate a referral for an x-ray?

  A. Joint effusion
  B. Limited ROM
  C. Palpable tenderness on the fibular head
  D. Positive posterior drawer test

18.2 Which of the following is the *best* indicator to advance an athlete through the next stage of a return-to-sport progression following PCL reconstruction?

  A. Pain-free response with current activities with no increase in joint effusion
  B. Proper technique with exercise
  C. Surgeon's rehabilitation guidelines
  D. Upcoming game or competition

ANSWERS

18.1 **C.** According to Ottawa Knee Rules, localized tenderness to the fibular head indicates a need for referral for x-ray imaging.

18.2 **A.** Although there will be many factors and indicators the physical therapist may follow in order to advance an athlete through the stages of return-to-play progression, the best indicator would be a pain-free response with current activities with no increase in joint effusion.[26]

REFERENCES

1. Manske RC, Hosseinzadeh P, Giangarra CE. Multiple ligament knee injury: complications. *N Am J Sports Phys Ther*. 2008;3:226-233.
2. Grassmayr MJ, Parker DA, Coolican MR, Vanwanseele B. Posterior cruciate ligament deficiency: biomechanical and biological consequences and the outcomes of conservative treatment. A systematic review. *J Sci Med Sport*. 2008;11:433-443.
3. Majewski M, Susanne H, Klaus S. Epidemiology of athletic knee injuries: a 10-year study. *Knee*. 2006;13:184-188.
4. Fanelli GC, Edson CJ. Posterior cruciate ligament injuries in trauma patients: part II. *Arthroscopy*. 1995;11:526-529.
5. Schulz MS, Russe K, Weiler A, Eichhorn HJ, Strobel MJ. Epidemiology of posterior cruciate ligament injuries. *Arch Orthop Trauma Surg*. 2003;123:186-191.
6. Janousek AT, Jones DG, Clatworthy M, Higgins LD, Fu FH. Posterior cruciate ligament injuries of the knee joint. *Sports Med*. 1999;28:429-441.

7. Dandy DJ, Pusey RJ. The long-term results of unrepaired tears of the posterior cruciate ligament. *J Bone Joint Surg Br*. 1982;64:92-94.

8. Cross MJ, Powell JF. Long-term followup of posterior cruciate ligament rupture: a study of 116 cases. *Am J Sports Med*. 1984;12:292-297.

9. Cooper DE, Warren RF, Warner JJ. The posterior cruciate ligament and posterolateral structure of the knee: anatomy, function and patterns of injury. *Instr Course Lect*. 1991;40:249-270.

10. Fanelli GC, Beck JD, Edson CJ. Current concepts review: the posterior cruciate ligament. *J Knee Surg*. 2010;23:61-72.

11. Rubinstein RA Jr, Shelbourne KD, McCarroll JR, VanMeter CD, Rettig AC. The accuracy of the clinical examination in the setting of posterior cruciate ligament injuries. *Am J Sports Med*. 1994;22:550-557.

12. Jakob RP, Hassler H, Staeubli HU. Observations on rotatory instability of the lateral compartment of the knee. Experimental studies on the functional anatomy and the pathomechanism of the true and the reversed pivot shift sign. *Acta Orthop Scand Suppl*. 1981;191:1-32.

13. Shelbourne KD, Benedict F, McCarroll JR, Rettig AC. Dynamic posterior shift test. An adjuvant in evaluation of posterior tibial subluxation. *Am J Sports Med*. 1989;17:275-277.

14. Daniel DM, Stone ML, Barnett P, Sachs R. Use of the quadriceps active test to diagnose posterior cruciate-ligament disruption and measure posterior laxity of the knee. *J Bone Joint Surg Am*. 1988;70:386-391.

15. Flynn TW, Cleland JA, Whitman JM. *Users' Guide to the Musculoskeletal Examination: Fundamentals for the Evidence-Based Clinician*. Louisville, KY: Evidence in Motion; 2008.

16. Stiell IG, Greenberg GH, Wells GA, et al. Derivation of a decision rule for the use of radiography in acute knee injuries. *Ann Emerg Med*. 1995;26:405-413.

17. Bachmann LM, Haberzeth S, Steurer J, ter Riet G. The accuracy of the Ottawa knee rule to rule out knee fractures: a systematic review. *Ann Intern Med*. 2004;140:121-124.

18. Beall DP, Googe JD, Moss JT, et al. Magnetic resonance imaging of the collateral ligaments and the anatomic quadrants of the knee. *Radiol Clin North Am*. 2007;45:983-1002.

19. Kocabey Y, Tetik O, Isbell WM, Atay OA, Johnson DL. The value of clinical examination versus magnetic resonance imaging in the diagnosis of meniscal tears and anterior cruciate ligament rupture. *Arthroscopy*. 2004;20:696-700.

20. Madhusudhan TR, Kumar TM, Bastawrous SS, Sinha A. Clinical examination, MRI and arthroscopy in meniscal and ligamentous knee Injuries - a prospective study. *J Orthop Surg Res*. 2008;3:19.

21. Richter M, Kiefer H, Hehl G, Kinzl L. Primary repair for posterior cruciate ligament injuries. An eight-year follow-up of fifty-three patients. *Am J Sports Med*. 1996;24:298-305.

22. Clancy WG Jr, Shelbourne KD, Zoellner GB, Keene JS, Reider B, Rosenberg TD. Treatment of knee joint instability secondary to rupture of the posterior cruciate ligament. Report of a new procedure. *J Bone Joint Surg Am*. 1983;65:310-322.

23. Keller PM, Shelbourne KD, McCarroll JR, Rettig AC. Nonoperatively treated isolated posterior cruciate ligament injuries. *Am J Sports Med*. 1993;21:132-136.

24. Allen CR, Kaplan LD, Fluhme DJ, Harner CD. Posterior cruciate ligament injuries. *Current Opin Rheumatol*. 2002;14:142-149.

25. Irrgang JJ, Anderson AF, Boland AL, et al. International Knee Documentation Committee. Responsiveness of the International Knee Documentation Committee Subjective Knee Form. *Am J Sports Med*. 2006;34:1567-1573.

26. Reinold MM, Carter CC, Wilk KE. Rehabilitation after PCL reconstruction. *Athletic Ther Today*. 2001;6:23-31.

27. Manal TJ, Snyder-Mackler L. Practice guidelines for anterior cruciate ligament rehabilitation: a criterion based rehabilitation progression. *Oper Tech Orthop*. 1996;6:190-196.

Postsurgical Rehabilitation After Knee Articular Cartilage Repair

Mathew Failla
David Logerstedt

CASE 19

A 21-year-old male is referred to physical therapy 4 weeks following an arthroscopic right knee microfracture procedure. The patient was injured 6 weeks prior to surgery when he planted and twisted his right knee during a rugby game. He had immediate pain and noticed swelling later that day. He was unable to continue playing and noticed grinding and catching symptoms in his knee. The team trainer referred him to an orthopaedic surgeon for evaluation. A magnetic resonance imaging (MRI) scan revealed a full thickness articular cartilage lesion ($2\ cm^2$) of the central medial femoral condyle. Long cassette radiographs revealed that the lesion was not in the path of the mechanical axis of the knee. The decision was made to undergo arthroscopic microfracture surgery. The surgery was uncomplicated and the patient was non-weightbearing (NWB) on the right lower extremity with bilateral axillary crutches for 2 weeks, followed by 2 weeks of progressive weightbearing from toe touch to partial weightbearing. At home, the patient is performing quadriceps sets and using a continuous passive motion (CPM) machine 6 to 8 hours daily. He has now been referred to physical therapy 4 weeks after surgery with a prescription reading "Evaluate and treat, begin weightbearing as tolerated." The patient presents with well-healed portal incisions. His past medical and surgical histories are otherwise unremarkable.

▶ What are possible complications interfering with physical therapy?
▶ What is his rehabilitation prognosis?
▶ What precautions should be taken during physical therapy examination and/or interventions?
▶ Describe a physical therapy plan of care based on each stage of the health condition.

KEY DEFINITIONS

ARTHROSCOPIC MICROFRACTURE PROCEDURE: Surgical procedure in which an awl is arthroscopically used to puncture small holes 2 to 3 mm deep into subchondral bone at a synovial joint with the goal of filling a cartilaginous lesion; the holes cause bleeding, which releases growth factors that stimulate chondrocyte production. This new cartilage growth, however, is not completely hyaline in nature, but rather a hybrid of hyaline and fibrocartilage.[1]

ARTICULAR CARTILAGE LESION: Partial or full thickness tears in the articular cartilage in a joint; partial thickness tears extend from the outer surface into the articular cartilage layer, whereas full thickness tears extend through the entire articular cartilage layer and expose underlying subchondral bone.

AUTOLOGOUS CHONDROCYTE IMPLANTATION (ACI): Procedure in which cartilage cells are taken from an individual, stimulated to proliferate in cultured cells in a laboratory, and are placed back into the cartilage lesion and covered with a periosteal patch to hold them in place

LONG CASSETTE RADIOGRAPHS: Radiographs taken in standing from the hip to the ankle to determine where the mechanical (weightbearing) axis falls within the knee joint; a cartilage lesion that falls within this axis will fail if a surgical procedure is performed and must be accompanied by a procedure that changes alignment in order to be successful.[2]

OSTEOCHONDRAL AUTOGRAFT TRANSPLANTATION (OATS): Osteochondral autografts (plugs) taken from an area of the knee joint with less degeneration and used to fill large articular cartilage defects

Objectives

1. Explain the different grades of articular cartilage injury.
2. Explain the factors that influence precautions and limitations after microfracture surgery.
3. Utilize and interpret functional and self-reported outcomes after microfracture surgery.

Physical Therapy Considerations

PT considerations during postoperative management of an individual following arthroscopic microfracture surgery of the knee:

- **General physical therapy plan of care/goals:** Increase active and passive range of motion (ROM); improve quadriceps strength and activation; restore full function without placing excessive load through healing articular cartilage
- **Physical therapy interventions:** Patient education regarding injury pathomechanics, tissue healing timeframes, and procedure-specific precautions; effusion

management; manual therapy and stretching for joint mobility and motion; progressive resistive exercise and neuromuscular electrical stimulation (NMES) for quadriceps strengthening; neuromuscular re-education and dynamic stabilization exercises to improve proprioception and neuromuscular control of the lower limb; home exercise program

▶ **Precautions during physical therapy:** Monitor pain, joint effusion, and muscle soreness during progression of treatment; timeframe of tissue healing guides the amount of load that should be placed through the healing structure

▶ **Complications interfering with physical therapy:** Less than optimal healing due to postoperative infection, poor tissue quality, and large lesion size; lesion location may limit ROM, especially during weightbearing; patient noncompliance with maintaining appropriate weightbearing status; arthrofibrosis may develop after a period of immobilization

Understanding the Health Condition

Articular cartilage covers the surfaces of synovial joints and consists of hyaline cartilage. While articular cartilage resists both shear and compressive loading of the joint, lesions can occur because of acute trauma or repeated microtrauma.[3] Full thickness articular cartilage lesions are more common after acute traumatic injury,[4] whereas partial thickness lesions can be because of either acute trauma or repetitive microtrauma.[3] Because of the avascularity of articular cartilage, lesions have poor healing potential.[5] Nonoperative rehabilitation is generally unsuccessful, especially in active young individuals with symptomatic focal lesions.[6] Articular cartilage lesions of the knee occur in 16% to 19% of the general population. In a systematic review of 11 studies with 931 athletes, the overall prevalence of full thickness articular lesions was 36%.[7] It has been estimated that articular cartilage lesions are also observed in 60% to 70% of knee arthroscopies.[8-10] In a 2007 study of 25,124 knee arthroscopies in the general population, 30% of articular cartilage lesions were isolated while the remaining 70% were non-isolated.[11] In non-isolated lesions, 36% were accompanied by ruptures of the anterior cruciate ligament and 37% were accompanied by medial meniscal injuries.[11] Traumatic injury caused by a non-contact mechanism resulted in 32% to 58% of lesions.[4,11] Articular cartilage lesions are most commonly found on the medial femoral condyle and the articular patellar surface.[11] The International Cartilage Repair Society (ICRS) has established a grading system for classifying articular cartilage lesions.[12] The classification system comprises 5 levels ranging from normal cartilage without defects (grade 0) to severe abnormality with full thickness osteochondral injury (grade 4).[12]

Physical Therapy Patient/Client Management

Patients presenting for rehabilitation following arthroscopic microfracture surgery can benefit from manual therapy, therapeutic exercise, neuromuscular re-education, and modalities (e.g., ice and electrical stimulation). The location and size of the lesion are critical in determining the speed of treatment progression as well as the extent to which excessive forces through the location of the defect should be limited. Knowledge of knee joint surface contact locations allows the therapist to prescribe safe ranges of motions and weightbearing limitations that limit undue stress through the healing tissue. **Progressive loading is beneficial to optimal healing of cartilage.**[3] In contrast, excessive load may damage the clotted lesion or new cartilage, so loads need to be carefully managed with respect to tissue healing timeframes. It is important for the therapist to note that an articular lesion on the central medial femoral condyle engages with the tibial plateau at around 90° of knee flexion. While all condylar surfaces bear weight throughout the complete arc of knee motion, tibiofemoral contact forces progressively increase during squatting.[13] At 90° of flexion, these contact forces can range from 2.7 to 4 times one's body weight.[14]

Examination, Evaluation, and Diagnosis

Preoperatively, articular cartilage lesions clinically present similar to meniscal injuries, with complaints of swelling, pain, and mechanical symptoms such as locking and catching.[10] The results from the physical examination are non-specific. Diagnosis must be made or confirmed using diagnostic imaging.[15] If the patient presents with mechanical locking symptoms, the physical therapist should make a referral to an orthopaedic surgeon.

Radiographs and computed tomography (CT) scans are both able to detect displaced osteochondral lesions. Less significant lesions (lower stages of ICRS classification) are more difficult to detect and do not provide the physician sufficient information about the stability of the defect. Because of this poor sensitivity, MRI is the gold standard for assessing osteochondral defects.[16] While MRI gives valuable information for planning specific procedures, arthroscopic evaluation is performed to confirm diagnostic imaging findings and evaluate the defect for depth or tunneling that may not have been apparent or clear on MRI, prior to continuing with the cartilage repair procedure.[16]

Postoperatively, ROM of both the involved and uninvolved limbs is important, paying close attention to limitations placed by the surgeon. ROM limitations are based on the location of the articular defect and are highly individualized. Open chain isometric quadriceps strength can usually be assessed in safer ranges of motion (i.e., where contact forces are limited over the repair) by using an electromechanical dynamometer (see Fig. 16-4). Studies have shown that deficits in quadriceps and hamstring muscle performance persist for up to 7 years after articular cartilage procedures.[17,18] Proximal and distal joint ROM and strength may also be evaluated within the confines of postoperative precautions.

Plan of Care and Interventions

Little is known about outcomes with nonsurgical rehabilitation after knee articular cartilage lesions. Wondrasch et al.[19] reported outcomes after a 3-month active rehabilitation program focusing on cardiovascular exercise, progressive resistance exercises of the hip and knee, proprioceptive exercises, and plyometric exercises in patients with full thickness articular cartilage lesions. Clinically significant improvements in muscle performance were achieved, and 65% of the sample postponed their surgical appointments at least in the short term. Significant clinical improvements were seen in the International Knee Documentation Committee (IKDC) Subjective Knee Evaluation Form 2000 scores and the Knee Injury and Osteoarthritis Outcome Score (KOOS) quality of life subscale. There have been no studies investigating long-term outcomes after conservative management of articular cartilage lesions or its relationship with the future development of knee osteoarthritis.

Four types of surgical procedures have emerged as the most commonly used for the treatment of articular cartilage lesions: microfracture, debridement, ACI, and OATS.[3] Although studies with high levels of evidence and long-term follow-ups are limited, no particular procedure has repeatedly shown clinically superior results and outcomes.[20,21] Microfracture surgery is the preferred procedure, especially for lesions less than 2 cm^2.[22-24] This preference is mostly based on the relative ease of the procedure and low cost.

Several rehabilitation protocols and practice guidelines have been published concerning management after microfracture surgery.[6,14,25-27] In 2010, Logerstedt et al.[28] reviewed the current literature and concluded that **early progressive knee motion, supervised rehabilitation, strength and functional training, and NMES** were beneficial interventions to increase quadriceps strength and endurance, hamstrings strength, and functional performance after cartilage procedures. Although the authors determined that opinions were conflicting regarding implementation of a progressive weightbearing protocol, recent evidence suggests that weightbearing after matrix-induced ACI may be accelerated, though the evidence specifically following microfracture procedures is lacking.[29] Impairments after microfracture surgery include pain, effusion, and deficits in ROM, strength, balance, and gait.

Rehabilitation after articular cartilage procedures is highly individualized based on size and location of the defect, the type of procedure that is performed, and the patient's goals. The rehabilitation protocol for this case patient was based on a 2-cm^2 full thickness articular cartilage lesion of the middle portion of the medial femoral condyle repaired by microfracture surgery 4 weeks ago. Appropriate mobilization is a critical factor after cartilage repair procedures. The precautions and restrictions for mobilization can vary greatly, depending if the lesion is on the anterior or middle femoral condyle versus the retropatellar femoral surface or the trochlea. Animal research suggests that immobilization and extended unloading periods are not advantageous because they lead to softening of the healing cartilage.[30] Progressive weightbearing and ROM improve mechanical properties and matrix production of human articular cartilage.[5] Passive ROM is performed immediately after surgery and is commonly done with a CPM machine. Continuous motion is thought to promote nutrient uptake, maintain a low friction environment, and reduce the risk of arthrofibrosis.[31] Following microfracture surgery for full thickness chondral defects, use of a CPM machine for 6 to 8 hours daily for 8 weeks resulted in significantly higher patient satisfaction outcomes compared to those who did not use a CPM machine.[32] Others have used isokinetic devices or stationary bikes for passive

ROM as long as weightbearing and ROM restrictions are well maintained.[6,25] As with the majority of knee surgeries, full knee extension ROM should be achieved as soon as possible following surgery. However, the sheer loading associated with active knee extension could be damaging to the healing cartilage prior to 8 weeks post-surgery. Therefore, *active* knee extension should be limited within the range of 90° to 45° without resistance for the first 4 weeks, with progression to full active knee extension by 8 weeks. At 4 weeks post-surgery, passive knee flexion ROM is gradually progressed to 125° and to full knee flexion by 8 weeks post-surgery. To help restore normal joint mobility, the physical therapist should perform patellofemoral joint mobilizations.

Weightbearing protocols that have evolved from bench research on animal and human cartilage suggest that compressive loads without shear stress may be beneficial to healing cartilage while shear or excessive compressive stresses are not beneficial.[5] Patients begin NWB postoperatively and weightbearing status systematically progresses (as early as 2 weeks after surgery) to partial weightbearing, commonly incremented as a percentage of body weight in kilograms. However, different opinions exist on how quickly to progress partial weightbearing.[28] In traditional protocols, full weightbearing can begin 11 weeks after surgery, whereas in accelerated protocols full weightbearing may begin 8 weeks post-surgery. There is limited literature evaluating weightbearing progression after microfracture procedures. Ebert et al.[29] compared traditional and accelerated weightbearing protocols following ACI procedures and reported similar gait characteristics and functional outcomes between protocols up to 2 years after surgery. Even after progression to full weightbearing, weightbearing motion ranges must be restricted because all condylar surfaces bear weight through the arc of knee motion.[13] A good way to implement restricted ROM in weightbearing is by using a progressive squatting depth exercise. This exercise can be safely incorporated to promote nutrient uptake into the cartilage for matrix production so the cartilage can withstand the forces acting upon it.[30] Current recommendations suggest progressive walking programs may begin around 10 weeks and running around 16 to 20 weeks. Notably, recent literature shows that articular cartilage is of lesser quality after anterior cruciate ligament surgery than matched controls at time of return to sport.[33] Further research is needed to determine when running is appropriate after articular cartilage procedures. Progression of weightbearing should be guided by pain, symptoms, effusion, tissue healing timeframes (based on the biological healing properties of cartilage), and size/location of the healing surface.

Knee joint effusion is common after surgical procedures involving articular cartilage. Uncontrolled joint effusion can lead to increased pain, loss of ROM, altered patellofemoral joint mobility, and it may impact cartilage and joint health. Cryotherapy combined with compression and elevation can be effective at reducing both pain and joint effusion.[34] Monitoring joint effusion is also helpful in determining treatment progression. **Effusion** can be monitored by performing the modified stroke test prior to, during, and after treatment. This test is performed by sweeping fluid proximally out of the medial sulcus of the knee, and then performing a distally directed sweep along the lateral knee and watching for a wave of fluid returning to the medial sulcus.[35] Grading ranges from no effusion to 3+, which is the inability to push all the effusion out of the sulcus. An increase in effusion following treatment that does not return back to baseline likely indicates that treatment progression was too aggressive. Treatment should not be progressed again until the effusion has returned to baseline. The modified stroke test (see Fig. 16-2) has been used clinically for more than 15 years and has demonstrated very good inter-rater reliability.[35]

Muscle strengthening (especially quadriceps) is very important after articular cartilage surgeries. Van Assche et al.[17] found quadriceps strength deficits of greater than 20% in one-third of patients 1 year after microfracture surgery and in more than one-quarter of patients 2 years after surgery. Early after microfracture surgery, strengthening goals should focus on achieving volitional quadriceps control. Because of restrictions in weightbearing status and ROM, **NMES** can be highly beneficial in improving quadriceps strength and activation. While no studies have been done to investigate the efficacy of NMES after microfracture surgery, there is a preponderance of evidence showing improved quadriceps strength with the use of NMES following other knee surgeries and injuries.[36] Specific exercises and ranges of motion are restricted based on lesion location and must be highly individualized and determined by both the physician and treating therapist. To minimize deconditioning, hip, ankle, and abdominal core exercises should also be incorporated. When incisions are well healed, aquatic therapy can be initiated. The buoyant properties of water at different depths may allow the patient to complete more functional, full body exercise (*e.g.*, water walking or jogging) while maintaining weightbearing restrictions. When full weightbearing is achieved, progressive resistance activities on land such as weight shifting, leg press, and mini-squats may be utilized when appropriate. Current recommendations allow patients to begin a gradual return to more high impact activity such as running, agility, and plyometric training after 16 to 20 weeks.[6]

Proprioceptive deficits have been reported following many types of knee surgeries.[37] Neuromuscular training can be utilized to restore dynamic knee stability and control. Initially, training may include weight shifting with progression to single-leg balance on stable and then on unstable surfaces. Standing on rollerboards or rockerboards, with incorporation of tasks or perturbations, can be used for higher-level proprioceptive training. A typical progression might begin with single-leg stance on a rockerboard. The therapist can increase difficulty by adding perturbations and progressing these by increasing the speed or amplitude of the perturbations (Fig. 19-1). When the patient is no longer being challenged, sport-specific tasks can be added to distract the patient from concentrating on his knee. When adding sport-specific tasks, such as a ball toss, the therapist should decrease the speed and amplitude of perturbations and begin the progression again.

Few studies have reported outcomes after microfracture surgery in the athletic population. Van Assche et al.[17] found that 30% of patients had more than 15% deficits in overall functional performance 2 years after surgery. Gobbi et al.[38] found that 20% of patients had 20% to 50% performance deficits at a mean of 6 years after microfracture surgery compared to their uninvolved limb in single-legged hop tests. Measures typically used to assess functional ability include single-legged hop tests and the 6-minute walk test. Validated self-reported outcome measures that are

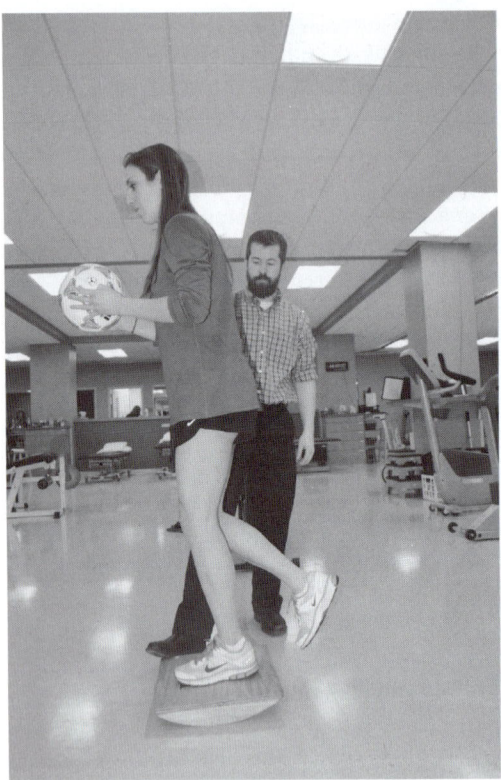

Figure 19-1. Neuromuscular control exercises using a rockerboard. The patient stands on rockerboard on the affected leg while the therapist provides external perturbations.

commonly used in research with individuals after knee surgery include the Knee Outcome Survey-Activities of Daily Living Scale (KOS-ADLS), the KOOS, the IKDC 2000, the Lysholm Knee Scale, the Cincinnati Knee Rating Scale, the Tegner Activity Level Scale, and the Marx Activity Level Scale. Logerstedt et al.[28] determined that clinicians should use validated general health questionnaires, activity scales, and patient-reported outcome scales in order to capture the complete functional picture of the individual after a cartilage procedure. For the athletic population, the KOOS and the KOS sports subscale are likely the most applicable self-report measures on outcomes after articular cartilage surgery, as well as the Marx or Tegner scales to monitor activity levels.

Evidence-Based Clinical Recommendations

SORT: Strength of Recommendation Taxonomy
A: Consistent, good-quality patient-oriented evidence
B: Inconsistent or limited-quality patient-oriented evidence
C: Consensus, disease-oriented evidence, usual practice, expert opinion, or case series

1. Early progressive knee motion and weightbearing, supervised rehabilitation, strength and functional training, and neuromuscular electrical stimulation (NMES) can be

used to increase quadriceps strength and endurance, hamstrings strength, and functional performance in individuals after cartilage procedures. **Grade B**

2. The modified stroke test can be used to monitor joint effusion and determine the aggressiveness of treatment progression. **Grade C**

3. After many types of knee surgery, quadriceps strength improves with NMES in conjunction with quadriceps exercises. **Grade A**

COMPREHENSION QUESTIONS

19.1 After surgery for an articular knee cartilage lesion, which of the following is *not* a consideration in an individualized rehabilitation protocol?
   A. Location of the lesion
   B. Sex of the patient
   C. Type of procedure
   D. Patient's goals

19.2 Which of the following statements is true?
   A. Articular cartilage lesions have poor vascularity and poor healing potential.
   B. Articular cartilage lesions have good vascularity and poor healing potential.
   C. Articular cartilage lesions have good vascularity and good healing potential.
   D. Articular cartilage lesions have poor vascularity and good healing potential.

19.3 Which articular cartilage procedure is the best for all types of lesions?
   A. Microfracture
   B. Osteochondral autograft transplantation (OATS)
   C. Autologous chondrocyte implantation (ACI)
   D. An overall best procedure has not been established at this time.

ANSWERS

19.1 **B.** Individualized rehabilitation should take into consideration the location and size of the articular lesion, the type of procedure performed, and the patient's goals. There is no evidence to support that the sex of the patient would alter a rehabilitation protocol.

19.2 **A.** Articular cartilage has poor vascularity and therefore poor healing potential.

19.3 **D.** The lack of consistent evidence from randomized controlled trials suggests that there is not a specific procedure recommended above others for all articular cartilage lesions. Instead, the procedure should be selected based on the patient's goals, lesion size, and lesion location.

REFERENCES

1. Bae DK, Yoon KH, Song SJ. Cartilage healing after microfracture in osteoarthritic knees. *Arthroscopy.* 2006;22:367-374.
2. Mina C, Garrett WE Jr, Pietrobon R, Glisson R, Higgins L. High tibial osteotomy for unloading osteochondral defects in the medial compartment of the knee. *Am J Sports Med.* 2008;36:949-955.
3. Bhosale AM, Richardson JB. Articular cartilage: structure, injuries and review of management. *Br Med Bull.* 2008;87:77-95.
4. Johnson-Nurse C, Dandy DJ. Fracture separation of articular cartilage in the adult knee. *J Bone Surg.* 1985;67B:42-43.
5. Buckwalter JA. Articular cartilage: injuries and potential for healing. *J Orthop Sports Phys Ther.* 1998;28:192-202.
6. Reinold MM, Wilk KE, Macrina LC, Dugas JR, Cain EL. Current concepts in the rehabilitation following articular cartilage repair procedures in the knee. *J Orthop Sports Phys Ther.* 2006;36:774-794.
7. Flanigan DC, Harris JD, Trinh TQ, Siston RA, Brophy RH. Prevalence of chondral defects in athletes' knees: a systematic review. *Med Sci Sports Exerc.* 2010;42:1795-1801.
8. Aroen A, Loken S, Heir S, et al. Articular cartilage lesions in 993 consecutive knee arthroscopies. *Am J Sports Med.* 2004;32:211-215.
9. Curl WW, Krome J, Gordon ES, Rushing J, Smith BP, Poehling GG. Cartilage injuries: a review of 31,516 knee arthroscopies. *Arthroscopy.* 1997;13:456-460.
10. Hjelle K, Solheim E, Strand T, Muri R, Brittberg M. Articular cartilage defects in 1,000 knee arthroscopies. *Arthroscopy.* 2002;18:730-734.
11. Widuchowski W, Widuchowski J, Trzaska T. Articular cartilage defects: study of 25,124 knee arthroscopies. *Knee.* 2007;14:177-182.
12. Brittberg M, Winalski CS. Evaluation of cartilage injuries and repair. *J Bone Joint Surg Am.* 2003;85-A(suppl 2):58-69.
13. Thambyah A, Goh JC, De SD. Contact stresses in the knee joint in deep flexion. *Med Eng Phys.* 2005;27:329-335.
14. Mithoefer K, Hambly K, Logerstedt D, Ricci M, Silvers H, Della Villa S. Current concepts for rehabilitation and return to sport after knee articular cartilage repair in the athlete. *J Orthop Sports Phys Ther.* 2012;42:254-273.
15. Buckwalter JA, Mankin HJ, Grodzinsky AJ. Articular cartilage and osteoarthritis. *Instr Course Lect.* 2005;54:465-480.
16. Galea A, Giuffre B, Dimmick S, Coolican MR, Parker DA. The accuracy of magnetic resonance imaging scanning and its influence on management decisions in knee surgery. *Arthroscopy.* 2009;25:473-480.
17. Van Assche D, Staes F, Van Caspel D, et al. Autologous chondrocyte implantation versus microfracture for knee cartilage injury: a prospective randomized trial, with 2-year follow-up. *Knee Surg Sports Traumatol Arthrosc.* 2010;18:486-495.
18. Loken S, Ludvigsen TC, Hoysveen T, Holm I, Engebretsen L, Reinholt FP. Autologous chondrocyte implantation to repair knee cartilage injury: ultrastructural evaluation at 2 years and long-term follow-up including muscle strength measurements. *Knee Surg Sports Traumatol Arthrosc.* 2009;17:1278-1288.
19. Wondrasch B, Aroen, A, Rotterud JH, Hoysveen T, Bolstad K, Risberg MA. The feasibility of a 3-month active rehabilitation program for patients with knee full-thickness articular cartilage lesions: the Oslo Cartilage Active Rehabilitation and Education Study. *J Orthop Sports Phys Ther.* 2013;43:310-324.
20. Magnussen RA, Dunn WR, Carey JL, Spindler KP. Treatment of focal articular cartilage defects in the knee: a systematic review. *Clin Orthop Relat Res.* 2008;466:952-962.

21. Jakobsen RB, Engebretsen L, Slauterbeck JR. An analysis of the quality of cartilage repair studies. *J Bone Joint Surg Am.* 2005;87:2232-2239.
22. Knutsen G, Engebretsen L, Ludvigsen TC, et al. Autologous chondrocyte implantation compared with microfracture in the knee. A randomized trial. *J Bone Joint Surg Am.* 2004;86-A:455-464.
23. Mithoefer K, McAdams T, Williams RJ, Kreuz PC, Mandelbaum BR. Clinical efficacy of the microfracture technique for articular cartilage in the knee: an evidence-based systematic analysis. *Am J Sports Med.* 2009;37:2053-2063.
24. Steadman JR, Briggs KK, Rodrigo JJ, Kocher MS, Gill TJ, Rodkey WG. Outcomes of microfracture for traumatic chondral defects of the knee: average 11-year follow-up. *Arthroscopy.* 2003;19:477-484.
25. Hurst JM, Steadman JR, O'Brien L, Rodkey WG, Briggs KK. Rehabilitation following microfracture for chondral injury in the knee. *Clin Sports Med.* 2010;29:257-265.
26. Irrgang JJ, Pezzullo D. Rehabilitation following surgical procedures to address articular cartilage lesions in the knee. *J Orthop Sports Phys Ther.* 1998;28:232-240.
27. Wilk KE, Macrina LC, Reinold MM. Rehabilitation following microfracture of the knee. *Cartilage.* 2010;1:96-107.
28. Logerstedt DS, Snyder-Mackler L, Ritter RC, Axe MJ. Knee pain and mobility impairments: meniscal and articular cartilage lesions. *J Orthop Sports Phys Ther.* 2010;40:A1-A35.
29. Ebert JR, Robertson WB, Lloyd DG, Zheng MH, Wood DJ, Ackland T. A prospective, randomized comparison of traditional and accelerated approaches to postoperative rehabilitation following autologous chondrocyte implantation: 2-year clinical outcomes. *Cartilage.* 2010;1:180-187.
30. Vanwanseele B, Lucchinetti E, Stussi E. The effects of immobilization on the characteristics of articular cartilage: current concepts and future directions. *Osteoarthritis Cartilage.* 2002;10:408-419.
31. Salter RB. The physiologic basis of continuous passive motion for articular cartilage healing and regeneration. *Hand Clin.* 1994;10:211-219.
32. Rodrigo JJ, Steadman JR, Silliman JF, Fulstone HA. Improvement of full-thickness chondral defect healing in the human knee after debridement and microfracture using continuous passive motion. *Am J Knee Surg.* 1994;7:109-116.
33. Ginckel AV, Verdonk P, Victor J, Witvrouw E. Cartilage status in relation to return to sports after anterior cruciate ligament reconstruction. *Am J Sports Med.* 2013;41:550-559.
34. Raynor MC, Pietrobon R, Guller U, Higgins LD. Cryotherapy after ACL reconstruction: a meta-analysis. *J Knee Surg.* 2005;18:123-129.
35. Sturgill LP, Snyder-Mackler L, Manal TJ, Axe MJ. Interrater reliability of a clinical scale to assess knee joint effusion. *J Orthop Sports Phys Ther.* 2009;39:845-849.
36. Bax L, Staes F, Verhagen A. Does neuromuscular electrical stimulation strengthen the quadriceps femoris? A systematic review of randomized controlled trials. *Sports Med.* 2005;35:191-212.
37. Roberts D, Friden T, Stomberg A, Lindstrand A, Moritz U. Bilateral proprioceptive defects in patients with a unilateral anterior cruciate ligament reconstruction: a comparison between patients and healthy subjects. *J Orthop Res.* 2000;18:565-571.
38. Gobbi A, Nunag P, Malinowski K. Treatment of full thickness chondral lesions of the knee with microfracture in a group of athletes. *Knee Surg Sports Traumatol Arthrosc.* 2005;13:213-221.

Early (Stages I and II) Posterior Tibial Tendon Dysfunction

Judy Gelber

CASE 20

A 40-year-old female is referred to an outpatient physical therapy clinic with a diagnosis of right posterior tibial tendon dysfunction (PTTD), stage II. The patient reports a gradual increase in pain over the previous 3 months that she attributes to an increase in her running regimen. She rates her pain at 7/10 with all weight-bearing activities and 1/10 with rest. Her physician has prescribed nonsteroidal anti-inflammatory drugs and has given her a prescription for a custom orthotic, which she has not yet obtained. She is referred to physical therapy to "evaluate and treat" for stage II PTTD. The patient's medical history is otherwise unremarkable.

- Based on the patient's diagnosis, what do you anticipate may be the contributing factors to her condition?
- What examination signs may be associated with this diagnosis?
- What are the most appropriate physical therapy interventions?
- Based on the patient's history, what is her prognosis with nonsurgical care?

KEY DEFINITIONS

ADULT ACQUIRED FLATFOOT DEFORMITY: Progressive lowering of the medial longitudinal arch that begins in adulthood

POSTERIOR TIBIAL TENDON DYSFUNCTION: Condition in which the posterior tibial tendon and associated ligaments and joints of the foot and ankle gradually lose their integrity; most common cause of adult acquired flatfoot deformity (the 2 terms are sometimes used interchangeably)

SINUS TARSI REGION: Cavity formed between the talus and the calcaneus; located immediately anterior and slightly distal to the lateral malleolus

Objectives

1. Describe PTTD.
2. Discuss signs and symptoms of a person with PTTD.
3. Describe options for external support for a person with PTTD.
4. Prescribe appropriate resistance exercises for a person with PTTD.

Physical Therapy Considerations

PT considerations during management of the individual with early stage PTTD:

- **General physical therapy plan of care/goals:** Decrease pain; increase ankle strength; support the medial longitudinal arch; increase ankle joint range of motion (ROM); increase muscle flexibility
- **Physical therapy interventions:** Patient education regarding foot and ankle anatomy and pathomechanics related to the diagnosis; modalities as needed to decrease pain; mobilization and stretching to decrease pain and improve joint mobility; ROM and flexibility exercises; resistance exercises to increase muscular strength and endurance; home exercise instruction
- **Precautions during physical therapy:** Monitor vital signs; avoid excessive walking if painful; address precautions or contraindications for exercise based on patient's pre-existing condition(s)
- **Complications interfering with physical therapy:** Patient noncompliance with exercise program; lifestyle issues that interfere with optimal tissue healing (e.g., smoking, excessive walking or standing)

Understanding the Health Condition

The posterior tibialis muscle originates along the proximal tibia, fibula, and the interosseus membrane and inserts primarily at the navicular tuberosity. Its actions include plantar flexion of the ankle and inversion of the foot. As the posterior tibialis contracts during stance phase of gait, it is uniquely positioned to provide a supinatory force to the midfoot, locking the transtarsal joint, and acting as a dynamic stabilizer of the medial longitudinal arch.[1]

PTTD is a condition that involves pathology of the posterior tibial tendon as well as surrounding ligaments and joints.[2-4] Initially, pain is localized to the posterior tibial tendon. As the condition progresses, it is characterized by medial longitudinal arch collapse, valgus position of the hindfoot, and abduction of the forefoot.[5] Over time, these deformities can become fixed. While the precise etiology of PTTD is unknown, it is often considered a degenerative condition associated with pronation.[6,7] Other proposed etiologies include inflammatory synovitis or acute trauma.[4,5] Patient-related factors associated with PTTD include the female sex, middle age, and obesity.[8,9]

Johnson and Strom[5] have described a 4-stage progression for PTTD. Stage I is marked by pain and swelling localized to the posterior tibial tendon with no associated deformity. Stage II is characterized by a flexible flatfoot deformity. In this stage, the tendon is lengthened and may show degeneration. However, the hindfoot is mobile and the foot demonstrates a flexible planovalgus.[3] Fixed deformity characterizes stage III, and the pain may transfer laterally because of impingement in the sinus tarsi region. Johnson and Strom[5] also proposed a stage IV, in which the deformity progresses to include valgus angulation of the talus. Stage IV was formally adopted several years later by Myerson.[4]

Nonsurgical treatment options for PTTD include bracing and physical therapy. Conservative care is indicated for patients who have a lower severity using the Johnson and Strom staging criteria, shorter duration of symptoms, and no history of prior cortisone injections or orthotic use.[10] Physical therapy interventions are indicated in the early stages (I and II) in which any associated deformity is flexible. Interventions include strengthening the supinators to improve midfoot stability and stretching the ankle plantar flexors to improve talocrural joint flexibility. Traditionally, medical management includes some form of external foot support via bracing.[11,12] Recent research has found that strengthening and stretching can augment a bracing program.[13,14] If a patient's symptoms have not resolved in 3 to 4 months of physical therapy, he/she should be referred to an orthopaedic physician for a surgical consultation. Indicators for physician referral include persistence of pain and/or continued need for bracing.[14]

Physical Therapy Patient/Client Management

Physical therapy is indicated for initial conservative management in early stages of PTTD. Given the wide variety of injuries associated with a pronated foot type, differential or additional diagnoses for which individuals with PTTD may be referred to physical therapy include posterior tibial tendonitis, pes planus, or a generic description such as "medial arch pain." The therapist should initiate interventions that support the injured structures, increase talocrural joint flexibility, and gradually strengthen the supinator muscles of the foot. The physical therapist may collaborate with an orthotist or pedorthist when customized bracing is indicated. If pain is not relieved or foot deformity progresses despite targeted intervention, the patient should be referred back to the orthopaedist for medical management, which may include advanced imaging, more aggressive offloading, and/or surgical consultation.

Examination, Evaluation, and Diagnosis

A physical therapy examination of the patient with suspected PTTD includes visual inspection and palpation of the feet, assessment of static foot alignment, ROM and accessory motion assessment, movement analysis, measurement of functional lower extremity strength, and gait analysis.

Pain and swelling are the primary characteristics of PTTD, particularly in stage I when there are no static alignment impairments.[5] Examination usually begins with a visual inspection of the foot and palpation of the posterior tibial tendon. Often, the leg is tender to palpation along the course of the posterior tibial tendon from behind the medial malleolus to its insertion on the navicular.

PTTD is associated with **static findings of a lower longitudinal arch and dynamic findings of ankle pronation**.[6,7,15,16] Static foot alignment can be measured and documented using a variety of methods. The "too many toes sign" is a common indicator of pronation during standing (Fig. 20-1).[5] The arch index is frequently used for

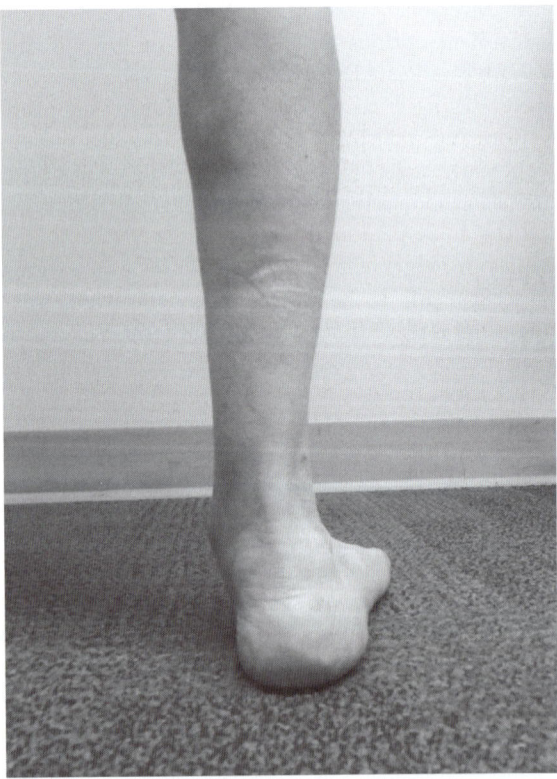

Figure 20-1. "Too many toes" sign. From a posterior view, a greater number of toes are seen laterally than medially. In this case, the great toe is not seen at all and the subject's toes are only visible laterally.

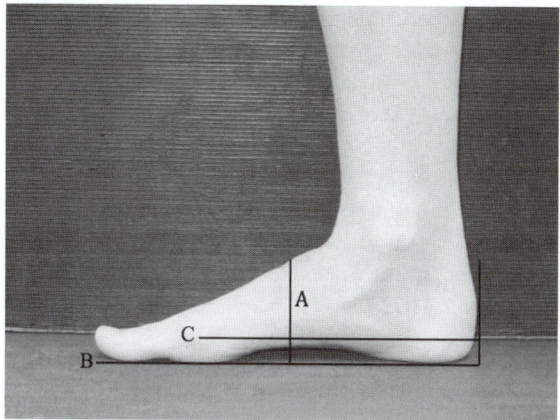

Figure 20-2. The arch index = A/C, where A represents the height of the foot at 50% of the total foot length (B), and C represents truncated foot length, measured from the head of the first metatarsal to the most posterior aspect of the heel.

static measurement of medial longitudinal arch height in this population. The arch index is measured as the height from the ground to the dorsal foot at 50% of the total foot length divided by the length from the posterior aspect of the heel to the first metatarsal (Fig. 20-2).[17] A higher arch index indicates a higher longitudinal arch, whereas an arch index less than 0.263 is considered to be a pronated foot type.[18] Researchers have found significant differences in standing arch height index in individuals with early stage PTTD relative to control subjects.[16,19] However, Rabbito et al.[6] found a difference in *seated* arch height index, but no differences in standing arch height index between individuals with stage I PTTD and controls. Thus, it may be beneficial for the physical therapist to measure the arch index of each foot in both seated and standing positions in order to clearly document non-weightbearing arch height and any change in a weightbearing position. While excessive pronation may be present bilaterally, PTTD is typically only observed unilaterally, with more severe pronation and a lower arch index accompanied by pain and loss of function on the involved side.

Given the static and movement findings associated with PTTD, foot and ankle ROM and accessory joint mobility must be assessed. Standard ROM measurements can be taken in prone or supine using a goniometer while keeping the ankle in subtalar joint neutral.[20] Calcaneal inversion and eversion must be measured to quantify hindfoot mobility. Great toe extension ROM values may also be valuable because passive toe extension engages the plantar fascia to assist in arch elevation during terminal stance and early push-off within the gait cycle.[21] Active and passive ankle dorsiflexion should be measured with the knee extended and flexed to assess for the contribution of gastrocnemius muscle shortness to limited ankle dorsiflexion. When the knee is extended and the ankle dorsiflexed, the gastrocnemius is maximally stretched because of the muscle's origin and insertion crossing the knee and the ankle. In an individual with gastrocnemius shortness, ankle dorsiflexion will be limited with the knee extended. If the measurement is repeated with the knee flexed, the gastrocnemius is no longer maximally stretched and an individual with isolated gastrocnemius shortness will exhibit increased ankle dorsiflexion range. Ankle dorsiflexion that is equally limited in both knee positions can be attributed to deficits in soleus length or to talocrural joint capsular stiffness. Accessory joint mobility testing at the talocrural joint is necessary to distinguish a muscular versus capsular restriction.

Adequate talocrural and subtalar joint mobility is also necessary for optimal foot mechanics. When talocrural joint mobility is limited, particularly into dorsiflexion, the calcaneus begins to evert and excessive valgus stress is placed at the subtalar joint. The pattern is cyclic; as the calcaneus everts, the gastrocnemius is placed in a shortened position.[3] Over time, the gastrocnemius can become shortened and the calcaneus may become fixed in an everted position.[5]

The actions of the posterior tibialis are hindfoot plantar flexion and inversion. Traditional manual muscle testing uses a break test at the end range of ankle plantar flexion and inversion.[22] However, it may also be beneficial to test each action individually. While Alvarez et al.[14] found ankle inversion weakness on the involved side in individuals with PTTD during isokinetic testing, Rabbito et al.[6] found no difference in ankle inversion strength (tested with dynamometry) in subjects with stage I PTTD compared to controls.

A functional assessment of the posterior tibialis tendon includes observation of the patient's ability to perform a heel rise. During a heel rise, the posterior tibial tendon inverts the hindfoot, which allows the triceps surae complex to plantar flex the ankle on a stable foot. In the presence of PTTD, the posterior tibialis is incompetent, resulting in hindfoot eversion during a single-leg heel rise or an inability to raise the heel off the ground.[19] Individuals with PTTD are often unable to perform a single heel rise.[5] Differences in forefoot motion have also been noted during the performance of a bilateral heel rise. In a study of foot kinematics during a bilateral heel rise task in subjects with stage II PTTD, Houck et al.[16] showed that forefoot plantar flexion on the hindfoot and metatarsophalangeal dorsiflexion were decreased. In the context of a thorough clinical examination, the physical therapist should assess both unilateral and bilateral heel rise, noting ankle plantar flexion range of motion, forefoot on hindfoot plantar flexion, as well as the presence or absence of hindfoot inversion (Fig. 20-3). If the individual is able to perform a unilateral heel rise with appropriate movement pattern and no substitutions, a repeated heel rise test is used to assess ankle plantar flexor performance. Normal strength of the ankle plantar flexors has been described as the ability to perform 25 unilateral heel rises through at least 50% of the height of an initial unilateral heel rise.[23]

While little is known about hip strength in this population, Kulig et al.[19] demonstrated that middle-aged females with early stage PTTD had decreased hip extension and abduction strength bilaterally compared to age-matched norms. Thus, hip muscle strength testing may be warranted on initial examination.

Initial examination also includes a gait analysis. The therapist must carefully observe motions of the feet during all phases of the gait cycle. In particular, the therapist should attempt to identify whether the affected foot has the following unwanted movements: excessive hindfoot eversion, forefoot dorsiflexion on the hindfoot, limited talocrural dorsiflexion and hallux dorsiflexion at terminal stance, and limited talocrural plantar flexion at push-off. Kinematic testing of individuals with stages I and II PTTD has shown increased hindfoot eversion throughout all

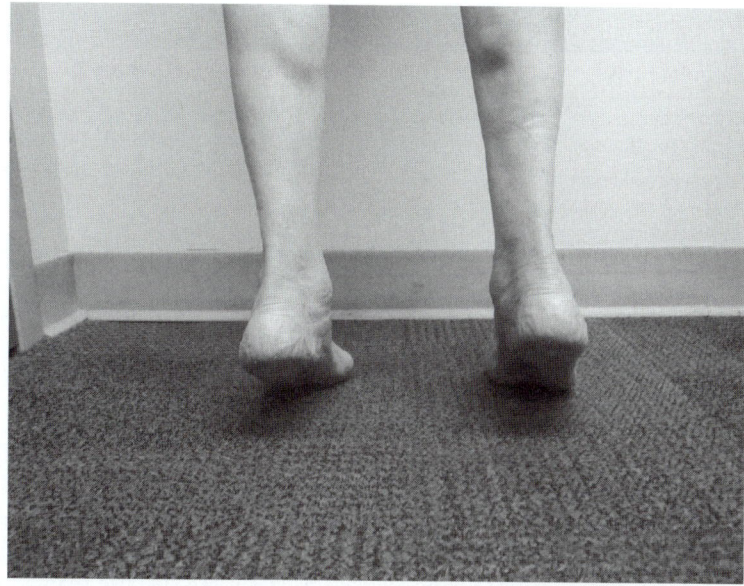

Figure 20-3. Bilateral heel rise. This individual exhibits limited ankle plantar flexion and an absence of hindfoot inversion bilaterally.

phases of stance,[6,7,24] less hindfoot dorsiflexion, and a forefoot that is more dorsiflexed compared to the hindfoot.[24] Decreased hallux extension has also been found throughout the gait cycle in individuals with PTTD.[24]

Plan of Care and Interventions

Bracing was the first strategy used in nonsurgical management for PTTD.[11,12,25] Neville and Lemley[26] found that **multiple styles of bracing** are effective in raising the medial longitudinal arch, and that custom articulated braces are the most effective at improving hindfoot inversion throughout stance relative to a no brace condition. Alvarez et al.[14] used a three-quarter length submalleolar foot orthosis for subjects who could walk greater than 1 block, perform a single-leg heel rise on the affected side, and had pain less than 3 months in duration. If any of these 3 conditions were not met, subjects were fit with a short (mid-leg) articulated ankle-foot orthosis (AFO). When pain subsided and strength was within 10% to 15% of the unaffected side, subjects were progressed from the AFO to the three-quarter length foot orthosis.[14] Bracing should be considered in conjunction with initial physical therapy in this patient population.

In recent years, the **addition of stretching and high repetition low-load strengthening to traditional bracing programs** in early stage PTTD has improved clinical outcomes.[13,14] Alvarez et al.[14] reported decreased pain and improved function in 83% of the 47 individuals studied. The rehabilitation program devised by Alvarez et al.[14] consisted of an initial treatment session (pre-treatment phase) followed by 3 progressive phases. During the pre-treatment phase, the patient was seen for 1 visit for home

Table 20-1	THERAPEUTIC EXERCISE PROGRAM FOR PTTD		
Pre-treatment Phase	**Phase 1**	**Phase 2**	**Phase 3**
"Sole-to-sole" exercise (Fig. 20-4): 25 repetitions per set Start with 4 sets, building to 12 sets and then toward 300 consecutive repetitions per day over the course of 2 weeks.	Theraband-resisted dorsiflexion, inversion, and eversion, building up to 200 repetitions per day	Double-leg heel rises progressing to single leg, building up to 50 repetitions Toe ambulation working toward 100 yards Achilles stretch, if muscular tightness is limiting full ankle dorsiflexion	Progression of phase 2 activities toward target repetitions and distances

exercise program instruction consisting of the sole-to-sole exercise. Table 20-1 shows examples of exercises in a 3-phase rehabilitation program for PTTD.[14]

Kulig et al.[27] have researched modes of exercise for recruiting the posterior tibialis muscle and concluded that in healthy individuals with a normal arch index, resisted foot adduction using an exercise band (Fig. 20-5) was more effective than a unilateral heel rise or band-resisted supination. In individuals with PTTD performing this

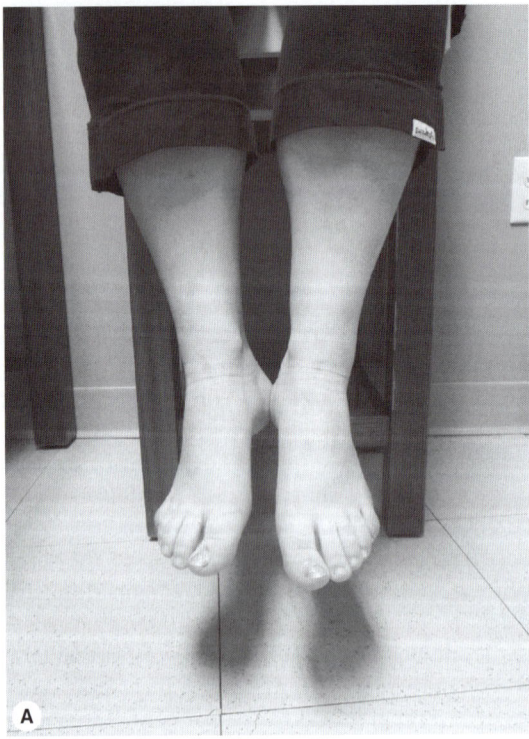

Figure 20-4. Sole-to-sole posterior tibialis strengthening exercise. **A.** With the ankles in slight plantar flexion and the heels together. **B.** The patient slowly inverts the feet so that the soles of the feet are facing and then returns to the starting position.

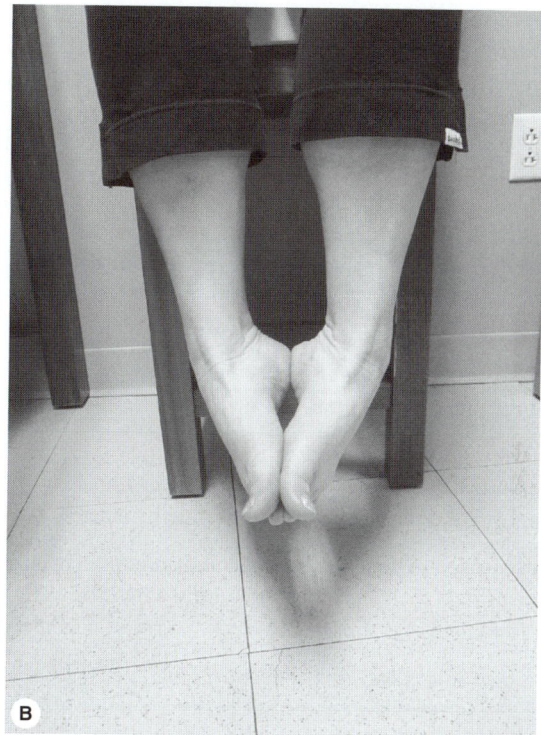

Figure 20-4. (*Continued*) Sole-to-sole posterior tibialis strengthening exercise. **B.** The patient slowly inverts the feet so that the soles of the feet are facing and then returns to the starting position.

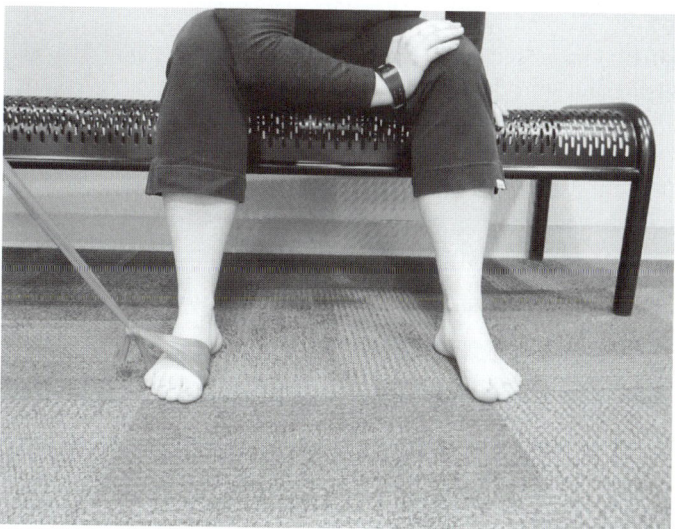

Figure 20-5. Resisted foot adduction exercise. With the band held at a 45° angle, and the leg to be exercised stabilized by the individual, the patient starts in an abducted foot position and adducts the right forefoot in the transverse plane while maintaining constant tension on the band.

foot adduction exercise, the same research team found that the tibialis posterior was most effectively activated with the concurrent use of an orthosis in a shoe.[28] In a comparison of eccentric and concentric tibialis posterior strengthening exercises in conjunction with foot orthoses, an eccentric strength protocol has been associated with the greatest improvements in pain and function; however, individuals in both strengthening groups improved more than individuals who used orthoses alone.[13]

Evidence-Based Clinical Recommendations

SORT: Strength of Recommendation Taxonomy
A: Consistent, good-quality patient-oriented evidence
B: Inconsistent or limited-quality patient-oriented evidence
C: Consensus, disease-oriented evidence, usual practice, expert opinion, or case series

1. Individuals with posterior tibial tendon dysfunction present with lower longitudinal arch height and dynamic findings of ankle pronation. **Grade A**

2. Bracing should be used to raise the medial longitudinal arch and prevent hindfoot eversion in individuals with PTTD, particularly when the individual is limited in the ability to ambulate or is unable to perform a single-leg heel rise. **Grade B**

3. Therapeutic programs that incorporate high-repetition and low-resistance strengthening exercises for the posterior tibialis and ankle plantar flexors decrease pain, increase posterior tibialis strength, and improve ambulation in individuals with PTTD. **Grade B**

COMPREHENSION QUESTIONS

20.1 A patient diagnosed with stage I PTTD reports pain particularly during squatting and stair descent. Visual analysis of squatting reveals neutral spine and femur position and a foot that progressively pronates with the depth of the squat. Which examination finding can *best* reveal the cause of foot pronation?
A. Arch height index
B. Gastrocnemius length
C. Hip abductor strength
D. Talocrural joint accessory mobility

20.2 An outpatient physical therapist evaluates a patient who was referred to physical therapy for stage II PTTD and an inability to perform a single-leg heel rise. Which exercise is *most* appropriate to add to the initial home program?
A. Double-leg heel rises
B. Eccentric Achilles strengthening off a step
C. Seated resisted plantar flexion with elastic band
D. "Sole-to-sole" ankle inversion

ANSWERS

20.1 **D.** Talocrural joint accessory mobility is used to assess the mobility of the ankle joint and is used to differentiate between capsular and muscular limitations. Because this patient's complaint occurs during a functional task in which the knee is flexed, the gastrocnemius is not maximally stretched, therefore gastrocnemius length is not the most likely contributor (option B).

20.2 **D.** "Sole-to-sole" ankle inversion is the exercise that best isolates the posterior tibialis muscle. In a patient who has stage II PTTD, the posterior tibialis tendon frequently is deficient at inverting the hindfoot, which is a prerequisite to plantar flexor strengthening. Alvarez et al.[14] have shown that a high-repetition, low-load program that begins with sole-to-sole exercises was effective in decreasing pain and increasing function in patients with PTTD.

REFERENCES

1. Thordarson DB, Schmotzer H, Chon J, Peters J. Dynamic support of the human longitudinal arch. A biomechanical evaluation. *Clin Orthop Relat Res*. 1995;316:165-172.
2. Deland JT, de Asla RJ, Sung IH, Ernberg LA, Potter HG. Posterior tibial tendon insufficiency: which ligaments are involved? *Foot Ankle Int*. 2005;26:427-435.
3. Geideman WM, Johnson JE. Posterior tibial tendon dysfunction. *J Orthop Sports Phys Ther*. 2000;30:68-77.
4. Myerson MS. Adult acquired flatfoot deformity: treatment of dysfunction of the posterior tibial tendon. *Instr Course Lect*. 1997;46:393-405.
5. Johnson KA, Strom DE. Tibialis posterior tendon dysfunction. *Clin Orthop Relat Res*. 1989;239:196-206.
6. Rabbito M, Pohl MB, Humble N, Ferber R. Biomechanical and clinical factors related to stage I posterior tibial tendon dysfunction. *J Orthop Sports Phys Ther*. 2011;41:776-784.
7. Neville C, Flemister A, Tome J, Houck J. Comparison of changes in posterior tibialis muscle length between subjects with posterior tibial tendon dysfunction and healthy controls during walking. *J Orthop Sports Phys Ther*. 2007;37:661-669.
8. Mann RA, Thompson FM. Rupture of the posterior tibial tendon causing flat foot. Surgical treatment. *J Bone Joint Surg Am*. 1985;67:556-561.
9. Johnson KA. Tibialis posterior tendon rupture. *Clin Orthop Relat Res*. 1983;140-147.
10. O'Connor K, Baumhauer J, Houck JR. Patient factors in the selection of operative versus nonoperative treatment for posterior tibial tendon dysfunction. *Foot Ankle Int*. 2010;31:197-202.
11. Chao W, Wapner KL, Lee TH, Adams J, Hecht PJ. Nonoperative management of posterior tibial tendon dysfunction. *Foot Ankle Int*. 1996;17:736-741.
12. Augustin JF, Lin SS, Berberian WS, Johnson JE. Nonoperative treatment of adult acquired flat foot with the Arizona brace. *Foot Ankle Clin*. 2003;8:491-502.
13. Kulig K, Reischl SF, Pomrantz AB, et al. Nonsurgical management of posterior tibial tendon dysfunction with orthoses and resistive exercise: a randomized controlled trial. *Phys Ther*. 2009;89:26-37.
14. Alvarez RG, Marini A, Schmitt C, Saltzman CL. Stage I and II posterior tibial tendon dysfunction treated by a structured nonoperative management protocol: an orthosis and exercise program. *Foot Ankle Int*. 2006;27:2-8.
15. Tome J, Nawoczenski DA, Flemister A, Houck J. Comparison of foot kinematics between subjects with posterior tibialis tendon dysfunction and healthy controls. *J Orthop Sports Phys Ther*. 2006;36:635-644.

16. Houck JR, Neville C, Tome J, Flemister AS. Foot kinematics during a bilateral heel rise test in participants with stage II posterior tibial tendon dysfunction. *J Orthop Sports Phys Ther*. 2009;39:593-603.
17. Williams DS, McClay IS. Measurements used to characterize the foot and the medial longitudinal arch: reliability and validity. *Phys Ther*. 2000;80:864-871.
18. Butler RJ, Hillstrom H, Song J, Richards CJ, Davis IS. Arch height index measurement system: establishment of reliability and normative values. *J Am Podiatr Med Assoc*. 2008;98:102-106.
19. Kulig K, Popovich JM Jr, Noceti-Dewit LM, Reischl SF, Kim D. Women with posterior tibial tendon dysfunction have diminished ankle and hip muscle performance. *J Orthop Sports Phys Ther*. 2011;41:687-694.
20. Martin RL, McPoil TG. Reliability of ankle goniometric measurements: a literature review. *J Am Podiatr Med Assoc*. 2005;95:564-572.
21. Neumann DA. *Kinesiology of the Musculoskeletal System. Foundations for Rehabilitation*. 2nd ed. St Louis, MO: Elsevier; 2010.
22. Kendall FP, McCreary EK, Provance PG, Rodgers MM, Romani WA. *Muscles: Testing and Function, With Posture and Pain*. 5th ed. Balitmore, MD: Lippincott Williams & Wilkins; 2005.
23. Lunsford BR, Perry J. The standing heel-rise test for ankle plantar flexion: criterion for normal. *Phys Ther*. 1995;75:694-698.
24. Ness ME, Long J, Marks R, Harris G. Foot and ankle kinematics in patients with posterior tibial tendon dysfunction. *Gait Posture*. 2008;27:331-339.
25. Lin JL, Balbas J, Richardson EG. Results of non-surgical treatment of stage II posterior tibial tendon dysfunction: a 7- to 10-year followup. *Foot Ankle Int*. 2008;29:781-786.
26. Neville C, Lemley FR. Effect of ankle-foot orthotic devices on foot kinematics in Stage II posterior tibial tendon dysfunction. *Foot Ankle Int*. 2012;33:406-414.
27. Kulig K, Burnfield JM, Requejo SM, Sperry M, Terk M. Selective activation of tibialis posterior: evaluation by magnetic resonance imaging. *Med Sci Sports Exerc*. 2004;36:862-867.
28. Kulig K, Burnfield JM, Reischl S, Requejo SM, Blanco CE, Thordarson DB. Effect of foot orthoses on tibialis posterior activation in persons with pes planus. *Med Sci Sports Exerc*. 2005;37:24-29.

Stress Fracture in Middle-Aged Runner

Kari Brown Budde

CASE 21

A 51-year-old male distance runner was referred to an outpatient physical therapy clinic with left shin pain. The patient started running 18 months ago to "lose weight." He reported enjoying running as his primary recreation. One year ago, the patient was treated by a physical therapist after experiencing an onset of left hip pain while running his first half marathon. The patient had been running approximately 30 miles per week. During that physical therapy episode of care, he underwent a video running gait analysis and participated in gait retraining modification and interventions to address hip mobility impairments. After 5 visits, he was able to return to his previous mileage and run in 5K and 10K races. The patient continued his training program of running 30 miles per week; however, he began experiencing left shin pain 8 months ago. Despite the pain, the patient continued to train because he wanted to run his first marathon. He completed the full marathon with a time of 5:23:29. His shin pain significantly worsened after the event. The patient saw his primary care physician (PCP) on multiple occasions over the last 6 months. One month ago, the PCP diagnosed a left tibial stress fracture, recommended running cessation, placed the patient in a walking boot with bilateral crutches and non-weightbearing status, and referred him to physical therapy. At the time of the initial physical therapy examination, the patient had not been running for 1 month. He had been ambulating with bilateral axillary crutches and non-weightbearing on the left leg until the week prior to physical therapy when he attempted to run a half mile after being released from his boot. Eight months after his initial shin pain symptoms, the patient still reports pain in the left shin during and after running. His premorbid functional status included pain-free running up to 30 miles per week. The patient's past medical history includes a right peroneal tendon tear 1 year ago, strained right hamstring 2 years ago, and a motocross accident 3 years ago that resulted in 5 fractured ribs, right acromioclavicular joint sprain, left wrist sprain, and left hip contusions. His surgical history includes a medial collateral ligament repair of the right knee 41 years ago and right arthroscopic knee surgery with debridement 3 years ago.

- ▶ Based on the diagnosis of tibial stress fracture, what do you anticipate may be the contributors to his activity limitations?
- ▶ What are the most appropriate physical therapy interventions and the safest way to progress the patient back to sport?
- ▶ What is his rehabilitation prognosis?

KEY DEFINITIONS

INSUFFICIENCY FRACTURE: Fracture that occurs because of normal loading placed on a bone with impaired healing capacity[1]

STRESS FRACTURE: Material fatigue failure of a bone; typically occurs in weightbearing lower extremity bones due to overuse or abnormal or high loading[2-7]

WOLFF'S LAW: Describes the normal, healthy remodeling process of bone after stress is applied; through adaptive response and remodeling, bone should be able to respond to crack initiation and loading by strengthening the bone for further loading.[3,4,8]

Objectives

1. Describe the classification system of stress fractures.
2. Describe the primary diagnostic tests for a stress fracture.
3. Describe how the physical therapist can determine when to treat a runner's stress fracture conservatively and when to refer to another healthcare provider.
4. Identify physical therapy interventions for a runner with a stress fracture.
5. Based on the examination and signs and symptoms, determine when to advise a client to cease running activities and perform cross-training activities.

Physical Therapy Considerations

PT considerations during management of the middle-age runner with tibial stress fracture:

- **General physical therapy plan of care/goals:** Decrease pain; increase ambulation ability with less pain for activities of daily living (ADLs); increase strength, dynamic control, and endurance for return-to-sport activities with decreased pain and risk of re-injury

- **Physical therapy interventions:** Patient education on diagnosis, prognosis, potential causes of injury, anticipated barriers or challenges to care, risks and benefits of physical therapy and anticipated outcomes; manual interventions to increase joint mobility, flexibility, and decrease pain; therapeutic exercise and neuromuscular re-education to decrease abnormal and dysfunctional movement patterns, increase strength, endurance and dynamic body control for return to running; home exercise instruction and education for best possible outcomes and safe return to running; video running gait analysis to assess and intervene with dysfunctional movement patterns that may increase stress to healing tissue

- **Precautions during physical therapy:** Monitor pain and abnormal movement patterns with gait and address precautions or contraindications for intervention based on patient's pre-existing conditions and goals

▶ **Complications interfering with physical therapy:** Inability to attend physical therapy sessions; noncompliance with physical therapist's recommendations; stress fracture size/stage; poor tissue quality; lower extremity mechanics and movement patterns that increase stress to affected tissue; patient's work activities that may interfere with healing

Understanding the Health Condition

In normal healthy bone, any stress or loading causes some deformation and microdamage.[3] Wolff's law states that healthy bone remodels in response to repetitive loading by laying down new bone tissue at the site of loading to resist the stress.[3,4,8] If the loading or stress to the bone in a specific site is greater or faster than the body can repair, the initial stage of a stress fracture can occur. Stress fractures are most commonly found in the lower extremities, particularly the tibia, of running and jumping athletes.[9] Stress fractures have 3 stages.[1,4,10] The first stage is crack initiation, which occurs at the site where the load stress is concentrated in a specific spot. The second stage is crack propagation that occurs when loading continues above the level at which bone can be repaired or new bone can be laid down. The final stage is a complete fracture with symptomatic presentation. Stress fractures are distinct from insufficiency fractures. An insufficiency fracture occurs when normal stress is applied to a bone that has *deficient* healing capacity and thus is unable to repair and remodel fast enough to prevent a fracture.[1] Insufficiency fractures represent impaired healing capacity that occurs in people with bone disorders, elderly females with low bone density, and in athletes with components of the female athlete triad (see Case 14). Differential diagnosis of an insufficiency fracture should be considered when assessing athletes with stress fractures because this diagnosis may predispose the athlete to future fractures and proper diagnosis is imperative to rehabilitation success.

Stress fractures occur when there is an imbalance between crack initiation and propagation and the body's ability to respond to these processes. Intrinsic risk factors for stress fractures include faulty static and dynamic biomechanics, abnormal bony alignment, and hormonal status.[11-16] Excessive forefoot varus, high longitudinal arch, and leg length inequality increase the risk of stress fractures.[13] Female runners, especially those with a history of menstrual irregularities, less lean mass in the lower extremities, leg length discrepancy, lower bone density, and a lower-fat diet, have an increased risk of lower extremity stress fractures.[9] Because estrogen and progesterone help calcium deposit into bone and maintain normal bone density, lower levels of these hormones in females have been associated with increased risk of lower extremity stress fracture.[11-13] Extrinsic risk factors for stress fractures include training errors, altered neuromuscular control, sport conditioning, and running form.[11-16]

Stress fractures are diagnosed by subjective history of symptoms during activity and through diagnostic imaging. The patient with a stress fracture typically describes pain only during activity. However, as the stress response progresses, the patient may feel pain at all times at the site of the injury.[17] At this stage, there is reproducible tenderness to palpation over the injured area on the bone. Radiographs and diagnostic ultrasound have not been reliable in diagnosing a stress fracture.[18-21] Bone scintigraphy has been reported to be nearly 100% sensitive for stress injuries of bone; however, it has lower specificity than magnetic resonance imaging (MRI).[22,23] MRI is currently considered the gold standard for diagnosing lower extremity stress fracture.[22,23]

The athlete's physical condition, neuromuscular control, and biomechanics all play a role in the stresses applied to the skeleton and the subsequent ability to dissipate these potentially injurious loads. Ideal neuromuscular control allows muscles to slowly absorb loads and dissipate ground reaction forces during activity. When muscles contract normally, they serve as shock absorbers that gradually place stress on bones, allowing healthy loading and reducing the risk of stress fracture.[3] If muscles are fatigued, they cannot effectively decrease the energy that is absorbed by the bones; this allows external forces to load the bone in a more abrupt manner, possibly leading to microtrauma.[10] Muscle fatigue and corresponding poor biomechanical and neuromuscular control may induce higher stress to the bones and lead to stress fractures.[3,10]

Physical Therapy Patient/Client Management

Patients often come to physical therapists with a general diagnosis from their PCP of "shin pain" or "leg pain." If the physical therapist suspects a stress fracture after the initial evaluation, referral back to the physician for diagnostic imaging must be made. Once a definitive diagnosis of a stress fracture has been determined through physical examination and bone scintigraphy and/or MRI, physical therapy interventions can ensue. Patients diagnosed with lower extremity stress fractures can benefit from physical therapy interventions including manual therapy, therapeutic exercise, and modalities. These interventions should fit into the overall plan of care agreed upon by patient and physician. Manual therapy techniques are performed to decrease pain and increase mobility of joints surrounding the fracture. Therapeutic exercises are prescribed to address muscular weakness and to promote proximal and distal joint stability. Modalities such as bone stimulation and cryotherapy are administered to promote healing and decrease pain.

Examination, Evaluation, and Diagnosis

Examination of an injured runner consists of a comprehensive assessment of the entire lower extremity including posture, range of motion, flexibility, strength, functional movement patterns, and gait (walking and running).

Beginning with the athlete standing, the therapist assesses foot type, posture, and lower extremity alignment to gain an appreciation of intrinsic alignment and stability. Gait assessment in bare feet and in the patient's chosen running footwear should be assessed at the patient's current level of function. The patient in this case has only recently started to walk without the use of the boot and an assistive device (crutches), so only walking should be assessed. A running gait analysis should only be performed when the referring physician has cleared the patient to return to sport.

Next, leg length and range of motion, joint mobility, and flexibility of the lower extremities are assessed. The best way to measure lower extremity limb length is to measure the distance from the patient's anterior superior iliac spine to the terminal portion of the medial malleolus. Limited or decreased joint mobility or flexibility can place uneven stress on the lower extremities and decrease the body's ability to absorb ground reaction forces.[24]

Strength assessment should be performed bilaterally for all lower extremity muscles to identify isolated muscle weakness. Hip muscle weakness can cause increased femoral internal rotation and hip adduction, leading to poor lower extremity control and increased valgus stress on the legs. Muscular weakness of the gluteus maximus and medius can increase the risk of stress fractures.[25,26] Ankle and foot strength are also important for the athlete to be able to limit excessive rear foot eversion angles.[25,26] Last, core strength should be assessed because running is a sport of balance and stability; proximal control helps with lower extremity coordination and helps with absorbing stresses.[27]

If the patient does not already have a confirmed diagnosis of a stress fracture, the physical therapist can perform special tests to rule in or rule out a stress fracture during the initial examination. These special tests include the heel tap test (also known as the percussion test), the fulcrum test, the squeeze test, and the tuning fork test (Table 21-1).[28] Reproduction of the patient's pain in these tests indicates a positive test. However, the therapist should be aware that the diagnostic utility of these tests is either limited or unknown.

A functional assessment of the lower extremities helps to determine if the athlete has poor lower extremity movement patterns including (but not limited to) a dynamic lower extremity posture often referred to as "miserable malalignment" that consists of knee valgus, femoral internal rotation, and hip adduction. Common functional tests that can be performed include single-leg balance, bilateral and unilateral squat, jumping, single-leg hopping, and the step-down test.[29] These functional tests often highlight gross movement dysfunction to help the physical therapist determine the need for neuromuscular retraining as part of the rehabilitation plan.

Running gait should be assessed before progression back to running. Running gait analysis is important to determine underlying biomechanical movement patterns that may increase the risk of stress fractures. This assessment enables the therapist to determine which dysfunctional movement patterns need to be addressed to help prevent continued stress to the healing fracture site when the patient is ready to return to activity. Patterns that can increase lower extremity stresses and risk of injury include stiffness of the knee in the sagittal plane, increased hip adduction moment, decreased cadence, and increased rearfoot eversion angles.[25,26,30,31]

Plan of Care and Interventions

A 3-phase (acute, subacute, and chronic) treatment approach is beneficial for patients with a lower extremity stress fracture. The acute phase focuses on rest and interventions to relieve symptoms, whereas the subacute phase focuses on progressing weightbearing tolerance.[32,33] Rest can range from complete rest (e.g., non-weightbearing on involved extremity and immobilization) to relative rest. Relative

Table 21-1	SPECIAL TESTS ASSOCIATED WITH STRESS FRACTURES
Test	Test Position
Heel tap (percussion test)	The patient is supine on treatment table. The therapist elevates involved lower extremity off the table. The therapist applies a forceful "tap" to the heel with the force directed along the long axis of the lower extremity.
Fulcrum test	The patient sits with lower extremities hanging off the end of a treatment table. The therapist stabilizes the involved leg by holding the ankle. The therapist applies a force with the opposite hand to create a fulcrum—in a medial direction followed by lateral direction to the injured region.
Squeeze test	The patient is supine on treatment table. The therapist compresses the tibia and fibula (squeezing them together) distal to injury site.
Tuning fork test	The patient is supine on treatment table with knee of affected extremity flexed to 90° and foot flat on the tabletop. The therapist strikes the tuning fork prior to applying it to the injury site.

rest describes avoiding the performance of activities that cause pain or replicate the pathomechanical loading of the bone. Relative rest is recommended for 4 to 6 weeks in individuals with suspected or confirmed diagnosis of a stress fracture. If pain resolves after the initial weeks of relative rest, the rehabilitation process can continue with weightbearing activities and strengthening to promote tissue healing and the patient can gradually return to sport or activity. However, if pain persists after the initial prescription of relative rest, complete rest (with or without immobilization) is recommended for an *additional* 4 to 6 weeks. If pain increases and the activity modification, rest, and immobilization are not adequate to decrease pain, surgical immobilization may be warranted.[17] For the patient in this case, running was restricted but walking and swimming were encouraged to maintain his cardiovascular fitness without stress to the injured bone.

The goal of the subacute phase is to progress to weightbearing strengthening and activities when the patient can tolerate these without reproduction of symptoms.[33] When developing strengthening exercises for runners with lower extremity stress fractures, **strengthening the lower extremities and core muscles should be initiated in non-weightbearing positions.** Strengthening exercises that require a high percentage of maximal voluntary isometric contraction (MVIC) are effective in targeting underlying weaknesses.[34] According to Boren et al.,[33] the best exercises for activating the gluteus medius are the side plank (Fig. 21-1), clamshell with internal rotation (Fig. 21-2), front plank with hip extension (Fig. 21-3), and sidelying abduction (Fig. 21-4). Activation of the gluteus maximus is highest with front plank with hip extension and side plank with hip abduction leg lift (Fig. 21-5).[35] Other lower extremity muscles that may help increase shock absorption include the quadriceps, hamstrings, and the muscles controlling the ankles. If weaknesses are identified in the examination, these muscles should be strengthened. Resisted ankle strengthening exercises can be performed in all directions (Fig 21-6). The physical therapist should tailor the strengthening exercise prescription to build muscular endurance, using low resistance and high repetitions.

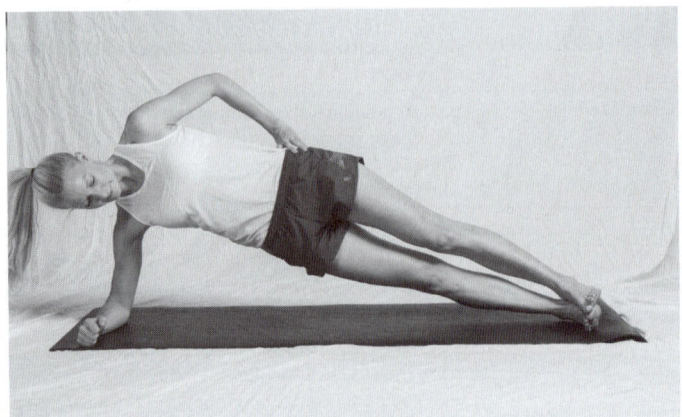

Figure 21-1. Side plank.

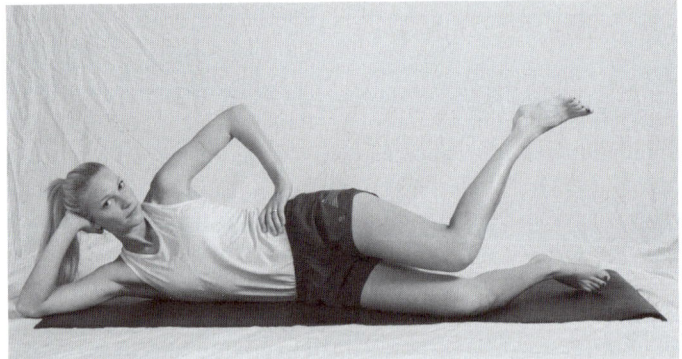

Figure 21-2. Clamshell with internal rotation (reverse clamshell).

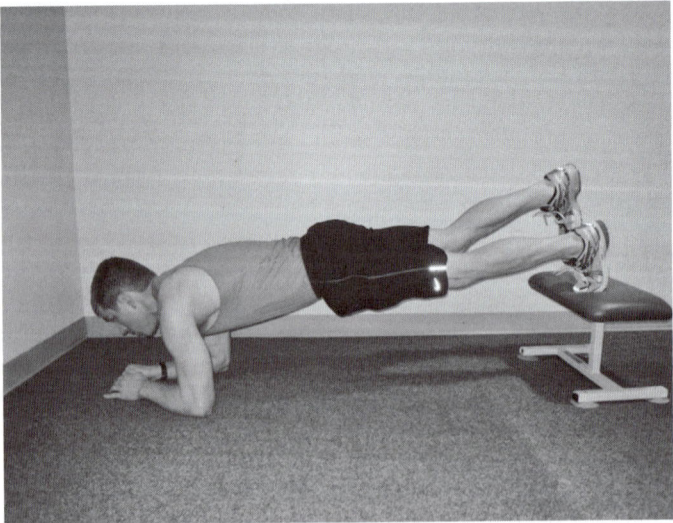

Figure 21-3. Front plank with hip extension.

SECTION III: CASE 21 357

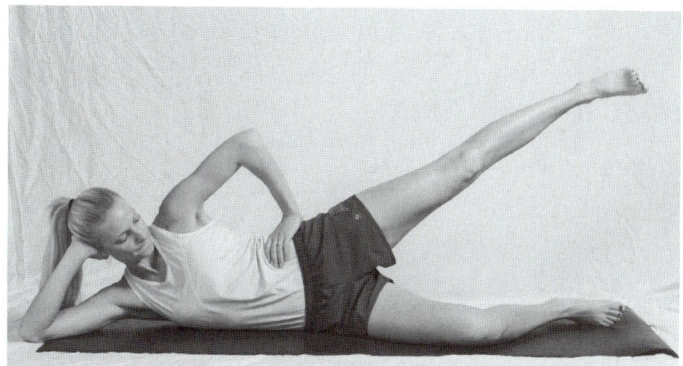

Figure 21-4. Sidelying hip abduction.

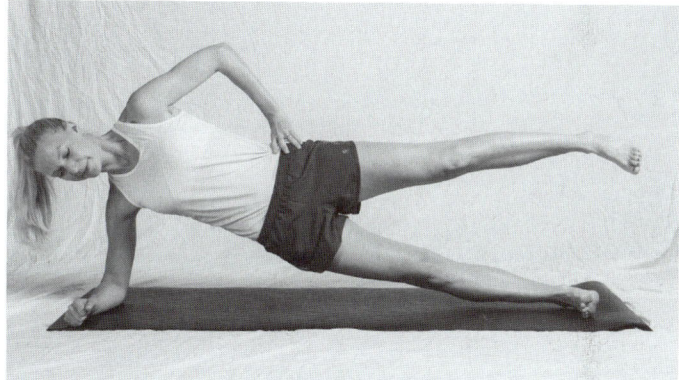

Figure 21-5. Side plank with hip abduction leg lift.

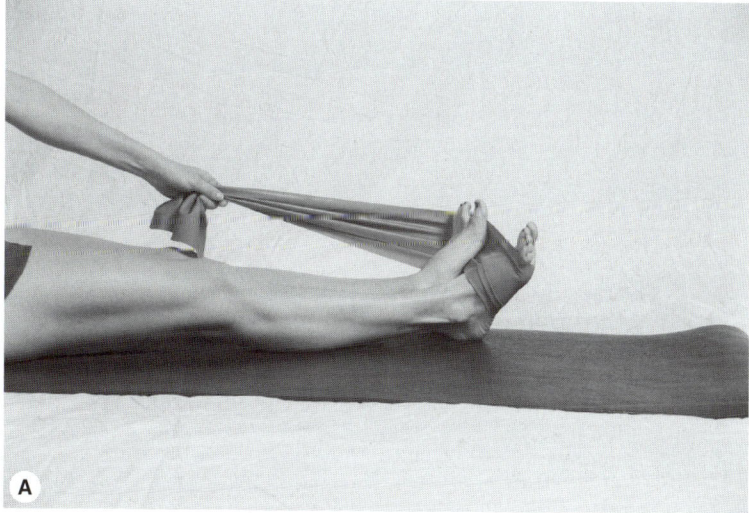

Figure 21-6. Ankle movement exercises with resistive tubing. **A.** Eversion.

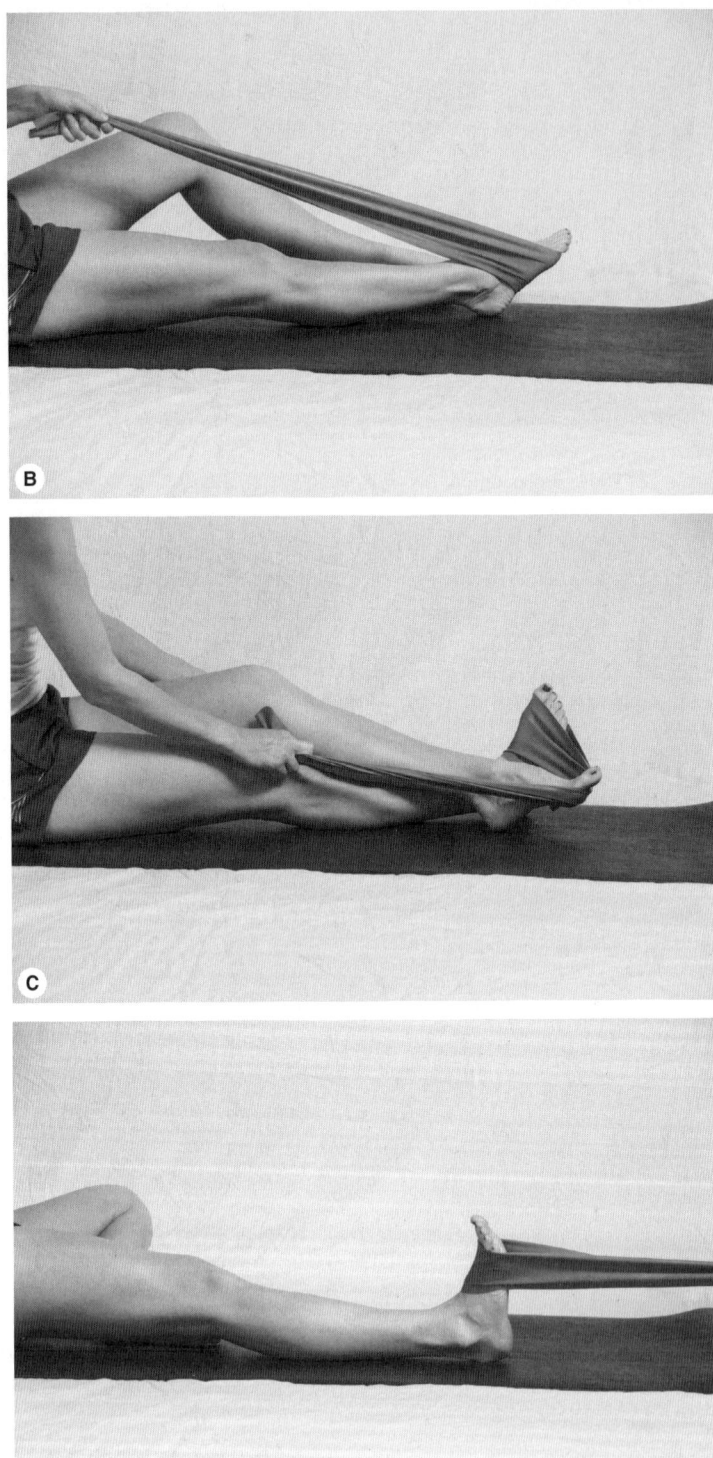

Figure 21-6. (*Continued*) Ankle movement exercises with resistive tubing. **B.** Plantar flexion. **C.** Inversion. **D.** Dorsiflexion.

The therapist can also begin to address decreased flexibility and joint hypomobility at this early stage in the healing process. Interventions such as soft tissue and joint mobilizations performed to increase flexibility and joint mobility must not increase pain at this stage in the healing process. Pain-eliciting manual treatments may delay the healing process.[33] During the loading response in gait, hip flexion, knee flexion, ankle dorsiflexion, and subtalar pronation help dissipate ground reaction forces and assist in keeping the center of gravity low.[36] Regaining strength and normalized movement patterns through strengthening and neuromuscular re-education can provide the patient with improved ground reaction loading and shock absorption to decrease stress and strain on the injured bone. Maintenance of cardiovascular fitness through non- or partial weightbearing aerobic activities, either through biking or swimming, can also be started at this stage. If available, deep water running or antigravity treadmill training may also be used in the first phase of rehabilitation to reintroduce the patient to running.[24] Reports of pain during or after cross-training is a sign that the fracture is not healed and the patient should stop cross-training at that point.[33] Other suggestions for the subacute phase of rehabilitation include addressing footwear and running training plans and how these may impact the injury. Referral to a dietician may be appropriate to address any nutritional concerns that may have played a role in the injury and in rehabilitation.

Strengthening is next progressed in more functional weightbearing positions. Based on the high percentage of MVIC that occurs during the single squat and the lateral step-up exercises, these are ideal to continue to address weakness in the gluteus maximus and medius muscles.[35] Distefano et al.[37] also recommend lateral band resisted walks (Fig. 21-7) for gluteus medius strengthening and the single-leg deadlift (Fig. 21-8) for gluteus medius and maximus strengthening. During the subacute stage, the running athlete should also be introduced to eccentric strengthening and functional movement exercises. Eccentric loading helps accustom the runner to the ground reaction forces that will be experienced during running. The prescription of functional movements can facilitate improvements in neuromuscular control and reduce abnormal movement patterns (*e.g.*, miserable malalignment). Maintenance of cardiovascular conditioning is also continued in this phase. The patient can begin cross-training on an elliptical or arc trainer in addition to the previously mentioned forms of cross-training. The athlete can also begin to improve walking endurance, with a goal of tolerating 30 minutes of vigorous walking without exacerbation of symptoms prior to progression into a return-to-running program.[38] An athlete should be able to walk and perform ADLs symptom-free for a minimum of 2 weeks prior to initiating a return to running program.

During the final functional phase of rehabilitation of stress fractures (> 10 weeks after injury), the athlete is gradually reintroduced to the sport.[33] Early in this phase, the athlete can be reintroduced to increasing ground reaction forces by implementing plyometric training.[39] Plyometric training should begin on bilateral lower extremities, focusing on equal weightbearing and adequate landing mechanics at the hip, knee, and ankle. Return to sport-specific activities is a gradual progression that must take into consideration multiple factors including medical and health status (*e.g.*, symptoms, signs, psychological state, laboratory tests), sport risk modifiers (*e.g.*, type of sport, competitive level), and decision modifiers (*e.g.*, pressure from athlete, external

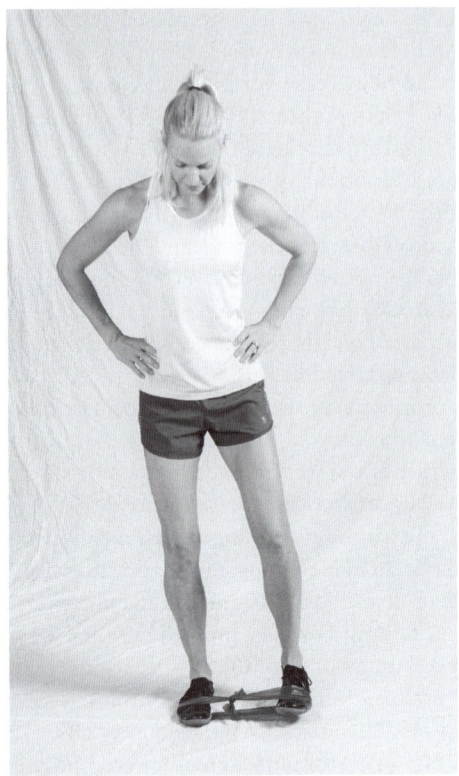

Figure 21-7. Lateral band walk.

pressure to participate in sport).[40] Progression continues from straight plane movements into multidirectional jumping and finally single-leg hopping. Based on clinical experience, the patient should be able to tolerate 300 to 400 foot contacts on the injured lower extremity without exacerbation of symptoms. Because running a mile requires approximately 750 foot contacts per leg, this would allow the patient to safely tolerate a 1/4 mile run.[39] A return-to-running program using a walk-jog progression or a gradual running progression to transition back to running is recommended to prevent re-injury.[38,39] Running should be resumed at a slower pace and shorter frequency than what was typical for the athlete. Distance and duration should be slowly increased first, followed by increased intensity, and only once the athlete is back to running typical distances.[24] Although not well supported by evidence, it is recommended that **runners should not progress their weekly mileage by more than 10% when training.**[24] It is important at this stage to continue with previous exercises addressing strengthening, flexibility, balance, neuromuscular control, and core stability to remediate identified underlying biomechanical impairments that may have led to the initial injury. Non-impact activities and cross-training should continue on days off from running to continue to address these impairments.[38]

The runner is gradually returned to running when he is asymptomatic, demonstrates restored strength and no biomechanical abnormalities, and when he is

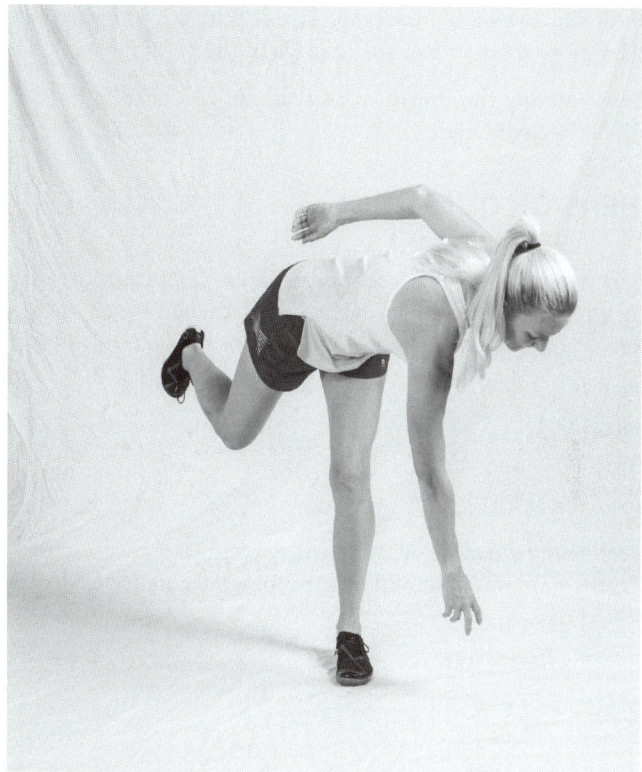

Figure 21-8. Single-leg deadlift.

allowed by the primary medical provider. If the patient experiences any pain during the return-to-running program, the program must be delayed until all activities are pain-free. Any asymmetries or abnormalities identified in the running gait analysis should be addressed by modifying the loading ability of the lower extremities to help prevent re-injury to the bone. **Techniques to decrease ground reaction forces on the bone** include increasing steps per minute[31] and modifying the impact load by providing visual feedback during real-time gait retraining.[41-43]

Evidence-Based Clinical Recommendations

SORT: Strength of Recommendation Taxonomy

A: Consistent, good-quality patient-oriented evidence
B: Inconsistent or limited-quality patient-oriented evidence
C: Consensus, disease-oriented evidence, usual practice, expert opinion, or case series

1. Strengthening exercises for the lower extremities and core muscles should be initiated in non-weightbearing positions for runners with lower extremity stress fractures. **Grade C**

2. For the individual with a history of stress fracture, running should not be increased by more than 10% of the mileage of the previous week. **Grade C**

3. Techniques to modify running form decrease the risk of re-injury once the stress fracture site is healed. **Grade C**

COMPREHENSION QUESTIONS

21.1 During the initial stages of a suspected stress fracture, which test could the physical therapist perform to determine if the shin pain is due to a stress fracture?

A. Bone scintigraphy

B. Squeeze test

C. MRI

D. Step-down test

21.2 When returning a patient with a history of tibial stress fracture to running, which is the best way to modify his running mechanics to decrease stress to the affected tissue?

A. Increasing heel strike

B. Decreasing steps per minute

C. Decreasing push off

D. Increasing steps per minute

ANSWERS

21.1 **B.** The squeeze test is a physical examination special test that the physical therapist can use to help determine if pain is reproduced by placing compression stress to the affected area of the tibia or fibula on the affected lower extremity.[30] MRI (option C) and bone scintigraphy (option A) are diagnostic imaging that have been used to diagnose stress fractures; however, physical therapists cannot perform these tests. MRI is the gold standard for diagnosing lower extremity stress fracture. Physical therapists often ask patients to perform the step-down test (option D). However, this is a functional test used to highlight movement dysfunction, especially in the lower extremities.

21.2 **D.** Heiderscheit et al.[31] reported that by increasing step rate during running, the ground reaction forces to the lower extremities can be significantly reduced.

REFERENCES

1. Koch JC. The laws of bone architecture. *Am J Anat.* 1917;21:177-298.

2. Baker J, Frankel VH, Burstein A. Fatigue fractures: biomechanical considerations. *J Bone Joint Surg.* 1972;54:1345-1346.

3. Jones BH, Harris JM, Vinh TN, Rubin C. Exercise-induced stress fractures and stress reactions of bone: epidemiology, etiology, and classification. *Exerc Sport Sci Rev.* 1989;17:379-422.
4. Keaveny TM, Hayes WC. Mechanical properties of cortical and trabecular bone. In: Hall BK, ed. *Bone.* Boca Raton, FL; CRC Press; 1993:285-344.
5. Alba E, Youngberg R. Occult fractures of the femoral neck. *Am J Emerg Med.* 1992;10:64-68.
6. Hulkko A, Orava S. Stress fractures in athletes. *Int J Sports Med.* 1987;8:221-226.
7. McBryde AM Jr. Stress fractures in athletes. *J Sports Med.* 1975;3:212-217.
8. Li GP, Zhang SD, Chen G, Chen H, Wang AM. Radiographic and histologic analyses of stress fracture in rabbit tibias. *Am J Sports Med.* 1985;13:285-294.
9. Bennell KL, Malcolm SA, Thomas SA, et al. Risk factors for stress fractures in track and field athletes. A twelve-month prospective study. *Am J Sports Med.* 1996;24:810-818.
10. Kaeding CC, Spindler KP, Amendola A. Management of troublesome stress fractures. *Instr Course Lect.* 2004;53:455-469.
11. Barrow GW, Saha S. Menstrual irregularity and stress fractures in collegiate female distance runners. *Am J Sports Med.* 1988;16:209-216.
12. Drinkwater BL, Nilson K, Chesnut CH 3rd, Bremner WJ, Shainholtz S, Southworth MB. Bone mineral content of amenorrheic and eumenorrheic athletes. *N Engl J Med.* 1984;311:277-281.
13. Korpelainen R, Orava S, Karpakka J, Siira P, Hulkko A. Risk factors for recurrent stress fractures in athletes. *Am J Sports Med.* 2001;29:304-310.
14. Greaney RB, Gerber FH, Laughlin RL, et al. Distribution and natural history of stress fractures in U.S. Marine recruits. *Radiology.* 1983;146:339-346.
15. Milgrom C, Giladi M, Stein M, et al. Stress fractures in military recruits. A prospective study showing an unusually high incidence. *J Bone Joint Surg Br.* 1985;67:732-735.
16. Sormaala MJ, Niva MH, Kiuru MJ, Mattila VM, Pihlajamaki HK. Bone stress injuries of the talus in military recruits. *Bone.* 2006;39;199-204.
17. Kaeding CC, Miller T. The comprehensive description of stress fractures: a new classification system. *J Bone Joint Surg Am.* 2013;95:1214-1220.
18. Diehl JJ, Best TM, Kaeding CC. Classification and return-to-play consideration for stress fractures. *Clin Sports Med.* 2006;25:17-28.
19. Romani WA, Perrin DH, Dussault RG, Ball DW, Kahler DM. Identification of tibial stress fractures using therapeutic continuous ultrasound. *J Orthop Sports Phys Ther.* 2000;30:444-452.
20. Fredericson M, Jennings F, Beaulieu C, Matheson GO. Stress fractures in athletes. *Top Magn Reson Imaging.* 2006;17:309-325.
21. Wilson ES Jr, Katz FN. Stress fractures: an analysis of 250 consecutive cases. *Radiology.* 1969;92:481-486.
22. Ishibashi Y, Okamura Y, Otsuka H, Nishizawa K, Sasaki T, Toh S. Comparison of scintigraphy and magnetic resonance imaging for stress injuries of bone. *Clin J Sports Med.* 2002;12:79-84.
23. Shin AY, Morin WD, Gorman JD, Jones SB, Lapinsky AS. The superiority of magnetic resonance imaging in differentiating the cause of hip pain in endurance athletes. *Am J Sports Med.* 1996;24:168-176.
24. Liem BC, Truswell HJ, Harrast MA. Rehabilitation and return to running after lower limb stress fractures. *Curr Sports Med Rep.* 2013;12:200-207.
25. Pohl MB, Mullineaux DR, Milner CE, Hamill J, Davis IS. Biomechanical predictors of retrospective tibia stress fractures in runners. *J Biomech.* 2008;41:1160-1165.
26. Milner CE, Hamill J, Davis IS. Distinct hip and rearfoot kinematics in female runners with a history of tibial stress fracture. *J Orthop Sports Phys Ther.* 2010;40:59-66.
27. Fredericson M, Moore T. Muscular balance, core stability and injury prevention for middle- and long-distance runner. *Phys Med Rehabil Clin N Am.* 2005;16:669-689.

28. Magee DJ. *Orthopedic Physical Assessment*. 5th ed. St. Louis, MO: Saunders; 2008.
29. Magrum E, Wilder RP. Evaluation of the injured runner. *Clin Sports Med*. 2010;29:331-345.
30. Milner CE, Hamill J, Davis I. Are knee mechanics during early stance related to tibial stress fracture in runners? *Clin Biomech*. 2007;22:697-703.
31. Heiderscheit BC, Chumanov ES, Michalski MP, Wille CM, Ryan MB. Effects of step rate manipulation on joint mechanics during running. *Med Sci Sports Exerc*. 2011;43:296-302.
32. Fredericson M, Jennings F, Beaulieu C, Matheson GO. Stress fractures in athletes. *Top Magn Reson Imaging*. 2006;17:309-325.
33. Dugan SA, Weber KM. Stress fractures and rehabilitation. *Phys Med Rehabil Clin N Am*. 2007;18:401-416.
34. Anderson LL, Magnusson SP, Nielsen M, Haleem J, Poulsen K, Aagaard P. Neuromuscular activation in conventional therapeutic exercises and heavy resistance exercises: implications for rehabilitation. *Phys Ther*. 2006;86:683-697.
35. Boren K, Conrey C, Le Cougic JL, Paprocki L, Voight M, Robinson TK. Electromyographic analysis of gluteus medius and gluteus maximus during rehabilitation exercises. *Int J Sports Phys Ther*. 2011;6:206-223.
36. Dugan SA, Bhat KP. Biomechanics and analysis of running gait. *Phys Med Rehabil Clin N Am*. 2005;16:603-621.
37. Distefano LJ, Blackburn JT, Marshall SW, Padua DA. Gluteal muscle activation during common therapeutic exercises. *J Orthop Sports Phys Ther*. 2009;39:532-540.
38. Harrast MA, Colonno D. Stress fractures in runners. *Clin Sports Med*. 2010;29:399-416.
39. Wilcox R. Running injury prevention tips & return to running program. The Brigham and Women's Hospital, Inc. Department of Rehabilitation Services. http://www.brighamandwomens.org/patients_visitors/pcs/rehabilitationservices/physical%20therapy%20standards%20of%20care%20and%20protocols/le%20-%20running%20injury%20prevention%20tips%20&%20return%20to%20running%20program.pdf. Accessed January 29, 2015.
40. Creighton DW, Shrier I, Shultz R, Meeuwisse WH, Matheson GO. Return-to-play in sport: a decision-based model. *Clin J Sport Med*. 2010;20:379-385.
41. Willy RW, Scholz JP, Davis IS. Mirror gait retraining for treatment of patellofemoral pain in female runners. *Clin Biomech*. 2012;27:1045-1051.
42. Noehren B, Scholz J, Davis I. The effect of real-time gait retraining on hip kinematics, pain and function in subjects with patellofemoral pain syndrome. *Br J Sports Med*. 2011;45:691-696.
43. Crowell HP, Davis IS. Gait retraining to reduce lower extremity loading in runners. *Clin Biomech*. 2011;9:78-83.

Lateral Ankle Sprain

Todd E. Davenport

CASE 22

A 52-year-old recreational athlete presented with chief concern of inversion mechanism right ankle sprain occurring 6 days ago. The injury occurred during an adventure run with the staff from his office. He slipped while traversing a muddy and wet balance beam that was inclined slightly downhill. The patient felt a "pop" in his lateral ankle and midfoot at the time of injury and was only able to bear weight for a few steps immediately afterward. He walked approximately ½ mile away from the adventure run course with the assistance of a fellow competitor until he reached the first aid tent. From the first aid tent, 2 friends drove him to an urgent care clinic in the small mountain community where the adventure run was held. The on-call primary care physician at the urgent care clinic evaluated the patient and provided him with a prescription for a nonsteroidal anti-inflammatory medication, a posterior splint, and bilateral axillary crutches. He was instructed to ice the ankle for 20 minutes every 2 hours with the right lower extremity elevated, to keep all of his weight off of the right lower extremity when ambulating, and to schedule an appointment with an orthopaedic surgeon for imaging studies. No more information about the medical evaluation conducted at the urgent care clinic was available at the time of physical therapy evaluation. The patient was able to obtain an appointment with a physical therapist before his appointment with the orthopaedic surgeon.

▶ What examination signs may be associated with this diagnosis?
▶ What are the most appropriate examination tests?
▶ What are the most appropriate physical therapy interventions?
▶ Describe a physical therapy plan of care based on each stage of the health condition.

KEY DEFINTIONS

FUNCTIONAL INSTABILITY: Disabling ankle pain and swelling primarily associated with decreased ankle/foot proprioception following a lateral ankle sprain. Tests of ankle ligament laxity (*e.g.*, anterior drawer test, talar tilt test) are most often negative.

LATERAL ANKLE INJURY: Injury created by forceful inversion, plantar flexion, and adduction of the ankle and foot (*i.e.*, "hyper-supination"); associated with disruption of bony, muscular, ligamentous, and/or cartilaginous structures

MECHANICAL INSTABILITY: Disabling ankle pain and swelling associated with disrupted ligamentous fibers that support the ankle following a lateral ankle sprain; tests of ankle ligament laxity (*e.g.*, anterior drawer test, talar tilt test) are often positive.

POSTERIOR SPLINT: Rigid device that supports the posterior aspect of the ankle and the plantar aspect of the foot and is fixed in place by an elastic wrap

Objectives

1. Describe the functional and surface anatomy of the ankle and foot as they relate to the examination of a patient/client with a lateral ankle injury.
2. Describe subjective and objective examination findings that would warrant referral of an individual with a lateral ankle injury to an orthopaedic physician.
3. Apply clinical practice guidelines for physical therapy management of lateral ankle injuries.

Physical Therapy Considerations

PT considerations during management of the individual with a suspected diagnosis of inversion mechanism ankle sprain:

- **General physical therapy plan of care/goals:** Use of the Ottawa Ankle Rules to exclude need for ankle and foot plain film radiographs; decrease pain; increase active and passive range of motion (ROM) of the ankle and midfoot joints; increase lower extremity strength; restore neuromuscular function and dynamic balance; facilitate full return to prior level of athletic function

- **Physical therapy interventions:** Patient education for weightbearing as tolerated; prescription of assistive device and/or bracing; cryotherapy to decrease edema and pain; manual therapy techniques to decrease pain and edema and increase ROM; light therapeutic exercise with progression to sport-specific training as appropriate for the specific phase of tissue healing

- **Precautions during physical therapy:** Mechanical instability; adjust therapeutic exercise dosage based on symptomatic and tissue response

▶ **Complications interfering with physical therapy:** Poor tolerance to weightbearing; excessive edema and pain; mechanical instability secondary to ligament rupture; concomitant involvement of other ankle and foot structures (*e.g.*, peroneal tendon tear, distal tibiofibular joint complex pathology); severe functional instability

Understanding the Health Condition

The most common mechanism of injury for lateral ankle sprains is when forefoot adduction, hindfoot internal rotation, ankle inversion in plantar flexion, and external rotation of the leg occur beyond anatomical constraints. This injury mechanism may result when stepping off a curb or step, stepping into a hole, landing from a jump, or landing on a competitor's foot during sport activities. The injury commonly results in damage to the lateral structures of the foot and ankle. Reflexive activation of the fibularis muscles in response to the end-range supinated position may result in a rapid reactive eversion of the ankle and foot complex. As a result, the anteromedial structures of the ankle and foot also may become injured.

The incidence of ankle sprains is 2.15 per 1000 person-years in the general population, and it is highest in individuals between 15 and 19 years of age (7.2 per 1000 person-years).[1,2] Ankle sprains occur with similar frequency in males and females; however, ethnic and racial differences have been noted. African-Americans and Caucasians have higher rates of ankle sprains compared to Latinos/Hispanics.[2] Physically active individuals, particularly those who participate in court and team sports such as basketball, are at a higher risk than the general population.[3-5] Nearly half of all ankle sprains occur during athletic activity, with basketball, football, and soccer associated with the highest percentage of ankle sprains.[2] The ankle joint accounts for up to one-third of all sport-related injuries with lateral ankle sprains comprising up to 83% of these injuries.[3] The overall incidence of lateral ankle sprains may be underestimated because approximately 50% of those sustaining an ankle sprain do not seek medical attention after injury.[5,6]

Most often, a lateral ankle sprain involves either partial or complete disruption of the lateral ankle ligaments: anterior talofibular ligament, calcaneofibular ligament, and/or posterior talofibular ligament (Fig. 22-1). Almost three-fourths of lateral ankle sprains involve an isolated injury to the anterior talofibular ligament.[7] Disruption of the posterior talofibular ligament may occur; however, this rarely occurs in isolation with an inversion mechanism of injury. Injury to other structures is also possible. For example, combined injuries to ligaments supporting the subtalar, medial, and/or syndesmotic joints can occur along with a lateral ankle sprain. Following a severe lateral ankle injury, lesions can occur in the lateral subtalar ligaments, fibular tendons, peripheral nerves, extensor and fibular retinacula, inferior tibiofibular ligament, and osteochondral regions.

The rate of lateral ankle sprain re-injury is important for physical therapists to consider.[8] Data from a systematic review indicate that re-injury occurs in up to one-third of patients, with a timeframe between initial injury and second injury ranging from within 2 weeks to 8 years.[9] The re-injury rate is greater in sports such as basketball, in which up to three-fourths of athletes sustaining a lateral ankle injury may become re-injured.[5]

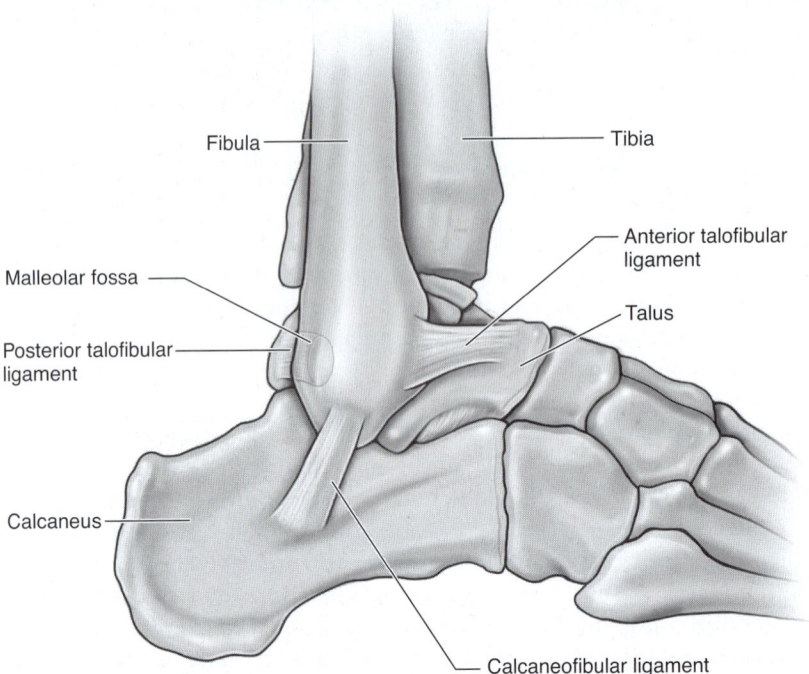

Figure 22-1. Articular anatomy of the foot and ankle showing relevant lateral ligaments. (Reproduced with permission from Morton DA, Foreman KB, Albertine KH. *The Big Picture: Gross Anantomy*. New York: McGraw-Hill Education; 2011. Figure 37-5B.)

Up to one-third of individuals continue to report symptoms 1 year after lateral ankle injury.[10] Individuals with long-term symptoms are commonly characterized as having chronic ankle instability, which can be further clinically characterized as mechanical or functional ankle instability.[11] Mechanical ankle instability has been used to describe a clinical presentation of excessive joint motion. Functional ankle instability describes normal articular motion but subjective instability that may be due to neuromuscular deficits.[12,13] Mechanical and functional instabilities involving the talocrural joint and other joints may co-exist.[14] The mechanisms and risk factors that potentially mediate the conversion from an acute lateral ankle sprain to chronic ankle instability are unknown.

Physical Therapy Patient/Client Management

This patient presented to physical therapy after consulting a primary care physician at a rural urgent care clinic. In this encounter, the physical therapist is evaluating the patient prior to consultation with a specialist, such as an orthopaedic surgeon. The physical therapist must determine the appropriateness of physical therapy, ascertain the extent and stage of the acute injury, create a plan of care, and provide appropriate initial intervention.

Examination, Evaluation, and Diagnosis

The first decision a physical therapist must make is to determine the appropriateness of physical therapy intervention,[15] even for a common orthopaedic trauma. During the examination and evaluation process, the therapist must consider competing or concomitant health conditions that may be responsible for the patient's presentation. For the patient in this case, diagnostic consideration should be broad, with the physical therapist specifically focusing on the following differential or concomitant diagnoses: iatrogenic deep vein thrombosis (DVT) from post-injury immobilization, ankle and/or foot fractures, and ligamentous laxity secondary to partial or complete ruptures.[15] The presence of one of these conditions could serve as either a contraindication or major predictor of prognosis with physical therapy interventions.

Orthopaedic trauma and subsequent immobilization are moderate to strong risk factors for the development of DVT. Wells et al.[16-18] have outlined the likelihood of a DVT based on the presence of risk factors including active cancer, immobilization of the involved extremity or paralysis/paresis, a "major" surgery within the last weeks or having been bedridden for more than 3 days, tenderness about the deep venous system, swelling of the involved lower extremity, swelling of the calf of the involved extremity that is more than 3 cm greater than the uninvolved extremity, pitting edema, and a presentation of collateral superficial veins. Using the Wells clinical prediction rule for DVT,[16-18] the patient received a score of "1" for the presence of each of the aforementioned criteria and a deduction of 2 points if an alternative diagnosis is at least as likely to account for symptom presentation. The likelihood of a person having a DVT can be predicted by the total score, with the probability being high if the score is 3 or more, moderate if the score is 1 to 2, and low if the score is 0 or less. For the current patient, the therapist added 1 point each for immobilization and pitting edema and subtracted 2 points for an alternative diagnosis (i.e., severe inversion mechanism ankle sprain). Thus, the therapist determined that the likelihood of a DVT was low based on his overall score of 0. Nevertheless, throughout the episode of care, the physical therapist will monitor the patient for symptoms and signs consistent with evolving DVT, such as severe calf tenderness, calf redness, and swelling of the calf, ankle, and foot. If symptoms and signs are present, the physical therapist should refer the patient to his primary care provider for D-dimer blood testing, venous ultrasonography, or both.[19]

Because the patient presented without any prior imaging performed on his ankle, the physical therapist must rule out the likelihood for fracture. The need for plain film radiographs of the ankle and foot can be determined on the basis of the patient's history and physical examination data. The **Ottawa Ankle Rules** comprise a clinical prediction rule that can be used to establish the need for radiographs.[20] According to the Ottawa Ankle Rules, an ankle series (anteroposterior, lateral, and oblique x-rays) may be indicated if there is tenderness along the tip of the posterior edge of the distal 6 cm of the lateral malleolus, tenderness along the medial malleolus, or if the patient is unable to bear weight for 4 steps after the injury (Fig. 22-2A).[20] A foot series may be indicated if there is tenderness at the base of the fifth metatarsal, tenderness over the navicular bone, or if the patient is unable to bear weight for 4 steps after the injury (Fig. 22-2B).[20] A large systematic review and meta-analysis

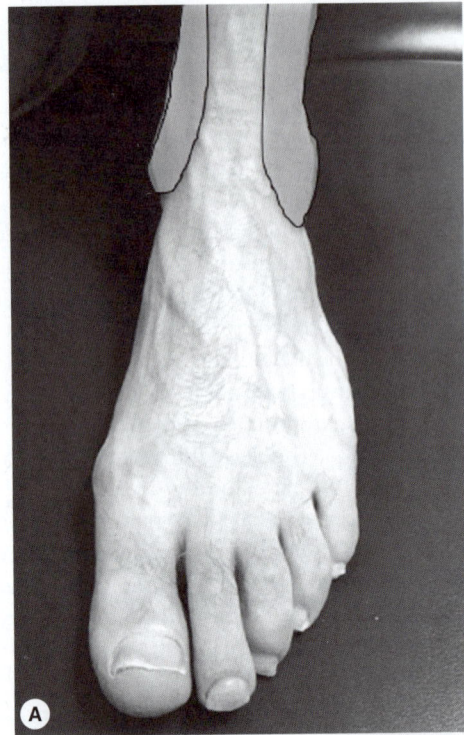

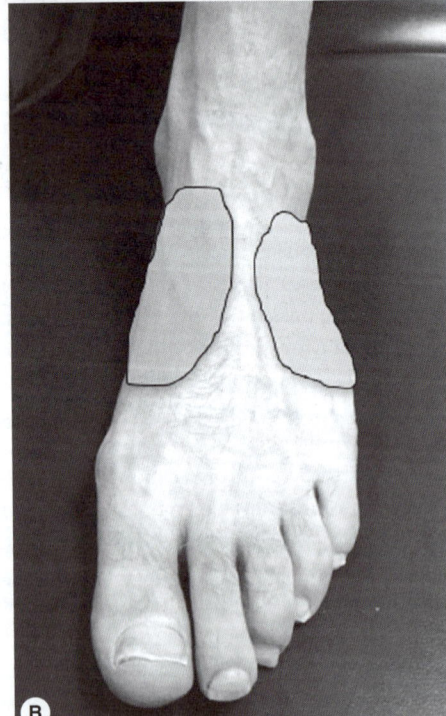

Figure 22-2. Areas of shading represent the zones of tenderness to palpation that may indicate the need for plain radiographs including an ankle series (A) and/or a foot series (B) based on the Ottawa Ankle Rules.[20]

demonstrated a negative likelihood ratio of less than 1.4%, so very few individuals with fractures are appropriately not directed to ankle and/or foot radiographs with application of these rules.[21] However, the specificity of the Ottawa Ankle Rules was found to be low to modest, suggesting a high false-positive rate. This finding means that a high proportion of individuals without fractures may receive ankle and/or foot radiographs. The high sensitivity and low specificity of the Ottawa Ankle Rules are acceptable in a screening examination, because the goal is to direct appropriate individuals toward additional necessary testing.

Last, the physical therapist needs to determine whether the patient has gross mechanical laxity secondary to ligament rupture. In the acute phase, this can be difficult to determine because elevated intracapsular pressure associated with injury-related joint effusion may limit the diagnostic accuracy of clinical tests designed to detect ligament tears. A negative anterior drawer test suggests an absence of damage to the anterior talofibular ligament, and a negative talar tilt test indicates the absence of calcaneofibular ligament involvement. Even if the anterior drawer test (Fig. 22-3 A and B) and talar tilt test (Fig. 22-3C) are negative in the acute phase of a lateral ankle

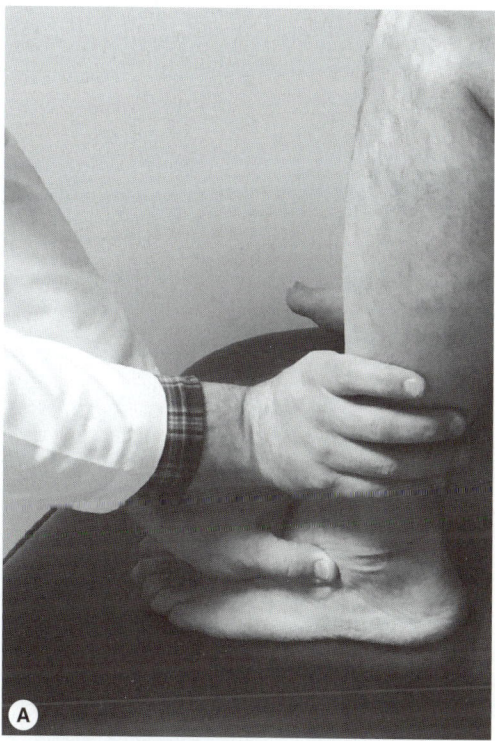

Figure 22-3. Tests for ligamentous laxity of the talocrural joint. **A.** Anterior drawer test with foot fixed on the table. The therapist provides a posteriorly directed force with the hand that is placed on the anterior aspect of the shin.

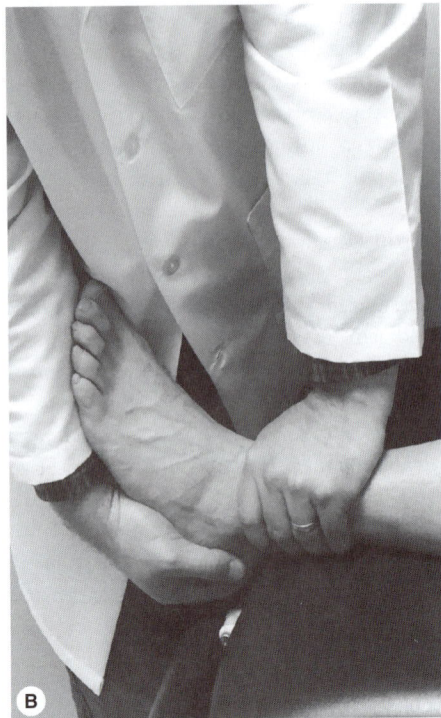

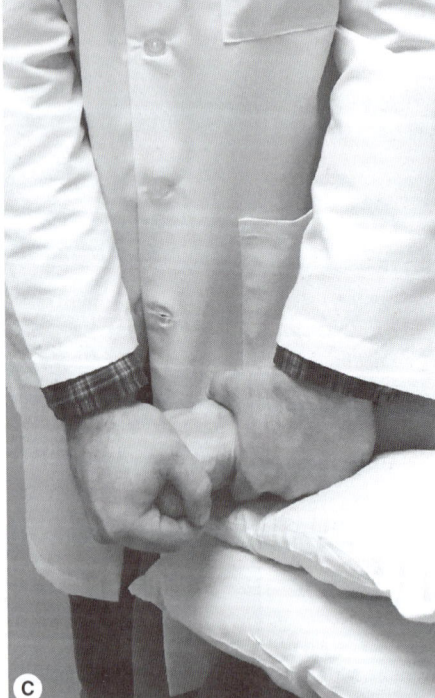

Figure 22-3. (*Continued*) Tests for ligamentous laxity of the talocrural joint. **B.** Anterior drawer test with foot stabilized by the therapist. With one hand stabilizing the leg just proximal to the ankle, the therapist provides an anteriorly directed force with the opposite hand cupped around the heel. **C.** Talar tilt test. The patient is sidelying (or seated) with ankle positioned in 10° to 20° of plantar flexion. With one hand, the therapist stabilizes the distal leg. With the other hand on the hindfoot, the therapist applies an inversion force.

injury, these tests should be repeated during the post-acute injury phases. Re-testing for ligamentous integrity is especially important if the patient presents with persistent instability during the rehabilitation process. In a study with 160 individuals with lateral ankle sprains in which physical examination was compared to arthrography, **a cluster of findings** that includes pain with palpation of the anterior talofibular ligament, lateral ankle hematoma, and a positive anterior drawer test 5 days after injury had a sensitivity of 100%, specificity of 75%, positive likelihood ratio of 4.13, and negative likelihood ratio of 0.01 to identify lateral ankle ligament rupture.[22] Inter-tester reliability of this cluster of examination findings ranged between moderate to perfect among 5 investigators.[23]

After ruling out the likelihood of a DVT (based on Wells clinical prediction rule for DVT) and the need for ankle/foot radiographs (based on the Ottawa Ankle Rules), the physical therapist determined that physical therapy was appropriate for this patient. Next, the physical therapist can quantify patient-reported activity limitations through a valid and reliable questionnaire. Regular use of questionnaires throughout the episode of care allows the therapist to track outcomes longitudinally and benchmark them with respect to other patients with similar conditions. There are several self-report questionnaires that have demonstrated validity and reliability in individuals with lower extremity injuries. The **Foot and Ankle Ability Measure (FAAM)** was designed to assess activity limitations and participation restrictions for individuals with general musculoskeletal foot and ankle disorders. Unlike many of the other self-report questionnaires, the FAAM has specifically been reported to be valid and reliable in individuals with ankle sprains.[24] It consists of a subscale for activities of daily living (ADLs; 21 items) and a subscale for sports (8 items). There is strong evidence supporting the content validity, construct validity, test-retest reliability, and responsiveness of the FAAM in individuals with general musculoskeletal foot and ankle disorders.[24] The minimal clinically important difference (MCID) was reported to be 8 and 9 points over a 4-week timeframe for the ADLs and sport subscales, respectively.[24] This finding means that physical therapists can use these scales to help identify clinically meaningful change for the patient. There is also evidence for validity in those with chronic ankle instability,[25] although these data may demonstrate limited generalization to acute lateral ankle injuries.

A thorough examination is conducted to characterize the body structure/function deficits and activity limitations that may contribute to restrictions in overall societal participation. The examination includes physical measurements for edema, ankle and foot ROM, weightbearing, and balance. The Figure-of-8 measurement is a common method to measure ankle and foot edema. It demonstrates high inter-tester reliability (ICC 0.93-0.099)[26-30] and intra-tester reliability (ICC 0.98-0.99),[26,27,29] and good concurrent validity with water displacement volumetry (the criterion standard).[28] To perform the Figure-of-8 measurement, the therapist should position the (non-weightbearing) ankle in a comfortably plantar flexed position. The tape should pass over the landmarks of the navicular and cuboid, and beneath the medial and lateral malleoli (Fig. 22-4). Non-weightbearing goniometric measurements of passive ROM at the ankle and foot are commonly used to quantify movement loss because of lateral ankle injury. Good intra-tester reliability (ICC range > 0.90) and fair inter-tester reliability (ICC range >0.70) for ankle dorsiflexion

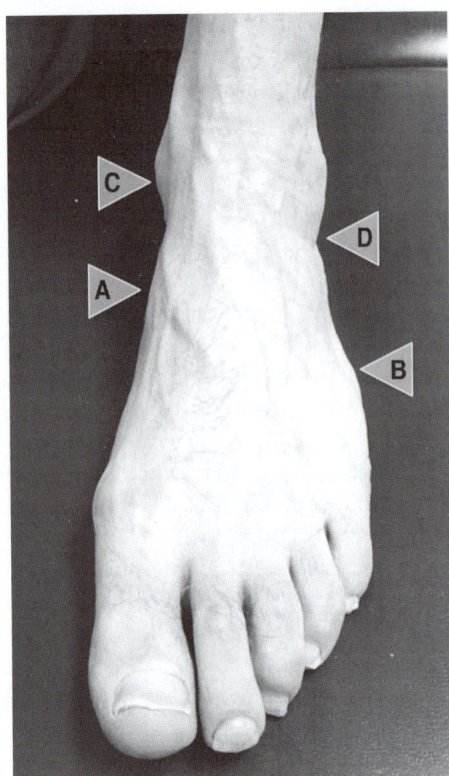

Figure 22-4. Sequential landmarks for Figure-of-8 ankle edema measurement, including the navicular body (A), styloid process of the fifth metatarsal (B), distal tip of the medial malleolus (C), and distal tip of the lateral malleolus (D). The tape is drawn from the distal tip of the lateral malleolus (D) back to the navicular body (A), and the measurement is read.

and plantar flexion measurements were established in a large systematic review and meta-analysis.[31] ROM should be measured for the subtalar joint, transverse tarsal joint, and metatarsophalangeal joints on both the involved and uninvolved sides. The physical therapist should also assess ROM at the knee and hip on both sides to exclude possible contributory movement restrictions at these joints. After the acute phase, single-limb balance should be assessed on the involved and uninvolved lower extremities. Evaluation and management of balance deficits are important to mitigate the conversion from an acute ankle injury to chronic ankle instability. Tests such as the Balance Error Scoring System,[32-34] single-limb balance test,[35] Star Excursion Balance Test (SEBT) and Y Balance Test (see Case 17),[36-40] and a variety of hop tests (see Case 23)[41-43] can be used to assess performance and potentially predict the risk for re-injury in the post-acute injury state. However, these tests would be inappropriate for acute lateral ankle sprains in which weightbearing is painful.

To establish a prognosis for an acute lateral ankle injury, objective injury grading from body structure/function findings may be important. Malliaropoulos and colleagues[44,45] identified a method to grade acute lateral ankle sprains. In this framework, Grade I injuries include no loss of function, no ligamentous laxity (e.g., negative anterior drawer and talar tilt tests), little or no hematoma, no point tenderness, and a minimal decrease in total ankle motion ($\leq 5°$) and mild edema

(≤0.5 cm) compared to the uninvolved side. Grade II injuries involve some loss of function, a positive anterior drawer test (suggesting anterior talofibular ligament involvement), a negative talar tilt test (indicating absence of calcaneofibular ligament involvement), hematoma, point tenderness, decreased total ankle motion greater than 5° but less than 10° compared to the uninvolved side, and edema greater than 0.5 cm but less than 2.0 cm compared to the uninvolved side. Grade III injuries are characterized by near total loss of function, positive anterior drawer and talar tilt tests, hematoma, extreme point tenderness, decreased total ankle motion greater than 10° compared to the uninvolved side, and edema more than 2 cm compared to the uninvolved side. Malliaropoulos and colleagues[45] further subdivided Grade III injuries according to stress radiography results, with IIIA injuries including anterior displacement of 3 mm or less and IIIB injuries involving greater than 3 mm of anterior displacement. This grading method demonstrates a satisfactory level of both internal validity and predictive validity for the number of days until return to sport, with more severe injuries involving significantly greater edema, radiographic evidence of laxity, and delayed return to sport.[44]

Plan of Care and Interventions

The primary goals of intervention in acute phase lateral ankle sprains are to reduce the acute inflammatory process, support optimal healing of damaged and inflamed structures, and reinforce adaptive weightbearing through the affected lower extremity. These goals can be achieved by specific evidence-based interventions.

Based on a systematic review and meta-analysis of 22 studies involving individuals with acute lateral ankle injuries, there are significant clinical benefits to weightbearing as tolerated compared to non-weightbearing cast immobilization.[46] In their analysis, Kerkhoffs and colleagues[46] compared the clinical benefit of various forms of external ankle support. Lace-up bracing led to significantly better short-term edema control than semi-rigid bracing. Semi-rigid ankle support was associated with significantly shorter time to return to activity and decreased incidence of subjective instability compared to an elastic wrap. External support from tape was associated with the most complications (*e.g.*, skin irritation) compared to an elastic wrap.[46] These results suggest that, when possible, a lace-up ankle brace is preferred to optimize outcomes and minimize potential adverse effects. In addition, assistive devices (*e.g.*, crutches, canes, walkers, etc.) must be selected to optimize safety and adaptive weightbearing.

The goal of intervention for acute, mechanically unstable ankles should be to improve mechanical instability as much as possible. **Individuals with severe lateral ankle injuries (*e.g.*, Grade IIIA and IIIB)** may benefit from cast immobilization.[12] In a study by Freeman et al.[12] including subjects with ligamentous injuries of the foot and ankle, recovery was quickest in the early mobilization group (average time to recovery = 12 weeks) compared to the immobilization group (average time to recovery = 22 weeks) and a surgical group (suturing of lateral collateral ligament) (average time to recovery = 26 weeks). However, immobilization and suturing were associated with improved mechanical stability on stress radiography. The findings of Freeman et al.[12] suggest that cast immobilization is clinically useful to optimize both ankle stability and recovery. A subsequent study found that dorsiflexion angles of 5° to 15° reduced the anterior talocrural subluxation in cadaver models, suggesting that this position may be most useful to reduce mechanical instability by bringing the talocrural joint into a closed pack position.[47] Thus, cast immobilization should be considered for mechanically unstable injuries, and the ankle should be immobilized in the maximal amount of dorsiflexion possible.

To address pain, edema, and ROM restrictions in the acute phase of healing after a lateral ankle injury, low-grade manual therapy procedures should be considered. Eisenhart and colleagues[48] found significant improvements in edema and pain in 28 individuals with acute ankle sprains who were randomized to receive a single session of osteopathic manual therapy in addition to standard of care intervention compared to 27 individuals who only received standard of care intervention in the emergency department.[48] The osteopathic manual therapy interventions included soft tissue mobilization, joint mobilization, isometric mobilization (*i.e.*, "muscle energy"), positional release, and lymphatic drainage procedures. Green and colleagues[49] found that individuals with acute lateral ankle sprains who received low-grade pain-free anteroposterior glides of the talus relative to the tibiofibular mortise (Fig. 22-5) in addition to rest, ice, compression, and elevation (RICE) achieved full ankle dorsiflexion and step symmetry within the first 2 to 3 treatments.[49]

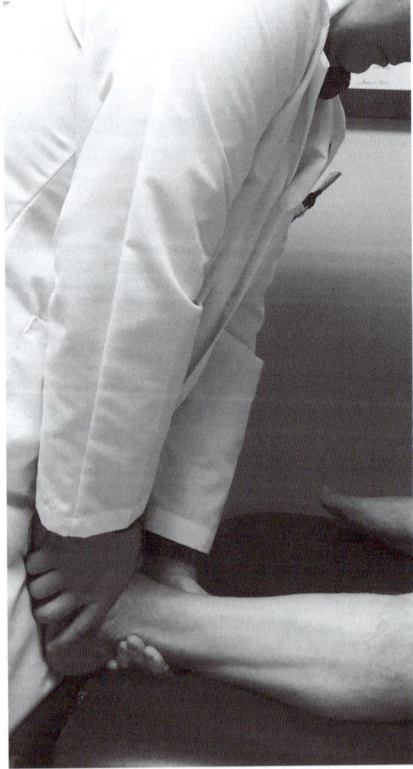

Figure 22-5. Posterior glide of the talus under the tibiofibular mortise in open chain position. The physical therapist's left hand supports the leg against the table, whereas the right hand provides a graded, posteriorly directed force to the head of the talus using the radial aspect of the second metacarpal head as the primary contact surface. The therapist stabilizes the patient's foot against his thigh. The physical therapist's elbow is extended, and his shoulders are oriented directly over the mobilizing hand to optimize his own body mechanics during the technique.

While many modalities have traditionally been used for clinical management of structural and functional deficits following acute lateral ankle injury, evidence for the use of **cryotherapy** is consistently the strongest. Evidence for the use of other physical agents is either equivocally supportive or clearly unsupportive. A systematic review by Bleakley and colleagues[50] concluded that there was marginal evidence favoring the use of ice in addition to exercise for the management of acute phase healing after lower extremity sprain and minor surgery. A longer duration of icing (20-30 minutes per session) appeared to be most beneficial. However, the optimal mode and dosage for ice application could not be identified from the reviewed studies. In 1978, Pasila and colleagues[51] found that individuals with acute lateral ankle injuries who received pulsed **shortwave diathermy** compared to a sham control experienced significant reduction in edema and gait deviations, though no improvement was noted in ROM or strength. An earlier report by Wilson[52] reported greater improvement in swelling, pain, and gait deviations in individuals with acute lateral ankle injuries who received pulsed **electrical stimulation** compared to placebo. In contrast, Man and colleagues[53] found no significant difference in ankle and foot volume, girth, and self-perceived functioning in individuals with acute lateral ankle injuries who received electrical stimulation at either motor or submotor intensity compared to sham treatment. **Low-level laser therapy** (LLLT) has been used for several years to treat sports injuries. Stergioulas[54] reported significant decreases in foot and ankle volume at 24, 48, and 72 hours following initiation of LLLT in individuals with acute ankle sprains. However, de Bie and colleagues[55] found no significant differences in pain and function between individuals with acute ankle sprains who received LLLT and those who received a placebo. Last, ultrasound has no significant effect on healing ankle sprains. Systematic reviews by van der Windt et al.[56] and van den Bekerom et al.[57] identified no significant differences between active **ultrasound** treatment and sham ultrasound following ankle sprains.

For more rapid functional recovery in individuals with **low-grade lateral ankle injuries,** therapy should include active and passive ROM exercises, strengthening, and progression of weightbearing as tolerated on the affected lower extremity.[58-62] Pain, redness, swelling, and reports of instability should be monitored carefully, because these may be signs of maladaptive overload. In a randomized trial by van Rijn et al.,[62] individuals with severe ankle sprains who received physical therapy and conventional medical treatment experienced significant functional improvement compared to controls that received only conventional medical treatment. Holme and colleagues[61] randomized 92 subjects with acute unilateral ankle sprains to receive either advice for early weightbearing (n = 46) or the same advice in addition to supervised physical therapy sessions (n = 46; two 1-hour sessions per week for 4 weeks). At 1-year follow-up, the group receiving supervised physical therapy demonstrated a significant decrease in 1-year recurrence rate compared to the group receiving advice only. Subsequently, Bassett and Prapavessis[60] have shown that both home- and clinic-based physical therapy intervention programs significantly improved self-reported ankle function, but there was no significant difference between groups. Thus, the appropriateness of a robust independent self-management and home exercise program should be considered for people with acute lateral ankle injuries.

There is moderate evidence supporting advancement of acute phase exercises such as progressive re-loading (static and dynamic balance training) to reduce the risk for subsequent lateral ankle injuries during the post-acute and chronic phases. In soccer players with a previous history of lateral ankle sprains, Tropp and colleagues[8] documented a 5-fold decrease in the proportion of recurrent sprains in those who received ankle disk training (*i.e.*, standing on an unstable surface) compared to those who used orthoses alone. Wester et al.[63] also documented a reduction in self-reported symptoms and decreased incidence of recurrent sprains after 12 weeks of wobble board training in a cohort of individuals with post-acute lateral ankle sprains. Despite the established positive effects of balance retraining on re-injury rates, the optimal training parameters for balance retraining and the specific mechanism/s for the improvement remains unclear.[64-66] Based on their systematic review of studies involving functional (weightbearing) rehabilitation strategies, Webster and Gribble[67] suggest that functional exercises and activities, especially those that utilize unstable surfaces, may improve dynamic postural control. Balance retraining should involve a progression of planes and movement/reaction speeds that replicate the patient's favored activities. The physical therapist should monitor the patient for signs of adverse overload and proceed with progression of interventions cautiously. The therapist may also consider training the patient in a lace-up ankle brace, especially in the early stages of balance training, in order to mitigate the likelihood of re-injury during the exercise program. In individuals with functional ankle instability, hip muscle recruitment patterns during perturbation are altered compared to non-disabled individuals.[68-70] Therapeutic exercises to address potential hip and trunk muscle deficits have an important role in rehabilitation for patients following lateral ankle injuries.

Evidence-Based Clinical Recommendations

SORT: Strength of Recommendation Taxonomy
A: Consistent, good-quality patient-oriented evidence
B: Inconsistent or limited-quality patient-oriented evidence
C: Consensus, disease-oriented evidence, usual practice, expert opinion, or case series

1. Use of clinical decision rules for the presence of deep vein thrombosis (Wells clinical prediction rule) and the need for imaging for ankle and foot fractures (Ottawa Ankle Rules), as well as physical examination clusters for mechanical instability, can help exclude conditions that may be worsened by physical therapy. **Grade A**

2. The use of valid and reliable self-report questionnaires (*e.g.*, Foot and Ankle Ability Measure) can identify and track patients' progress throughout the episode of care. **Grade A**

3. For individuals with severe ankle sprains (*e.g.*, Grade IIIA and IIIB), ankle cast immobilization in maximal ankle dorsiflexion optimizes mechanical stability. **Grade C**

4. Cryotherapy decreases pain, reduces edema, and restores functional deficits in individuals with lateral ankle injuries. **Grade A**

5. Short-wave diathermy, electrotherapy, and low-level laser therapy may reduce acute phase pain, swelling, and improve functional deficits in individuals with lateral ankle injuries. **Grade B**

6. The use of therapeutic ultrasound does not contribute to significantly better clinical outcomes than placebo ultrasound in individuals with lateral ankle injuries. **Grade A**

7. For individuals with Grade I or Grade II ankle sprain injuries, recovery time may be reduced with early mobilization (active and passive ROM exercises) and supported weightbearing as tolerated. **Grade A**

COMPREHENSION QUESTIONS

22.1 According to the best available evidence, which of the following is a risk factor for lateral ankle sprains?

A. No prior ankle sprain
B. Sedentary lifestyle
C. Playing basketball
D. General deconditioning

22.2 Supported weightbearing and early mobilization appear *most* appropriate for lateral ankle injuries that include which of the following?

A. Ligament ruptures
B. Mild to moderate ligament sprains
C. Chronic ankle instability
D. Ankle and foot fractures

22.3 Which modality does the evidence *most* strongly support for use in treating acute lateral ankle sprains?

A. Ultrasound therapy
B. Low-level laser therapy
C. Cryotherapy
D. Electrotherapy

ANSWERS

22.1 **C.** Participation in non-contact sports that involve frequent cutting such as basketball are documented risk factors for lateral ankle injuries.

22.2 **B.** Supported weightbearing and early mobilization are best utilized for early-phase mild to moderate lateral ankle injuries. Early mobilization for a chronically unstable ankle would be inappropriate (option C). For ligament ruptures and resultant mechanical instability, an approach involving immobilization would promote optimal results for joint stability, but at the potential expense of recovery speed (option A). If an ankle or foot fracture is suspected, supported weightbearing is not preferable (option D). Rather, the patient should be directed to appropriate plain film radiography.

22.3 **C.** Evidence is strongest for the use of cryotherapeutic modalities, although the best method of delivery has yet to be elucidated. Grade B evidence exists for the use of electrotherapy and low-level laser therapy (options B and D).[52-55] Grade A evidence exists *against* the use of therapeutic ultrasound, based on a preponderance of high-quality placebo-controlled studies (option A).[56,57]

REFERENCES

1. Waterman BR, Belmont PJ Jr., Cameron KL, Deberardino TM, Owens BD. Epidemiology of ankle sprain at the United States Military Academy. *Am J Sports Med*. 2010;38:797-803.
2. Waterman BR, Owens BD, Davey S, Zacchilli MA, Belmont PJ Jr. The epidemiology of ankle sprains in the United States. *J Bone Joint Surg Am*. 2010;92:2279-2284.
3. Fong DT, Hong Y, Chan LK, Yung PS, Chan KM. A systematic review on ankle injury and ankle sprain in sports. *Sports Med*. 2007;37:73-94.
4. McKay GD, Goldie PA, Payne WR, Oakes BW, Watson LF. A prospective study of injuries in basketball: a total profile and comparison by gender and standard of competition. *J Sci Med Sport*. 2001;4:196-211.
5. McKay GD, Goldie PA, Payne WR, Oakes BW. Ankle injuries in basketball: injury rate and risk factors. *Br J Sports Med*. 2001;35:103-108.
6. Bahr R, Karlsen R, Lian O, Ovrebo RV. Incidence and mechanisms of acute ankle inversion injuries in volleyball. A retrospective cohort study. *Am J Sports Med*. 1994;22:595-600.
7. Forkin DM, Koczur C, Battle R, Newton RA. Evaluation of kinesthetic deficits indicative of balance control in gymnasts with unilateral chronic ankle sprains. *J Orthop Sports Phys Ther*. 1996;23:245-250.
8. Tropp H, Askling C, Gillquist J. Prevention of ankle sprains. *Am J Sports Med*. 1985;13:259-262.
9. van Rijn RM, van Os AG, Bernsen RM, Luijsterburg PA, Koes BW, Bierma-Zeinstra SM. What is the clinical course of acute ankle sprains? A systematic literature review. *Am J Med*. 2008;121:324-331.
10. Gerber JP, Williams GN, Scoville CR, Arciero RA, Taylor DC. Persistent disability associated with ankle sprains: a prospective examination of an athletic population. *Foot Ankle Int*. 1998;19:653-660.
11. Hertel J. Functional anatomy, pathomechanics, and pathophysiology of lateral ankle instability. *J Athl Train*. 2002;37:364-375.
12. Freeman MA, Dean MR, Hanham IW. The etiology and prevention of functional instability of the foot. *J Bone Joint Surg Br*. 1965;47:678-685.
13. Hertel J. Sensorimotor deficits with ankle sprains and chronic ankle instability. *Clin Sports Med*. 2008;27:353-370.
14. Hertel J, Denegar CR, Monroe MM, Stokes WL. Talocrural and subtalar joint instability after lateral ankle sprain. *Med Sci Sports Exerc*. 1999;31:1501-1508.
15. Davenport TE, Kulig K, Sebelski CA, Gordon J, Watts HG. *Diagnosis for Physical Therapists: A Symptom-Based Approach*. Philadelphia, PA: F.A. Davis; 2012.
16. Wells PS, Hirsh J, Anderson DR, et al. A simple clinical model for the diagnosis of deep-vein thrombosis combined with impedance plethysmography: potential for an improvement in the diagnostic process. *J Intern Med*. 1998;243:15-23.

17. Wells PS, Hirsh J, Anderson DR, et al. Accuracy of clinical assessment of deep-vein thrombosis. *Lancet.* 1995;345:1326-1330.
18. Wells PS, Anderson DR, Bormanis J, et al. Value of assessment of pretest probability of deep-vein thrombosis in clinical management. *Lancet.* 1997;350:1795-1798.
19. Riddle DL, Wells PS. Diagnosis of lower-extremity deep vein thrombosis in outpatients. *Phys Ther.* 2004;84:729-735.
20. Stiell IG, Greenberg GH, McKnight RD, Wells GA. Ottawa ankle rules for radiography of acute injuries. *N Z Med J.* 22 1995;108:111.
21. Bachmann LM, Kolb E, Koller MT, Steurer J, ter Riet G. Accuracy of Ottawa ankle rules to exclude fractures of the ankle and mid-foot: systematic review. *BMJ.* 2003;326:417.
22. van Dijk CN, Lim LS, Bossuyt PM, Marti RK. Physical examination is sufficient for the diagnosis of sprained ankles. *J Bone Joint Surg Br.* 1996;78:958-962.
23. Landis JR, Koch GG. The measurement of observer agreement for categorical data. *Biometrics.* 1977;33:159-174.
24. Martin RL, Irrgang JJ, Burdett RG, Conti SF, Van Swearingen JM. Evidence of validity for the Foot and Ankle Ability Measure (FAAM). *Foot Ankle Int.* 2005;26:968-983.
25. Carcia CR, Martin RL, Drouin JM. Validity of the Foot and Ankle Ability Measure in athletes with chronic ankle instability. *J Athl Train.* 2008;43:179-183.
26. Rohner-Spengler M, Mannion AF, Babst R. Reliability and minimal detectable change for the figure-of-eight-20 method of measurement of ankle edema. *J Orthop Sports Phys Ther.* 2007;199-205.
27. Pugia ML, Middel CJ, Seward SW, et al. Comparison of acute swelling and function in subjects with lateral ankle injury. *J Orthop Sports Phys Ther.* Jul 2001;31:384-388.
28. Mawdsley RH, Hoy DK, Erwin PM. Criterion-related validity of the figure-of-eight method of measuring ankle edema. *J Orthop Sports Phys Ther.* 2000;30:149-153.
29. Petersen EJ, Irish SM, Lyons CL, et al. Reliability of water volumetry and the figure of eight method on subjects with ankle joint swelling. *J Orthop Sports Phys Ther.* 1999;29:609-615.
30. Tatro-Adams D, McGann SF, Carbone W. Reliability of the figure-of-eight method of ankle measurement. *J Orthop Sports Phys Ther.* 1995;22:161-163.
31. Martin RL, McPoil TG. Reliability of ankle goniometric measurements: a literature review. *J Am Podiatr Med Assoc.* 2005;95:564-572.
32. Riemann B, Guskiewicz KM, Shields EW. Relationship between clinical and forceplate measures. *J Sport Rehabil.* 1999;8:71-82.
33. Finnoff JT, Peterson VJ, Hollman JH, Smith J. Intrarater and interrater reliability of the Balance Error Scoring System (BESS). *PM R.* 2009;1:50-54.
34. Valovich McLeod TC, Perrin DH, Guskiewicz KM, Shultz SJ, Diamond R, Gansneder BM. Serial administration of clinical concussion assessments and learning effects in healthy young athletes. *Clin J Sport Med.* 2004;14:287-295.
35. Chrintz H, Falster O, Rood J. Single-leg postural equilibrium test. *Scand J Med Sci Sports.* 1991;1:244-246.
36. Olmsted LC, Carcia CR, Hertel J, Shultz SJ. Efficacy of the Star Excursion Balance tests in detecting reach deficits in subjects with chronic ankle instability. *J Athl Train.* 2002;37:501-506.
37. Gribble PA, Hertel J, Denegar CR, Buckley WE. The effects of fatigue and chronic ankle instability on dynamic postural control. *J Athl Train.* 2004;39:321-329.
38. Hertel J, Braham RA, Hale SA, Olmsted-Kramer LC. Simplifying the star excursion balance test: analyses of subjects with and without chronic ankle instability. *J Orthop Sports Phys Ther.* 2006;36:131-137.
39. Akbari M, Karimi H, Farahini H, Faghihzadeh S. Balance problems after unilateral lateral ankle sprains. *J Rehabil Res Dev.* 2006;43:819-824.

40. Hubbard TJ, Kramer LC, Denegar CR, Hertel J. Contributing factors to chronic ankle instability. *Foot Ankle Int.* 2007;28:343-354.
41. Buchanan AS, Docherty CL, Schrader J. Functional performance testing in participants with functional ankle instability and in a healthy control group. *J Athl Train.* 2008;43:342-346.
42. Caffrey E, Docherty CL, Schrader J, Klossner J. The ability of 4 single-limb hopping tests to detect functional performance deficits in individuals with functional ankle instability. *J Orthop Sports Phys Ther.* 2009;39:799-806.
43. Wikstrom EA, Tillman MD, Chmielewski TL, Cauraugh JH, Naugle KE, Borsa PA. Self-assessed disability and functional performance in individuals with and without ankle instability: a case control study. *J Orthop Sports Phys Ther.* 2009;39:458-467.
44. Malliaropoulos N, Ntessalen M, Papacostas E, Longo UG, Maffulli N. Reinjury after acute lateral ankle sprains in elite track and field athletes. *Am J Sports Med.* 2009;37:1755-1761.
45. Malliaropoulos N, Papacostas E, Papalada A, Maffulli N. Acute lateral ankle sprains in track and field athletes: an expanded classification. *Foot Ankle Clin.* 2006;11:497-507.
46. Kerkhoffs GM, Rowe BH, Assendelft WJ, Kelly KD, Struijs PA, van Dijk CN. Immobilisation for acute ankle sprain. A systematic review. *Arch Orthop Trauma Surg.* 2001;121:462-471.
47. Smith RW, Reischl S. The influence of dorsiflexion in the treatment of severe ankle sprains: an anatomical study. *Foot Ankle.* 1988;9:28-33.
48. Eisenhart AW, Gaeta TJ, Yens DP. Osteopathic manipulative treatment in the emergency department for patients with acute ankle injuries. *J Am Osteopath Assoc.* 2003;103:417-421.
49. Green T, Refshauge K, Crosbie J, Adams R. A randomized controlled trial of a passive accessory joint mobilization on acute ankle inversion sprains. *Phys Ther.* 2001;81:984-994.
50. Bleakley C, McDonough S, MacAuley D. The use of ice in the treatment of acute soft-tissue injury: a systematic review of randomized controlled trials. *Am J Sports Med.* 2004;32:251-261.
51. Pasila M, Visuri T, Sundholm A. Pulsating shortwave diathermy: value in treatment of recent ankle and foot sprains. *Arch Phys Med Rehabil.* 1978;59:383-386.
52. Wilson DH. Treatment of soft-tissue injuries by pulsed electrical energy. *Br Med J.* 1972;2:269-270.
53. Man IO, Morrissey MC, Cywinski JK. Effect of neuromuscular electrical stimulation on ankle swelling in the early period after ankle sprain. *Phys Ther.* 2007;87:53-65.
54. Stergioulas A. Low-level laser treatment can reduce edema in second degree ankle sprains. *J Clin Laser Med Surg.* 2004;22:125-128.
55. de Bie RA, de Vet HC, Lenssen TF, van den Wildenberg FA, Kootstra G, Knipschild PG. Low-level laser therapy in ankle sprains: a randomized clinical trial. *Arch Phys Med Rehabil.* 1998;79:1415-1420.
56. van der Windt DA, van der Heijden GJ, van den Berg SG, ter Riet G, de Winter AF, Bouter LM. Ultrasound therapy for musculoskeletal disorders: a systematic review. *Pain.* 1999;81:257-271.
57. van den Bekerom MP, van der Windt DA, ter Riet G, van der Heijden GJ, Bouter LM. Therapeutic ultrasound for acute ankle sprains. *Cochrane Database Syst Rev.* 2011;(6):CD001250.
58. Bleakley CM, O'Connor SR, Tully MA, et al. Effect of accelerated rehabilitation on function after ankle sprain: randomised controlled trial. *BMJ.* 2010;340:c1964.
59. Hale SA, Hertel J, Olmsted-Kramer LC. The effect of a 4-week comprehensive rehabilitation program on postural control and lower extremity function in individuals with chronic ankle instability. *J Orthop Sports Phys Ther.* 2007;37:303-311.
60. Bassett SF, Prapavessis H. Home-based physical therapy intervention with adherence-enhancing strategies versus clinic-based management for patients with ankle sprains. *Phys Ther.* 2007;87:1132-1143.
61. Holme E, Magnusson SP, Becher K, Bieler T, Aagaard P, Kjaer M. The effect of supervised rehabilitation on strength, postural sway, position sense and re-injury risk after acute ankle ligament sprain. *Scand J Med Sci Sports.* 1999;9:104-109.

62. van Rijn RM, van Heest JA, van der Wees P, Koes BW, Bierma-Zeinstra SM. Some benefit from physiotherapy intervention in the subgroup of patients with severe ankle sprain as determined by the ankle function score: a randomised trial. *Aust J Physiother*. 2009;55:107-113.
63. Wester JU, Jespersen SM, Nielsen KD, Neumann L. Wobble board training after partial sprains of the lateral ligaments of the ankle: a prospective randomized study. *J Orthop Sports Phys Ther*. 1996;23:332-336.
64. Kaminski TW, Buckley BD, Powers ME, Hubbard TJ, Ortiz C. Effect of strength and proprioception training on eversion to inversion strength ratios in subjects with unilateral functional ankle instability. *Br J Sports Med*. 2003;37:410-415.
65. Coughlan G, Caulfield B. A 4-week neuromuscular training program and gait patterns at the ankle joint. *J Athl Train*. 2007;42:51-59.
66. van der Wees PJ, Lenssen AF, Hendriks EJ, Stomp DJ, Dekker J, de Bie RA. Effectiveness of exercise therapy and manual mobilisation in ankle sprain and functional instability: a systematic review. *Aust J Physiother*. 2006;52:27-37.
67. Webster KA, Gribble PA. Functional rehabilitation interventions for chronic ankle instability: a systematic review. *J Sport Rehabil*. 2010;19:98-114.
68. Beckman SM, Buchanan TS. Ankle inversion injury and hypermobility: effect on hip and ankle muscle electromyography onset latency. *Arch Phys Med Rehabil*. 1995;76:1138-1143.
69. Bullock-Saxton JE, Janda V, Bullock MI. The influence of ankle sprain injury on muscle activation during hip extension. *Int J Sports Med*. 1994;15:330-334.
70. Bullock-Saxton JE. Local sensation changes and altered hip muscle function following severe ankle sprain. *Phys Ther*. 1994;74:17-31.

Preseason Testing to Assess Athletic Readiness and Risk of Injury in a Soccer Player

Phil Plisky

CASE 23

A collegiate Division III female soccer player presents to an outpatient physical therapy clinic for a musculoskeletal evaluation prior to the start of her season. Her past medical history includes multiple ankle sprains and occasional low back pain (LBP). Several of her teammates had anterior cruciate ligament (ACL) injuries over the past few years, and she is extremely concerned about experiencing an ACL tear. She would like you to determine whether she is ready to start the season from an injury prevention perspective.

- What are the most appropriate examination tests?
- What are the examination priorities?
- How will you know if your injury prevention measures are successful?

KEY DEFINITIONS

POST-INJURY MOTOR CONTROL CHANGES: Neuromuscular changes that can occur distant from the site of a previous injury; for example, after frequent ankle sprains, gluteal musculature timing and firing can be altered, which may increase the individual's risk of future injury.

PREPARTICIPATION PHYSICAL EXAMINATION: Compilation of medical history and physical tests typically administered prior to the start of the sports season to determine an athlete's readiness for sport by identifying current or potential problems

Objectives

1. Describe the key risk factors for injury in sport and relate them to test selection in the preparticipation examination.
2. Select evidence-based screens and tests most appropriate for preseason musculoskeletal physical screening.
3. Identify the passing criteria for preparticipation tests and develop a follow-up plan based on outcomes.

Physical Therapy Considerations

PT considerations during examination of a healthy Division III athlete prior to the start of the sports season:

- ▶ **General physical therapy plan of care/goals:** Evidence-based preparticipation physical examination that clears the musculoskeletal system; identify if athlete possesses modifiable risk factors for injury; develop a plan to mitigate injury risks

- ▶ **Physical therapy interventions:** Efficient and effective history and examination that clears the musculoskeletal system and identifies athletes at risk of injury; patient education regarding risk factors for ACL sprain and other lower-quadrant traumatic injuries; functional tests (*e.g.*, Functional Movement Screen, Star Excursion/Y Balance Test, hop testing, and jump landing); joint-specific examination procedures, depending on results of other tests and/or insurance or liability requirements (*e.g.*, if the university requires ligamentous testing as part of annual preparticipation examinations to identify pre-existing conditions); specific interventions to mitigate identified risk factors which may include corrective exercises, manual therapy techniques, and neuromuscular training program; appropriate outcome measures to determine effectiveness of interventions

- ▶ **Precautions during physical therapy:** Review athlete's medical history and current injury status to ensure that there are no contraindications to testing; monitor vital signs; discontinue testing if athlete experiences pain or instability episodes

▶ **Complications interfering with physical therapy:** Internal and external pressures on the athlete and healthcare provider for the athlete to participate in sports regardless of athlete's health status

Understanding the Health Condition

The goals of the preparticipation physical examination are to determine the athlete's readiness for sport and to identify risk factors that place the athlete at greater risk of injury. To clear the athlete for athletic participation, it is important to note that depending on the particular sport and athlete, multiple systems may need to be assessed including the cardiovascular, pulmonary, genitourinary, gastrointestinal, integumentary, lymphatic, endocrine, and neuromuscular.

A thorough history is essential because it may provide some of the most relevant information since past injuries and medical conditions can highlight areas needing more detailed examination. When considering risk factors for future injury, some of the modifiable intrinsic risk factors identified by prospective cohort studies include body mass index, dynamic balance, faulty movement patterns, knee alignment with landing, and training load.[1-11] Previous injury is not frequently included in that list because it is considered non-modifiable. However, previous injury is the most robust risk factor for future injury as identified by numerous prospective cohort studies.[3,12-14]

Motor control changes can persist even after the completion of a rehabilitation program. For example, individuals with a history of ankle sprain (the most common sport-related injury) have shown delayed onset times for ankle, hip, and hamstring muscles when transitioning from double-limb to single-limb stance compared to those individuals without history of ankle sprain.[15] Researchers have also found that individuals with chronic ankle instability (i.e., multiple ankle sprains), exhibit significant gluteus medius activation latency differences when an inversion perturbation was applied.[16] Another study reported delayed onset of gluteus maximus activation in previously injured subjects when compared with controls.[17] These data suggest that an altered motor control strategy persists following ankle sprains and that the deficits are identifiable even during low-level activities without an external load applied (e.g., landing from a jump).

Previous LBP also affects motor control. In athletes with a history of LBP who were pain-free at the time they were tested, researchers found altered activation of outer core muscles (i.e., rectus abdominis, external and internal obliques, latissimus dorsi, thoracic and lumbar erector spinae).[18,19] In a prospective study of 277 collegiate athletes, Zazulak et al.[11] used a logistic regression model to determine that trunk displacement measured after an unexpected perturbation, decreased trunk proprioception, and history of LBP predicted future knee ligament injury with 91% sensitivity and 68% specificity. Given the extensive amount of research demonstrating the persistence of motor control changes after injury and that these changes can increase the risk of future injury, it seems prudent to include post-injury motor control changes in the list of modifiable injury risk factors.

Physical Therapy Patient/Client Management

There are 2 critical times when the physical therapist can significantly impact an athlete's musculoskeletal health by identifying potential risk factors for injury. The first is during rigorous and systematic testing prior to physical therapy discharge to help ensure that any modifiable motor control changes that occurred after injury have normalized (see Case 17). The second is during the preparticipation examination in which the therapist identifies risk factors through an individual's history and simple-to-perform clinical tests. After preparticipation testing, the therapist must design a comprehensive program to correct any identified modifiable risk factors. The athlete should be reassessed during a follow-up testing session to determine whether the modifiable risk factors have been mitigated. Performing the reassessment is the most frequently omitted step in injury prevention management.

Examination, Evaluation, and Diagnosis

Efficiency and efficacy are of utmost importance in all physical therapy practice, but particularly in this case. While there are numerous tests and measures that a physical therapist could perform in the preseason, it is important to consider the goals for testing. In this case, the physical therapist is trying to clear the musculoskeletal system, identify an athlete at risk of injury to determine readiness for sports participation, and implement meaningful injury reduction measures. Typically, the therapist may have 1 hour to take a history, perform an examination, interpret and explain the results, and develop a mitigation plan. Given virtually unlimited tests that could be performed, a hierarchical approach should be used. For example, even if the therapist had time to measure range of motion (ROM) and strength at every joint and found no significant deficits, that does not imply that the player can use that motion to perform a deep squat without demonstrating a valgus collapse at the knee. However, if an athlete is able to perform a full deep squat without compensation, the therapist does not necessarily have to measure knee and hip flexion ROM. By starting with whole body movements, areas that may require additional specific testing can be identified. Each test or measure chosen should also be reliable, predictive, modifiable, and clinically feasible.

The goal of preparticipation screens is to clinically identify motor control deficits through movement testing. While biomechanics laboratories provide voluminous amounts of data regarding movement, most clinicians have neither the access nor the time to complete full biomechanical assessment. Clinical movement testing can be difficult to perform in a reliable manner. One option reported in the literature to help objectify and quantify movement testing is the **Functional Movement Screen (FMS)**. The FMS is reliable,[20-23] modifiable,[24] and predictive of injury in professional football players,[6] marine officer candidates,[25] female collegiate athletes,[26] and firefighters.[27] The purpose of the FMS is to screen for major movement pattern dysfunction and asymmetry.[28] An additional benefit of the FMS is that it takes most joints to their end range, thereby "clearing" those joints (i.e., full, pain-free ROM) from a musculoskeletal screening perspective. The FMS consists of

7 fundamental movements that are each scored on a scale of 0, 1, 2, or 3. A score of 0 indicates that there was pain with the movement pattern or clearing test; a score of 1 means the person is unable to perform the movement; 2 indicates the ability to perform the movement pattern with a compensation; and 3 indicates the ability to perform the movement according to the specified criteria.[28] The 7 movements are deep squat (Fig. 23-1A), hurdle step (Fig. 23-1B), inline lunge (Fig. 23-1C), active

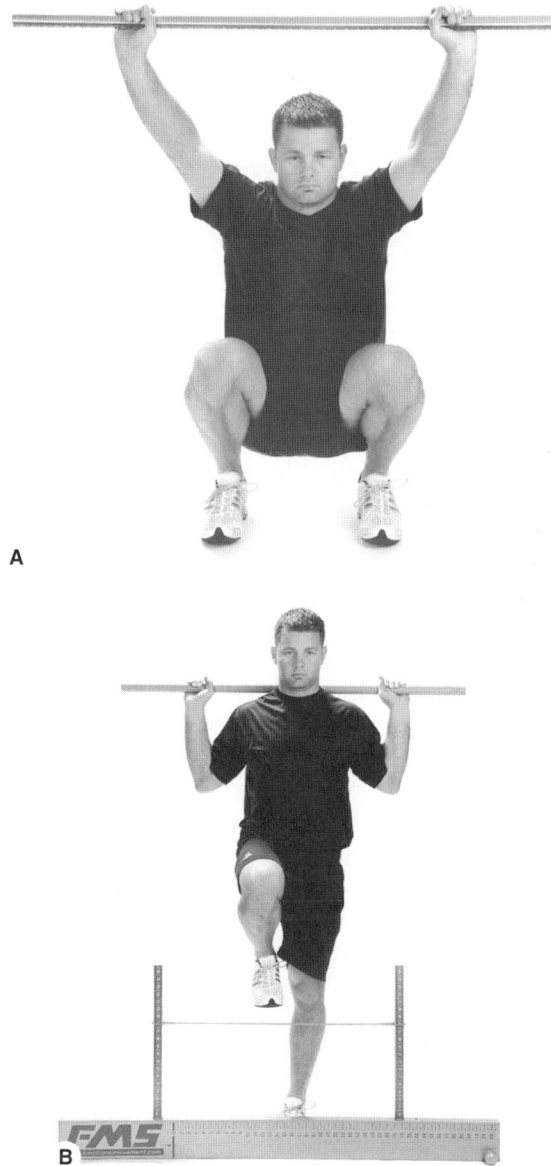

Figure 23-1. Components of Functional Movement Screen. **A.** Deep squat. **B.** Hurdle step.

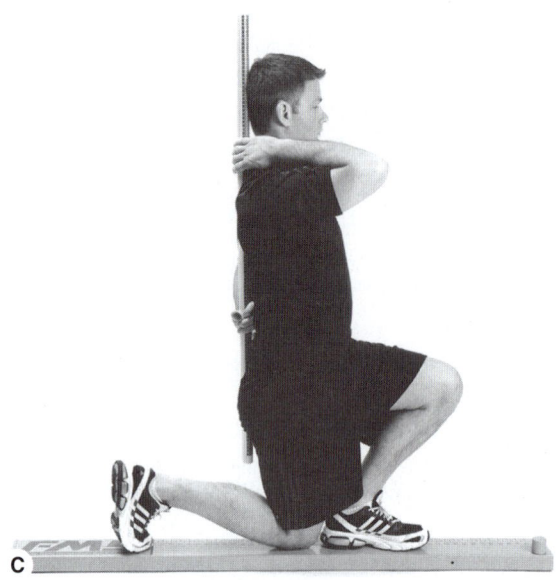

Figure 23-1. (*Continued*) Components of Functional Movement Screen. **C.** Inline lunge.

straight leg raise, shoulder mobility, trunk stability push-up, and rotary stability.[28] In addition, there are 3 clearing tests (shoulder impingement, prone press-up, and lumbar flexion).

Interpreting the results of the FMS can be confusing. While the FMS composite score was initially used in injury prediction research[6] to establish the cut point for injury risk, analyzing the score on the individual tests may be more important. In a prospective cohort study, Lehr et al.[8] utilized not only the composite score on the FMS, but also the presence of any 0s (pain) or 1s (unable to perform) on any individual test in an injury prediction model. They found that if the athlete had a composite score greater than 14 (which coincides with having at least a score of 2 on each of the 7 movement patterns), but had 0s or 1s on any individual test, she is still at greater risk of injury.[8] The FMS attempts to identify players who have pain with movement or the inability to perform a simple movement. If the athlete has pain on any test, she should have further evaluation and interventions from the rehabilitation provider. If she scores a 1 on any of the tests or presents with side-to-side asymmetries, these can likely be managed outside the rehabilitation process (*e.g.*, the athlete could be given corrective exercises and then follow-up with the school's strength and conditioning specialist for re-screening).

The **Star Excursion Balance Test (SEBT) and Y Balance Test–Lower Quarter (YBT-LQ)** are dynamic balance tests performed in single-leg stance that require adequate strength, flexibility, core control, and proprioception. The YBT-LQ is a simplified version of the SEBT in which only 3 reach directions are performed using a specific testing protocol and device to improve reliability and ease of administration.[30] In a systematic review and subsequent prospective cohort studies of the SEBT and YBT-LQ, researchers concluded that these are reliable tests of dynamic balance, predictive of injury, able to identify balance deficits after injury, and modifiable.[1,8,29] Researchers have suggested including either of these tests in screening prior to activity participation. The YBT-LQ incorporates 3 movement directions (anterior, posteromedial, and posterolateral; Fig. 23-2) instead of the original 8 directions within the SEBT. The goal of the YBT-LQ is to maintain single-limb stance while reaching as far as possible with the contralateral leg.[30] Because limb length is a small, but significant factor in how far someone reaches, limb length needs to be measured (from most inferior aspect of the anterior superior iliac spine to the inferior distal surface of the medial malleolus of the ankle to the nearest 0.5 cm).[29] To administer the test, 6 practice trials are performed. Next, 3 trials in each of the 3 directions for each foot (for a total of 9 trials on each limb) are collected and the maximum reach in each direction is included for analysis.[30]

The predictive ability of the SEBT and YBT has been examined by Plisky et al.[10] and Lehr et al.[8] These authors noted that high school and collegiate athletes with asymmetries of greater than 4 cm between the right and left reach distance in the anterior direction as well as a composite score below the age, sex, and sport risk cutoff had an increased risk of lower extremity injury. The composite score is the sum

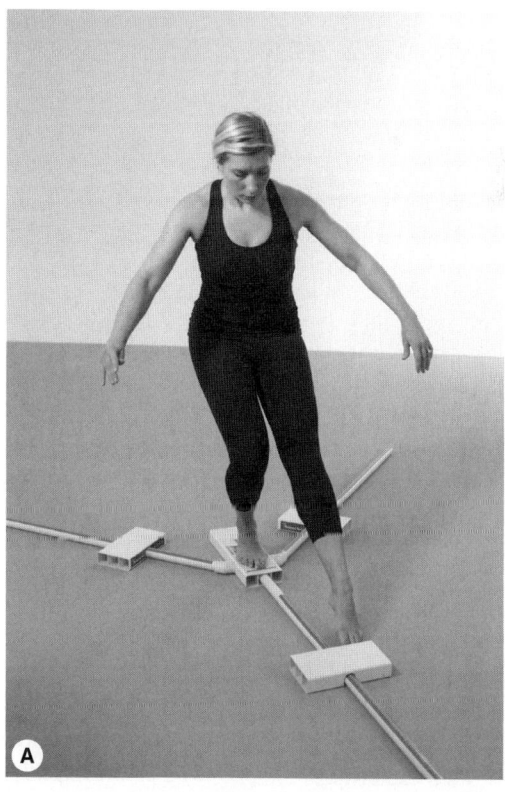

Figure 23-2. Y Balance Test–Lower Quarter (YBT-LQ). Goal is to maintain single-limb stance while reaching as far as possible with the contralateral leg. **A.** Anterior reach.

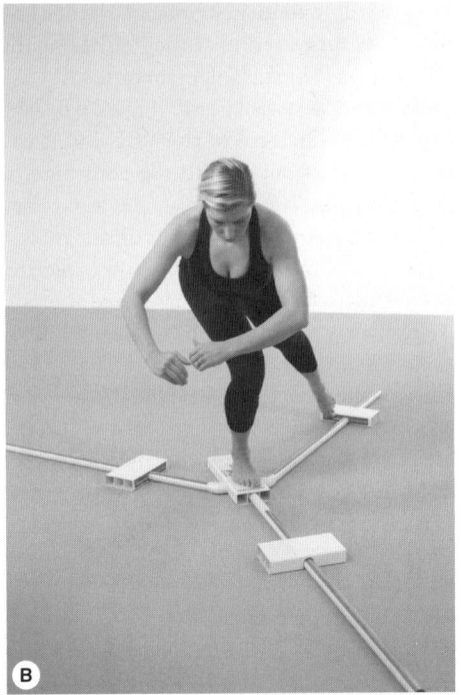

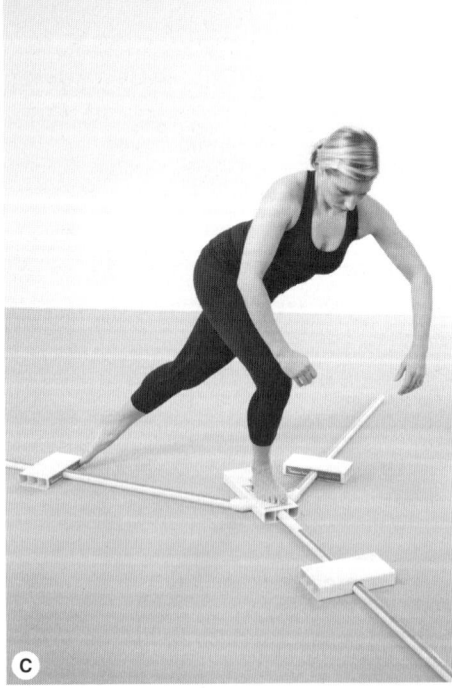

Figure 23-2. (*Continued*) Y Balance Test–Lower Quarter (YBT-LQ). Goal is to maintain single-limb stance while reaching as far as possible with the contralateral leg. **B.** Posteromedial reach. **C.** Posterolateral reach.

of the greatest reach in each of the 3 directions (anterior, posteromedial, posterolateral) divided by 3 times the limb length, and then multiplied by 100. Male and female high school basketball players with anterior asymmetry of greater than 4 cm were at increased risk of injury and females with a composite score (94%) in the bottom third of their peers were 6 times more likely to get injured.[10] In collegiate football, players with a composite score of less than 89% were more likely to get injured. Thus, because the injury risk cut point is different in each population, the composite score should not be less than the cut points that are specific for the age, sex, and sport of the athlete.[1,8,10] In another study in active college students, those with posterolateral reach of less than 80% of limb length had an increased risk of ankle sprain, whereas those who had posterolateral reach of greater than 90% were protected from ankle sprain.[31] Finally, improving the SEBT can reduce injury risk. In a randomized controlled trial with 226 youth female soccer players, researchers found that if performance on the SEBT is improved, injury risk is reduced.[32]

Many biomechanical laboratory studies have documented that landing in a knee valgus collapse position is a risk factor for ACL tear[5] and re-tear.[33] Two methods for clinically assessing high-risk landing positions are the **tuck jump assessment and the Landing Error Scoring System.** While the reliability, clinical feasibility, and predictive validity of these measures are debated,[34-37] it is apparent from the biomechanical literature that some form of clinical assessment of landing position is warranted once the athlete has passed lower-level tests (*e.g.*, fundamental movement, balance, etc.).

Hop testing is often used in preparticipation testing. Unilateral hop tests that are reliable, valid, clinically feasible, and modifiable include single-leg hop for distance, 6-m timed hop, triple hop, and triple crossover hop (see Case 16).[38-40] While little research has been performed using hop testing for injury prediction, hop testing has demonstrated discriminant validity (*i.e.*, the ability to distinguish between healthy and injured individuals). Interestingly, one study found that female athletes with an asymmetrical single-hop score were at increased risk of injury and that male athletes with increased hop distance compared to their peers were at increased risk of injury.[41] It could be hypothesized that these men may be "overpowered," meaning they did not have the fundamental movement competency to handle the power that they developed in their body. For example, if these males did not have the basic stability or mobility to perform certain movements (*e.g.*, in a squat, lunge, active straight leg raise), then they may have had to compensate somewhere else. When more load is applied by hopping, sprinting, or cutting, even greater compensation may occur that may stress and consequently injure the musculoskeletal system. Further study in this area is needed. Given the scant research on hop testing, hop testing should only be implemented if the athlete passes lower-level testing (FMS, SEBT, YBT-LQ).

Once all the preparticipation testing is completed, the interaction of the results of individual tests needs to be considered. Because injury risk is multifactorial, current trends in injury prevention are to categorize athletes using multiple risk factors. Lehr et al.[8] screened Division III college athletes in the preparticipation physical examination and followed them for an entire competitive season. At the start of the season, 183 collegiate athletes across multiple sports (including soccer) were interviewed about their injury history and tested on the YBT-LQ and FMS. Scores were entered into an algorithm to classify the athlete into 1 of 4 risk categories.[8] The algorithm calculated and weighted the composite FMS score, individual FMS test scores, results of FMS clearing tests, presence of asymmetry on any of the 5 bilateral FMS movements, pain during testing, previous injury, YBT-LQ asymmetry, and YBT-LQ composite score less than the risk threshold for the individual athlete. The YBT-LQ composite score risk threshold was determined by the software based on competition level (*i.e.*, junior high, high school, college, and professional), sport, and sex of the athlete.[1,8,10] If athletes were in the moderate or substantial risk category, they were 3.4 times (95% confidence interval, 2.0-6.0) more likely to get injured during that season. Not one athlete in the normal category got injured; in a subsequent unpublished analysis, there were 4 non-contact ACL injuries (3 in the high-risk group and 1 in the slightly increased risk group).[42]

Plan of Care and Interventions

After testing is completed, the results of the individual's tests should be examined starting with the FMS. If any scores of 0 are found (*i.e.*, pain with any testing), local testing of the painful area should be performed including any additional ROM, strength, or special tests to attempt to determine the cause of the pain. If scores of 1 or asymmetries are found, specific corrective strategies should be implemented to correct those movement dysfunctions. If scores on all FMS tests are more than 2 and performance is symmetrical, it would be beneficial to have the athlete perform a general injury prevention program. Examples of evidenced-based injury prevention programs can be found in the literature.[32,43-46] In the case of this athlete, it would be beneficial to have her perform the FIFA 11+ or similar injury prevention program because it has been extensively studied in female soccer players.[32,43,45] The therapist should be certain that there are no underlying movement dysfunctions prior to prescribing a general program. For example, if this athlete's FMS indicates an asymmetrical lunge pattern (*e.g.*, score of 1 on the left and 2 on the right) and a score of 1 on the deep squat, performing a plyometric jump training program would likely further ingrain the compensations already present in lower-demand movement patterns.

Test results in relation to other tests can be very insightful. For example, if the player has scored 2 on each component of the FMS, except for a score of 1 with the deep squat and a score of 1 on the left and 2 on the right on the lunge pattern and demonstrated 7 cm of asymmetry on the anterior reach on the YBT-LQ, the physical therapist should examine the ankle joint further through testing of closed kinetic chain dorsiflexion.

A key component in successful injury prevention is a **reassessment after risk factors have been identified** and an intervention plan to mitigate the risk factors has been implemented. While some benefit may be gained by providing corrective exercises, a true change in injury risk factors (and therefore injury risk) cannot be assured unless indicated by re-test. For example, Steffen et al.[32] found that those who had high compliance to the FIFA 11+ program had improved performance on the SEBT and decreased injury rate. Those with low compliance did not improve on the SEBT and did not decrease their injury rate.

Evidence-Based Clinical Recommendations

SORT: Strength of Recommendation Taxonomy
A: Consistent, good-quality patient-oriented evidence
B: Inconsistent or limited-quality patient-oriented evidence
C: Consensus, disease-oriented evidence, usual practice, expert opinion, or case series

1. Functional movements and dynamic balance can be tested with the Functional Movement Screen, Star Excursion Balance Test (SEBT), and Y Balance Test–Lower Quarter (YBT-LQ) tests, which are reliable, predictive of injury, modifiable, and clinically feasible. **Grade A**

2. Once an athlete has passed lower-level preparticipation tests, the tuck jump assessment and the Landing Error Scoring System are clinical tools that can be used to assess high-risk landing positions. **Grade B**

3. If injury risk factors are identified, a reassessment needs to be performed after mitigation strategies have been implemented to ensure that modifiable risk factors have been removed. **Grade C**

COMPREHENSION QUESTIONS

23.1 You are asked by the local university team physician to be part of an injury prevention task force. What is the *most* consistently reported risk factor for future injury in sports?
   A. Valgus collapse
   B. Poor balance
   C. Previous injury
   D. Flexibility asymmetry

23.2 When performing a preparticipation screen for a soccer player, which of the following would be considered a "pass" of the Functional Movement Screen (FMS) component tests?
   A. Overhead deep squat score of 1 (unable to perform the movement with compensation)
   B. Pain in lumbar spine with the inline lunge
   C. Trunk stability push-up score of 2 (able to perform movement with compensation)
   D. Asymmetrical active straight leg raise (score of 1 on the left and 3 on the right)

23.3 Which of the following is true regarding the Star Excursion Balance Test (SEBT) and Y Balance Test–Lower Quarter (YBT-LQ)?
   A. They identify people with chronic ankle instability and anterior cruciate ligament (ACL) deficiency.
   B. They are predictive of injury.
   C. Scores on these tests improve after training, but improving the SEBT score does not change injury rate.
   D. The reliability of the YBT-LQ has not been established.

ANSWERS

23.1 **C.** Previous injury is the most consistently reported risk factor identified by more than 25 prospective studies. While valgus collapse is a risk factor identified by 2 prospective studies (option A) and poor and asymmetrical balance have been identified as risk factors for future injury by multiple studies (option B), these are not the most consistently reported risk factors. There are a few prospective studies that identify flexibility asymmetry as a risk factor for injury; however, general poor flexibility is not consistently reported as a risk factor for injury (option D).

23.2 **C.** A passing score on the FMS is 2 or greater without asymmetry. Pain (score of 0) on any test in the FMS is considered a failure (option B). Given the research regarding pain affecting motor control as well as pain on the FMS predicting injury, any scores of 0 or 1 are considered a failure. Asymmetrical (score of 1) means unable to perform movement without compensation (option D). This is also not considered passing.

23.3 **B.** Both the SEBT and YBT-LQ have been shown to be predictive of injury in high school basketball players, collegiate athletes, and active college students. Multiple studies indicate that the SEBT identifies people with chronic ankle instability and ACL deficiency (option A). Those who underwent an injury prevention program were able to improve their score and additional research has found that those who improved their score also reduced their injury rate (option C). Two studies have established both inter-rater and test-retest reliability of the YBT-LQ to be good to excellent (option D).

REFERENCES

1. Butler RJ, Lehr ME, Fink ML, Kiesel KB, Plisky PJ. Dynamic balance performance and noncontact lower extremity injury in college football players: an initial study. *Sports Health*. 2013;5:417-422.
2. Dahle LK, Mueller MJ, Delitto A, Diamond JE. Visual assessment of foot type and relationship of foot type to lower extremity injury. *J Orthop Sports Phys Ther*. 1991;14:70-74.
3. de Visser HM, Reijman M, Heijboer MP, Bos PK. Risk factors of recurrent hamstring injuries: a systematic review. *Br J Sports Med*. 2012;46:124-130.
4. Gomez JE, Ross SK, Calmbach WL, Kimmel RB, Schmidt DR, Dhanda R. Body fatness and increased injury rates in high school football linemen. *Clin J Sport Med*. 1998;8:115-120.

5. Hewett TE, Myer GD, Ford KR, et al. Biomechanical measures of neuromuscular control and valgus loading of the knee predict anterior cruciate ligament injury risk in female athletes: a prospective study. *Am J Sports Med*. 2005;33:492-501.
6. Kiesel K, Plisky PJ, Voight ML. Can serious injury in professional football be predicted by a pre-season functional movement screen? *N Am J Sports Phys Ther*. 2007;2:147-158.
7. Kiesel KB, Butler RJ, Plisky PJ. Prediction of injury by limited and asymmetrical fundamental movement patterns in american football players. *J Sport Rehabil*. 2014;23:88-94.
8. Lehr ME, Plisky PJ, Butler RJ, Fink ML, Kiesel KB, Underwood FB. Field-expedient screening and injury risk algorithm categories as predictors of noncontact lower extremity injury. *Scand J Med Sci Sports*. 2013;23(4):e225-e232.
9. Paterno MV, Schmitt LC, Ford KR, et al. Biomechanical measures during landing and postural stability predict second anterior cruciate ligament injury after anterior cruciate ligament reconstruction and return to sport. *Am J Sports Med*. 2010;38:1968-1978.
10. Plisky PJ, Rauh MJ, Kaminski TW, Underwood FB. Star excursion balance test as a predictor of lower extremity injury in high school basketball players. *J Orthop Sports Phys Ther*. 2006;36:911-919.
11. Zazulak BT, Hewett TE, Reeves NP, Goldberg B, Cholewicki J. Deficits in neuromuscular control of the trunk predict knee injury risk: a prospective biomechanical-epidemiologic study. *Am J Sports Med*. 2007;35:1123-1130.
12. Hagglund M, Walden M, Ekstrand J. Previous injury as a risk factor for injury in elite football: a prospective study over two consecutive seasons. *Br J Sports Med*. 2006;40:767-772.
13. Walden M, Hagglund M, Ekstrand J. High risk of new knee injury in elite footballers with previous anterior cruciate ligament injury. *Br J Sports Med*. 2006;40:158-162.
14. Wright RW, Magnussen RA, Dunn WR, Spindler KP. Ipsilateral graft and contralateral ACL rupture at five years or more following ACL reconstruction: a systematic review. *J Bone Joint Surg Am*. 2011;93:1159-1165.
15. Van Deun S, Staes FF, Stappaerts KH, Janssens L, Levin O, Peers KK. Relationship of chronic ankle instability to muscle activation patterns during the transition from double-leg to single-leg stance. *Am J Sports Med*. 2007;35:274-281.
16. Beckman SM, Buchanan TS. Ankle inversion injury and hypermobility: effect on hip and ankle muscle electromyography onset latency. *Arch Phys Med Rehabil*. 1995;76:1138-1143.
17. Bullock-Saxton JE, Janda V, Bullock MI. The influence of ankle sprain injury on muscle activation during hip extension. *Int J Sports Med*. 1994;15:330-334.
18. Cholewicki J, Greene HS, Polzhofer GK, Galloway MT, Shah RA, Radebold A. Neuromuscular function in athletes following recovery from a recent acute low back injury. *J Orthop Sports Phys Ther*. 2002;32:568-575.
19. Cholewicki J, Silfies SP, Shah RA, et al. Delayed trunk muscle reflex responses increase the risk of low back injuries. *Spine*. 2005;30:2614-2620.
20. Minick KI, Kiesel KB, Burton L, Taylor A, Plisky P, Butler RJ. Interrater reliability of the functional movement screen. *J Strength Cond Res*. 2010;24:479-486.
21. Schneiders AG, Davidsson A, Horman E, Sullivan SJ. Functional movement screen normative values in a young, active population. *Int J Sports Phys Ther*. 2011;6:75-82.
22. Teyhen DS, Shaffer SW, Lorenson CL, et al. The functional movement screen: a reliability study. *J Orthop Sports Phys Ther*. 2012;42:530-540.
23. Frohm A, Heijne A, Kowalski J, Svensson P, Myklebust G. A nine-test screening battery for athletes: a reliability study. *Scand J Med Sci Sports*. 2012;22:306-315.
24. Kiesel K, Plisky P, Butler R. Functional movement test scores improve following a standardized off-season intervention program in professional football players. *Scand J Med Sci Sports*. 2011;21:287-292.
25. O'Connor FG, Deuster PA, Davis J, Pappas CG, Knapik JJ. Functional movement screening: predicting injuries in officer candidates. *Med Sci Sports Exerc*. 2011;43:2224-2230.

26. Chorba RS, Chorba DJ, Bouillon LE, Overmyer CA, Landis JA. Use of a functional movement screening tool to determine injury risk in female collegiate athletes. *N Am J Sports Phys Ther*. 2010;5:47-54.
27. Butler RJ, Contreras M, Burton LC, Plisky PJ, Goode A, Kiesel K. Modifiable risk factors predict injuries in firefighters during training academies. *Work*. 2013;46:11-17.
28. Cook G, Burton L, Hoogenboom B. Pre-participation screening: the use of fundamental movements as an assessment of function - part 2. *N Am J Sports Phys Ther*. 2006;1:132-139.
29. Gribble PA, Hertel J, Plisky P. Using the star excursion balance test to assess dynamic postural-control deficits and outcomes in lower extremity injury: a literature and systematic review. *J Athl Train*. 2012;47:339-357.
30. Plisky PJ, Gorman PP, Butler RJ, Kiesel KB, Underwood FB, Elkins B. The reliability of an instrumented device for measuring components of the star excursion balance test. *N Am J Sports Phys Ther*. 2009;4:92-99.
31. de Noronha M, Franca LC, Haupenthal A, Nunes GS. Intrinsic predictive factors for ankle sprain in active university students: a prospective study. *Scand J Med Sci Sports*. 2013;23:541-547.
32. Steffen K, Emery CA, Romiti M, et al. High adherence to a neuromuscular injury prevention programme (FIFA 11+) improves functional balance and reduces injury risk in Canadian youth female football players: a cluster randomised trial. *Br J Sports Med*. 2013;47:794-802.
33. Paterno MV, Rauh MJ, Schmitt LC, Ford KR, Hewett TE. Incidence of contralateral and ipsilateral anterior cruciate ligament (ACL) injury after primary ACL reconstruction and return to sport. *Clin J Sport Med*. 2012;22:116-121.
34. Onate J, Cortes N, Welch C, Van Lunen BL. Expert versus novice interrater reliability and criterion validity of the landing error scoring system. *J Sport Rehabil*. 2010;19:41-56.
35. Padua DA, Boling MC, Distefano LJ, Onate JA, Beutler AI, Marshall SW. Reliability of the landing error scoring system-real time, a clinical assessment tool of jump-landing biomechanics. *J Sport Rehabil*. 2011;20:145-156.
36. Padua DA, Marshall SW, Boling MC, Thigpen CA, Garrett WE Jr, Beutler AI. The landing error scoring system (less) is a valid and reliable clinical assessment tool of jump-landing biomechanics: the JUMP-ACL study. *Am J Sports Med*. 2009;37:1996-2002.
37. Smith HC, Johnson RJ, Shultz SJ, et al. A prospective evaluation of the landing error scoring system (less) as a screening tool for anterior cruciate ligament injury risk. *Am J Sports Med*. 2012;40:521-526.
38. Munro AG, Herrington LC. Between-session reliability of four hop tests and the agility T-test. *J Strength Cond Res*. 2011;25:1470-1477.
39. Myer GD, Schmitt LC, Brent JL, et al. Utilization of modified NFL combine testing to identify functional deficits in athletes following ACL reconstruction. *J Orthop Sports Phys Ther*. 2011;41:377-387.
40. Reid A, Birmingham TB, Stratford PW, Alcock GK, Giffin JR. Hop testing provides a reliable and valid outcome measure during rehabilitation after anterior cruciate ligament reconstruction. *Phys Ther*. 2007;87:337-349.
41. Brumitt J, Heiderscheit BC, Manske RC, Niemuth PE, Rauh MJ. Lower extremity functional tests and risk of injury in division iii collegiate athletes. *Int J Sports Phys Ther*. 2013;8:216-227.
42. Butler RJ, Lehr M, Kiesel KB, Queen RM, Garrett WE, Plisky PE. An economical model for ACL injury screening in college athletes. Southern Orthopaedic Association Annual Meeting. 2013.
43. Gilchrist J, Mandelbaum BR, Melancon H, et al. A randomized controlled trial to prevent non-contact anterior cruciate ligament injury in female collegiate soccer players. *Am J Sports Med*. 2008;36:1476-1483.
44. Hewett TE, Lindenfeld TN, Riccobene JV, Noyes FR. The effect of neuromuscular training on the incidence of knee injury in female athletes. A prospective study. *Am J Sports Med*. 1999;27:699-706.

45. Mandelbaum BR, Silvers HJ, Watanabe DS, et al. Effectiveness of a neuromuscular and proprioceptive training program in preventing anterior cruciate ligament injuries in female athletes: 2-year follow-up. *Am J Sports Med.* 2005;33:1003-1010.
46. Myklebust G, Engebretsen L, Braekken IH, Skjolberg A, Olsen OE, Bahr R. Prevention of anterior cruciate ligament injuries in female team handball players: a prospective intervention study over three seasons. *Clin J Sport Med.* 2003;13:71-78.

Concussion

Christopher J. Ivey
Jonathan Warren
Anthony G. Schneiders

CASE 24

A 20-year-old collegiate ice hockey player presents to physical therapy 2 days after sustaining a suspected concussion in a high impact collision (*i.e.*, body check) with an opposing player during a game. At the time of impact, the player was wearing standard protective equipment including a helmet and mouthguard. The initial sideline examination was performed by the team physical therapist. The therapist's assessment of concussion-related symptoms, postural control, and neurocognitive function was consistent with a concussion injury, and the athlete was not permitted to return to the game. During the post-game injury clinic, the team physician confirmed the diagnosis of a concussion and referred the player for physical therapy.

- ▶ What are the most appropriate goals for physical therapy?
- ▶ What precautions should be taken during the physical therapy examination and interventions?
- ▶ What are possible complications associated with physical therapy?
- ▶ How effective is protective equipment at reducing concussion injury risk?

KEY DEFINITIONS

CONCUSSION: Complex pathophysiologic process affecting the brain, induced by biomechanical forces. Mechanisms and sequelae include (1) injury caused by either a direct blow to the head, face, neck, or elsewhere on the body resulting in an "impulsive" force transmitted to the head; (2) rapid onset of short-lived impairment of neurologic function that resolves spontaneously; (3) possible resultant neuropathologic changes; however, acute clinical symptoms largely reflect functional change rather than structural injury such that no abnormality is seen on standard neuroimaging studies; (4) graded set of clinical symptoms that may or may not involve loss of consciousness (LOC). Resolution of clinical and cognitive symptoms typically follows a sequential course; however, in some cases, symptoms may be prolonged.[1]

POST-CONCUSSION SYNDROME: Symptoms of a prolonged nature that occur following a concussion; symptoms lasting for 3 months or more following a concussion are classified as persistent post-concussion syndrome.[2]

SECOND IMPACT SYNDROME: Condition that is suggested to occur within minutes of a concussion in someone who is still experiencing symptoms from a prior brain injury that may have occurred earlier during the same event. Vascular engorgement can lead to an increase in intracranial pressure and brain herniation, which can result in severe brain damage or death.[2] There is some debate regarding whether and to what degree the intracranial swelling occurs.[3]

Objectives

1. Discuss appropriate components of the examination of the athlete with a potential concussion.
2. Describe potential complications during the early recovery period and over an extended period of time.
3. Identify reliable and valid outcome tools to measure an athlete's readiness for return to play (RTP) after concussion.
4. Describe the phases of rehabilitation in concussion management.
5. Discuss prevention equipment to reduce the risk of injury.

Physical Therapy Considerations

PT considerations for management of the individual with a diagnosis of concussion:

- **General physical therapy goals:** Monitoring of the athlete for signs and symptoms that indicate any potential neurologic decline warranting further medical evaluation; sequential progression of rehabilitation, based on athlete's symptom resolution
- **Physical therapy interventions:** Patient education regarding common signs and symptoms of post-concussion syndrome; implementation of a progressive rehabilitation

program commencing with physical and cognitive rest and progressing to aerobic exercise, resistance exercise, sport-specific exercise, non-contact training drills, full contact practice, and return to play

▶ **Precautions during physical therapy interventions:** Recovery course is longer with slower progressions for younger athletes; advancement in the rehabilitation stage is not recommended for an individual with post-concussion symptoms.

▶ **Complications interfering with physical therapy:** Persistent symptoms associated with post-concussion syndrome alter progression of the rehabilitation stages and may affect the return-to-play timeline.

Understanding the Health Condition

It is estimated that 1.6 to 3.8 million people sustain a traumatic brain injury (TBI) during sports activities each year in the United States.[4,5] The majority of these injuries are categorized as mild traumatic brain injuries (mTBIs). Many are classified as concussions. Children have the highest annual incidence, with concussions occurring in 692 of every 100,000 American children younger than 15 years.[6] The epidemiological data are most likely conservative, given that a LOC is not a requirement for a diagnosis of concussion and a large number of individuals do not seek medical attention following this type of injury. With increasing numbers of sports participants and improved awareness of mTBI, the number of diagnosed concussions will likely increase.

Concussions are a common occurrence in sport, and these injuries occur in both sports that require wearing a helmet as well as those sports that do not.[7] Several epidemiological studies have been performed researching the incidence of concussion by sport, age, and sex. The trend from these studies demonstrates that sports with the highest concussion injury rate in the United States are football, wrestling, girls' and boys' soccer, and girls' basketball; in addition, collegiate athletes had a higher rate of concussion injury when compared to high school athletes.[8] In male and female sports, such as basketball and soccer, female athletes had a higher incidence of concussion when compared to their male counterparts.[9] The rates of concussion injury are higher during competition than in practice in all sports with the exception of cheerleading.[10]

The incidence of concussion in collegiate ice hockey has been reported as 0.41/1000 exposures and 0.91/1000 exposures for male and female athletes, respectively.[10] By comparison, the incidence rate of concussion in collegiate football is 0.54/1000 exposures.[7] The concussion incidence in ice hockey has *increased* since the introduction of helmet standards. It has been suggested that this increase is due to a heightened awareness and recognition of concussion and more aggressive play.[11] There is also debate regarding the age that body checking should be introduced in ice hockey. It has been reported that the risk of injury and concussion is more than 3-fold higher in a Pee Wee league (ages 11-12 years) that allows body checking compared to a Pee Wee league that does not allow bodychecking.[12]

Much of the research regarding the pathophysiology associated with concussion has been performed on animal models. After a concussion, a sudden release of the excitatory neurotransmitter glutamate occurs with a resulting rapid loss of intracellular potassium and influx of calcium.[13,14] In order to restore the normal resting membrane potential of injured neurons, the sodium-potassium pump works overtime, which increases cerebral glucose metabolism.[13,14] Unfortunately, this increase in cerebral glucose metabolism occurs during a time of diminished cerebral blood flow, creating a cellular energy crisis.[13] Furthermore, the influx of calcium disrupts oxidative metabolism within injured neurons, thereby inhibiting mitochondrial activity and increasing the mismatch of energy supply and demand.[14] This mismatch may increase vulnerability to a second insult during the recovery process, possibly leading to a more serious head injury.[2] After the initial period of increased glucose metabolism, there is a much longer period (~7-10 days) of decreased aerobic metabolism of glucose in the injured neurons.[15] In animal models, this neurometabolic cascade following a concussion represents a *functional* change in the nervous system rather than structural damage. This evidence from animal models is consistent with the findings that plain film radiographs or magnetic resonance imaging scans are of little value in diagnosing concussions.

Many signs and symptoms associated with concussion are not specific to this condition. There are 4 main categories that include physical, cognitive, emotional, and sleep disturbances. An individual diagnosed with a concussion can experience symptoms in 1 or more of these categories. While LOC can occur with this type of injury, less than 10% of diagnosed concussions result in LOC.[16] The common concussion signs and symptoms are listed in Table 24-1.[17]

While concussion symptoms generally improve in a predictable pattern within 7 to 10 days, some individuals have persistent symptoms.[18] These symptoms can be vague and nonspecific, which can make diagnosis difficult. The World Health Organization established a definition of postconcussional syndrome (post-concussion syndrome) as the presence of 3 or more of the following symptoms persisting for up to 4 weeks following a head injury: headache, dizziness, fatigue, irritability, difficulty with concentrating and performing mental tasks, impairment of memory, insomnia, and reduced tolerance to stress, alcohol, or emotional excitement.[19]

Table 24-1 COMMON SIGNS AND SYMPTOMS ASSOCIATED WITH CONCUSSION[17]

Physical	Cognitive	Emotional	Sleep
Headache	Feeling mentally "foggy"	Irritability	Drowsiness
Nausea	Feeling slowed down	Sadness	Sleeping less or more than usual
Vomiting	Difficulty concentrating	More emotional	Trouble falling asleep
Balance problems	Difficulty remembering	Nervousness	
Dizziness	Forgetful of recent information or conversations		
Visual problems	Confused about recent events		
Fatigue	Answers questions slowly		
Sensitivity to light	Repeats questions		
Sensitivity to noise			
Numbness/tingling			
Dazed or stunned			

Symptoms that last 3 months or longer following a concussion are classified as relating to persistent post-concussion syndrome.[2]

Returning to play following a concussion is an area that requires qualified assessment. It is not recommended that individuals RTP if they are still symptomatic. Athletes who have a history of concussion have an increased risk of having further concussions.[16] The prolonged or persisting neurocognitive effects of repetitive concussions were initially recognized in boxers in a syndrome classified as dementia pugilistica (punch drunk syndrome). In addition, parkinsonism (pugilistic parkinsonism) can also be associated with this type of repetitive injury.[19] As evidence of the neurocognitive effects of repetitive concussions has accumulated, it has become apparent that the cumulative effects of head injury are not specific to boxing. The term chronic traumatic encephalopathy (CTE) has been used to describe a similar phenomenon and has become more widely used in sports including football and wrestling. The first autopsy report from a professional football player demonstrating the effects of CTE was in 2005.[20] CTE is defined as a progressive neurodegenerative disease resulting from cumulative brain trauma. Generally, the initial signs and symptoms are not thought to manifest until decades after the trauma, usually in the fifth or sixth decade of life. The incidence and prevalence of CTE is unknown[21] because the condition is diagnosed on autopsy by distinctive immunoreactive stains for tau protein in the brain. However, this is not the same disease as Alzheimer's disease.[2] The typical signs and symptoms of CTE include a decline in recent memory and executive function, mood and behavioral disturbances such as depression, aggressiveness, and suicidal behavior, with progression to dementia.[2] A small subset of individuals with CTE have been thought to develop chronic traumatic encephalomyopathy, a progressive motor neuron disease similar to amyotrophic lateral sclerosis characterized by profound weakness, atrophy, spasticity, and fasciculation.[2]

As many as 25 sets of criteria to grade concussions have been developed; however, none have been fully validated.[22] The current recommendations advise abandoning management of concussion based on these grading scales.[18] Therefore, RTP criteria should rely on symptoms as a guide through the rehabilitation process rather than on a timeline based on grading.[23]

Physical Therapy Patient/Client Management

Concussion requires a multidisciplinary approach for effective management. The medical professional involved in the sideline assessment depends on who is present at the sporting event. The initial evaluation of the athlete may be performed by a sports physical therapist, athletic trainer, physician, or an emergency medical technician (EMT). Early recognition of concussion symptoms is imperative, and the **athlete should not RTP on the same day.**[1,2] A physician should confirm the diagnosis, and this generally occurs in the post-game injury clinic or during an office visit the following day. When available, results from baseline neurocognitive and balance tests performed during the preparticipation examination should be compared to the results of those tests following the injury. The initial treatment recommendations following the diagnosis of a concussion emphasize rest with a gradual and monitored return to activity. As the athlete progressively increases his activity, the physical therapist is often involved to monitor and safely progress his RTP. Once the athlete has completed the graduated RTP protocol, a physician who is trained in concussion management should be involved in the final RTP decision.

Examination, Evaluation, and Diagnosis

Several healthcare providers may be involved in the initial examination and ongoing reassessment of the injured athlete. The identification of a concussion is perhaps the most difficult component of the assessment because most athletes often do not inform medical personnel of concussion symptoms due to fear that they will be removed from the game or event.[24] While LOC is a readily identifiable sign of a possible concussion injury, less than 10% of athletes have an identifiable episode of LOC.[16] The immediate assessment of an unconscious athlete is the primary survey, which can occur on the field of play. If an athlete is unconscious, a cervical spine injury should be suspected until proven otherwise with the appropriate precautions maintained. First, the level of unconsciousness must be determined and the duration should be recorded. The Glasgow Coma Scale (GCS) can be used to assess the level of unconsciousness.[25] The primary survey continues with an assessment of the athlete's airway, breathing, and circulation. Once the athlete regains consciousness, he can be taken to the sidelines for further evaluation provided that the probability of more severe injuries, such as injuries to the cervical spine, is low.[26] Balance problems or unsteadiness may be noted during transfer from the field of play to the sidelines. If the athlete does not regain consciousness, immediate transportation to the nearest medical facility is mandatory.

The initial sideline evaluation includes an assessment of the athlete's symptoms, a neurologic examination, and an evaluation of cognition. Several sideline assessment tools are available, including a graded system checklist, the Maddocks questions, the **Standardized Assessment of Concussion (SAC), the Modified Balance Error Scoring System (BESS), and the Sport Concussion Assessment Tool 3 (SCAT3)**.[27] The SCAT3 is an updated version of 2 previous versions (SCAT and SCAT2), and it includes the majority of accepted sideline assessments in one comprehensive evaluation. The SCAT3 was designed to be administered by healthcare professionals. The SCAT3 contains sections for a graded system checklist, GCS, Maddocks Score, SAC, and modified BESS. The SCAT3 has not been independently validated; however, it contains a section to calculate the SAC, which has been validated in detecting mental status changes after a concussion injury in athletes.[28] The SCAT3 is available for free download.[29]

While Table 24-1 lists numerous signs and symptoms that can occur with a concussion, the graded system checklist allows the examiner to track symptoms *over time*. The athlete should complete this checklist at the initial evaluation and at each follow-up assessment until all signs and symptoms have cleared at rest and during physical exertion.[30] The symptoms are scored on a scale of 0 to 6, where 0 = not present, 1 = mild, 3 = moderate, and 6 = most severe. The graded system checklist has been shown to have a sensitivity of 64% to 89% and a specificity of 91% to 100%.[31]

The examiner must be aware that the standard orientation questions such as time, place, and person have been shown to be *unreliable* in assessing for concussion in athletes during sport when compared to a more complete memory assessment.[32] For that reason, brief neuropsychological (NP) tests such as the Maddocks questions and the SAC can be utilized as practical and effective evaluation tools.[33] The Maddocks questions are a qualitative measure used to evaluate the orientation of short- and long-term memory related to the sport and current game.[32] An athlete's inability to answer Maddocks questions correctly should raise suspicion for the presence of a concussive injury. For the current case patient, two particularly relevant Maddocks questions are "what venue are we at today?" and "which half is it now?" The SAC is a brief screening tool used to assess neurocognition. The SAC does not require training in psychometric testing to administer or interpret.[34] The SAC requires approximately 5 minutes to perform; orientation, immediate memory, concentration, and delayed recall are measured.[34,35] Because multiple variations of the SAC are used, little to no practice effect occurs.[28] In other words, the use of multiple variations prevents the athlete from memorizing the answers to the SAC in advance or with repeated testing. The results of the sideline assessment can be compared to those from a baseline assessment performed earlier in the season or preseason. Any decrease from the baseline SAC score has been shown to be 95% sensitive and 76% specific for a concussion.[36]

Balance disruption is common with concussion. The modified BESS is an assessment of postural stability that is easy to administer, inexpensive, and requires approximately 5 to 7 minutes to complete. It was developed to provide healthcare professionals with an inexpensive and objective way to assess postural stability outside the laboratory.[37] Much like the SAC, the results of the modified BESS test can be compared to a baseline assessment. Three stances (narrow double-leg stance, single-leg stance, and tandem stance) and two standing surfaces (firm surface/floor or medium-density foam) are used. Each stance is held, with hands on hips and eyes closed, for 20 seconds. Point deductions are given for specific errors including opening eyes, lifting hands off hips, stepping, stumbling, falling, moving stance hip into more than 30° of flexion or abduction, lifting forefoot or heel, or remaining out of the testing position for more than 5 seconds.[38] There is a maximum score of 60 points if both floor surfaces are used, or 30 points if only one surface is used. It is important to note that the BESS, from which the modified test is derived, seems to have a practice effect resulting in improved scores from repeatedly performing the same test.[39] In addition, the BESS can be influenced by fatigue.[37] The BESS has been validated against the Sensory Organization Test in the concussion population.[38] The intra-tester and inter-tester reliability for the BESS ranges from 0.6 to 0.92 and 0.57 to 0.85, respectively, and the test-retest reliability is moderate.[40] The specificity of the BESS ranges from 0.91 to 0.96 from days 1 to 7 following a concussion injury; however, the sensitivity of the BESS is poor with 0.34 the highest value at the time of injury.[40] Thus, the BESS would not be a good tool to rule out a concussion. Athletes experiencing impaired postural stability following concussion typically return to their baseline BESS scores within 3 to 5 days following injury.[40] The SCAT3 utilizes a modified BESS that is performed on one surface (which should match the surface from the baseline test). At present, no reported reliability, sensitivity, or specificity studies are available for the modified BESS. Thus, it should be noted that repeated testing using the modified BESS results in an as yet unquantified training effect. The SCAT3 also incorporates the timed Tandem Gait test, which is a new test for measuring dynamic balance and coordination. While this test has excellent reliability in the normal population, it has yet to be formally validated in a concussive population.[41]

Neuropsychological testing in athletes began in the 1980s as a tool to identify cognitive impairment and assist in documenting recovery from a concussive injury.[38] With the availability of computerized neuropsychological (CNP) testing, the use of NP testing has expanded. Several CNP testing programs are currently utilized, including ANAM (Automated Neuropsychological Assessment Metrics), CogState, HeadMinder, and ImPACT. The CNP test can be performed in a computer laboratory monitored by a qualified medical professional such as a sports physical therapist, athletic trainer, or physician who is familiar with the software.[42] In addition, NP testing can be administered by a neuropsychologist and performed via paper and pencil testing. Cognitive impairments may last longer than subjective symptoms, and while NP testing has not been validated as a diagnostic tool for concussion, it has the ability to identify cognitive impairments in the otherwise asymptomatic athlete.[43,44] The interpretation of the tests should be performed by a neuropsychologist or physician who is experienced with the test and concussion management. Additional research is needed to create evidenced-based guidelines or validated protocols concerning *when* to administer CNP tests following a concussion.

Plan of Care and Interventions

The immediate treatment of the post-concussive individual should emphasize education to the athlete as well as to the coach, parents, spouse, and/or caregivers. Education includes the signs and symptoms that should be monitored that would indicate any potential decline warranting further medical evaluation. The typical recovery process should also be discussed. When individuals who had sustained a concussion injury were provided education about concussion injury and treatment, they experienced fewer sleep disturbances and less anxiety and psychological stress compared to those who did not receive the education.[45]

Current guidelines recommend rest, both physical and cognitive, for the treatment of concussion.[46] As previously mentioned, an earlier RTP could have serious adverse effects such as second impact syndrome.[2] Physical rest includes removal from the competitive sport as well as other aerobic activities and resistance training. The athlete should avoid these activities until symptoms are no longer present when the athlete is at rest. This rest period is followed by a gradual increase in physical activity. If symptoms occur during the gradual increase in physical activity, the athlete should return to the previous level at which he was symptom-free. Cognitive rest is achieved by minimizing activities that require concentration and attention, including reading, schoolwork, video games, text messaging, and working online.[46] Academic accommodations should be considered during the recovery process. These accommodations facilitate cognitive rest and may preserve the patient's grades, which are likely to be affected during the recovery process.

Table 24-2 GRADUATED RETURN-TO-PLAY PROTOCOL[1,36,47]

Rehabilitation Stage	Functional Exercise at Each Stage of Rehabilitation	Objective of Each Stage
1. No activity	Complete physical and cognitive rest	Recovery
2. Light aerobic exercise	Walking, swimming, or stationary cycling (keeping intensity at 70% of age-predicted maximum heart rate) No resistance training	Increase heart rate
3. Sport-specific exercise	Skating drills in ice hockey, running drills in soccer. No head impact activities	Add movement
4. Non-contact training drills	Progression to more complex training drills (*e.g.*, passing drills in football and ice hockey) May start progressive resistance training	Exercise, coordination, and cognitive load
5. Full contact practice	Following medical clearance, participate in normal training activities	Restore confidence and assess functional skills by coaching staff
6. Return to play	Normal game play	

Guidelines for RTP should also follow a gradual progression. Table 24-2 presents the gradual progression of activity that is supported by the American Medical Society for Sports Medicine and the National Athletic Trainers Association.[1,36,47] Each rehabilitation stage should take approximately 24 hours, and the general rehabilitation protocol takes approximately 1 week.[2] The recovery course is longer for younger athletes than for collegiate and professional athletes and warrants a more conservative approach.[48] If any symptoms occur with advancement in the rehabilitation stage, the athlete should return to the previous asymptomatic stage. Progression to the next stage is attempted after the next 24-hour rest has occurred.

Prevention of injury during sport is still considered the best intervention strategy, and many sports (including ice hockey) have mandated equipment changes such as helmets and mouthguards in hopes of decreasing concussion injury risk. The use of helmets is standard practice in ice hockey. Although protective equipment has decreased the incidence of severe TBI in sport, the extent that this equipment is able to limit or minimize lower-impact collisions responsible for concussion injury remains unclear.[1,11] Biomechanical studies have demonstrated reduced impact forces to the brain when wearing helmets and headgear, but the incidence of concussion injury has increased. This most likely represents a better understanding and reporting of concussion injury. However, there has been a suggestion that protective equipment can result in risk compensation[4] in which athletes may feel encouraged to have a more aggressive style of play with a false sense of security from the protective equipment. Education of athletes is vital to address this potential problem. Mouthguards were implemented in many sports including ice hockey in the 1960s and 1970s.[11] While these do have a role in the prevention of dental and orofacial injuries, there is no good clinical evidence that they prevent concussion.[1]

Education of the athlete in terms of fair play and respect of the opposition, combined with correct sporting techniques, is vital to help prevent concussion. The complex condition of concussion requires all personnel involved with sport, including parents and healthcare providers, to be educated on the detection, treatment, and principles of safe RTP.[1]

Evidence-Based Clinical Recommendations

SORT: Strength of Recommendation Taxonomy
A: Consistent, good-quality patient-oriented evidence
B: Inconsistent or limited-quality patient-oriented evidence
C: Consensus, disease-oriented evidence, usual practice, expert opinion, or case series

1. Athletes diagnosed with a concussion should not return to play on the same day. **Grade C**

2. Athletes' performance on sideline tests such as the Standardized Assessment of Concussion (SAC), Balance Error Scoring System (BESS), and Sport Concussion Assessment Tool 3 (SCAT3) should be compared to their performance on pre-injury baseline tests. **Grade C**

3. To decrease the likelihood of serious adverse effects such as second impact syndrome, an athlete should not engage in physical or cognitive activities that increase symptoms during the early stages of concussion recovery. **Grade B**

4. Return to play after a concussion should be individualized, gradual, and progressive. **Grade C**

COMPREHENSION QUESTIONS

24.1 The sideline assessment for concussion should include which of the following tests?
   A. Standard orientation questions such as time, place, and person
   B. Computerized neuropsychological testing
   C. Maddocks questions
   D. Sensory Organization Test

24.2 A physical therapist is working with an athlete who sustained a concussion injury 4 days ago. As the athlete progressed to stage 3 of the graduated return-to-play protocol, she reported the onset of a headache. Given this situation, what recommendations should the physical therapist make to this athlete?
   A. Continue the current treatment with a reassessment of symptoms the following day.
   B. Have the athlete stop stage 3 and continue with stage 2.
   C. Progress the athlete to stage 4.
   D. Have the athlete stop stage 3 and continue with stage 1.

ANSWERS

24.1 **C.** Maddocks questions are a qualitative measure used to evaluate orientation as well as short- and long-term memory related to the sport and current game. Standard orientation questions such as time, place, and person have been shown to be unreliable in assessing concussion in athletes during sport (option A). Computerized neuropsychological testing and Sensory Organization Test are not practical assessments for the sideline examination (options B and D). The Standardized Assessment of Concussion (SAC) and Balance Error Scoring System (BESS) tests should also be considered as sideline assessments.

24.2 **B.** If symptoms occur with advancement in the rehabilitation stage, the athlete should return to the previous asymptomatic stage. Progression to the next stage is attempted after the next 24-hour rest has occurred.

REFERENCES

1. McCrory P, Meeuwisee WH, Aubry M, et al. Consensus statement on concussion in sport: the 4th International Conference on Concussion in Sport held in Zurich, November 2012. *Br J Sports Med*. 2013;47:250-258.
2. Herring SA, Cantu RC, Guskiewicz KM, et al; American College of Sports Medicine. Concussion (mild traumatic brain injury) and the team physician: a consensus statement-2011 update. *Med Sci Sports Exerc*. 2011;43:2412-2422.
3. McCrory P, Davis G, Makdissi M. Second impact syndrome or cerebral swelling after sporting head injury. *Curr Sports Med Rep*. 2012;11:21-23.
4. Hagel B, Meeuwisse W. Risk compensation: a "side effect" of sport injury prevention? *Clin J Sport Med*. 2004;14:193-196.
5. Langlois JA, Rutland-Brown W, Wald MM. The epidemiology and impact of traumatic brain injury: a brief overview. *J Head Trauma Rehabil*. 2006;21:375-378.
6. Guerrero JL, Thurman DJ, Sniezek JE. Emergency department visits associated with traumatic brain injury: United States, 1995-1996. *Brain Inj*. 2000;14:181-186.
7. Hootman JM, Dick R, Agel J. Epidemiology of collegiate injuries for 15 sports: summary and recommendations for injury prevention initiatives. *J Athl Train*. 2007;42:311-319.
8. Gessel LM, Fields SK, Collins CL, Dick RW, Comstock RD. Concussions among United States high school and collegiate athletes. *J Athl Train*. 2007;42:495-503.
9. Lincoln AE, Caswell SV, Almquist JL, Dunn RE, Norris JB, Hinton RY. Trends in concussion incidence in high school sports: a prospective 11-year study. *Am J Sports Med*. 2011;39:958-963.
10. Schultz MR, Marshall SW, Meuller FO, et al. Incidence and risk factors for concussion in high school athletes, North Carolina. *Am J Epidemiol*. 2004;160:937-944.
11. Daneshvar DH, Baugh CM, Nowinski CJ, McKee AC, Stern RA, Cantu RC. Helmets and mouth guards: the role of personal equipment in preventing sport-related concussions. *Clin Sports Med*. 2011;30:145-163.
12. Emery CA, Kang J, Shrier I, et al. Risk of injury associated with body checking among youth ice hockey players. *JAMA*. 2010;303:2265-2272.
13. Giza CC, Hovda DA. The neurometabolic cascade of concussion. *J Athl Train*. 2001;36:228-235.
14. DeLellis SM, Kane S, Katz K. The neurometabolic cascade and implications of mTBI: mitigating risk to the SOF community. *J Spec Oper Med*. 2009;9:36-42.

15. Giza CC, DiFiori JP. Pathophysiology of sports-related concussion: an update on basic science and tranlational research. *Sports Health*. 2011;3:46-51.
16. Guskiewicz KM, McCrea M, Marshall SW, et al. Cummulative effects associated with recurrent concussion in collegiate football players: the NCAA concussion study. *JAMA*. 2003;290:2549-2555.
17. US Department of Health and Human Services, Centers for Disease Control and Prevention. Heads Up: Facts for physicians about mild traumatic brain injury (MTBI). http://www.cdc.gov/concussion/headsup/pdf/Facts_for_Physicians_booklet-a.pdf. Accessed February 10, 2015.
18. Brooks D, Hunt BM. Current concepts in concussion diagnosis and managment in sports: a clinical review. *BCMJ*. 2006;48:453-459.
19. The ICD-10 Classification of Mental and Behavioural Disorders Diagnositic criteria for research. The World Health Organization. http://www.who.int/classifications/icd/en/GRNBOOK.pdf. Accessed February 11, 2015.
20. DeKosky ST, Ikonomovic, MD, Gandy S. Traumatic brain injury—football, warfare, and long-term effects. *N Engl J Med*. 2010;363:1293-1296.
21. Omalu BI, DeKosky ST, Minster RL, Kamboh MI, Hamilton RL, Wecht CH. Chronic traumatic encephalopathy in a National Football League player. *Neurosurgery*. 2005;57:128-134.
22. McCrory P. The eighth wonder of the world: the mythology of concussion management. *Br J Sports Med*. 1999;33:136-137.
23. Johnston KM, Bloom GA, Ramsay J, et al. Current concepts in concussion rehabilitation. *Curr Sports Med Rep*. 2004;3:316-323.
24. McCrea M, Hammeke T, Olsen G, Leo P, Guskiewicz K. Unreported concussion in high school footballl players: implications for prevention. *Clin J SportMed*. 2004;14:13-17.
25. Jones C. Glasgow coma scale. *Am J Nurs*. 1979;79:1551-1557.
26. Broglio SP, Guskiewicz KM. Concussion in sports: the sideline assessment. *Sports Health*. 2009;1:361-369.
27. Guskiewicz KM, Register-Mihalik J, McCrory P, et al. Evidence-based approach to revising the SCAT2: introducing the SCAT3. *Br J Sports Med*. 2013;47:289-293.
28. McCrea M, Kelly JP, Randolph C, Cisler R, Berger L. Immediate neurocognitive effects of concussion. *Neurosurgery*. 2002;50:1032-1042.
29. SCAT3 Sport Concussion Assessment Tool- 3rd Edition. Concussion in sport group. 2013. http://bjsm.bmj.com/content/47/5/259.full.pdf. Accessed February 11, 2015.
30. Guskiewicz KM, Bruce SL, Cantu RC, et al. National Athletic Trainers' Association position statement: managment of sport-related concussion. *J Athl Train*. 2004;39:280-297.
31. Giza CC, Kutcher JS, Ashwal S, et al. Summary of evidence-based guideline update: evaluation and management of concussion in sports: report of the Guideline Development Subcommittee of the American Academy of Neurology. *Neurology*. 2013;80:2250-2257.
32. Maddocks DL, Dicker GD, Saling MM. The assessment of orientation following concussion in athletes. *Clin J Sport Med*. 1995;5:32-35.
33. McCrory P, Meeuwisee W, Johnston K, et al. Consensus statement on concussion in Sport: the 3rd International Conference on Concussion in Sport held in Zurich, November 2008. *Br J Sports Med*. 2009;43:i76-i90.
34. McCrea M, Kelly JP, Randolph C. *Standardized Assessment of Concussion (SAC): Manual for Administration, Scoring and Interpretation*. 2nd ed. Waukesha, WI: CNS Inc; 2000.
35. McCrea M. Standardized mental status testing on the sideline after sport-related concussion. *J Athl Train*. 2001;36:274-279.
36. Harmon KG, Drenzer JA, Gammons M, et al. American Medical Society for Sports Medicine position statement: concussion in sport. *Br J Sports Med*. 2013;47:15-26.
37. Wilkins JC, Valovich McLeod TC, Perrin DH, Gansneder BM. Performance on the Balance Error Scoring System decreases after fatigue. *J Athl Train*. 2004;39:156-161.

38. Guskiewicz KM, Ross SE, Marshall SW. Postural stability and neuropsychological deficits after concussion in collegiate athletes. *J Athl Train.* 2001;36:263-273.
39. Valovich TC, Perrin DH, Gansneder BM. Repeat administration elicits a practice effect with the Balance Error Scoring System but not with the Standardized Assessment of Concussion in high school athletes. *J Athl Train.* 2003;38:51-56.
40. Bell DR, Guskiewicz KM, Clark MA, Padua DA. Systematic review of the balance error scoring system. *Sports Health.* 2011;3:287-295.
41. Schneiders AG, Sullivan SJ, Gray AR, Hammond-Tooke GD, McCrory PR. Normative values for three clinical measures of motor performance used in the neurological assessment of sports concussion. *J Sci Med Sport.* 2010;13:196-201.
42. ImPACT. ImPACT training overview. https://www.impacttest.com/training/. Accessed February 10, 2015.
43. McCrea M, Barr WB, Guskiewicz K, et al. Standard regression-based methods for measuring recovery after sport-related consussion. *J Int Neuropsychol Soc.* 2005;11:58-69.
44. Makdissi M, Darby D, Maruff P. Natural history of concussion in sport: markers of severity and implications for management. *Am J Sports Med.* 2010;38:464-471.
45. Ponsford J, Willmott C, Rothwell A, et al. Impact of early intervention on outcome following mild head injury in adults. *J Neurol Neurosurg Psychiatry.* 2002;73:330-332.
46. Meehan WP 3rd. Medical therapies for concussion. *Clin Sports Med.* 2011;30:115-124.
47. McCory P, Meeuwisee WH, Aubry M, et al. Consensus statement on concussion in sport: the 4th International Conference on Concussion in Sport, Zurich, November 2012. *J Athl Train.* 2013;48:554-575.
48. Halstead ME, Walter KD; Council on Sports Medicine and Fitness. American Academy of Pediatrics. Clinical report—sports-related concussion in children and adolescents. *Pediatrics.* 2010;126:597-615.

Peripheral Neuropathic Pain

William I. Rubine

CASE 25

A 27-year-old right-hand dominant male golfer presents to an outpatient physical therapy clinic in a Comprehensive Pain Center with a referral for left-sided neck and shoulder pain. He complains of left shoulder and arm pain, left upper extremity paresthesia, and neck pain. He thinks his problem started after a car accident 4 years ago. His symptoms improved for 2 years, later worsening again for no apparent reason. He now finds himself unable to play golf or ride his motorcycle. He describes his current pain as burning and shooting. His pain increases when he stretches his arm or "really uses it all." The pain decreases when he holds his arm at his side and does not use it. An electromyogram (EMG) of the upper quarter was normal and the patient's primary care physician reported that the patient's cervical magnetic resonance imaging (MRI) scan showed "nothing of concern." However, the patient worries that he has some rare condition that cannot be cured. He has been treated over the past 3 months by a chiropractor and massage therapist; both clinicians told him that his condition was "weird."

- Based on the patient's suspected diagnosis, what do you anticipate may be the contributing factors to his condition?
- What are the most appropriate physical therapy interventions?
- What are possible complications interfering with physical therapy?
- Identify topics for interprofessional discussion that should be addressed with other team members in the Comprehensive Pain Center.

KEY DEFINITIONS

ADVERSE RESPONSE TO NEURAL TENSION: Pain, sensory changes, and/or tension along the course of a peripheral nerve, provoked by strain placed on the nerve by active or passive lengthening of the nerve bed

ALLODYNIA: Painful response to normally innocuous stimuli such as light touch or a brush stroke

CENTRAL SENSITIZATION: Alteration of pre- and postsynaptic processes of high threshold and wide-dynamic-range neurons in the dorsal horn of the spinal cord; manifested as increased receptor field size and increased responsiveness and/or decreased threshold to innocuous or noxious stimuli[1]

DYSESTHESIA: Spontaneous or evoked unpleasant abnormal sensation[1]

DYSESTHETIC PAIN: Spontaneous or evoked pain (burning, tingling, or lancinating) due to abnormal firing of damaged or regenerating nociceptive afferent fibers

HYPERALGESIA: Increased response to a stimulus that is normally painful[1]

MECHANOSENSITIVITY: Tendency of neural tissue to produce impulses that are perceived as pain or paresthesia in response to mechanical forces such as compression, tension, or shear[2,3]

NERVE SLIDER: Multi-joint movement that combines one motion that lengthens the nerve bed with another motion at a different part of the body that shortens the nerve bed causing nerve excursion toward the segment that is being lengthened[2-6]

NERVE TENSIONER: Uni- or multi-joint movement at one or both ends of a nerve bed that increases strain in the nerve[2-6]

NERVE TRUNK PAIN: "Deep and aching" pain from mechanically or chemically sensitized nociceptors in the nervi nervorum[7]

NERVI NERVORUM: Plexus of unmyelinated nerves that invests and innervates tissues within a peripheral nerve trunk; responsive to mechanical, thermal, and chemical stimuli,[8] which can result in nociception as well as vasodilation of the vaso nervorum, contributing to inflammation within the nerve[2]

NEUROGENIC INFLAMMATION: Release of proinflammatory neuropeptides by injured peripheral nerves into their target tissues, sometimes contributing to musculoskeletal conditions that do not resolve within the expected timeframe[7]

NEUROPATHIC PAIN: Pain arising as a direct consequence of a lesion or disease affecting the somatosensory system[1]

NOCICEPTION: Perception of actual or potential tissue damage that may or may not be interpreted by the individual as pain

RADICULAR PAIN: Lancinating pain typically down a limb in a narrow band, indicating ectopic discharges from a dorsal root or its ganglion[9]

RADICULOPATHY: Conduction block along a spinal nerve or its roots, resulting in diminished reflexes; when sensory fibers are blocked, numbness occurs in a dermatomal pattern and when motor fibers are blocked, weakness occurs in a myotomal pattern[9]

STRUCTURAL DIFFERENTIATION: Clinical assessment for a change in symptoms in one area of the body by active or passive alteration of nerve strain in the same nerve in a remote area of the body

VASA NERVORUM: Small interlacing blood vessels that provide blood supply to peripheral nerves

Objectives

1. Describe peripheral neuropathic pain (PNP).
2. Recognize signs and symptoms that characterize PNP and musculoskeletal conditions perpetuated by peripheral neurogenic inflammation.
3. Discuss the patient education and cognitive behavioral techniques physical therapists can provide to individuals with neuropathic pain.
4. Prescribe evidence-based manual techniques to decrease muscle guarding and improve intraneural blood flow that can encourage resolution of peripheral nerve mechanosensitivity and its consequent pain.
5. Prescribe evidence-based mobility exercises to improve intraneural blood flow and restore mobility to affected limbs.
6. Prescribe evidence-based resistance exercises to restore strength, endurance, and motor control to muscles affected by pain and/or disuse and to restore patients' confidence in their ability to perform normal activities.

Physical Therapy Considerations

PT considerations during management of the individual with PNP:

- **General physical therapy plan of care/goals:** Decrease pain and peripheral nerve mechanosensitivity; improve cervical, upper thoracic, and upper extremity mobility; increase rotator cuff and scapular stabilizer muscle strength; improve function in activities of daily living and sport

- **Physical therapy interventions:** Patient education regarding neurophysiology of pain and nerve mechanosensitivity; physical agents to decrease muscle guarding and facilitate mobilization of sensitive tissues; passive mobilization to decrease mechanosensitivity and improve upper-quarter mobility; upper extremity nerve sliders and tensioners to manage symptoms and improve mobility; resistance exercises to address impairments in muscular strength and endurance; sport-specific exercises to facilitate return to sport

- **Precautions during physical therapy:** Avoid painful stretching of irritated nerves (*i.e.*, nerves that are sensitive to palpation and/or demonstrate adverse response to neural tension); monitor vital signs; address precautions or contraindications for exercise based on patient's pre-existing condition(s)

▶ **Complications interfering with physical therapy:** Catastrophization, passive pain coping mechanisms, poor pacing, noncompliance with exercise program, sleep difficulties, nerve compression that is unresponsive to conservative management

Understanding the Health Condition

There are several possible mechanisms for neck and arm pain in athletes, including PNP. PNP has been defined as "pain caused by a lesion or disease of the peripheral part of the somatosensory nervous system."[10] The signs and symptoms of PNP are consequences of increased peripheral nerve sensitivity and neurogenic inflammation that can result from mechanical or chemical irritation of a peripheral nerve trunk. This is not uncommon in sport, where repetitive, loaded, and end-range movements challenge the physical tolerance of peripheral nerves and their surrounding soft tissues.[7,11] Compressive, shear, vibrational, or tensile forces can injure or irritate a peripheral nerve, usually in anatomically narrow areas such as the spinal foramina, thoracic outlet, cubital tunnel, or carpal tunnel. Chemical irritation of a peripheral nerve can result from exposure to inflammatory exudate from nearby injured tissues such as an extruded nucleus pulposus or another inflamed nerve. PNP can also result from chemotherapy, radiation therapy, viral infection (*e.g.*, shingles), or metabolic conditions such as diabetes. Common sites of peripheral nerve injury in the upper quarter include the cervical nerve roots in the cervical foramina, the brachial plexus in the neck and thoracic outlet, and any of the nerves of the upper extremity including the ulnar nerve at the cubital tunnel and the median nerve at the carpal tunnel. While musculoskeletal presentations of PNP and their physical therapy management have been described since at least 1980,[12] the condition has had several names including peripheral nerve sensitization,[1] peripheral neurogenic pain,[4] neck pain with radiating pain,[13] cervicobrachial pain syndrome,[14,15] and, most recently, "nerve-related neck and arm pain."[16]

Individuals with a lesion or disease in a peripheral nerve may experience two types of pain: dysesthetic pain and/or nerve trunk pain. Dysesthetic pain is an unpredictable burning, electric, or crawling pain. Nerve trunk pain is typically more predictable and described as aching ("like a toothache"[12]) along the course of the nerve trunk. In addition to pain, patients with PNP may complain of paresthesia, dysesthesia, numbness, weakness, or spasm. Often, the pain and other symptoms present in a dermatomal or peripheral nerve distribution.[17] Some individuals with peripheral nerve injuries report neither dysesthetic nor nerve trunk pain, but rather report seemingly common musculoskeletal injuries that have persisted far beyond the expected healing timeframe. Upon examination, these conditions are often found to be related to increased peripheral nerve mechanosensitivity due to an unnoticed injury in one or more places along the course of the nerve innervating the involved tissue. It is believed that these conditions are perpetuated by the production of inflammatory factors within the injured nerve[7] that are transported down the nerve and into the innervated tissue (*i.e.*, "neurogenic inflammation").

To better understand the proposed mechanisms underlying PNP, a brief review of sensory nerve fiber types, connective tissue, and blood supply to peripheral nerves is helpful. A peripheral nerve is composed of individual nerve fibers (axons), connective tissue, the vasa nervorum (blood vessels), and the nervi nervorum (small unmyelinated nerves that innervate the connective tissue and vasa nervorum). Sensory neurons in the dorsal horn generate action potentials because of activation of mechano- and chemosensitive ion channels in their nerve endings. These ion channels have a half-life of hours or days, meaning they are continuously replaced as the nervous system adapts to its environment.[3] The 3 main types of sensory afferent fibers are A-beta, A-delta, and C. The myelinated A-beta fibers encode touch, stretch, and kinesthesia. A-delta fibers are also myelinated and transmit sharp localized nociception. Last, unmyelinated C fibers encode dull unlocalized nociception.[1] Schwann cells are responsible for producing and maintaining myelin sheaths around individual A-beta and A-delta fibers. While Schwann cells surround groups of type C fibers, they do not produce myelin.

The connective tissue of a peripheral nerve has 3 layers: endoneurium, perineurium, and epineurium. The endoneurium surrounds individual axons. The perineurium surrounds groups of axons (bundled in fascicles), protecting them from chemical insult and maintaining intraneurial fluid pressure. The perineurium also provides some tensile strength. The outermost epineurium forms the external sheath around the nerve that provides it a "cord-like structure,"[18] protecting it from compression and allowing it to slide and glide within the surrounding tissues. Collectively, the connective tissue comprises 30% to 85% of the total tissue of the nerve trunk.[18]

Peripheral nerves require significant oxygen, glucose, and other nutrients to function.[3] The vasa nervorum—coiled and anastomosing blood vessels running within and among the fasciculi—is responsible for supplying oxygen and other nutrients to the nerves. Blood flow to nerves is critical because nerve ischemia can cause positive symptoms such as paresthesia and mechanosensitivity. In addition, venous stasis and endoneurial edema can degrade myelin and axon structure.[7,19] Two major factors drive blood flow through the vasa nervorum: the pressure gradient between the arterioles and venules and the transient pressure changes from constriction, dilation, uncoiling and recoiling of the blood vessels and nerve tissues that occur during movement. Thus, blood flow within a peripheral nerve can decrease with extraneural compression, intraneural edema, and lack of movement. Conversely, blood flow can increase with gentle repetitive movement.

Many investigators have studied the process by which the nervous system generates pain and other symptoms in response to mechanical or chemical injury of peripheral nerves or surrounding tissues.[2,7,12] A concise summary starts with the mechanical damage to nerve fibers and connective tissues that leads to venous congestion, decreased intraneural circulation, decreased axoplasmic flow, breakdown of endoneurial capillary membranes, and hypoxia. A complex inflammatory response follows in the nerve and dorsal root ganglion (DRG). Glial cells, Schwann cells, and immune cells release immune mediators such as cytokines and histamine that contribute to an edematous and irritating "inflammatory soup" that forms within and around the fasciculi. This "soup" can persist in the fasciculi because of the perineural diffusion barrier. Chemical irritants from inflamed tissues adjacent to the nerve can also contribute to inflammation within a nerve at this stage.[7]

Inflammation has several negative effects on nerves.[7,19,20] Nociceptors in the nervi nervorum in the connective tissue become sensitized. Connective tissue becomes fibrotic, reducing the nerve's extensibility so that innocuous movement places additional mechanical load on the nociceptors. Neurons increase their production of mechano- and chemosensitive ion channels. If endoneurial edema is severe and persistent, myelin and axons may be damaged, possibly impairing the ability of the nerve to conduct impulses.[19] Ion channels may randomly insert themselves into the axonal membrane within areas of damaged myelin and begin to spontaneously generate abnormal (ectopic) impulses. These areas are termed abnormal impulse generating sites (AIGS)[7] because they form in the middle of the axon where impulses are not normally generated. Depending on the type of ion channels that have been inserted, the trigger for a particular AIGS might be temperature, an immune mediator, a stress-related hormone, or a mechanical force.[3] Ectopic impulses produced by AIGS can travel orthodromically (toward the spinal cord), similar to normal action potentials traveling in sensory nerves. However, impulses from AIGS can also travel antidromically (toward the tissues innervated by the sensory nerve). These antidromic impulses trigger the release of proinflammatory chemicals such as substance P and C-reactive protein into the innervated tissues.[2,3,7] This is believed to be the cause of the "neurogenic inflammation" that contributes to and perpetuates musculoskeletal injuries such as shoulder pain, frozen shoulder, lateral epicondylitis, medial knee pain, chronic ankle sprain, and other chronic conditions that do not resolve in the expected timeframe.[7]

PNP is usually accompanied by changes at higher levels of the nervous system. Prolonged nociceptive input (which can result from neurogenic inflammation) stimulates the central nervous system (CNS) to become more sensitive to nociceptive signals by increasing neuronal excitability in central nociceptive pathways. For example, some type A-beta neurons are diverted to nociceptive pathways in the dorsal horn, and endogenous pain inhibition in the spinal cord is reduced.[21] Collectively, these adaptations are termed central sensitization. Multiple adaptations also occur within the brain in response to peripheral nerve injuries. In human subjects with PNP, functional MRI studies have found that the somatosensory cortex becomes reorganized.[17]

Individuals with PNP may present with maladaptive psychosocial responses to pain such as catastrophization, depression, improper conceptualization of pain, and fear of re-injury.[3,20] These issues can worsen symptoms by triggering stress-related endocrine and immune responses that increase pain, interfere with sleep, decrease compliance and adherence to a home exercise program, and impede recovery. To some extent, central sensitization and psychosocial responses may represent normal responses to injury; however, the responses to neuropathic pain may be much more pronounced than those following musculoskeletal injury.[21] When these responses persist or dominate the clinical presentation, they may produce signs and symptoms that baffle patients and clinicians alike. The contribution of central sensitization and psychosocial issues varies from patient to patient. Criteria have been posited for determining the contribution of PNP, central sensitization, and psychosocial issues to individual patients.[20] Characteristics of PNP include pain in a dermatomal or peripheral nerve distribution, cold sensitivity, and flare-ups that are delayed for days after the provoking stimulus. Characteristics of central sensitization include provocation by certain stimuli at some times but not at others, multiple areas of sensitivity, spreading pain, flare-ups that occur days after the provoking stimuli, allodynia, cold sensitivity, and pain lasting longer than 3 months. Pain that is influenced by meaning, mood, or social context suggests a strong contribution by psychosocial issues. Physical therapists and other healthcare providers must appreciate the impact of central sensitization and psychosocial issues in managing individuals with PNP. Additional treatment modalities such as patient education, coaching, and cognitive behavioral therapy should be incorporated as adjuncts to the treatment of the mechanical aspects of the health condition.[3,7,20]

Examination of a patient with a suspected lesion or disease of the peripheral nervous system requires assessment of more than just pain. Clinical tests of muscle strength, sensation, and deep tendon reflexes (DTRs) are also performed. The signs and symptoms of peripheral nerve injury are commonly divided into positive and negative symptoms[7,22] or gains and losses of function.[17] Positive symptoms (gains of function) are those that represent an increased responsiveness or decreased threshold to stimuli. These include spontaneous pain, hyperalgesia, allodynia, paresthesia, hypoesthesia, and increased DTRs. Negative symptoms (losses of function) result from impaired impulse conduction. These include hypoesthesia or anesthesia, weakness, and decreased DTRs. Identification of negative symptoms, if present, can help determine the course of treatment.

Electrodiagnostic tests (*e.g.*, EMG, nerve conduction velocity [NCV]) can also be performed to confirm the findings of the clinical examination. However, it is important to note that EMG and NCV tests are only sensitive to changes in the large-diameter motor and A-beta fibers and not to changes in the A-delta or C fibers that are responsible for nociception.[17] This means that patients can have PNP and improve with physical therapy interventions, despite having normal results on electrodiagnostic tests.

Physical Therapy Patient/Client Management

A multidisciplinary pain clinic (MPC) is a specialized facility in which a team of clinicians (physicians, psychologists, physical therapists) collaborate in the care of patients with persistent or complex pain conditions. Specific interventions vary, but usually include 4 elements: medication, behavioral therapy, physical conditioning, and education.[23] The goals of treatment are to identify and treat unresolved medical issues, provide appropriate (and eliminate inappropriate) medications, improve coping skills and psychological well-being, educate the patient about the neurophysiology of pain, establish realistic goals, and restore function.[23] Primary care physicians often refer individuals who seem to lack identifiable physical causes for their persistent pain to MPCs. Accordingly, individuals with inflammatory PNP who have negative electrodiagnostic tests and present without negative symptoms in their neurologic examinations are often referred to MPCs because their peripheral nerve injury is undetected. For the patient presented in this case, the physician at the MPC screened the patient for serious illness that may have been missed by the referring provider and considered the potential for a procedural intervention such as an epidural glucocorticoid injection or nerve block. It was determined that the best course for this patient was an initial trial of physical therapy prior to other interventions. The psychologist evaluated the patient for psychosocial issues such as depression, catastrophization, and poor coping skills and determined that the patient was coping well with his condition. The psychologist instructed him in breathing and relaxation techniques, and discussed the need to use pacing and return gradually to sport. The majority of this patient's management was provided by the physical therapist.

Physical therapy management of PNP is commonly divided into 6 parts:[4] patient education and coaching, mobilization of non-neural tissues (possibly including spinal traction), neural desensitization techniques, graded mobilization of neural tissue, strength training, and functional restoration. Several mechanical and physiologic mechanisms have been postulated to support the effectiveness of these interventions including restoration of the mechanical extensibility of the tissues surrounding the nerve, restoration of normal oxygenation via improved intraneural circulation and axoplasmic flow, desensitization of the AIGS through normalization of the ion channel distribution in the axonal plasma membrane, desensitization of neurons in the DRG and CNS, and improved representation of the affected areas in the CNS.[3,24]

Examination, Evaluation, and Diagnosis

The diagnosis of PNP is based on history and clinical examination. The physical therapist should gather information regarding onset, character, and distribution of the patient's symptoms, as well as aggravating and easing factors and a description of the patient's basic lifestyle and work- or family-related responsibilities. The therapist should also inquire about the patient's preference for ice or heat, the efficacy of anti-inflammatories, if the patient has flare-ups, and how long they typically last. A patient's history and symptom distribution may be enough for a diagnosis of possible PNP.[25] While this information may be used to make a general clinical diagnosis,[10,25,26] it is not enough information to create a specific treatment plan. If the subjective examination supports the likelihood of PNP, the clinical examination must determine if increased neural mechanosensitivity is present, the radicular or peripheral nerve distribution of the symptoms, specific dysfunctions within non-neural tissues that may be perpetuating the condition, and whether negative symptoms are present to indicate that nerve impulse conduction has been altered.

Patients with PNP often complain of burning or stinging pain, electrical pain, or a deep ache.[27] They may also complain of numbness and tingling. The distribution of PNP often follows a pattern consistent with the involved nerve, though it may not.[17] PNP is worsened by positions that lengthen or compress the nerve, and is eased by positions that unload the nerve such as holding the hand at the chest or over the head. Ice often worsens PNP, whereas heat often lessens it. While nociceptive pain typically increases in response to mechanical provocation of the involved tissue and decreases immediately or shortly after the provocation stops, PNP often changes unpredictably and spontaneously in the tissue innervated by the affected nerve with an intensity that seems out of proportion to the stimulus. In this case, the patient reported burning and shooting pain in multiple sites from the shoulder to the hand and along the ulnar nerve course and intermittent numbness and tingling in the arm and hand. He also reported that his condition had not improved over the course of 4 months. These comments alerted the therapist to suspect either PNP or central sensitization. The therapist considered PNP more likely than central sensitization for 3 reasons: (1) a dominant case of central sensitization would be uncommon among avid athletes and motorcycle riders; (2) the pain had not spread to multiple body sites; and (3) while the pain seemed unpredictable to the patient because it occurred at various sites on the arm at different times, it was *predictably* triggered by activities that stressed the major nerves of the upper extremity and their surrounding structures and it was always perceived somewhere along a nerve course.

The basic elements of the clinical examination include postural observation, active and passive movement of the upper quarter (including upper-limb nerve tension tests [ULNTs]), nerve palpation, examination of innervated tissues, examination of non-neural structures anatomically related to the involved nerve (also known as the "mechanical interface"[2]) and clinical assessment of nerve conduction via myotomal strength testing, sensory testing, and DTRs. There are 3 clinical subtypes of PNP: inflammatory, compressive, and mixed. Inflammatory cases generally demonstrate only positive signs and symptoms, whereas compressive cases demonstrate negative signs and symptoms, and mixed cases present with both. The therapist identifies which subtype best describes the patient's presentation. The physical therapist also attempts to categorize the patient's presentation based on the condition of the neural structures, mechanical interface, and innervated tissues.[2] Patients often present with multiple impairments. After the clinical examination, the therapist should have a fairly complete idea of the impairments limiting the patient's return to normal activities. Very often, it makes the most sense to manage the PNP first, especially in cases in which nerve trunk or dysesthetic pain clearly predominate and in musculoskeletal cases that have not previously responded to usual care.

The physical examination begins with posture. The therapist should observe posture from anterior, posterior, and lateral views. Typical deviations in the upper quarter include cervical lateral tilt either toward or away from the affected side and scapular elevation, elbow flexion, and/or clawing of the fingers on the affected side. Patients unconsciously adopt these positions to protect the affected nerve or nerves, either by shifting toward the affected side to decrease nerve tension, or by leaning away from the affected side to reduce compression placed on the nerves by adjacent tissues. The patient in this case preferred to hold his symptomatic arm at his side and tilt his head slightly toward it, effectively decreasing the strain on the nerves of the affected upper extremity (Fig. 25-1).

After posture, the therapist examines active range of motion (AROM) of the cervical spine and upper extremity. Up to this point, this is the same examination that a physical therapist would conduct for most patients with pain in the upper quarter. In cases of upper-quarter PNP, the therapist should expect to find decreased AROM on the affected side in the cervical spine, shoulder, elbow, forearm, wrist, and/or hand, depending on the site of the impairment. The patient in this case had decreased left cervical rotation with pain and tingling in his left arm and medial

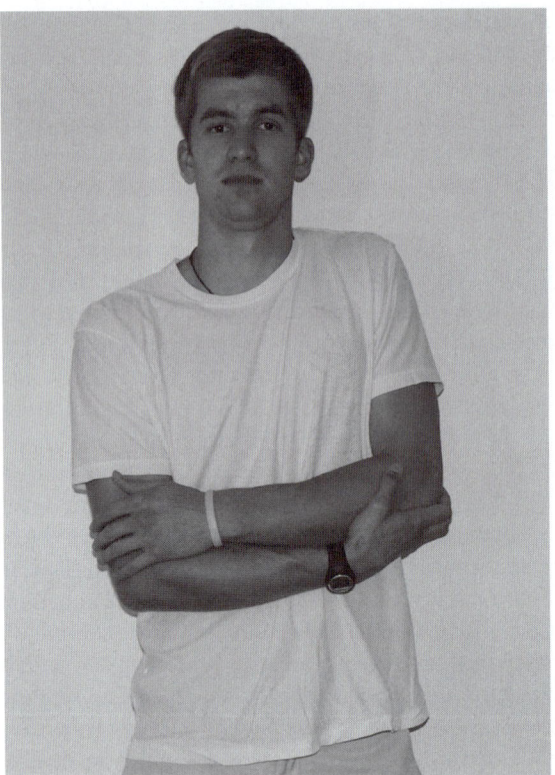

Figure 25-1. Protective posturing for the left upper quarter.

hand with shoulder elevation over 60°. Combined with the patient's subjective history and posture, these signs supported PNP, though which nerve was involved still had to be determined. Three "quick tests" of active upper extremity movements have been developed to screen for increased nerve trunk mechanosensitivity in the 3 major nerves of the upper extremity (median, radial, ulnar).[5] Each test applies preferential strain to one of the nerves; if symptoms arise, the strain is altered to determine if there is a predictable effect on the symptoms. The process of altering symptoms by adjusting strain on a nerve at an area remote from those symptoms is called structural differentiation.[2,3] Positive tests reproduce some aspect of the patient's symptoms and demonstrate structural differentiation.[2,3,5] Table 25-1 shows the median, ulnar, and radial quick tests, as well as the movements used for structural differentiation. These active quick tests are very similar to passive ULNTs. ULNTs are commonly used by experts[13,27] and have been found to be plausible tests for detecting PNP with "moderate to substantial" reliability though their diagnostic validity remains unconfirmed.[26] If the patient's history strongly suggests neuropathic pain, but quick tests are negative, the next step would be for the patient to actively demonstrate a movement or position that provoked his symptoms. Then the therapist would try to perform structural differentiation in that position via the principles outlined in Table 25-1.

Table 25-1 ACTIVE QUICK TESTS FOR THE PRESENCE OF INCREASED NEURAL MECHANOSENSITIVITY IN THE UPPER EXTREMITY[5]

Name of Test	Image of Final Position	Position of Patient	Positive Test
Median nerve quick test		Patient elevates shoulder with wrist and elbow straight. If the symptoms are distal to the elbow, structural differentiation is performed by side bending the neck away from the affected side. If the symptoms are proximal to the elbow, structural differentiation is performed by extending the wrist.	Patient's symptoms are reproduced by moving toward the final position *and* worsened with addition of contralateral cervical side bending or wrist extension.
Radial nerve quick test		Patient makes a fist with the thumb inside the hand. With elbow extended, the patient internally rotates shoulder and pronates forearm so thumb points away from body. Next, the patient depresses shoulder and extends shoulder a few degrees. Last, he side bends neck away from the involved side. If symptoms are distal to the shoulder, structural differentiation is performed by elevating scapula or returning neck to neutral position. If symptoms are in the shoulder or neck, structural differentiation is performed by returning wrist and fingers to neutral.	If patient's symptoms are reproduced by moving toward the final position *and* relieved by returning the cervical spine to a neutral position or returning the wrist to neutral.

(Continued)

Table 25-1. ACTIVE QUICK TESTS FOR THE PRESENCE OF INCREASED NEURAL MECHANOSENSITIVITY IN THE UPPER EXTREMITY[5] (CONTINUED)

Name of Test	Image of Final Position	Position of Patient	Positive Test
Ulnar nerve quick test		Patient puts his hand on his ear with fingers pointing down and lifts elbow up and out to side. Structural differentiation is performed by returning wrist to neutral position or by decreasing shoulder abduction.	If patient's symptoms are reproduced by moving toward the final position *and* relieved by returning wrist position to neutral or by decreasing shoulder abduction.

For this patient, only the ulnar nerve quick test reproduced his symptoms. In addition, the therapist was able to reduce the paresthesia in the patient's hand by decreasing shoulder abduction and reduce the shoulder pain by flexing the patient's wrist. This structural differentiation suggested that the patient may be experiencing PNP from an injury to the ulnar nerve or one of its roots. The therapist could now consider this as a case of probable PNP with some evidence of positive symptoms (paresthesia with positive structural differentiation), but further testing was required to know how to structure the treatment plan.

The next step of the examination is assessment of passive range of motion (PROM) of the involved body segments, both individually and in combination (via ULNTs). In cases of possible PNP, any of the noted limitations in *active* motion of the cervical spine and upper extremity might be due to myofascial dysfunction (*e.g.*, shortened or inflamed muscles or tendons), articular dysfunction, increased neural mechanosensitivity, or any combination of the three. Assessing the PROM of the involved body segments helps to distinguish between each of these potential causes. For example, decreased PROM resulting from restricted myofascial tissue (*i.e.*, tight muscles and fascia) should correspond to specific myofascial structures and may span 1 or more joints, but should *not* be affected by changes in the position of segments 2 or more joints *removed* from the area in question. Decreased PROM resulting from articular dysfunction occurs in a single joint in 1 or more directions, is usually accompanied by corresponding changes in the accessory motion of the joint, and is also unaffected by the position of remote segments. Impaired PROM due to increased neural mechanosensitivity can be identified by the end feel and the quality of the symptoms provoked (dysesthetic or nerve trunk pain). However, the most distinguishing and reliable indicator of increased neural mechanosensitivity is that the end ROM changes depend on the position of remote segments of the body (*i.e.*, structural differentiation is possible).[10]

ULNTs utilize specific sequences of passive movements of the upper extremities to selectively and progressively apply mechanical strain to the brachial plexus and each of the 3 major nerve trunks of the upper limb.[26] Smart et al.[27] reported that **ULNTs are the most commonly used objective test for neural mechanosensitivity.** ULNT 1 (median nerve) is included in current guidelines for evaluating patients with neck and upper extremity pain[13] and in clinical prediction rules to identify patients with neck pain likely to benefit from cervical traction and exercise.[28] There are different definitions of a "positive" response to an ULNT in the literature; however, the most current definition is that the test reproduces some aspect of the patient's symptoms and those symptoms should be altered during structural differentiation.[10] There is fair to moderate inter-rater reliability among examiners using ULNTs for detecting increased neural mechanosensitivity associated with conditions such as cervical radiculopathy, carpal tunnel syndrome, or cubital tunnel syndrome.[10,26] In a systematic review of the diagnostic accuracy of several provocative tests for diagnosing cervical radiculopathy, ULNT 1 demonstrated high sensitivity and low specificity.[29] A more recent review concluded that there was not enough evidence to determine the validity of using ULNTs to detect PNP because more work must be done to define a reference standard.[10]

Table 25-2 describes the standard versions of the 4 basic ULNTs as they are typically performed[10,26] and examples of ways to perform structural differentiation.

Table 25-2 BASIC SEQUENCES OF UPPER-LIMB NERVE TENSION TESTS FOR PATIENT WITH SUSPECTED PNP[3]

Test	Sequential Movements of Patient's Upper Extremity by Therapist	Starting Position	Final Position
ULNT 1 (median nerve)	90° elbow flexion and 110° shoulder abduction with wrist/finger extension, (thumb abducted and extended) Forearm supination Shoulder external rotation Elbow extension Cervical side bends away from symptomatic extremity		Perform structural differentiation by returning cervical spine to neutral or by releasing wrist from extension. If remote symptoms are altered by these changes of position, then nerve mechanosensitivity is probably responsible.
ULNT 2a (median nerve bias)	With patient positioned with shoulder just over the edge of the table: Shoulder girdle depression Elbow extension Shoulder external rotation and forearm supination Wrist and finger extension Shoulder abduction		If the symptoms are proximal to elbow, assess for structural differentiation by releasing wrist extension. If the symptoms are distal to elbow, assess for structural differentiation by releasing scapular depression.

ULNT 2b (radial nerve bias)	With patient positioned with shoulder just over the edge of the table: Shoulder girdle depression Elbow extension Whole-arm internal rotation Wrist flexion		If the symptoms are proximal to elbow, assess for structural differentiation by releasing wrist and finger flexion. If the symptoms are distal to elbow, assess for structural differentiation by releasing scapular depression.
ULNT 3 (ulnar nerve)	With patient positioned with shoulder just over the edge of the table: Depress shoulder girdle Abduct shoulder Externally rotate shoulder Flex elbow Extend wrist and fingers Pronate forearm		If the symptoms are proximal to elbow, perform structural differentiation by releasing wrist extension. If the symptoms are distal to elbow, perform structural differentiation by releasing scapular depression.

ULNT 1 tests the median nerve; ULNT 2a and ULNT 2b test the median nerve and radial nerves, respectively. ULNT 3 tests the ulnar nerve. For each test, the patient is positioned in a comfortable supine position. For simplicity and reproducibility, the physical therapist can perform the test movements in the manner and sequential order presented in Table 25-2. However, cadaver studies show that during an ULNT, the mechanical effects on the nerve are greatest in the immediate vicinity of the joint that moves first.[24] The authors suggested clinical options for altering the sequence of movements when the examiner wishes to challenge a specific segment of the nerve. The starting position, order of movements, ROM, posture, and load on the limb can all be adapted. The details of how and when to alter these variables are beyond the scope of this case, but are covered in several books on the clinical management of PNP.[2,3,5]

Before beginning an ULNT, the physical therapist should explain to the patient that the objective of the test is to attempt to reproduce at least some of his symptoms such as pain or paresthesia. A stretching sensation, which is a common response to ULNTs, does not indicate pathology[10] and this should be communicated to the patient. The explanation should be as nonthreatening as possible because research has found that when ULNTs are described as "nerve tests," patients allow less motion and report more symptoms. In contrast, when the tests are described as tests of "circulation" or "mobility," the patients allow more motion and report fewer symptoms.[3,30]

To familiarize the patient with the test and to give the therapist an idea of potentially normal neural mobility, it is generally better to test the uninvolved upper extremity first. The physical therapist should prompt the patient to report when symptoms *begin* to emerge, not when he cannot tolerate the symptoms anymore. It is important to remember that these neurodynamic tests are *provocation* tests, not tolerance tests. When performing the test, the therapist should stop the movement immediately if the patient begins to experience adverse symptoms (*i.e.*, reproduction of his symptoms or symptoms beyond a stretching sensation) and ask about the location of the symptoms. The therapist then performs structural differentiation by making small changes in the patient's position at a site remote from the symptoms that decrease mechanical strain on the affected nerve. If this alters the patient's symptoms, it demonstrates that neural mechanosensitivity contributes to the symptoms in question.

Myofascial and articular examination can be combined with ULNTs to assess the effect of neural tension on those structures. The details of such an examination are outside the scope of this case, but are discussed in textbooks.[2,3]

In this patient's case, ULNT 3 reproduced his proximal symptoms, which were altered when the therapist released wrist extension. The ULNT 2b was negative, and the ULNT 1 produced fewer symptoms than the ULNT 3. The combined results of these tests suggested increased mechanical sensitivity to strain in the ulnar nerve compared to the radial and median nerves. While positive active quick tests and passive ULNTs are highly suggestive of peripheral nerve injury, they are not conclusive and they do not indicate the location of the injury responsible for perpetuating the symptoms.

Nerve palpation helps to confirm increased mechanosensitivity suggested by the active and passive tests. The therapist performs this technique by gently

Table 25-3 GUIDE TO PALPATION OF NERVES OF UPPER QUARTER[3,26]

Neural Structure	Location
Upper trunk of brachial plexus	Posterior triangle at the interscalene cleft
Lower trunk of brachial plexus	Supraclavicular fossa
Ulnar nerve	Posteromedial elbow proximal and distal to ulnar groove Medial arm along the brachial artery Guyon's canal at the wrist
Radial nerve	Spiral groove of humerus about 3 fingers below deltoid insertion Distal forearm about 4 fingers width proximal to radial stylus
Median nerve	Bicipital groove alongside the brachial artery Antecubital fossa medial to biceps tendon Carpal tunnel
Axillary nerve	Between posterior deltoid and teres minor
Suprascapular nerve	Supraspinous and infraspinous fossas, about 2/3 of the way distal along the spine of the scapula

strumming with a single finger across the suspected nerve. The therapist should not press too hard because inflamed or irritated nerves can be very tender. This patient was tender to palpation along the ulnar and median nerves and the lower trunk of the brachial plexus. At this point in the examination, there was strong evidence that this patient was experiencing PNP of the ulnar nerve and/or its contributors in the nerve roots of the brachial plexus. Table 25-3 lists the easiest locations to palpate upper-quarter peripheral nerves.

Although many patients demonstrate impairments in neurodynamic tests, that does not necessarily indicate that their condition will benefit from manual therapy,[22] because individuals with PNP secondary to diabetes or tumor infiltration can also have positive neurodynamic tests. To provide a target for manual therapy, there should be one or more identifiable mechanical dysfunctions, such as altered passive accessory mobility or tissue quality in the mechanical interface somewhere along the course of the nerve. Localization of mechanical dysfunction maximizes the mechanical, physiologic, and neurophysiologic effects of the intervention.[4]

The therapist should examine the spine, especially at the levels from which the involved nerve originates.[2-4,31] Vertebral segments can be examined via central posterior to anterior mobilizations (PAs), unilateral PAs, lateral translations, and 3-dimensional testing. In the cervical spine, manual therapists have demonstrated excellent inter-rater reliability in the identification of symptomatic joints.[13,32] In a study of neural tissue management for individuals with PNP, a spinal segment was defined as symptomatic if it was hypomobile and provoked pain greater than 2/10 on a numeric pain scale, though reliability of this test was not assessed.[6]

Common sites of nerve entrapment and/or irritation in the upper quarter such as the thoracic outlet, cubital and carpal tunnels, and radial groove should also be examined.[2] Several well-established special tests can function as tests of the neural interface for patients with suspected cervical radiculopathy,[29] thoracic outlet syndrome,[33]

Table 25-4 CUTANEOUS TISSUES RELATED TO CERVICAL NERVE ROOTS

C4	Posterior/lateral neck, trapezius, posterior deltoid
C5	Posterior trapezius, posterior deltoid, posterior/lateral neck
C6	Posterior/lateral arm, posterior and anterior deltoids, posterior trapezius, dorsal radial forearm, superior periscapular area
C7	Posterior deltoid, posterior trapezius, posterior shoulder, lateral arm, dorsal aspect of radial forearm; dorsal radial aspects of hand, index finger, and third finger
C8	Posterior deltoid, posterior medial arm, posterior lateral arm, dorsal ulnar forearm, dorsal ulnar hand

cubital tunnel syndrome,[34] and carpal tunnel syndrome.[35,36] Many are provocation tests (rather than motion tests), so they may not readily guide the therapist in localizing treatment. Special tests useful for identifying cervical radiculopathy include cervical compression, cervical distraction, and Spurling's test.[37] In this case, the therapist noted hypomobility in PA glides of C6 and C7 on the left as well as segmental hypomobility between T1 and T4, and an elevated first rib on the left.

Because injured peripheral nerves release proinflammatory chemicals into their innervated tissues, tissues innervated by the affected nerve/s should be carefully palpated to determine if the tissue is tender.[2,3,7] Table 25-4 lists areas that were most often affected by cervical nerve root irritation in a study of pain referral from fluoroscopy guided stimulation of cervical nerve roots.[38]

Last, the therapist must perform a clinical assessment of nerve conduction via myotomal strength testing, sensory testing (light touch and pinprick), and DTRs. If the physical examination indicates mechanical hyperalgesia of one or more peripheral nerves and the neurologic examination shows no signs of decreased nerve conduction, then the patient's condition should be classified as inflammatory PNP. If the physical examination does not indicate mechanical hyperalgesia of one or more peripheral nerves, but signs of decreased nerve conduction are present, then the patient's condition should be classified as compressive PNP. If the patient has mechanical hyperalgesia of one or more peripheral nerves and signs of decreased nerve conduction, then the patient's condition should be classified as mixed. Table 25-5 summarizes the signs and symptoms that are more consistent with compressive or inflammatory PNP.

Table 25-5 SIGNS AND SYMPTOMS SUGGESTIVE OF COMPRESSIVE OR INFLAMMATORY PNP[4]

Compressive	Inflammatory
Loss of reflexes	Possibly hyper-reflexive
Hypoesthesia	Hyperesthesia
Loss of strength	Symptoms provoked by positions that increase strain on the nerve
Symptoms peripheralized by positions that increase pressure on the nerve from the mechanical interface	Tender points in tissues innervated by the involved nerve
Hair loss	Mechanical hyperalgesia
Nonspecific results from electrodiagnostic tests (results can be positive or negative)	Negative results from electrodiagnostic tests

To summarize the examination and results in this patient's case, the therapist assessed posture, AROM, PROM, ULNTs, tenderness of suspected involved nerve/s and innervated tissue, condition and mobility of the mechanical interface, and performed a neurologic examination. The therapist found signs of increased mechanosensitivity in the ulnar nerve, and to a lesser degree in the median nerve by the results of the ulnar nerve quick test (validity unexamined), ULNT 3 (kappa for inter-examiner reliability 0.36[10]), and palpation of the ulnar nerve at the cubital fossa (kappa 0.59[26]). Mechanical dysfunction of the nerve interface was found in the cervical and thoracic spines via unilateral PAs, contralateral cervical lateral glides, and spring testing of the first rib (reliability and diagnostic validity undetermined[6]). The patient demonstrated no signs of impaired nerve conduction via the results of manual muscle tests (kappa 0.68[26]), sensory testing (kappa 0.53[26]), and DTRs (kappa 0.61-0.74 for upper extremity[39]). The clinical examination was consistent with the patient's history of neuropathic symptoms in the neck, shoulder, and medial hand.

Plan of Care and Interventions

Ideally, management of PNP begins with therapy 2 to 3 times per week for the first 6 visits.[2] It is not uncommon for the patient's pain to be worsened by the initial evaluation. Therefore, some clinicians elect to begin treatment on the second visit, rather than at the end of the evaluation, so that the patient does not perceive that his pain was increased by treatment. No general rule can be drawn on this topic; clinical judgment should be used based on the apparent irritability of the patient's condition.

When treatment does begin, the therapist starts the patient with education and physical agents such as moist heat or possibly transcutaneous electrical nerve stimulation (TENS), if the pain is severe. When a patient shows signs of nerve compression, the first priority is decompression. This can be attempted via spinal traction,[28] manual mobilization,[34,40] and/or postural exercise.[28] Each of these interventions must be carefully provided to avoid further irritation of the nerve tissue or peripheralization of symptoms. As an individual with a compressive PNP improves, normalization of segmental strength or DTRs are the signs used by many clinicians to reclassify the patient from compressive to inflammatory.[4] Occasionally, nerve symptoms will be worsened by traction. If positive or negative signs and symptoms worsen with cervical traction, it may be better to start with mobilization of the thoracic spine, desensitization techniques such as heat and TENS, or to refer the patient back to the physician for adjustment of medication.

If the patient has been classified (or reclassified) by the therapist as having inflammatory PNP without signs of nerve compression, treatment also begins with education and physical agents, but then proceeds with passive mobilization of the nerve tissue. As the patient demonstrates maintenance of gains from one treatment session to the next, the therapist can add graded active movement. For example, the therapist progresses the patient from "sliders" to "tensioners" as he demonstrates that he is able to tolerate and manage the exercises without overdoing them. As soon as possible, usually coincident with the addition of sliders to the home exercise program, the therapist should add muscle-specific strengthening exercises, generally beginning in the upper quarter with craniocervical flexion. Craniocervical flexion helps strengthen the deep cervical flexors, provides gentle traction to the cervical spine, promotes endoneurial blood flow, and has been shown to decrease pain in the cervical spine.[41-43] Craniocervical flexion exercises have been used either alone or as part of combined movement with the scapula in multiple studies on the treatment of upper-quarter PNP.[13,28,44] Once the patient is able to manage his symptoms and is independent with a home program, physical therapy visits decrease in frequency. As mobility and strength improve further, the patient can gradually return to normal activities, including sport.

Patient education and coaching reduce patients' fear of movement and make therapy more effective.[6,20,45-47] Nee et al.[16] emphasized two points in the education of patients with PNP of the upper quarter. First, sensitized nerves become overly sensitive to movement. Second, gentle, pain-free movement reduces that sensitivity. Clear explanation of neural mechanosensitivity, rationale for treatment, and self-management of symptoms have been shown to decrease protective muscle hyperactivity and pain and help patients cooperate and follow through with their therapy.[7,16,48] For this patient, education had a large effect. When the therapist told the patient at the initial evaluation "this is not such a weird condition," the patient expressed surprise and then relief, and appeared much more confident and relaxed in his movement.

Moist heat and/or TENS have been found to decrease tension and muscle guarding in patients with PNP.[1,49] While not necessary, these modalities can help prepare patients to tolerate mobilization of the affected tissues and mechanical interface. Soft tissue and/or joint mobilization techniques should be applied to restricted tissues in the spine or along the course of the involved nerve.[3,5,31,34] Manual mobilization or manipulation decreases pain and improves function in patients with cervical radiculopathy,[13] cubital tunnel syndrome,[34] and carpal tunnel syndrome.[40] Specific targets for treatment must be identified during the examination. Treatment should be gentle; it may be painful at the site of restriction, but it should not provoke an increase in the referred pain lasting longer than a few moments. The patient's most limited ULNTs can be reassessed between interventions to ascertain the effectiveness of the particular intervention.[3,7,31] However, the therapist should be careful in some situations not to over-test.[3] In this case, mobilization of the patient's thoracic spine and left ribs provoked transient paresthesia in the left hand and a marked improvement in left shoulder elevation and ULNT 3.

Cervical lateral glides decrease muscle guarding, restore endoneurial circulation, and decrease mechanosensitivity through gentle oscillatory motions.[2,4,6,14] Three sets of 10 repetitions or 3 bouts of 30 seconds are typically performed in 1 treatment session.[4,6] The therapist should initially perform cervical lateral glides with the patient's symptomatic upper extremity in a position of comfort (Fig. 25-2A). The lateral glides should be localized, as much as possible, to the level of dysfunction identified during the examination. During this technique, motion is taken up to the first sensation of resistance (*i.e.*, when the therapist feels the patient start to develop tension in response to the lateral glide), but not into that resistance,[2] although this may take some practice to appreciate. Remember that the object of this treatment is *desensitization* rather than mobilization. Pushing through resistance can result in a flare-up for the patient. The therapist should increase the excursion of the technique as the resistance recedes. Increased numbness should not be provoked.[7] Between sets, the therapist should reassess the ULNT that was most positive during the examination. As the patient progresses (*i.e.*, lateral glides can be taken further without provoking symptoms or the post-treatment ULNT demonstrates increased symptom-free range), the therapist can position the patient with the involved upper extremity in positions of greater nerve excursion, usually in the directions of the motions that were most limited in the active and passive motion tests (Figs. 25-2B and C).[2,6]

Another mobilization technique for the nerves of the upper extremity is shoulder girdle elevation and depression on the symptomatic side while the patient simultaneously performs active craniocervical flexion and extension (Fig. 25-3). The therapist should initially have the patient perform this technique with his involved arm in a position of comfort, typically with his hand on his stomach. Three sets of 10 repetitions are performed with re-tests of the ULNT between sets.[6] Again, the therapist must take care not to push past any resistance when moving the shoulder girdle. As the patient improves, the involved upper extremity can be placed in positions of increased nerve strain, typically moving toward the position of the ULNT that was most restricted. Remember that the most nerve excursion occurs near the joint that is moved first.[24] In this case, the patient's shoulder was abducted first, so the greatest ulnar nerve excursion occurred at the shoulder.

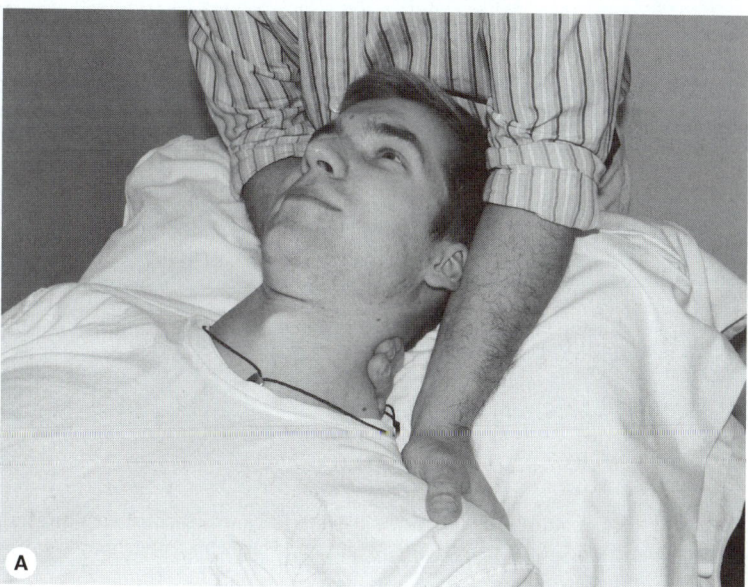

Figure 25-2. Contralateral cervical lateral glides. The therapist's left hand provides scapular stabilization and slight depression while the right hand (using a lumbrical grip) holds the patient's neck. The therapist shifts his weight to the right in order to gently mobilize the neural tissue and mechanical interface in the cervical spine. By using more weight shift and less shoulder motion, a more relaxed manual contact is promoted than if the therapist just pulls with his arm. **A.** Symptomatic extremity in a position of comfort.

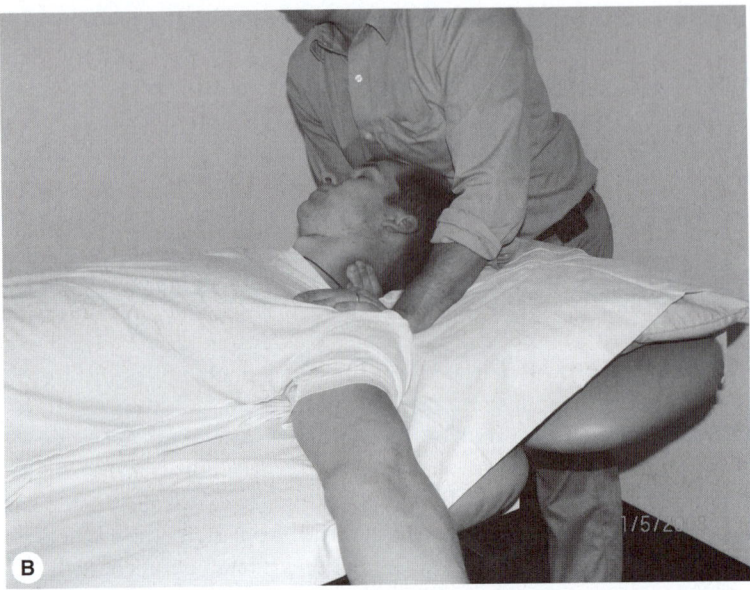

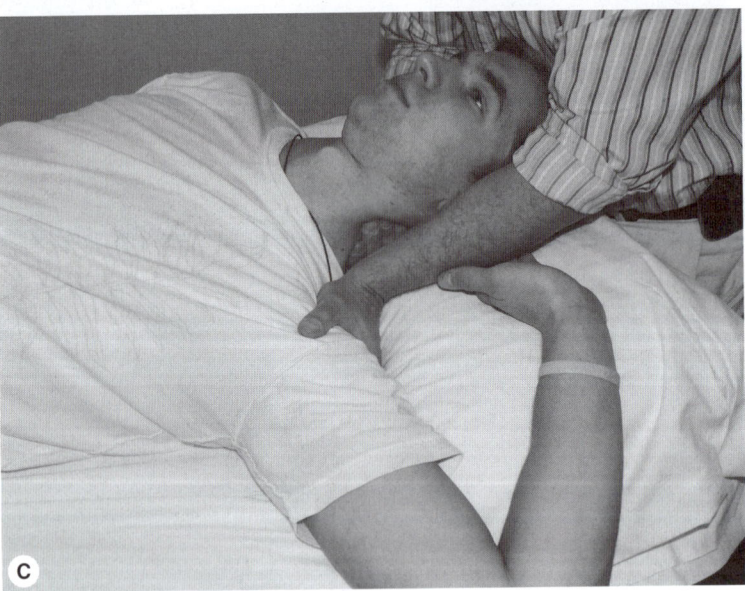

Figure 25-2. *(Continued)* Contralateral cervical lateral glides. **B.** Symptomatic extremity in a position of moderate ulnar nerve strain. **C.** Symptomatic extremity in a position of maximal ulnar nerve strain.

Sliders and tensioners are multi-joint movements intended to encourage motion in the affected area and improve endoneurial blood flow. Sliders shorten the nerve bed at one end while lengthening it at the other. Tensioners lengthen the nerve bed at both ends. Either exercise can be performed actively or passively. Gentle passive tensioners are typically performed between sets of lateral glides or shoulder girdle oscillations. Ten repetitions of tensioners in a symptom-free range

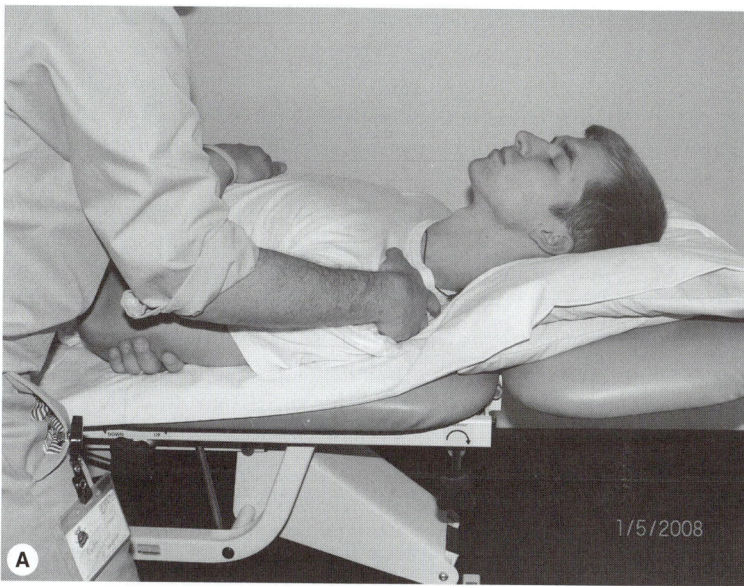

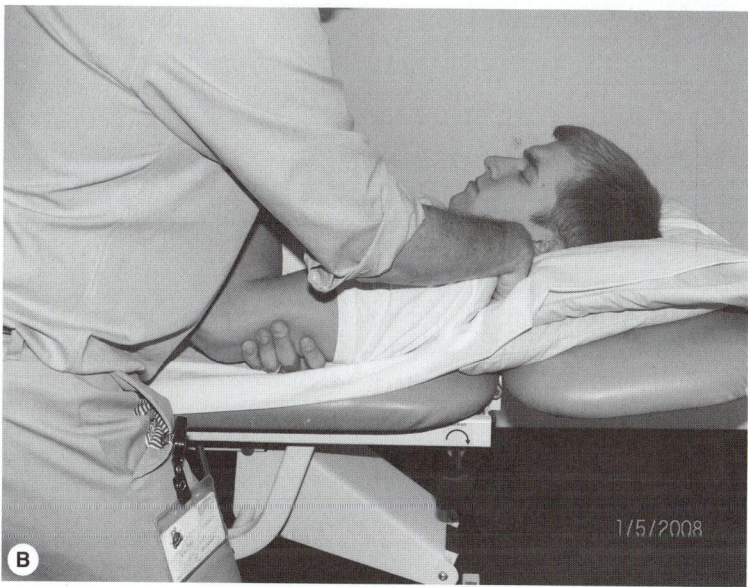

Figure 25-3. Combined passive scapular elevation and active craniocervical flexion and extension. **A.** The therapist provides scapular depression and slight downward rotation which provides a distal excursion to the brachial plexus and surrounding tissues while the patient performs craniocervical extension which shortens the tissues from above and so prevents the development of strain. **B.** The therapist then provides scapular elevation and slight upward rotation, providing a proximal excursion to the brachial plexus and surrounding tissues while the patient performs craniocervical flexion, lengthening the same tissues from above, promoting endoneurial circulation and tissue extensibility.

generally suffice. Active sliders and tensioners are typically prescribed as a home program once a patient demonstrates increased range of symptom-free movement or decreased intensity of symptoms because of passive treatment, and maintains these gains through 2 treatment sessions. Initially, the therapist may suggest 1 set of 10 to 15 repetitions, 2 to 3 times per day, though many patients perform more if these provide symptomatic relief. The therapist must remind the patient that active techniques in a home program should not elicit numbness or any lasting increase in symptoms.[3,7] Sliders and tensioners can be varied based on the segment of the nerve that is to be targeted, the position or symptom severity of the patient, or other factors.[2,3,5,26] Table 25-6 illustrates a progression of 3 active sliders that were used for the current patient with left ulnar nerve PNP. Note that the patient's left upper extremity is passively supported in an elevated position; this unloads the neural structures and makes it much easier for the patient to perform sliders in a symptom-free manner. By the time the patient progresses to tensioners, this modification is usually not necessary.

Table 25-7 illustrates 3 variations of an ulnar nerve tensioner. Note that the difficulty increases as shoulder abduction is increased. Good patient handouts for sliders and tensioners are publicly available on the Internet. One good source is the website of the International Spine and Pain Institute.[50]

Many combined upper extremity movements have been developed as alternatives to the tensioner exercise pictured in Table 25-7 for self-management techniques for PNP.[5] Figures 25-4 through 25-6 show the final positions for 3 alternative movements designed to restore the ability to tolerate ulnar nerve strain. For each of these, the patient moves the arm from a position of comfort toward one of these end-range positions, staying in a pain-free range. Clinical experience has shown that these are sometimes quicker to learn than the classic sliders and tensioners illustrated in Tables 25-6 and 25-7.

PNP commonly leads to inhibition of slow motor units and consequent weakness and fatigability of postural muscles.[51] Multiple studies have shown that muscle-specific training of the deep cervical flexors is effective for treating neck pain[41-43] and that treatment programs consisting of strengthening and endurance exercises as well as manual therapy lead to more improvement in pain, strength, endurance, and ROM than programs consisting of manual therapy alone.[52,53] Once the patient has made stable gains in pain-free mobility and is able to manage his own symptoms, the physical therapist should test the strength and/or motor control of the muscles of the upper quarter. Where indicated, specific strengthening exercises should be initiated. The testing and training of muscles commonly inhibited by PNP of the upper quarter are described in Table 25-8. Once the patient has been able to progress to general strengthening and conditioning, he is no longer, strictly speaking, an individual with a primary PNP injury. Rehabilitation can then follow evidence-based guidelines for individuals with postural impairment, impaired motor control, or upper-quarter weakness.

In addition to isolating and retraining specific muscles, it is important to "put it all together" for the patient as he transitions back to sport. This should begin when the patient's pain is mostly resolved and self-managed and he has demonstrated the necessary mobility and strength required for at least brief bouts of activity. In this case, the patient was unable to ride his motorcycle or play golf without neck and

Table 25-6 THREE ULNAR SLIDERS FOR PATIENT WITH LEFT ULNAR PNP

	Starting Position		Ending Position
Least provocative	Cervical spine in neutral with left scapula elevated and arm in position of comfort		Cervical rotation to left
	Cervical side bends to left with left shoulder abducted 45° and externally rotated, elbow flexed, forearm pronated, and wrist extended		Cervical side bends to right with shoulder abducted 45° with arm in position of comfort
Most provocative	Cervical side bends to left; shoulder abducted 90° and externally rotated, elbow flexed, forearm pronated, and wrist extended		Cervical side bends to right with shoulder abducted 90° with arm in position of comfort

Table 25-7 THREE VARIATIONS OF ULNAR NERVE TENSIONER FOR PATIENT WITH LEFT ULNAR PNP

Starting Position	Ending Position 1	Ending Position 2	Ending Position 3
	Cervical side bends to right with left shoulder abducted 45° and externally rotated, elbow flexed, forearm pronated, wrist and fingers extended	Same as ending position 1, except left shoulder abducted 60°	Same as ending position 1, except left shoulder abducted 100°

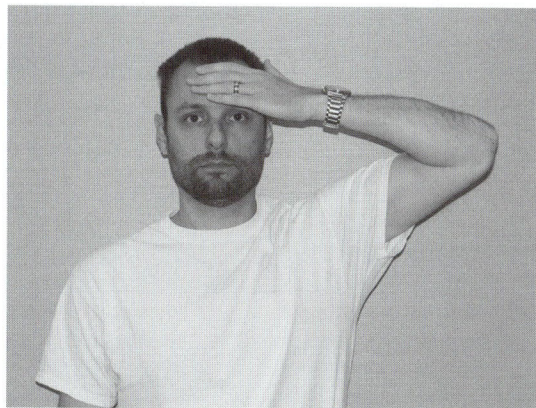

Figure 25-4. "Oye vey" exercise. This exercise places minimal strain[5] on the ulnar nerve and its mechanical interface.

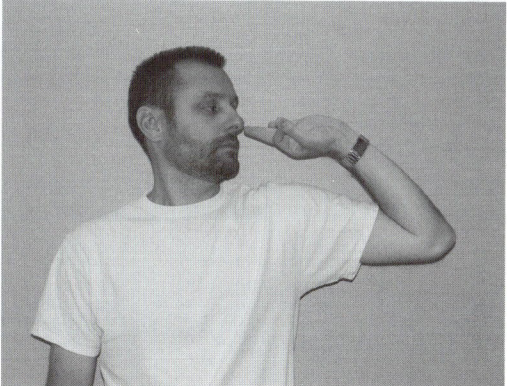

Figure 25-5. "Smoking" exercise. This exercise places moderate strain[5] on the ulnar nerve and its mechanical interface.

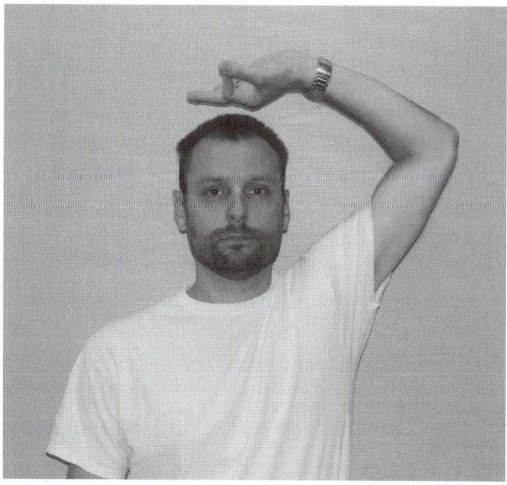

Figure 25-6. "Make a Halo" exercise. This exercise places maximal strain[5] on the ulnar nerve and its mechanical interface.

Table 25-8 TESTS AND EXERCISES FOR POSTURAL MUSCLES OF THE UPPER QUARTER

Muscle or Muscle Group	Tests	Exercise
Deep neck flexors	Craniocervical flexion test[13] Cervical flexion endurance test[13]: isometric holds for 15 sec each for 2 repetitions should "look and feel easy"	Supine chin tuck Hold head ~1 inch off table for 10 seconds. Perform 10 times.
Dorsal neck muscles	Prone cervical extension: isometric holds for 15 sec × 2 repetitions should "look and feel easy"	Prone cervical hold. Hold head ~1 inch off table for 10 seconds. Perform 10 times.
Global neck muscles		Cervical isometrics: hold head and neck in good alignment. The patient applies manual or external force at side of head in the direction of craniocervical extension, right and left rotation, and flexion and resists each force with a 10-sec isometric hold for up to 10 repetitions in each direction.
Trapezius	MMT for middle and lower trapezius	Rows Prone Is, Ts, and Ys
Serratus anterior	In quadruped: unilateral UE weightbearing with protracted scapulae for 15 sec × 2 repetitions should "look and feel easy"	In quadruped: unilateral UE weightbearing with protracted scapulae: 10-sec isometric holds and weight shifts × 10 repetitions

shoulder pain or upper extremity paresthesia. Functional activity training began with short rides on his "easier" motorcycle (lighter weight), gradually increasing the duration, and progressing to rides on his "harder" motorcycle. The patient also resumed playing golf by first swinging a club through several repetitions, then hitting several buckets of balls. The therapist advised him to begin with an amount of activity he could do without lasting symptom provocation, slowly progress, and use his home exercises (sliders and tensioners) to control any symptoms that arose. In the final phase of rehabilitation, the therapist should provide guidelines for the patient to return to golf. Similar to preparation to participate in any sport, the patient should perform an active warm-up and stretch before training. Ellenbecker et al.[54] have recommended an interval program to assist individuals in returning to golf after shoulder injuries. Guidelines specific to the golfer include paying attention to the mechanics of the golf swing and allowing 1 day of rest between sessions. Ellenbecker et al.[54] recommend that the golfer returning from a shoulder injury should perform the program as outlined in Table 25-9. Each task within each workout should be completed without increased symptoms before advancing to the next. Although some intermittent discomfort is expected, swinging the golf club should not cause pain. If pain and/or swelling persist, the program should be discontinued until the patient is examined by a medical professional.

Table 25-9 INTERVAL GOLF PROGRAM[54]

	Day 1	Day 3	Day 5
Week 1	10 putts 10 chips (with pitching wedge) Rest 5-10 minutes 15 chips	15 putts 15 chips Rest 5-10 minutes 25 chips	20 putts 20 chips Rest 5-10 minutes 20 puts 20 chips Rest 5-10 minutes 10 chips 10 short irons (with W, 9, or 8 irons)
Week 2	20 chips 10 short irons Rest 5 minutes 10 short irons	20 chips 15 short irons Rest 5 minutes 10 short irons 15 chips	15 short irons 10 med irons (with 7, 6, or 5 irons) Rest 5 minutes 20 short irons 15 chips
Week 3	15 short irons 10 med irons Rest 5 minutes 5 long irons (with 4, 3, or 2 irons) 15 short irons Rest 20 chips	15 short irons 10 med irons 10 long irons Rest 5 minutes 10 short irons 10 med irons 5 long irons 5 woods (3, 5 woods)	15 short irons 10 med irons 10 long irons Rest 5 minutes 10 short irons 10 med irons 10 long irons 10 woods
Week 4	15 short irons 10 med irons 10 long irons 10 drives Rest 5 minutes Repeat above	Play 9 holes	Play 9 holes
Week 5	Play 9 holes	Play 9 holes	Play 18 holes

Reproduced with permission from Ellenbecker TS, Wilk, KE, Reinold, MM, Murphy TF, Paine RM. Use of Interval Return Programs for Shoulder Rehabilitation. In: Ellenbecker TS, ed. *Shoulder Rehabilitation: Non-Operative Treatment*. New York: Thieme; 2006:139–165.

Evidence-Based Clinical Recommendations

SORT: Strength of Recommendation Taxonomy
A: Consistent, good-quality patient-oriented evidence
B: Inconsistent or limited quality patient-oriented evidence
C: Consensus, disease-oriented evidence, usual practice, expert opinion, or case series

1. For individuals with pain in the neck and upper extremity, particularly pain described as burning, shooting, or lancinating, upper-limb neural tension tests (ULNTs) can help confirm the presence of increased peripheral nerve mechanosensitivity. **Grade C**

2. For individuals with peripheral neuropathic pain, education that includes an explanation of neural mechanosensitivity, rationale for treatment, and self-management of symptoms can decrease muscle hyperactivity and pain, reduce fear of movement, and help patients follow through with therapy. **Grade A**

3. In patients with PNP in the neck and arm, upper-quarter mobilizations such as cervical lateral glides and nerve mobilization procedures decrease mechanosensitivity and reduce pain. **Grade B**

COMPREHENSION QUESTIONS

25.1 Which of the following findings does *not* contribute to the diagnosis of peripheral neuropathic pain of the upper quarter?
   A. Pain can be reproduced by passive positioning of the limb that puts mechanical strain on the suspected nerve.
   B. The suspected peripheral nerve is unusually tender to gentle palpation.
   C. Cervical rotation toward the unaffected side is decreased.
   D. Pain provoked by mechanical strain on the suspected nerve can be altered by removal of the strain at a site remote from the location of the pain.

25.2 What is the *best* order of interventions within a single treatment session of a patient with peripheral neuropathic pain (PNP) in the upper extremity?
   A. Coaching and patient education; moist heat and possibly transcutaneous electrical nerve stimulation (TENS); mobilization of the interface; gentle mobilization of the affected nerves
   B. Postural education, strength training, and ice
   C. Coaching and education, desensitization, mobilization, strength training, functional activity training, and return to sports
   D. Moist heat, mobilization of the interface, tensioners, and strength training

ANSWERS

25.1 **C.** Decreased cervical rotation toward the unaffected side does not indicate or suggest PNP in the upper extremity. The diagnosis of PNP is suggested by physical tests of mechanical neurosensitivity including pain with passive positioning which puts strain on peripheral nerves (option A), mechanical hyperalgesia of peripheral nerves (option B), and the presence of structural differentiation (option D).

25.2 **A.** In the early phase for a patient with PNP, coaching and patient education with moist heat and possibly TENS to the affected area, followed by mobilization of the interface and gentle mobilization of the affected nerves is a good course of treatment. Option B is too aggressive, does not take into account the principles of neurodynamics, and includes ice, which is often irritating to these patients. Option C is a good overview of the whole treatment paradigm, but all these could not reasonably be covered in a single session, particularly in the early phase of treatment. Option D leaves out patient education and coaching, which is often vital in allowing the patient to effectively follow through with his symptom management and home exercise program.

REFERENCES

1. Sluka K. *Mechanisms and Management of Pain for the Physical Therapist*. Seattle, WA: IASP Press; 2009:24.
2. Shacklock M. *Clinical Neurodynamics: A New System of Neuromusculoskeletal Treatment*. Adelaide, Australia: Elsevier Inc.; 2005.
3. Butler D. *The Sensitive Nervous System*. Adelaide, Australia: NOIgroup Publications; 2000.
4. Stagge JM. The upper quarter pain puzzle-differential diagnosis and treatment of the orthopedic patient with upper quarter radicular symptoms. International Manual Therapy Seminar. 2012.
5. Butler D. *Neurodynamic Techiques*. Adelaide, Australia: NOIgroup Publications; 2005.
6. Nee RJ, Vicenzino B, Jull GA, Cleland JA, Coppieters MW. A novel protocol to develop a prediction model that identifies patients with nerve-related neck and arm pain who benefit from the early introduction of neural tissue management. *Contemp Clin Trials*. 2011;32:760-770.
7. Nee RJ, Butler D. Management of peripheral neuropathic pain: integrating neurobiology, neurodynamics, and clinical evidence. *Phys Ther Sport*. 2006;7:36-49.
8. Bove GM, Light AR. The nervi nervorum. *Pain Forum*. 1997;6:181-190.
9. Bogduk N. On the definitions and physiology of back pain, referred pain, and radicular pain. *Pain*. 2009;147:17-19.
10. Nee RJ, Jull GA, Vicenzino B, Coppieters MW. The validity of upper-limb neurodynamic tests for detecting peripheral neuropathic pain. *J Orthop Sports Phys Ther*. 2012;42:413-424.
11. Feinberg JH, Nadler SF, Krivickas LS. Peripheral nerve injuries in the athlete. *Sport Med*. 1997;24:385-408.
12. Elvey RL. Brachial plexus tension tests and the pathoanatomical origin of arm pain. *Proceedings: Aspects Of Manipulative Therapy*. Melbourne, Australia: Lincoln Institute of Health Sciences; 1979:105-110.
13. Childs JD, Cleland JA, Elliott JM, et al. Neck Pain: clinical practice guidelines linked to the International Classification of Functioning, Disability, and Health From the Orthopaedic Section of the American Physical Therapy Association. *J Orthop Sports Phys Ther*. 2008;38:A1-A34.
14. Allison GT, Nagy BM, Hall T. A randomized clinical trial of manual therapy for cervico-brachial pain syndrome—a pilot study. *Man Ther*. 2002;7:95-102.
15. Cowell IM, Phillips DR. Effectiveness of manipulative physiotherapy for the treatment of a neurogenic cervicobrachial pain syndrome: a single case study—experimental design. *Man Ther*. 2002;7:31-38.
16. Nee RJ, Vicenzino B, Jull GA, Cleland JA, Coppieters MW. Neural tissue management provides immediate clinically relevant benefits without harmful effects for patients with nerve-related neck and arm pain: a randomised trial. *J Physiother*. 2012;58:23-31.
17. Schmid AB, Nee RJ, Coppieters MW. Reappraising entrapment neuropathies—mechanisms, diagnosis and management. *Man Ther*. 2013;18:449-457.
18. Sunderland SS. The anatomy and physiology of nerve injury. *Muscle Nerve*. 1990;13:771-784.
19. Rempel D, Dahlin L, Lundborg G. Pathophysiology of nerve compression syndromes: response of peripheral nerves to loading. *J Bone Jt Surg Am*. 1999;81:1600-1610.
20. Louw A, Puentedura E. *Therapeutic Neuroscience Education: Teaching Patients About Pain, A Guide for Clinicians*. Minneapolis, MN: OPTP; 2013.
21. Latremoliere A, Woolf CJ. Central sensitization: a generator of pain hypersensitivity by central neural plasticity. *J Pain*. 2009;10:895-926.
22. Hall TM, Elvey RL. Nerve trunk pain: phsyical diagnosis and treatment. *Man Ther*. 1999;4:63-73.
23. Loeser J, Turk D. Multidisciplinary pain management. In: Loeser JD, Butler SH, Chapman, R, Turk DC, eds. *Bonica's Management of Pain*. 3rd ed. Baltimore, MD: Lippincott Williams & Wilkins; 2001:2069-2079.

24. Topp KS, Boyd BS. Structure and biomechanics of peripheral nerves: nerve responses to physical stresses and implications for physical therapist practice. *Phys Ther.* 2006;86:92-109.
25. Treede RD, Jensen TS, Campbell JN, et al. Neuropathic pain: redefinition and a grading system for clinical and research purposes. *Neurology.* 2008;70:1630-1635.
26. Schmid AB, Brunner F, Luomajoki H, et al. Reliability of clinical tests to evaluate nerve function and mechanosensitivity of the upper limb peripheral nervous system. *BMC Musculoskelet Disord.* 2009;10:11.
27. Smart KM, Blake C, Staines A, Doody C. Clinical indicators of "nociceptive", "peripheral neuropathic" and "central" mechanisms of musculoskeletal pain. A Delphi survey of expert clinicians. *Man Ther.* 2010;15:80-87.
28. Raney NH, Petersen EJ, Smith TA, et al. Development of a clinical prediction rule to identify patients with neck pain likely to benefit from cervical traction and exercise. *Eur Spine J.* 2009;18:382-391.
29. Rubinstein SM, Pool JJ, van Tulder MW, Riphagen II, de Vet HC. A systematic review of the diagnostic accuracy of provocative tests of the neck for diagnosing cervical radiculopathy. *Eur Spine J.* 2007;16:307-319.
30. Coppieters MW. The impact of neurodynamic testing on the perception of experimentally induced muscle pain. *Man Ther.* 2005;10:52-60.
31. Jacobs DP. http://www.dermoneuromodulation.com/. Accessed May 9, 2013.
32. Jull G, Treleaven J, Versace G. Manual examination: is pain provocation a major cue for spinal dysfunction? *Aust Physiother.* 1994;40:159-165.
33. Donahue DM, Illig KA. Neurogenic TOS for the primary care team: when to consider the diagnosis? In: Illig KA, Thompson RW, Freischlag JA, Donahue DM, Jordan SE, Edgelow PI, eds. *Thoracic Outlet Syndrome.* London: Springer 2013.
34. Kearns G, Wang S. Medical diagnosis of cubital tunnel syndrome ameliorated with thrust manipulation of the elbow and carpals. *J Man Manip Ther.* 2012;20:90-95.
35. MacDermid JC, Wessel J. Clinical diagnosis of carpal tunnel syndrome: a systematic review. *J Hand Ther.* 2004;17:309-319.
36. Boland RA, Kiernan MC. Assessing the accuracy of a combination of clinical tests for identifying carpal tunnel syndrome. *J Clin Neurosci.* 2009;16:929-933.
37. Wainner RS, Fritz JM, Irrgang JJ, Boninger ML, Delitto A, Allison S. Reliability and diagnostic accuracy of the clinical examination and patient self-report measures for cervical radiculopathy. *Spine.* 2003;28:52-62.
38. Slipman CW, Plastaras CT, Palmitier RA, Huston CW, Sterenfeld EB. Symptom provocation of fluoroscopically guided cervical nerve root stimulation: are dynatomal maps identical to dermatomal maps? *Spine.* 1998;23:2235-2242.
39. Litvan I, Mangone CA, Werden W, et al. Reliability of the NINDS myotatic reflex scale. *Neurology.* 1996;47:969-972.
40. Maddali-Bongi S, Signorini M, Bassetti M, Del Rosso A, Orlandi M, De Scisciolo G. A manual therapy intervention improves symptoms in patients with carpal tunnel syndrome: a pilot study. *Rheumatol Int.* 2013;33:1233-1241.
41. O'Leary S, Falla D, Hodges PW, Jull G, Vicenzino B. Specific therapeutic exercise of the neck induces immediate local hypoalgesia. *J Pain.* 2007;8:832-839.
42. Jull G, Falla D, Treleaven J, Hodges P, Vicenzino B. Retraining cervical joint position sense: the effect of two exercise regimes. *J Orthop Reseach.* 2007;25:404-412.
43. Chiu TT, Lam TH, Hedley AJ. A randomized controlled trial on the efficacy of exercise for patients with chronic neck pain. *Spine.* 2005;30:E1-E7.
44. Neblett R, Cohen H, Choi Y, et al. The Central Sensitization Inventory (CSI): establishing clinically significant values for identifying central sensitivity syndromes in an outpatient chronic pain sample. *J Pain.* 2013:14:438-445.

45. Nijs J, Roussel N, Paul van Wilgen C, Köke A, Smeets R. Thinking beyond muscles and joints: therapists' and patients' attitudes and beliefs regarding chronic musculoskeletal pain are key to applying effective treatment. *Man Ther.* 2013;18:96-102.
46. Meeus M, Nijs J, Van Oosterwijck J, Van Alsenoy V, Truijen S. Pain physiology education improves pain beliefs in patients with chronic fatigue syndrome compared with pacing and self-management education: a double-blind randomized controlled trial. *Arch Phys Med Rehabil.* 2010;91:1153-1159.
47. Moseley GL, Nicholas MK, Hodges PW. A randomized controlled trial of intensive neurophysiology education in chronic low back pain. *Clin J Pain.* 2004;20:324-330.
48. Hall AM, Ferreira PH, Maher CG, Latimer J, Ferreira ML. The influence of the therapist-patient relationship on treatment outcome in physical rehabilitation: a systematic review. *Phys Ther.* 2010;90:1099-1110.
49. DeSantana JM, Walsh DM, Vance C, Rakel BA, Sluka KA. Effectiveness of transcutaneous electrical nerve stimulation for treatment of hyperalgesia and pain. *Curr Rheumatol Rep.* 2008;10:492-499.
50. Louw A, Puentedura E. Free information. http://www.ispinstitute.com/FreeInfo.aspx. Accessed February 3, 2015.
51. Hodges PW, Tucker K. Moving differently in pain: a new theory to explain the adaptation to pain. *Pain.* 2011;152:S90-S98.
52. Bronfort G, Evans R, Nelson B, Aker PD, Goldsmith CH, Vernon H. A randomized clinical trial of exercise and spinal manipulation for patients with chronic neck pain. *Spine.* 2001;26:788-798.
53. Evans R, Bronfort G, Nelson B, Goldsmith CH. Two-year follow-up of a randomized clinical trial of spinal manipulation and two types of exercise for patients with chronic neck pain. *Spine.* 2002;27:2383-2389.
54. Ellenbecker TS, Wilk KE, Reinold MM, Murphy TF, Paine RM. Use of interval return programs for shoulder rehabilitation. In: Ellenbecker TS, ed. *Shoulder Rehabilitation: Non-Operative Treatment.* New York, NY: Thieme; 2006:139-165.

Iron Deficiency in an Endurance Athlete

Kari Brown Budde

CASE 26

A 48-year-old male currently attending physical therapy for left knee pain complains of fatigue, difficulty concentrating, weakness, and general malaise throughout the day. The patient noted declining performance and increased fatigue approximately 1 month prior to attending physical therapy while he was training for a marathon. At that time, he was increasing his overall running mileage per week, which he thought was attributing to his general fatigue. On his initial physical therapy evaluation, he was seen for the onset of left knee pain. He mentioned the general fatigue as a presumed symptom of his marathon training at that point. The patient's medical history was otherwise unremarkable. The patient is an avid runner, running approximately 40 miles per week. He participates in 3 marathons per year and either a 10-km race or half marathon each month. The patient was treated for approximately 6 weeks with a full cessation of left knee pain with running, allowing him to resume training for the upcoming marathon. However, throughout his time in physical therapy, the patient complained of feeling increasingly fatigued, started having shortness of breath with all activity, and had a new onset of abdominal pain unrelated to meals. The physical therapist performed a re-evaluation secondary to his change in medical status and referred him to his family physician. The family physician ordered a series of blood tests including a complete blood count (CBC) and platelet and ferritin levels. The patient was found to have low hemoglobin (Hb, 11.9 g/dL), hematocrit (Hct, 35.5%), and ferritin levels (9 ng/mL); he was diagnosed with iron-deficiency anemia (IDA). The patient was instructed by his family physician to increase his intake of foods high in iron and to monitor fatigue levels while training for the marathon.

▶ Based on the patient's diagnosis of IDA, what do you anticipate may be the contributors to his activity limitations?
▶ What are the most appropriate physical therapy interventions and the safest way to progress the patient back to sport?
▶ What is his rehabilitation prognosis?

KEY DEFINITIONS

FERRITIN: Intracellular protein in which iron is stored in the body[1,2]

IRON DEFICIENCY (ID): Diminished iron stores due to a chronic negative iron balance in which iron stores no longer meet the needs of normal iron turnover and the appropriate amount of iron cannot be delivered to body tissues[3]

IRON-DEFICIENCY ANEMIA (IDA): Diminished iron stores coupled with diminished hemoglobin levels[3]

IRON STATUS: Described on a continuum from IDA to ID without anemia to normal iron status with varying amounts of stored iron to excessive iron or iron overload[1,2]

SERUM FERRITIN: Amount of ferritin released into the plasma; can be used to determine the total amount of iron stores in the body in the absence of inflammation[1,2]

Objectives

1. Describe the signs and symptoms that would help the physical therapist recognize anemia.
2. Describe how the physical therapist can determine dosage and progression of interventions in an individual with IDA.
3. Identify precautions for physical therapy interventions in an individual with IDA.
4. Determine appropriate interdisciplinary team consultation and referral if the physical therapist suspects an individual has anemia.
5. Use the results of laboratory values for hemoglobin, hematocrit, and ferritin in patient/client management.

Physical Therapy Considerations

PT considerations during management of the middle-aged athlete with IDA:

- **General physical therapy plan of care/goals:** Decrease fatigue levels; increase activity level and decrease rating of perceived exertion (RPE) with physical activity
- **Physical therapy interventions:** Therapeutic exercise and neuromuscular re-education to re-introduce the patient to prior level of physical activity including muscular strength, endurance, joint range of motion and flexibility; improve lower extremity and full-body dynamic control; decrease dysfunctional movement patterns that may lead to injury and pain; manual interventions to increase flexibility, mobility, and assist with improving lower extremity and full-body movement patterns; education in diagnosis, prognosis, treatment plan, and risks and benefits of physical therapy as well as return to prior level of sport progression

- **Precautions during physical therapy:** Assess for fatigue and dysfunctional movement patterns due to fatigue and lack of neuromuscular control and endurance; assess heart rate response to interventions
- **Complications interfering with physical therapy:** Fatigue; monitor progress and risk factors based on patient's function and pre-existing conditions

Understanding the Health Condition

Iron is an essential trace element and serves critical functions in the body. As the central atom of the heme group within hemoglobin, iron binds oxygen in lung capillaries and delivers it to all the cells in the body that require oxygen to perform their functions. The human body contains only a few grams of iron, the majority of which is stored in hemoglobin. Other sources of iron in the body include myoglobin, proteins within the electron transport chain, serum protein ferritin, and within the bone marrow. Iron stores are regulated by intestinal iron absorption.[4] **Iron is not synthesized in the body and therefore must be consumed in the diet for proper body functions.** Two forms of dietary iron exist: heme and non-heme. Heme iron is derived from hemoglobin and is found in animal products that contain hemoglobin. These animal products include fish, red meat, and poultry.[5] Non-heme iron sources such as broccoli, beans, and spinach are not absorbed as well as heme iron sources. Other non-heme iron sources include fortified foods like oatmeal and bread.[5]

Iron absorption affects iron regulation. Iron absorption can be influenced by storage levels of iron, type of dietary iron consumed, and type of accompanying foods ingested with the iron consumed.[4,6-14] A person with high levels of iron stores will not absorb as much iron as someone with low levels of iron stores. This regulation allows individuals with low levels of iron to absorb more iron from their food to meet their needs and protects those with high levels from excessive iron and potentially harmful effects of absorbing too much iron.[6,8,11] Absorption is most efficient from the heme iron consumed in meats and animal products and less efficient from non-heme foods.[4,6] Absorption of iron can be enhanced by eating meat and may be enhanced by eating vitamin C along with non-heme iron-containing foods.[8,9] Non-heme iron absorption is decreased when ingested with calcium, tannins (found in teas), phytates (found in whole grains, nuts, and seeds), and polyphenols (from fruits, tea, coffee, and red wine).[10-15] If the diet is deficient in iron or an individual loses iron stores in any other way, he may demonstrate symptoms including fatigue, reduced immunity, and poor athletic performance.[16-18]

Once iron stores have been depleted over an extended time, the stores no longer meet the needs of normal iron turnover and cannot deliver appropriate amounts of iron to body tissues. This state of diminished iron stores is known as iron deficiency (ID).[2,3] In an iron-deficient state, new red blood cells contain less hemoglobin. After the hemoglobin level drops below 2 standard deviations of the normal mean, an iron-deficient person is now considered to have iron-deficiency anemia (IDA).[2] To diagnose ID or IDA, serum ferritin is measured. Serum ferritin is the amount of ferritin (or iron stores) that has been released into the plasma.[1] ID is the most common nutritional deficiency in the world.[19,20] Up to 50% of people worldwide have ID.[19] ID is more prevalent in females; in developed nations, up to 15% of females have ID and 4% have IDA.[3] In adult males, the prevalence is only 2% and 1% for ID and IDA, respectively.[21,22] **Long-term exercisers have a higher prevalence of ID compared to non-athletes.**[23]

Typical causes of ID include inadequate iron intake or absorption, iron loss through menstruation in females, and gastrointestinal bleeding. The recommended amount of iron in a person's diet varies by age and sex. Recommended dietary allowances suggest 15 mg per day for females 14 to 18 years old and 18 mg per day for females 19 to 50 years old. Males from 14 to 18 years old should ingest 11 mg per day and once older than 18 years, males should ingest 8 mg per day of iron.[20] Decreased iron absorption may also be caused by inflammation from excessive physical activity through expression of proinflammatory cytokines and hepcidin, a peptide hormone that regulates iron homeostasis.[3,24] Iron deficiency may range from transient ID to sustained IDA. Transient ID can occur during and after exercise.

Common signs and symptoms of IDA include feeling weak and tired, decreased mental performance, delayed cognitive and social maturation during childhood, reduced thermoregulation, and decreased immunity.[25] Other symptoms include dizziness, headaches, shortness of breath, tinnitus, restless leg syndrome, spoon nail, glossitis (swollen tongue), blue sclera, pale conjunctivae, and pallor.[26] Symptoms of IDA that commonly affect male athletes include decreased physical and mental performance, excessive fatigue, reduced temperature regulation, and decreased immune function. Without the ability to regulate temperature, an athlete can overheat or be unable to increase workload without becoming more fatigued. With decreased mental and physical performance, an athlete will not be able to train or compete at his previously trained level. Without proper immune function, the athlete may suffer from chronic illness that will negatively impact training and competition.

Once IDA is suspected, specific tests help confirm the diagnosis. The first steps are taking a CBC and measuring the hematocrit, which is the ratio of the volume of red blood cells to the total volume of blood. Once anemia has been diagnosed based on normative hematocrit levels, further testing for IDA is required. Measuring serum ferritin is the most accurate initial test for IDA.[21] Normal and diagnostic values for IDA are shown in Table 26-1.

Table 26-1 LABORATORY MEASUREMENTS FOR DIAGNOSING IRON-DEFICIENCY ANEMIA[20,21,26]

Population	Indicator	Normal Range	IDA Diagnostic Range
Males	Hematocrit	38%-50%	< 39.9%
Menstruating females	Hematocrit	35%-45%	< 35.9%
Males	Hemoglobin	13.5-17.5 g/dL	< 13 g/dL
Menstruating females	Hemoglobin	12-15.5 g/dL	< 12 g/dL
Males	Serum ferritin	> 100 ng/mL	< 25 ng/mL
Menstruating females	Serum ferritin	> 100 ng/mL	< 25 ng/mL

Hormone activity, inflammation, gastrointestinal bleeding, hematuria (blood in the urine), sweating, and hemolysis (breakdown of red blood cells) are variable components of exercise that can cause lower levels of iron in the body.[27] Exercise decreases visceral blood flow and increases gastrointestinal bleeding. High-intensity exercise can cause impact stress to the bladder that may lead to bleeding and hematuria. Athletes also lose iron through sweating; increased frequency and/or duration of sweating causes more iron loss. Last, distance runners may have an increased destruction of red blood cells due to impact forces from repetitive foot striking during running, a phenomenon known as foot strike hemolysis.[22,27-29] **Endurance athletes, specifically distance runners, demonstrate a higher prevalence of ID and IDA**, most likely due to the longer and more cumulative bouts of exercise and the risk factors of increased sweating, gastrointestinal bleeding, and foot strike hemolysis.[27-30] One additional factor that may affect distance runners more than other types of athletes or non-athletes is dietary concerns. Endurance athletes are lean athletes who often place significant importance on their diet and weight for competition. Distance runners with IDA consume lower amounts of iron, especially heme sources of iron.[31]

Physical Therapy Patient/Client Management

Any individual with systemic signs and symptoms that lead the physical therapist to suspect ID or IDA should be thoroughly evaluated and referred to a primary care physician for diagnostic testing to rule out or confirm ID or IDA. The patient may also benefit from further functional activity testing using a scale to measure RPE to assess current functional and performance ability. Beneficial physical therapy interventions may include the development of a graded exercise progression that correlates with the patient's overall functional ability and fatigue levels as well as repeated blood testing by the physician. Restoring full range of motion, mobility, strength, and endurance as well as neuromuscular control and normalized movement patterning may help the patient return to full sport participation as well as reduce the risk of injury due to fatigue, loss of neuromuscular control, endurance, and sport-specific skill and ability.

Examination, Evaluation, and Diagnosis

Highlights of the systems review for the athlete with a recent change in medical status include diet, consistent assessment of vital signs and RPE during activity/exercise, and subjective report of fatigue levels. ID and IDA are not diagnoses made by a physical therapist. However, it is vital for a physical therapist to be able to identify the signs and symptoms of suspected ID or IDA for appropriate referral. When evaluating an endurance athlete, the physical therapist should consider ID and IDA as a possible differential or additional diagnosis.

The patient in this case noted a decline in performance and increased fatigue for approximately 1 month prior to attending physical therapy. Because he was increasing his overall running mileage per week, he assumed this was the cause of his fatigue and mentioned his suspicion to the physical therapist during his initial physical therapy evaluation. After 6 weeks of physical therapy, the patient reported no left knee pain with running. However, his fatigue was progressively increasing, he was experiencing shortness of breath with all activity, and he reported new abdominal pain. The physical therapist performed a re-evaluation (6 weeks after the initial evaluation) secondary to the patient's change in medical status.

Heart rate and blood pressure were within normal limits. Diet was assessed through subjective report. The patient reported eating a "well-balanced" diet that included heme and non-heme iron sources. The patient reported that his typical running exertion prior to the onset of fatigue symptoms was approximately 13 on the Borg RPE scale (6-20). In contrast, over the past 2 weeks, the patient reports a Borg RPE of 16 to 17 during the same training runs.[32]

The physical examination included assessment of strength, mobility, flexibility, range of motion, stability, endurance, dermatomes, reflexes, and posture. Sport-specific analysis and other weightbearing functional testing were performed to assess lower extremity biomechanics. The majority of the findings were normal. The only abnormal findings are shown in Table 26-2.

The primary physical examination findings of the re-evaluation were bilateral hip and quadriceps weakness and inflexibility in the left tensor fascia latae/iliotibial band. The patient demonstrated improved hip strength with manual muscle testing since his initial evaluation. However, during functional testing with the single-leg squat and video running analysis, he still demonstrated genu valgus and bilateral Trendelenburg sign, indicating hip weakness and lack of stability during sport. The physical therapist initially determined a physical therapy diagnosis of left patellofemoral pain syndrome secondary to muscle weakness and abnormal movement

Table 26-2 MUSCULOSKELETAL EXAMINATION FINDINGS		
Tests/Measures	**Initial Examination**	**Re-evaluation**
Hip abduction MMT	4/5 bilaterally	4+/5 bilaterally
Hip extension MMT	4/5 bilaterally	4+/5 bilaterally
Hip external rotation MMT	4/5 bilaterally	4+/5 bilaterally
Hip internal rotation MMT	4+/5 bilaterally	4+/5 bilaterally
Knee extension MMT	4/5 bilaterally	4+/5 bilaterally
Ober test	Positive on left for TFL and ITB	Negative bilaterally
Single-leg squat /small knee bend	Genu valgus Bilateral Trendelenburg sign	Genu valgus Bilateral Trendelenburg sign
Palpation	TTP over left medial PFJ	No TTP
Video gait running analysis	Decreased hip extension, excessive Trendelenburg, genu valgus, and femoral IR, left > right	Decreased hip extension, excessive Trendelenburg, genu valgus, and femoral IR, left > right

Abbreviations: IR, internal rotation; ITB, iliotibial band; MMT, manual muscle test; PFJ, patellofemoral joint; TFL, tensor fasciae latae; TTP, tenderness to palpation.

Table 26-3 TREATMENT FOR PATELLOFEMORAL PAIN SYNDROME AND CASE-SPECIFIC FINDINGS

Tests/Measures	Initial Examination	Interventions
Hip abduction MMT	4/5 bilaterally	Sidelying hip abduction with straight leg
Hip extension MMT	4/5 bilaterally	Single-leg bridges
Hip external rotation MMT	4/5 bilaterally	Clamshells
Hip internal rotation MMT	4⁺/5 bilaterally	Reverse clamshells
Knee extension MMT	4/5 bilaterally	Single-leg squats
Ober test	Positive on left for TFL and ITB	Foam rolling over TFL and ITB Manual myofascial release
Single-leg squat /small knee bend	Genu valgus Bilateral Trendelenburg sign	Single-leg squat
Palpation	TTP over left medial PFJ	Improve movement patterns during functional activities to reduce irritation to PFJ
Video gait running analysis	Decreased hip extension, excessive Trendelenburg, genu valgus, and femoral IR, left > right	Cueing to increase hip extension and decrease genu valgus during gait

Abbreviations: IR, internal rotation; ITB, iliotibial band; MMT, manual muscle test; PFJ, patellofemoral joint; TFL, tensor fasciae latae; TTP, tenderness to palpation.

patterns and biomechanics that increase stress to the affected tissues during running. Altered running mechanics may increase force through the patient's lower extremities, specifically to the patellofemoral joint, resulting in knee pain and soft tissue breakdown due to the repetitive nature of long distance running.[33,34] Table 26-3 outlines treatment guidelines and specific exercises for each identified impairment.

Findings from the re-evaluation indicated that the patient was improving and meeting initial physical therapy goals for increased strength, flexibility, decreased pain, and increased functional ability. The patient reported he was no longer experiencing knee pain throughout the day or with running. Despite the patient's improvements, he continued to complain of increasing fatigue, weakness, difficulty concentrating, shortness of breath, and abdominal pain. Therefore, the physical therapist referred the patient back to his family physician for further medical testing. Table 26-4 shows the test results from the patient's primary care physician.

Table 26-4 RESULTS FROM PRIMARY CARE PHYSICIAN TESTING[20,21,26]

Indicator	Normal Range in Males	IDA Diagnostic Range	Current Patient's Findings
Hematocrit	38%-50%	< 39.9%	35.5%
Hemoglobin	13.5-17.5 g/dL	< 13 g/dL	11.9 g/dL
Serum ferritin	> 100 ng/mL	< 25 ng/mL	9 ng/mL

Plan of Care and Interventions

The patient's family physician diagnosed him with IDA based on the results from his blood tests (Table 26-4). The physical therapist hypothesized that as the patient continued to run in an iron-deficiency state, he suffered from the common symptoms of fatigue, decreased aerobic capacity, and shortness of breath, consistent with ID and eventually IDA. Subsequently, he was unable to train at his previous performance level and with his continued fatigue, he started to demonstrate aberrant movement patterns during running that finally resulted in musculoskeletal injury.[26,31,32] Initial rehabilitation and medical treatment for ID focuses on dietary recommendations to increase dietary intake of heme and non-heme iron and iron supplementation.[26] After the systemic concerns are treated through diet and supplementation based on recommendations from the patient's primary care physician, physical therapy interventions can be resumed to focus on the remaining musculoskeletal and aerobic endurance concerns. In conjunction with the physician, the physical therapist should work with the athlete in a guided running progression while using RPE as a monitor of intensity.

Evidence-Based Clinical Recommendations

SORT: Strength of Recommendation Taxonomy
A: Consistent, good-quality patient-oriented evidence
B: Inconsistent or limited-quality patient-oriented evidence
C: Consensus, disease-oriented evidence, usual practice, expert opinion, or case series

1. Iron is not synthesized by the body and therefore must be consumed for proper body functions. **Grade A**

2. Long-term exercisers have a higher prevalence of iron deficiency compared to non-athletes. **Grade B**

3. Endurance athletes, specifically distance runners, have a higher prevalence of iron deficiency and iron-deficiency anemia, most likely due to the longer and more cumulative bouts of exercise and the risk factors of increased sweating, gastrointestinal bleeding, and foot strike hemolysis. **Grade B**

COMPREHENSION QUESTIONS

26.1 What are signs or symptoms to anticipate in the *initial* stages of suspected iron deficiency?

A. Stress fracture

B. Musculoskeletal injury

C. Fatigue

D. Difficulty breathing

26.2 Why are distance runners more likely than non-athletes to have iron deficiency or iron-deficiency anemia?

A. They may suffer from foot strike hemolysis.
B. They have more injuries than non-athletes.
C. They are more likely to consume heme iron sources.
D. They absorb more iron from their bone marrow than non-athletes.

26.3 When a patient presents to a physical therapist with a musculoskeletal injury and systemic symptoms, what should the initial plan of care include?

A. Treat the musculoskeletal diagnosis first.
B. Treat the systemic diagnosis first.
C. Treat the musculoskeletal diagnosis at the same time as the system diagnosis.
D. Refer the patient to his/her primary care physician for diagnosis and appropriate treatment of the systemic symptoms and then treat the musculoskeletal injury.

ANSWERS

26.1 **C.** Fatigue is one of the first symptoms found in people with ID. Difficulty breathing (option D) and musculoskeletal injury (options A and B) may happen in later stages of ID or IDA.[16-18]

26.2 **A.** Distance runners may have an increased destruction of red blood cells due to impact forces from repetitive foot striking during running, a phenomenon known as foot strike hemolysis.[22,27-29]

26.3 **D.** Initial rehabilitation and treatment for iron deficiency should focus on diet recommendations and iron supplementation by the primary care physician.[26] After the systemic concerns are treated through diet and supplementation based on recommendations from the patient's primary care physician, physical therapy interventions can be resumed to focus on the musculoskeletal concerns.

REFERENCES

1. World Health Organization. Serum ferritin concentrations for the assessment of iron status and iron deficiency in populations. Vitamin and Mineral Nutrition Information System. http://www.who.int/vmnis/indicators/ferritin/en/. Accessed January 27, 2015.
2. World Health Organization. Iron deficiency anaemia: assessment, prevention, and control, a guide for programme managers. http://www.who.int/nutrition/publications/en/ida_assessment_prevention_control.pdf. Accessed January 27, 2015.
3. McClung JP. Iron status and the female athlete. *J Trace Elem Med Biol*. 2012;26:124-126.
4. Miret S, Simpson RJ, McKie AT. Physiology and molecular biology of dietary iron absorption. *Annu Rev Nutr*. 2003;23:283-301.

5. Hurrell RF. Preventing iron deficiency through food fortification. *Nutr Rev.* 1997;55:210-222.
6. Monson ER. Iron and absorption: dietary factors which impact iron bioavailability. *J Am Dietet Assoc.* 1988;88:786-790.
7. Tapiero H, Gate L, Tew KD. Iron: deficiencies and requirements. *Biomed Pharmacother.* 2001;55:324-332.
8. Hunt JR, Gallagher SK, Johnson LK. Effect of ascorbic acid on apparent iron absorption by women with low iron stores. *Am J Clin Nutr.* 1994;59:1381-1385.
9. Siegenberg D, Baynes RD, Bothwell TH, et al. Ascorbic acid prevents the dose-dependent inhibitory effects of polyphenols and phytates on nonheme-iron absorption. *Am J Clin Nutr.* 1991;53:537-541.
10. Samman S, Sandstrom B, Toft MB, et al. Green tea or rosemary extract added to foods reduces nonheme-iron absorption. *Am J Clin Nutr.* 2001;73:607-612.
11. Brune M, Rossander L, Hallberg L. Iron absorption and phenolic compounds: importance of different phenolic structures. *Eur J Clin Nutr.* 1989;43:547-557.
12. Hallberg L, Rossander-Hulthen L, Brune M, Gleerup A. Inhibition of haem-iron absorption in man by calcium. *Br J Nutr.* 1993;69:533-540.
13. Hallberg L, Brune M, Erlandsson M, Sandberg AS, Rossander-Hulten L. Calcium: effect of different amounts on nonheme- and heme-iron absorption in humans. *Am J Clin Nutr.* 1991;53:112-119.
14. Minihane AM, Fairweather-Tair SJ. Effect of calcium supplementation on daily nonheme-iron absorption and long-term iron status. *Am J Clin Nutr.* 1998;68:96-102.
15. Cook JD, Reddy MB, Burri J, Juillerat MA, Hurrell RF. The influence of different cereal grains on iron absorption from infant cereal foods. *Am J Clin Nutr.* 1997;65:964-969.
16. Nielsen, P, Nachtigall D. Iron supplementation in athletes: current recommendations. *Sports Med.* 1998;26:207-216.
17. Shaskey DJ, Green GA. Sports haematology. *Sports Med.* 2000;29:27-38.
18. Landry GL, Bernhardt DT. *Essentials of Primary Care Sports Medicine.* Champaign, IL: Human Kinetics; 2003:174.
19. Sandström G, Börjesson M, Stig Rödjer S. Iron deficiency in adolescent female athletes—is iron status affected by regular sporting activity? *Clin J Sport Med.* 2012;22:495-500.
20. Institute of Medicine. *Iron. Dietary Reference Intakes.* http://iom.nationalacademies.org/~/media/Files/Activity%20Files/Nutrition/DRIs/DRI_Elements.pdf.
21. Killip S, Bennett J, Chambers M. Iron deficiency anemia. *Am Fam Physician.* 2007;75:671-678.
22. Sinclair L, Hinton PS. Prevalence of iron deficiency with and without anemia in recreationally active men and women. *J Am Diet Assoc.* 2005;105:975-978.
23. Beard J, Tobin B. Iron status and exercise. *Am J Clin Nutr.* 2000;72:594-597.
24. Latunde-Dada G. Iron metabolism in athletes–achieving a gold standard. *Eur J Haematol.* 2013;90:10-15.
25. National Institute of Health, Office of Dietary Supplements. http://ods.od.nih.gov/factsheets/list-all/. Accessed January 27, 2015.
26. University of Minnesota, School of Public Health. Iron deficiency anemia. http://www.epi.umn.edu/let/pubs/img/NMPA_37-46.pdf. Accessed January 27, 2015.
27. Ottomano C, Franchini M. Sports anaemia: facts or fiction? *Blood Transfus.* 2012;10:252-254.
28. Miller BJ, Pate RR, Burgess W. Foot impact force and intravascular hemolysis during distance running. *Int J Sports Med.* 1988;9:56-60.
29. Lippi G, Schena F, Salvagno GL, Aloe R, Banfi G, Guidi CG. Foot-strike haemolysis after a 60-km ultramarathon. *Blood Transfus.* 2012;10:377-383.
30. Robertson JD, Maughan RJ, Davidson RJ. Faecal blood loss in response to exercise. *Br Med J.* 1987;295:303-305.
31. Malczewska J, Raczynski G, Stupnicki R. Iron status in female endurance athletes and in non-athletes. *Int J Sport Nutr Exerc Metab.* 2000;10:260-276.

32. Chen MJ, Fan X, Moe ST. Criterion-related validity of the Borg ratings of perceived exertion scale in healthy individuals: a meta-analysis. *J Sports Sci*. 2002;20:873-899.
33. Dierks TA, Manal KT, Hamill J, Davis I. Lower extremity kinematics in runners with patellofemoral pain during a prolonged run. *Med Sci Sports Exerc*. 2011;43:693-700.
34. Dierks TA, Davis IS, Hamill J. The effects of running in an exerted state on lower extremity kinematics and joint timing. *J Biomech*. 2010;43:2993-2998.

INDEX

NOTE: Page numbers followed by an *f* indicate figures; page numbers followed by a *t* indicate tables.

A

A-beta fibers, 419
Abnormal impulse generating sites (AIGS), 420
Active assisted range of motion (AAROM), 60, 81
Active knee extension test, 169*f*, 170*f*
Active quadriceps test, 314*t*
Active range of motion (AROM), 60, 64, 81, 423
Active straight leg raise (ASLR), 128
Adductor longus, 141
Adductor squeeze test, 144–145, 144*f*
Adductor strains, 168*t*
A-delta fibers, 419
Adult acquired flatfoot deformity, 338
Adverse response to neural tension, 416
Allodynia, 416
Alternative lumbar manipulation technique, 131, 131*f*
AMBRI, 61
Amenorrhea
  primary, 242
  secondary, 240, 242
American Medical Society for Sports Medicine, 409
American Shoulder and Elbow Surgeons Standardized Shoulder Assessment Form, 17–18
Angle of peak torque, 164
Ankle
  articular anatomy of, 368*f*
  Foot and Ankle Ability Measure (FAAM), 373
  lateral ankle injury, 366
  lateral ankle sprains, 365–383

  movement exercises, with resistive tubing, 357*f*, 358*f*
  Ottawa Ankle Rules, 369, 370*f*
Ankylosing spondylitis, 125*t*
Anterior cruciate ligament
  anatomy of, 279, 279*f*
  injury, 261–275
    case overview, 261
    clinical recommendations for, 272
    contact, 279
    examination, evaluation and diagnosis of, 263–266
    health condition in, 262–263
    incidence of, 279
    in-season warm-up program, 271*t*
    patient/client management in, 263
    physical therapy considerations in, 262
    plan of care and interventions for, 266–272, 267*f*, 268*f*, 269*f*, 270*f*, 271*f*, 271*t*
    screening examination, 264*t*
    statistics, 279
  reconstruction, 277–295
    case overview, 277
    clinical recommendations for, 291
    definition of, 278
    examination, evaluation and diagnosis of, 281–283
    health condition in, 279–280
    hop tests, 289*f*, 289*t*
    modified soreness rules in, 288*t*
    patient/client management in, 281

Anterior cruciate ligament, reconstruction (*Cont.*):
  physical therapy considerations in, 278–279
  plan of care and interventions for, 283–291
  return-to-sport testing after, 297–307
  running progression, 287*t*
  statistics, 280
  University of Delaware Rehabilitation Practice Guidelines for, 283, 284*t*
Anterior drawer test, 371, 371*f*, 372*f*
Anterior load and shift test, 46–47, 46*f*
Anterior shoulder dislocation, first-time, 41–58
  case studies, 41
  clinical recommendations for, 56*f*
  examination, evaluation and diagnosis of, 44–49
  health condition in, 43
  patient/client management in, 43–44
  physical therapy considerations in, 42–43
  plan of care and interventions for, 49–56, 50*t*, 51*t*
  rehabilitation in, 50*t*, 51*t*
Anterior superior iliac spine (ASIS), 126, 132
Anterior talofibular ligament, 367, 368*f*
Anterior thigh contusion. *See* Quadriceps, contusion
Apprehension test, 47–48, 48*f*
Arthroscopic microfracture procedure, 326
Articular cartilage lesion, 326
Athletic pubalgia, 139–151
  case overview, 139
  clinical recommendations for, 148
  definition of, 140
  differential diagnosis of, 145*t*
  examination, evaluation and diagnosis of, 142–145
  health condition in, 141–142
  patient/client management in, 142
  physical therapy considerations in, 140–141
  plan of care and interventions for, 145–148
Autograft, 278
Autoimmune diseases, 125*t*
Autologous chondrocyte implantation (ACI), 326
Automated Neuropsychological Assessment Metrics (ANAM), 408
Axillary nerve, 431*t*
Axons, 419

B
Back pain, low, 121–138
  case overview, 121
  clinical recommendations for, 134
  differential diagnosis of, 125*t*
  examination, evaluation and diagnosis of, 125–129
  examination of, 125*t*
  health condition in, 123–124
  incidence of, 123
  patient/client management in, 125
  physical therapy considerations in, 123
  plan of care and interventions for, 129–134, 130*f*
Balance Error Scoring System (BESS), 374, 406–407
Bankart lesion, 43, 61, 62*f*
Bankart repair, 60
Baseball players
  superior labrum anterior to posterior repair in, 75–90
  ulnar collateral ligament reconstruction in, 91–106
Basketball player, anterior cruciate ligament reconstruction in, 297–307
Beighton's hypermobility index, 10, 14

Biceps tenodesis, 60
Bike, 233t. *See also* Cyclists
  anatomy of, 217f
  cleats, 233, 234f
  fitting, 233–234
Bilateral heel rise, 343f
Bird dog exercise, 115f, 146, 147f
  with opposite arm and leg in push-up opposition, 116f
Bone mineral density (BMD), 242–243
Bone scintigraphy, 353
Boston overlapping brace, 112, 112f
Bounding exercise, 269, 269f
Brachial plexus, 431t
Broad jump and hold exercise, 268, 268f

C
C fibers, 419
Cadence (cycling), 216
Calcaneofibular ligament, 367, 368f
Cancer, 125t
Case studies
  anterior cruciate ligament, 261–275
  anterior cruciate ligament reconstruction, 277–295
  anterior first-time shoulder dislocation, 41–58
  athletic pubalgia, 139–151
  concussion, 401–413
  glenohumeral joint dislocation, 59–73
  hamstring strain, acute, 163–185
  hamstring tendinopathy, 187–201
  iron deficiency in endurance athlete, 449–459
  knee articular cartilage repair, 325–335
  lateral ankle sprains, 365–383
  overuse shoulder injury, 9–40
  patellar tendinosis in volleyball player, 239–259
  patellofemoral pain in cross-country runner, 203–213
  patellofemoral pain in cyclist, 215–237
  peripheral neuropathic pain, 415–447
  posterior tibial tendon dysfunction, 337–348
  preseason testing of athletic readiness, 385–399
  quadriceps contusion, 153–161
  return to rugby after PCL reconstruction, 309–323
  return-to-sport after ACL reconstruction, 297–307
  spondylolysis, 107–119
  stress fracture in middle-aged runner, 349–364
  superior labrum anterior to posterior repair, 75–90
  ulnar collateral ligament reconstruction, 91–106
Central sensitization, 416
Centralization, 122
Cervical nerve roots, 432t
Chronic traumatic encephalopathy (CTE), 405
Cincinnati Knee Rating Scale, 332
Clamshell exercise, 146, 146f
Clamshell with internal rotation, 355, 356f
Cleat (cycling), 233, 234f
Clinical prediction rule (CPR), 122, 129
Clipless pedals (cycling), 216
Closed kinetic chain (CKC) exercises, 69–70, 70f, 193, 285–286
Closed-chain dorsiflexion, 221, 222f
CogState, 408
Compartment syndrome, 156t, 157
Compression fractures, 125t
Computed tomography (CT), 111
  in diagnosis of hip, groin and abdominal pain, 145t
  of glenohumeral dislocation, 49
  in knee articular cartilage repair, 328
  of spondylolysis, 111

Computerized neuropsychological (CNP) testing, 408
Concussion, 401–413
  case overview, 401
  definition of, 402
  examination, evaluation and diagnosis of, 406–408
  health condition in, 403–415
  incidence of, 403
  patient/client management in, 405–406
  physical therapy considerations in, 402–403
  plan of care and interventions for, 408–410
  return to play protocol in, 409t
  signs and symptoms, 404t
Continuous passive motion (CPM), 325
Contract-relax adduction stretch, 33, 33f
Contralateral cervical lateral glides, 434, 435f, 436f
Coxa saltans, 156t, 157
Crank arm length (bike), 224, 224t
C-reactive protein, 420
Cross-arm adduction, 16, 17f
Cross-arm adduction stretch, 31, 32f, 34f
Cross-country runner, patellofemoral pain in, 203–213
"C"-shaped scapular stabilization method, 15–16, 16f
Cyclists
  bike fitting for, 233–234
  categories of, 216
  patellofemoral pain in, 215–237
Cyclocross, 188

D

Deep friction massage (DFM), 253
Deep neck flexors, 442t
Deep squat, 389f
Deep tendon reflexes (DTRs), 420, 432, 433
Deep vein thrombosis (DVT), 369, 373
Degenerative disc disease (DDD), 125t
Dementia pugilistica, 405
Digital inclinometer, 16, 17f
Discitis, 125t
Donkey kicks, 251f
Dorsal neck muscles, 442t
Dorsal root ganglion (DRG), 419
Dorsiflexion self-mobilization, 228, 229f
Double-kneeling hold exercise, 270, 270f
Double-leg lawnmower, 84f
Double-leg squat, 220, 220f, 244
Drop vertical jump (DVJ), 266
Dynamic lower extremity valgus, 265–266, 265f
Dynamic stabilization, 42, 92
Dynamic stabilizers, 216
Dysesthesia, 416
Dysesthetic pain, 416, 418

E

Eccentric contraction, 164
Eccentric loading, 194
Eccentric strengthening, 173
Effusion, 278
Elbow
  extension lag, 92
  flexion angle, 225
  ulnar collateral ligament reconstruction of, 91–106
    case overview, 91
    health condition in, 92–94
    patient/client management in, 94–95
    physical therapy considerations in, 92
Ely's test, 243
Endurance athlete, 449–459
ER strengthening with elastic resistance, 27
ER/IR strength ratio, 26–27
External oblique, 141
External rotation with scapular retraction, 22f
Extracorporeal shock wave therapy (ESWT), 242

F

FABER test, 140, 143
Facet joint arthropathy, 125t
FADIR test, 140, 143
Fear-Avoidance Beliefs Questionnaire (FABQ), 126
Fear-Avoidance Beliefs Questionnaire Work (FABQW), 126
Female athlete triad, 240, 242
Female Athlete Triad Coalition Screening Questionnaire, 244, 245f, 247f, 248f
Femoral acetabular impingement (FAI), 140, 141, 144, 145t
Femoral neck stress fractures, 145t
Ferritin, 450, 451
Fibromyalgia, 125t
Flip sign, 10
Foot, articular anatomy of, 368f
Foot and Ankle Ability Measure (FAAM), 373
Foot strike hemolysis, 453
Football player
  anterior shoulder dislocation in, 41–58
  glenohumeral joint dislocation in, 59–73
Force closure, 122
Form closure, 122
Front plank exercises
  with elbow extended, 116f
  on forearms, 114f
  with hip extension, 356f
  with leg lift hip extension, 255f
Fulcrum test, 355t
Functional instability, 366
Functional Movement Screen (FMS), 302, 388–390, 389f, 390f, 394

G

Gait analysis, 206, 283
Gastrointestinal (GI) conditions, 125t
Gillet test, 128
Giving way episode, 278
Glasgow Coma Scale (GCS), 406
Glenohumeral instability, 42
Glenohumeral joint, 77–78
Glenohumeral joint dislocation, 59–73
  case overview, 59
  clinical recommendations for, 71
  examination, evaluation and diagnosis of, 64
  health condition in, 61–63
  patient/client management in, 63–64
  physical therapy considerations in, 60–61
  physical therapy guidelines, 66t, 67t, 68t
  plan of care and interventions for, 65–71
  statistics, 62
Glenohumeral joint internal rotation deficit (GIRD), 10, 11, 16, 78
Glenohumeral ligaments, 77–78
Glenoid labrum, 77
Global neck muscles, 442t
Global Rating Scale of Perceived Function (GRS), 290
Glucocorticoids, 124
Golfers
  interval program for, 443t
  peripheral neuropathic pain in, 415–447
Gymnast, spondylolysis in, 107–119

H

Half-kneeling lifts, 230, 232f
HamSprint program, 173
Hamstring
  strain, acute, 163–185
  case overview, 163–185
  clinical recommendations for, 179–180
  definition of, 164
  differential diagnosis of posterior thigh pain, 168t, 169f, 170f
  examination, evaluation and diagnosis of, 167–170
  in football players, 165

Hamstring, strain, acute (*Cont.*):
   health condition in, 165–166
   incidence of, 165
   patient/client management in, 167
   physical therapy considerations in, 164–165
   plan of care and interventions for, 170–179, 172*f*, 173*f*, 174*f*, 175*f*, 176*f*, 177*f*, 178*f*
   prognosis factors for recovery time in, 171*t*
   risk factors for, 166
  stretching in doorjamb, 249*f*
  tendinopathy, 187–201
   examination, evaluation and diagnosis of, 190–191, 192*f*, 192*t*
   health condition in, 189–190
   patient/client management in, 190
   physical therapy considerations in, 188–189
   plan of care and interventions for, 192–196, 195*f*, 196*f*, 197*f*, 198*f*
   postoperative rehabilitation protocol for, 193*t*
  tendon autografts, 280–281
  tendon avulsion, 168*t*
Handlebar reach (cycling), 216, 224, 224*f*
HeadMinder, 408
Heel tap, 355*t*
Helmets, 409
Hematocrit, 455*t*
Hematoma, 154
Hematuria, 453
Hemoglobin, 455*t*
Hemolysis, 453
Herniated lumbar disc, 125*t*
Herpes zoster, 125*t*
High hurdle lateral step-overs, 198*f*
Hill-Sachs lesions, 49, 60, 61–62, 61*f*, 62*f*
Hinged brace, 95*f*

Hip
  abduction MMT, 454*t*
  adductors, 141
  extension MMT, 454*t*
  internal rotation MMT, 454*t*
  snapping, 156*t*, 157
  strengthening exercises, 209
Home exercise program (HEP), 131–133
Hurdle step, 389*f*
Hyperalgesia, 416

I

Ice hockey
  concussion in, 401–413
  helmets, 409
Iliac crest (IC), 126
Iliopsoas strain, differential diagnosis for, 156*t*
ImPACT, 408
Impulse Trainer, 25*f*
Inclinometer, digital, 16, 17*f*
In-line surge, 390*f*
Inseam of cyclist, 216, 224*t*
Instability, 76
Insufficiency fractures, 351
Internal impingement, 76
Internal oblique, 141
International Cartilage Repair Society, 327
International Knee Documentation Committee (IKDC), 329
International Spine and Pain Institute, 438
Iron deficiency, 451
  case overview, 449
  clinical recommendations for, 456
  definition of, 450
  in endurance athlete, 449–459
  examination, evaluation and diagnosis of, 453–455, 454*t*, 455*t*
  health condition in, 451–452
  patient/client management in, 453
  physical therapy considerations in, 450–451

plan of care and interventions for, 456
prevalence of, 452
recommended dietary allowances and, 452
signs and symptoms, 452
Iron status, 450
Iron-deficiency anemia, 450, 451, 452t
Ischial apophyseal avulsions, 168t
Isokinetic shoulder internal/external rotation, 26f
Isometric shoulder external rotation exercise, 53f
Isometric strengthening, 208

J
Jobe subluxation/relocation test, 14, 15f
Jogging, 327
Joint hypermobility, 42
Jumper's knee. *See* Patellar tendinosis

K
Kerlan-Jobe Orthopaedic Clinic Shoulder and Elbow Score, 17
Kibler scapular dyskinesis, type I, 13f
Knee
  active knee extension test, 169f, 170f
  anterior cruciate ligament, 261–275
  articular cartilage repair, 325–335
    case overview, 325
    examination, evaluation and diagnosis of, 328–332
    health condition in, 327
    incidence of, 327
    patient/client management in, 327–328
    physical therapy considerations in, 326–327
    plan of care and interventions for, 328–329, 328f
    statistics, 327
  Cincinnati Knee Rating Scale, 332
  effusion grading scale of, 281t
  extension MMT, 454t

  patellar tendinosis of, 239–259
    case overview, 239
    clinical recommendations for, 256
    examination, evaluation and diagnosis of, 243–249
    health condition in, 241–243
    patient/client management in, 243
    physical therapy considerations in, 240–241
    plan of care and interventions for, 249–256
  patellofemoral pain of, 203–213, 215–237
  primary ligaments of, 279f
  range of motion, 206, 223, 223t
  valgus collapse, 207f, 226f
Knee Injury and Osteoarthritis Outcome Score (KOOS), 329, 332
Knee Outcome Survey-Activities of Daily Living Scale (KOS-ADLS), 290, 332

L
Labral tear, 145t
Labrum, 76
Lachman test, 278
Landing Error Scoring System, 303, 393
Lateral ankle injury, 366
Lateral ankle sprains, 365–383
  case overview, 365
  clinical recommendations for, 378–379
  examination, evaluation and diagnosis of, 369–375, 370f, 371f, 374f
  health condition in, 367–368
  patient/client management in, 368
  physical therapy considerations in, 366–367
  plan of care and interventions for, 375–378, 376f
Lateral band walks, 359, 360f

Lawnmower scapular exercise, 18, 21f
Limb symmetry index (LSI), 290, 298, 303
Long cassette radiographs, 326
Loss of consciousness (LOC), 402, 403
Low back pain, 121–138
    case overview, 121
    clinical recommendations for, 134
    differential diagnosis of, 125t
    examination, evaluation and diagnosis of, 125–129
    examination of, 125t
    health condition in, 123–124
    incidence of, 123
    patient/client management in, 125
    physical therapy considerations in, 123
    plan of care and interventions for, 129–134, 130f
Low row exercise, 18, 20f
Lower Extremity Functional Scale (LEFS), 303
Low-level laser therapy, 377
Lumbar strain or sprain, 125t
Lysholm Knee Scale, 332

M

Maddocks Score, 406
Magnetic resonance imaging (MRI)
    in acute hamstring strain, 170, 171t, 179, 181
    of anterior cruciate ligament injury, 277
    in athletic pubalgia, 145
    of hamstring tendinopathy, 187, 191, 194
    of knee articular cartilage, 325
    in low back pain, 124
    of overuse shoulder injury, 22
    of patellar tendinosis, 241
    in patellofemoral pain, 206
    in peripheral neuropathic pain, 415, 420
    of posterior cruciate ligament injury, 313, 315, 328
    in spondylolysis, 111
    of stress fracture, 353
    of stress fractures, 353
    of ulnar collateral ligament injury, 93
"Make a Halo" exercise, 441f
Manual muscle testing (MMT), 191, 222, 223, 223t, 454t
Maximum voluntary contraction, 216
Maximum voluntary isometric contraction (MVIC), 285–286, 316, 319f
Mechanical instability, 366
Mechanical interface, 423
Mechanisms of injury, 315
Mechanosensitivity, 416, 425t, 426t
Median nerve, 431t
Mild traumatic brain injuries (mTBIs), 403
Minimal clinically important difference (MCID), 373
Modifiable risk factors, 262, 298
Modified Balance Error Scoring System (BESS), 406–408
Modified stroke test, 282f
Motor control, 298
Mouthguards, 409
Mulligan mobilization with movement (MWM), 227, 227f
Multidirectional instability, 14
Multidisciplinary pain clinic (MPC), 421
Muscle energy techniques (METs), 124, 131–132, 133t
Myositis ossificans, 154, 156t, 157

N

National Athletic Trainers Association, 409
Negative provocation SIJ test, 122
Nerve slider, 416
Nerve tensioner, 416
Nerve trunk pain, 416, 418
Nervi nervorum, 416
Neurogenic inflammation, 416, 418
Neuromuscular control, 42

Neuromuscular electrical stimulation
 (NMES), 112, 114f, 284–285,
 316–317, 327
Neuromuscular training, 331, 332f
Neuropathic pain, 416
Neuropsychological (NP) testing, 408
90-90 muscle length test, 192f
90/90 plyometric drop exercise,
 27, 27f
90/90 reverse catch plyometric
 exercise, 27, 28f, 29f
Nociception, 416
Non-modifiable risk factors, 262
Nordic hamstring curl exercise,
 194, 195f

O
Ober test, 243, 454t
Oligomenorrhea, 242
One repetition maximum (1RM)
 testing, 285
Open kinetic chain (OKC) exercises,
 285–286
Osteitis pubis, 140, 145t
Osteoarthritis, 145t
Osteochondral autograft
 transplantation (OATS),
 326, 329
Osteomyelitis, 125t, 156t
Osteotendinous avulsion, 188
Oswestry Disability Questionnaire
 (ODQ), 126, 130
Ottawa Ankle Rules, 369, 370f
Ottawa Knee Rules, 313
Overuse shoulder injury, 9–40
 case overview, 9
 clinical recommendations for, 35
 evaluation of, 12–18
 examination, evaluation and
  diagnosis of, 12–18, 12f, 14f,
  15f, 16f, 17f
 health condition in, 11
 passive shoulder range of motion
  and, 17t
 patient/client management in,
  11–12

 physical therapy considerations in,
  10–11
 plan of care and interventions for,
  18–35, 19f, 20f, 21f, 22f, 23f,
  25f, 26f, 27f, 28f, 29f, 30f, 31f,
  33f, 34f
 statistics, 11
"Oye vey" exercise, 441f

P
Pain
 dysesthetic, 416, 418
 low back, 121–138
 nerve trunk, 416, 418
 neuropathic, 416
 patellofemoral, 203–213, 215–237
 peripheral neuropathic, 415–447
 posterior thigh, 168t, 169f, 170f
PAINT lesion, 76, 78
Pallof press, 229, 231f
Palpation, 454t
Parkinsonism, 405
Passive flexion, 317
Passive range of motion (PROM), 60,
 64, 79, 317, 427
PASTA lesion, 76, 78
Patellar tendinosis
 case overview, 239
 clinical recommendations for, 256
 examination, evaluation and
  diagnosis of, 243–249
 health condition in, 241–243
 patient/client management in, 243
 physical therapy considerations in,
  240–241
 plan of care and interventions for,
  249–256
 in volleyball player, 239–259
Patellar-pubic percussion (PPP) test,
 143
Patellofemoral pain
 in cross-country runner, 203–213
  case overview, 203
  clinical recommendations for,
   210–211
  definition of, 204

Patellofemoral pain, in cross-country runner (*Cont.*):
  examination, evaluation and diagnosis of, 206–208
  health condition in, 205
  patient/client management in, 206
  physical therapy considerations in, 204
  plan of care and interventions for, 208–209
 cycling related, 215–237
  case overview, 215
  clinical recommendations for, 234
  examination, evaluation and diagnosis of, 220–226, 220*f*, 221*f*, 222*f*, 223*t*, 224*t*, 225*f*, 226*f*
  health condition in, 218–219
  manual muscle testing in, 223*t*
  patient/client management in, 219–220
  physical therapy considerations in, 216
  plan of care and interventions for, 226–234, 227*f*, 229*f*, 230*f*, 231*f*, 232*f*
  range of motion in, 223*t*
 syndrome, 205, 455*t*
Pedal stroke (cycling), 216, 226*f*
Pee Wee league, 403
Peel-off injury, 311
Pelvic conditions, 125*t*
Pelvic fracture, 168*t*
Percussion test, 355*t*
Peripheral nerve, 419
Peripheral neuropathic pain, 415–447
 case overview, 415
 causes of, 418
 clinical recommendations for, 443–444
 examination, evaluation and diagnosis of, 422–433, 423*f*, 425*t*, 426*t*, 428*t*, 429*t*, 431*t*, 432*t*
 health condition in, 418–421
 patient/client management in, 421–422
 physical therapy considerations in, 417–418
 plan of care and interventions for, 433–442, 435*f*, 436*f*, 437*f*, 439*f*, 440*f*, 441*f*, 442*t*, 443*t*
 signs and symptoms, 432*t*
 sites of, 418
Peripheralization, 122
Pes planus, 204
Plyometric exercises, 42
Plyometric upper extremity exercise, 27
Post-concussion syndrome, 402
Posterior cruciate ligament (PCL), 311
 injuries, 312
Posterior cruciate ligament reconstruction, 309–323
 case overview, 309
 clinical recommendations for, 321
 examination, evaluation and diagnosis of, 314–315
 health condition in, 314–315
 patient/client management in, 312–313
 physical therapy considerations in, 311–312
 plan of care and interventions for, 315–321
 postoperative rehabilitation protocol for, 319*t*, 320*t*
 special tests for PCL injuries in, 314*t*
Posterior drawer test, 314*t*, 315*f*
Posterior splint, 366
Posterior superior iliac spine (PSIS), 126, 128, 132
Posterior talofibular ligament, 367, 368*f*
Posterior thigh pain, 168*t*, 169*f*, 170*f*
Posterior tibial tendon dysfunction (PTTD), 332*f*
 case overview, 337
 clinical recommendations for, 346

definition of, 339
examination, evaluation and
 diagnosis of, 340–343, 340f,
 341f, 343f
four-stage progression for, 339
health condition in, 338–339
nonsurgical treatment of, 339
patient/client management in,
 339–340
physical therapy considerations in,
 338
plan of care and interventions for,
 343–346, 344f, 345f
therapeutic exercises for, 344t
Posterolateral corner, 311, 313
Post-injury motor control changes,
 386
Prednisone, 124
Preparticipation physical examination,
 386
Preseason testing of athletic readiness,
 385–399
case overview, 385
clinical recommendations for, 395
examination, evaluation and
 diagnosis of, 388–394
patient/client management in, 388
physical therapy considerations in,
 386–387
plan of care and interventions for,
 394–395
Progressive agility and trunk
 stabilization (PATS), 171, 173,
 194
Prone dial test, 314t, 315f
Prone external rotation exercise, 23f
Protective equipment, 409
Proximal hamstring tendinopathy,
 168t
Psoas major muscles, 145t
Pugilistic parkinsonism, 405
Punch drunk syndrome, 405

Q
Q-angle, 204
Quad lag, 283

Quad set exercise, 154, 159f, 244, 283
Quadriceps
 activation test, 314t
 contusion, 153–161
  case overview, 153
  clinical recommendations
   for, 159
  differential diagnosis for, 156t
  examination, evaluation and
   diagnosis of, 155–157
  grading system for, 156t
  health condition in, 154–155
  patient/client management in,
   155
  physical therapy considerations
   in, 154
  plan of care and interventions for,
   157–158
  rehabilitation protocol, 158t
 index (QI), 285, 311
 isokinetic testing of, 319f
 strain, differential diagnosis for,
  156t
 strengthening exercises for,
  209, 252
Quadruped arm and leg lift exercise,
 229, 230f

R
Radial nerve, 431t
Radiculopathy, 416
Radiography
 of anterior first-time shoulder
  dislocation, 48
 of femoral acetabular impingement,
  145t
 of glenohumeral joint dislocation,
  59, 62
 of ischial apophyseal avulsions, 168t
 of knee articular cartilage repair,
  325, 328
 in knee articular cartilage repair,
  328
 of lateral ankle sprains, 369, 370f,
  371
 long cassette, 326

Radiography (Cont.):
    of overuse shoulder injury, 9
    of pelvic fracture, 168t
    of posterior cruciate ligament, 313
    of quadriceps contusion, 157
    of sacroiliac joint, 129
    of spondylolysis, 109, 111
    of stress fractures, 352–353
Rapid ankle-weighted kicks, 196f
Rectus abdominis, 141, 144
Red flags, 122
Referred posterior thigh pain, 168t
Regional interdependence, 204, 216
Renal conditions, 125t
Resisted external rotation walkout, 83f
Resisted foot adduction exercise, 345f
Return to play (RTP) protocol, 409–410, 409t
Return-to-sport
    after ACL reconstruction, 297–307
        case overview, 299
        checklist in testing for, 301t
        clinical recommendations for, 304
        examination, evaluation and diagnosis of, 300–301
        health condition in, 299–300
        patient/client management in, 300
        physical therapy considerations in, 298–299
        plan of care and interventions for, 301–304
    after PCL reconstruction, 309–323
        case overview, 309
        clinical recommendations for, 321
        examination, evaluation and diagnosis of, 314–315
        health condition in, 312
        patient/client management in, 312–313
        physical therapy considerations in, 311–312
        plan of care and interventions for, 315–321
        postoperative rehabilitation protocol for, 319t, 320t
        special tests for PCL injuries in, 314t
    preseason testing of athletic readiness, 385–399
    return to play protocol, 409–410, 409t
    time, 164
Reverse clamshell exercise, 356f
Reverse pivot shift, 314t
Rhythmic stabilization with exercise ball, 19, 24f
"Robbery" scapular exercise, 18, 19f
Rockerboard, 332f
Rotating side plank exercise, 172f, 173f
Rotator cuff tendonitis, 11
Rugby player
    posterior cruciate ligament reconstruction in, 309–323
    return to, after posterior cruciate ligament reconstruction, 309–323
Rugby Sevens, 311, 321
Runner
    cross-country, 203–213
    iron deficiency in, 449–459
    patellofemoral pain in, 203–213
    stress fracture in, 349–364
Russian hamstrings curls, 271, 271f

S

Sacroiliac joint dysfunction
    differential diagnosis for, 125t
    pathology, 122
    plan of care and interventions for, 129–134
    tests for, 126–129
Saddle (bike seat), 216, 223–224
scapular assistance test (SAT), 13, 14f
Schwann cells, 419
Seat height (bike), 216
Second impact syndrome, 402
Secondary amenorrhea, 240

Sensory afferent fibers, 419
Serratus anterior, 442t
Serum ferritin, 450, 451, 455t
Sevens Rugby, 311, 321
Short foot intrinsic strengthening, 228, 229f
Shoulder
  anterior dislocation, 41–58
    case studies, 41
    clinical recommendations for, 56f
    examination, evaluation and diagnosis of, 44–49
    health condition in, 43
    patient/client management in, 43–44
    physical therapy considerations in, 42–43
    plan of care and interventions for, 49–56, 50t, 51t
    rehabilitation in, 50t, 51t
  elevation in scapular plane, 55f
  external rotation, 24f
  external rotation with resistive band, 54f
  flexion, 52f
  glenohumeral instability, 42
  glenohumeral joint dislocation, 59–73
    case overview, 59
    clinical recommendations for, 71
    examination, evaluation and diagnosis of, 64
    health condition in, 61–63
    patient/client management in, 63–64
    physical therapy considerations in, 60–61
    physical therapy guidelines, 66t, 67t, 68t
    plan of care and interventions for, 65–71
    statistics, 62
  glenohumeral joint internal rotation deficit (GIRD), 10, 11, 16, 78
  instability, 60, 61
  internal and external rotation, 53f
  sling for, 49, 52f
Side plank exercise, 115f, 229, 230f, 355, 356f
  with hip abduction, 117f
Side plank with hip abduction leg lift, 355, 357f
Sidelying clamshell exercise, 229f
Sidelying hip abduction, 254f, 357f
Single-leg deadlifts, 361f
Single-leg hamstring strengthening, 255f
Single-leg lawnmower, 85f
Single-leg squat, 220–221, 221f, 454t
Single-leg windmills with opposite reaches, 174f, 175f
Single-leg X-hop, 269, 269f
Single-limb balance test, 374
Single-limb chair-bridge, 176f
Single-limb dead lift, 177f
Single-limb squat
  on 25-degree decline board, 252f
  on unstable surface, 253f
Single-photon emission computed tomography (SPECT), 111
Sinus tarsi region, 338
SLAP lesion, 62
Sleeper stretch, 31, 31f
Sliders, 437–438, 439t, 442
Slings, 63f
Small knee bend, 454t
"Smoking" exercise, 441f
Snapping hip, 157
  differential diagnosis for, 156t
Soccer players
  anterior cruciate ligament reconstruction in, 277–295
  anterior cruciate ligament ruptures in, 261–275
  athletic pubalgia in, 139–151
  preseason testing of, 385–399
  quadricep contusion in, 153–161
Soft tissue management (STM), 129, 133
"Sole-to-sole" exercise, 344t

Sole-to-sole posterior tibialis strengthening exercise, 344f, 345f
Spinal stenosis, 125t
Spondylolisthesis, 108, 125t
Spondylolysis, 107–119, 108, 125t
   case overview, 107
   classification of, 109t
   clinical recommendations for, 117
   definition of, 108
   examination, evaluation and diagnosis of, 110–111
   health condition in, 109–110
   imaging in, 111
   patient/client management in, 110
   physical therapy considerations in, 108–109
   plan of care and interventions for, 111–117, 114f, 113t, 115f, 116f, 117f
   therapeutic exercises for, 114f, 113t, 115f, 116f, 117f
Spondylosis, 108
Sport Concussion Assessment Tool 3 (SCAT3), 406, 407
Sports hernia. See Athletic pubalgia
Squeeze test, 355t
Standardized Assessment of Concussion (SAC), 406–407
Standing quadriceps stretching with a chair, 250f
Star Excursion Balance Test (SEBT), 207, 299, 302, 374, 390–393
Static stabilizers, 216
"Statue of Liberty" exercise, 25, 25f
Stem rise (bike), 216
Straight leg raise (SLR) test, 143, 169f, 170f, 283, 318f
Stress fractures, 354–361
   case overview, 349–350
   clinical recommendations for, 361
   definition of, 108, 351
   examination, evaluation and diagnosis of, 353–354, 356f, 357f, 358f, 361f
   health condition in, 352–353
   in middle-aged runner, 349–364
   patient/client management in, 353
   physical therapy considerations in, 351–352
   plan of care and interventions for, 354–361
   special tests associated with, 355t
Stress reaction, 108
Structural differentiation, 417
Subacromial decompression, 76
Substance P, 420
Sulcus sign, 45f
Superior labral tear, 62
Superior labrum anterior to posterior (SLAP) repair, 75–90
   case overview, 75
   clinical recommendations for, 86
   examination, evaluation and diagnosis of, 79–80, 81f, 82f, 83f, 84f, 85f, 86f
   health condition in, 77–79
   patient/client management in, 79
   physical therapy considerations in, 76–77
   plan of care and interventions for, 80–81
Supine bent knee walk out, 177f, 178f
Supine dead bug exercise, 146, 147f
Supine lumbopelvic manipulation technique, 129–130, 130f
Supine straight leg cable eccentric exercise, 197f
Suprascapular nerve, 431t

T

Talar tilt test, 371, 372f
Tegner Activity Level Scale, 332
Tendinopathy, 188, 240
Tendinosis, 240
Tennis player, overuse shoulder injury in, 9–40
Tensioners, 437–438, 440t, 442
Theraband, 228
Thomas test, 244
Throwing, phases of, 94
Throwing progression, 92

Tibiofemoral joint, 311
Timed hop, 290, 290f
"Too many toes" sign, 340f
Total rotation range of motion (TROM), 10, 29
Trainer (bike), 216, 225f
Transcutaneous electrical nerve stimulation (TENS), 433
Transversus abdominis, 141, 144
Trapezius, 442t
Traumatic brain injury (TBI), 403, 409
Trunk angle (cycling), 225
TUBS, 42, 61
Tuck jump, 268–269, 268f, 303
Tuck jump assessment, 393
Tuning fork test, 355t

U
Ulnar collateral ligament reconstruction, 91–106
  case overview, 91
  health condition in, 92–94
  patient/client management in, 94–95
  physical therapy considerations in, 92
Ulnar nerve, 431t
Ulnar nerve tensioner, 437–438, 440t
Ulnar sliders, 437–438, 439t
Ultrasonography
  for adduction strain/tendinopathy, 145t
  for lateral ankle sprains, 377
  for patellar tendinosis, 241
  for psoas major pathology, 145t
University of Washington's Simple Shoulder Test, 18
Upper limb neural tension gliding, 82f
Upper-limb nerve tension tests (ULNTs), 424, 427, 428t, 429t, 430, 432t, 434–435

V
Valgus collapse, 207f, 226f
Valsava maneuver, 144–145
Vasa nervorum, 417, 419
Video gait running analysis, 454t
Volleyball player, patellar tendinosis in, 239–259

W
Wall ball dribbles, 86f
Wall jump exercise, 267, 267f
Water walking, 327
Wolff's law, 351

Y
Y Balance Test, 302, 374
Y Balance Test–Lower Quarter (YBT-LQ), 303, 390–391, 391f, 392f, 394